HEALTH TEACHING IN SECONDARY SCHOOLS

W. B. Saunders Company: West Washington Square
Philadelphia, PA 19105

1 St. Anne's Road
Eastbourne, East Sussex BN21 3UN, England

833 Oxford Street
Toronto, Ontario, M8Z 5T9, Canada

Library of Congress Cataloging in Publication Data

Willgoose, Carl E

Health teaching in secondary schools.

1. Health education (Secondary)   I. Title. [DNLM:
   1. Health education.   2. School health. QT200 W714ha]
LB1587.A3W5 1977   613'.07'12   76–8587
ISBN 0–7216–9370–9

Health Teaching in Secondary Schools   ISBN 0-7216-9370-9

Last digit is the print number: 9   8   7   6   5   4   3   2   1

PREFACE
to the Second Edition

When Jean Mayer, the able and dynamic nutritionist from Harvard, became president of Tufts University he was asked if he intended to influence his undergraduate and graduate students so that they would sharpen their nutritional practices. His answer to this was stated clearly and simply, namely, that the purpose of an educational institution is to provide students with *choices*.

The purpose of this new edition is to give teachers of health education the means for providing their students with choices in life styles and selected patterns of living that will somehow advance well-being and permit a rich and full existence. Indeed, this can be done, and done well, today as more and more attention is being given to preventive medicine by health associations and medical specialists, and by citizens and educators, alike, who are pooling their legislative and other community efforts to bolster the need for comprehensive health education.

Although this edition gives space to the needs, issues, and trends in health education, the primary thrust is directed toward curriculum improvement, alternative programs, and more effective student responses generated from a variety of tested teaching techniques. In short, the text represents an attempt to prepare a better health educator—one who keeps an open mind about health science, demonstrates some creativity, and firmly believes that what is being taught is a significant dimension in the total educational program for the last quarter of the twentieth century.

Carl E. Willgoose

PREFACE

This book was written for middle and secondary school teachers. Although the total school health program is referred to, the real emphasis is on health teaching and how it can be carried out in a fascinating and exciting manner.

More specifically, this is a source book for curriculum development. It is designed to help the teacher organize the major health topics in such a way that students will embrace the essential health concepts, make decisions for their own health and for the well-being of others, and form the kind of value judgments that will promote the rich and full life. This is a formidable expectation. It is also a distinct possibility—providing, of course, that one aims high and communicates reasonably well with both colleagues and students. How much more can one hope to achieve?

Carl E. Willgoose

CONTENTS

Chapter 1

Hope, Health and Strategies for the Future

Somewhere in the deep strata of human awareness breathes a voice 'This is not good enough.' At moments there comes to people a painful sense of the nearness of richer and broader human fulfillment—and yet a feeling that some relentless, invisible, but not quite insurmountable barrier bars the way to a vastly better life. The clearness and vividness of this sense of the better possibility varies in different minds. In many it never breaks through at all to full consciousness. But in a few minds it becomes a dominant mood. It has been called the voice of Prometheus.[1]

The case for hope has never rested on provable facts or rational assessment. It is independent of the machinery of logic. What gives hope its power is the Promethean voice triggering the release of human energies in search of something better. It is this capacity for hope, says Norman Cousins, that gives human beings a sense of destination and the energy to get started. More specifically, "It enlarges sensitivities. It gives values to feelings as well as to facts."[2] It can provide men and women who are near despair with trust in their individual visions and in their own potentials.

Although hope and health have been clearly associated with one another from the days of Pope and Schopenhauer, not everyone in today's world is voicing optimism about human aspirations and the potentialities of a fully aware human being. Only recently the President of France, Valéry Giscard d'Estaing, spoke at length about an unhappy world that does not know where it is going, and senses that if it knew, it would discover that it was headed for disaster.

The crisis facing the world is a permanent one. In recognizing this situation d'Estaing reminded his listeners that the population buildup, the need for raw materials and energy, severe food shortages, and financial deficits are problems that will not change. In fact, because of their ongoing nature, the ultimate health of all human beings is at stake. There is little need to dramatize this conclusion, for it should be relatively easy to discern the relationship between sociopolitical shortcomings associated with worldwide competition for food and services and the mental, physical, and spiritual well-being of the citizenry.

---

[1]William H. Sheldon, *Prometheus Revisited*, Cambridge, Mass.: Schenkman Publishing Co., Inc., 1975, p.7.

[2]Norman Cousins, "Hope and Practical Realities," *Saturday Review/World*, December 14, 1974, p.5.

1

THE INEVITABILITY OF CHANGE

Almost two decades ago Rene Dubos wrote in *Mirage of Health* that life is an adventure in a world where nothing is static, "... where unpredictable and ill-understood events constitute dangers that must be overcome... where man himself... has set in motion forces that are potentially destructive and may someday escape his control."[3] This message represents one more anxious call to do something about forces bearing on illness and disease. It is one more summons to stimulate society to execute needed changes in support of the sensitivities and the fragilities of life.

During the past few years the President's Committee on Health Education has shown that it is now imperative to *educate* people about healthful living, for it is no longer possible to stem human illness and despair with improved medical and surgical techniques, more hospitals and social workers, and more sophisticated health care centers. The committee's message is a signal for a significant change — a call for prevention.

The new and spectacular forms of medicine and therapy should continue to excite an admiring public, as victims of maladies formerly deemed hopeless are rescued, and the catalogue of lifesaving strategies is extended. But it is the new dimension of health education (preventive medicine) that will help control the costly upkeep of elaborate medical facilities, complex technology, and highly trained health care personnel, and make a telling contribution to the prolongation of productive, enjoyable life. This can be accomplished with an adventurous, broad-spectrum approach to all human illness and health, from birth defects, cancer, and aging to the less sophisticated realms of ignorance, superstition, and indifference.

THE DANGERS OF TOLERANCE

The need to educate for health is not a new concept. It is the emphasis that is new. It is a twentieth century phenomenon that goes beyond political conflicts and astonishing technical inventions; in the words of Arnold Toynbee, it dares "... to think of the health of the whole human race as a practical objective."

The danger is that society will simply go along as it has in the past by tolerating illness and epidemics as somewhat inevitable in a highly populated and complex civilization. It is not likely that the citizenry is going to destroy itself, but it may well move to tolerate conditions that will weaken the quality of life. Dubos raises this warning very clearly:[4]

> Experience shows that people tend to tolerate bad conditions, if they have been *conditioned* to regard these conditions as normal during their formative years. Adults do not miss seeing the stars or the Milky Way if they have grown up in cities where the air is so polluted that they have never had the opportunity to learn to enjoy the exciting brilliance of a night sky.

Few people manage, in their adult years, to escape from early conditioning. For this reason alone, conditioning for health behavior is necessary in the formative years if one is to mature with appropriate living skills and understanding about the ecology of health.

One asks at this point: What specific happenings are relevant? What should one teach today? Are we not asking the old Spencerian question, "What knowledge is of

---

[3]Rene I. Dubos, *Mirage of Health,* New York: Doubleday and Co., Inc., 1960.
[4]Rene I. Dubos, "The Dangers of Tolerance," *Journal of School Health,* 44:182–185, April, 1974.

most worth?" Moreover, doesn't health education go beyond science and medicine to include a concern for housing, transportation, and finance? *In short, what is relevant in the seventies is a concern with the health system—a concern that becomes coterminous with concern about the total society.*

THE ECOLOGY OF HEALTH

"In Malaysia recently, in an effort to kill off mosquitoes, American technologists sprayed woods and swamplands with DDT. Result? Cockroaches which ate poisoned mosquitoes were so slowed in their reactions that they could be eaten by a variety of tree-climbing lizard, which promptly died of insecticide poisoning. The cats having died, the rat population began to increase; as rats multiplied, so did fleas; hence the rapid spread of bubonic plague in Malaysia. But this is not all. The tree-climbing lizards, having died, could no longer eat an insect which consumed the straw thatching of the natives' huts. So as Malaysians died of plague, their roofs literally caved in above their heads."[5]

—Peter A. Gunther

There is little to be accomplished in talking about Malaysia or any other society and its health, except in terms of the human environment and the standards that make living desirable. Human ecology, therefore, is concerned with the relationship between individ-

---

[5]Peter A. Gunther, "Mental Inertia and Environmental Decay: The End of an Era," *The Living Wilderness,* 34:3–5, Spring, 1970.

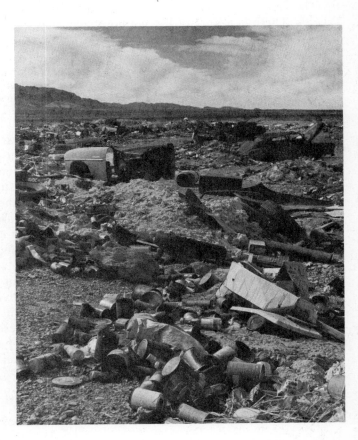

Figure 1–1 Land pollution near Las Vegas, Nevada. (Courtesy of Bureau of Land Management, U.S. Dept. of the Interior)

uals and their environment. The full scope of ecology goes beyond the boundaries of a discipline to the whole nature and meaning of life. Ecology views the whole earth as a living organism, "... of which man is simply a part, in exactly the same sense that the myriad organisms that participate in a single man's physical life processes are a part. Just as some of those organisms can be synergistically involved in promoting and prolonging creative, energetic survival of both themselves and their 'host', so can man be in relation to *his* host, the earth, or more precisely, the air and water and soil and sunlight that make up the tough and fragile and exceedingly precious envelope around it."[6]

The issue at hand is the quality of life in America. It is dead fish in polluted waters; it is eyes that smart from the city smog; it is DDT in robin eggs; it is a 95-decibel subway train and a roaring jet takeoff blasting in our ears and a host of other ecological disasters.

Human ecology embraces a great deal more than a calamitous view of the relationship between man and his environment. The nature of man is molded by the action of all physical, biological, and social forces in a constant process; this bears out the certainty of the World Health Organization definition of health: "Health is a state of complete physical, mental and social well-being and not merely an absence of disease or infirmity." Health, therefore, is more than a state; it is a potentiality.

It is this potentiality that will be embraced when greater attention is paid to the positive and beneficial effects of the environment than its pathogenic effects. In an attempt to advance these "beneficial effects," it is necessary to stress the word *equilibrium* as a fundamental concept in the study of ecology. Simply stated, an individual survives—and indeed a civilization survives—when it fashions an equilibrium with its ecosystem. Robert Russell, who wields a dynamic pen in support of ecology and health education, writes that life for any species is maintained best if that species is in equilibrium with other species. There is a kind of life harmony here that Russell nicely illustrates by quoting some lines used by Dubos from the Tao of Lao-Tzu:

> Those who flow as life flows
> Feel no wear, feel no tear
> Need no mending, no repair.[7]

Lines such as the above convey the connotation that human ecology and health education are inseparable. Health, like ecology, is both a multidimensional and multidisciplinary topic. It is as much an error to limit a discussion of a health item to the physical aspects as it is to study the mobility of an automobile strictly in terms of its wheels. An education for health, therefore, seeks ways to utilize the untapped resources of human beings. The concern is for all forces affecting man—anthropological, biological, psychological, and economic. And even the political dimension must be added, especially when one recalls the old English adage: "Where indeed is illness bred—in the heart or in the head—or in the body politic?"

There is one other particular on the ecological front that has meaning to the field of health science. This is conservation. It relates to individuality, to population and automation, to psychological stress and mental health, and to recreation. Man is a consumer of water, minerals, food, fibre—or of wilderness, for which there is no possible technological substitute. As wilderness, and even the partially open and wooded lands near the cities, declines in both total acreage and natural quality, man is the loser. A

---

[6]Russell E. Train, "Prescription for a Planet," *American Journal of Public Health,* 60:433–440, March, 1970.

[7]Robert D. Russell, "Toward a Functional Understanding of Ecology for Health Education," *Journal of School Health,* 39:702–708, December, 1969.

fresh conception of the relation of the human species to nature is needed. Like all other organisms, man performs a role within nature; he must learn that he is part of the whole, and that the ramifications of his total well-being are at times subtle and at other times forceful, but always something with which to reckon.[8]

THE HEALTH CARE DIMENSION

Schools, family life, and other facets of society are profoundly influenced by the health maintenance organizations (HMOs). In keeping with the nature of their operations and social philosophies, they are slowly integrating health education into their structures. There is also an economic logic that indicates that health benefits can match costs. This provides a compelling argument in favor of patient education in a variety of medical care settings—from hospitals and clinics to prepaid group practice plans.[9] Noteworthy group practice plans that include health education programs are the Health Insurance Plan of Greater New York (HIP), the Group Health Cooperative of Puget Sound, and the Kaiser Foundation. Common characteristics include periodic health examinations, immunizations, and other measures for the prevention and detection of disease. Thus, for their prepaid premiums, subscribers can expect full and continuous care, both medical and educational. Unfortunately, there is still a long way to go before health education becomes a significant part of the health care operation.

Another aspect of the health care dimensions concerns the preparation of the adult to handle what Herbert Klemme of the Menninger Foundation calls the "mid-life crisis"—a crisis that begins in the late twenties and extends through the forties. Klemme suggests that accidents, traumatic neuroses, physical illnesses, drug addiction, alcoholism, mild and severe depressions, suicide, and other self-destructive behavior in the middle years may be symptomatic of an inability to work through the mid-life crisis. It is the inability to face up to stress-related situations that reduce the effectiveness of the young leader and bring on high blood pressure and other significant items such as poor sexual functioning, which intensify the mid-life crisis by interfering with work productivity and home life, and by lowering self-esteem.[10]

There has been a growing effort to overcome the failure to comprehend long term adverse health effects that can result from living in a highly industrial and technological age by putting into practice comprehensive health planning. This kind of community-wide health planning was advanced under 1966 federal legislation known as the Comprehensive Health Planning and Public Health Services Act. It provides for the establishment of state and regional agencies with the expertise to bring all health personnel together. The consumer is involved in health planning and helps educate the public about existing health problems and resources. In Tecumseh, Michigan, an epidemiologic study of health and disease involved the whole community.[11] The effort was a total one, in which school children as well as adults were examined, studied, and counseled with

[8]For a more in-depth discussion of this topic see Carl E. Willgoose, "Health Aspects of the Conservation-Recreation Effort," *Journal of School Health*, 38:359–365, June, 1968.

[9]See especially L. W. Green and I. Figa-Talamancia, "Suggested Designs for Evaluation of Patient Education Programs." *Health Education Monographs*, Society of Public Health Educators, 2:54–71, 1974. See also Irving S. Shapiro, "HMOs and Health Education," *American Journal of Public Health*, 65:469–472, May, 1975.

[10]This theme is particularly well developed by the social worker Martha Stein in her book *Lovers, Friends, Slaves,* New York: G. P. Putnam's Sons, 1974, p. 325

[11]Henry J. Montoye, *Physical Activity and Health: An Epidemiologic Study of an Entire Community,* Englewood Cliffs, N.J.: Prentice-Hall, Inc., 1975.

respect to occupational and leisure time activities, physical exercise, weight, blood pressure, heart attacks, stress, smoking, cholesterol, and other comparable items. Such observational studies of populations in a community illustrate the complicated interplay of many genetic and environmental factors; they provide a superb opportunity to educate the inhabitants. Although they are not free of difficulties, other communities are doing similar activities. For example, in North Carolina, where two thirds of the population does not receive any regular dental care, there is a Ten Year Preventive Dentistry Plan to attain a major reduction in the prevalence of dental diseases by 1983. Dental epidemiologists have thoroughly mapped the state and there is every reason to believe that large numbers of individuals will become responsible for their own dental health.

CONTROLLING THE POPULATION

Progress in health care and health understanding would be more significant if the population on the earth would stabilize. It simply is not doing this. In fact, by the year 1980 the population of the United States will rise to 228 million people, and at a growth rate only two per cent less than in the preceding decade.[12] Actual growth will, of course, depend on the future levels of births, deaths, and net immigration.

About 75 per cent of all Americans are crammed together in metropolitan areas—a situation which breeds social and economic degradation to a high degree. Controlling the population becomes a concern of city planners, family partners, and schoolteachers alike. Mature students as well as adults must discuss such suggestions for control as social pressures and tax incentives for having fewer children, liberalized abortion laws, better contraceptive techniques, and improved sex education programs.

From a health and welfare viewpoint, the crowding of more and more people into a small space results in problems of transportation, housing, crime, air and water pollution, alcoholism, drug addiction, venereal disease, and a tendency for many people to become dehumanized and lost in the maze of the megalopolitan structure.

The health teaching implications here are numerous. There are very few other topics more relevant to modern education than the health concerns of urban areas. Research indicates that as people are crowded together they are more prone to violence. The U.S. homicide rate of 10 per 100,000 people is high when compared to Sweden's rate of 2.3 per 100,000 and England's 0.7 per 100,000. Moreover, individuals with low flash points for violence, of whom there are estimated to be several million, are likely to be triggered when crowded. Schizophrenia is far more prevalent in crowded urban areas than elsewhere. As privacy is threatened, humans squabble and fight back, frequently against unseen forces. They suffer the stresses of apprehension and anxiety, of fear and anger, and either resign themselves to their fate in apathy or rise in rebellion. Research at the National Institute of Mental Health indicates that when a population of laboratory rats is allowed to increase in a confined space, the rats develop acute abnormal patterns of behavior that can even lead to the extinction of the population.

The specter of starvation does not threaten very many people in the United States right now, but it is quite possible that real problems will arise in the lifetime of our grandchildren. Limiting the growth of population is an urgent and sensible demand upon the wealthiest as well as the poorest societies. Knowledge or technology alone cannot save mankind; only a change in values can.

An additional health factor is linked to the problem of overpopulation. It has to do with the unwanted child who becomes an unhappy child and ultimately a burden on both

---

[12]For details see *Statistical Bulletin* of Metropolitan Life Insurance Company, 55:9–11, November, 1974.

family and society. It is not uncommon in big city clinics to see the sad, unending and unyielding evidence of children being cuffed and beaten, being neither loved nor cared for—as vivid a ravagement as a virulent cancer. This "battered child syndrome" involves over 10,000 children a year in the U.S.—undoubtedly a conservative estimate.

To teach one to live in a highly populated area is no small task, yet it is a task that must be accomplished by the combined efforts of educators, parents, and community leaders.

ECONOMICS, POVERTY AND ILL HEALTH

Economists have become successors to Merlin, together with public opinion pollsters, as the seers of the technological age. Unfortunately, they frequently disagree with each other—even to being contradictory or, perhaps more accurately, fragmented. It is difficult, therefore, to predict just where the Gross National Product will be in the next several years. The same can be said for industrial production, unemployment, and poverty.

Poverty is a fact of life and poor families have more health problems than families with greater economic means. This has been demonstrated in a number of studies, including the United States National Health Survey. Internationally it has been shown over and over that intellectual and educational development of the individual is most difficult, if at all possible, when the body is chronically drained of its energy by lack of proper nutrition, illness, and parasites. The cycle of disease breeds poverty, and poverty in turn breeds additional disease; this occurs throughout the world (see Figure 1–2).[13] The solution is not found by attacking health problems alone. Rather, it is found by reducing illiteracy, achieving political stability, and integrating broad social and eco-

---

[13]From, *Strand IV Environmental and Community Health*, Curriculum Guide, Grades 7, 8, and 9, Albany, N.Y.: The State Education Department, 1970, p.28.

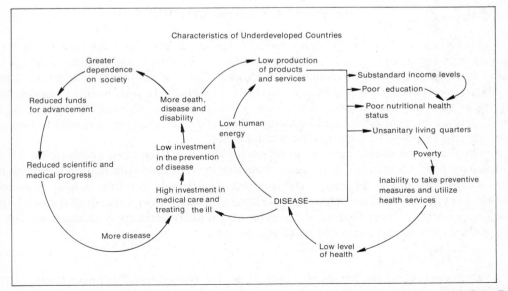

Figure 1–2 The vicious cycle of poverty, economics and ill health. (Courtesy of New York State Department of Education)

nomic reforms. Associated remedies involve better geographical distribution of physicians and other health manpower, and the use of physicians' assistants and neighborhood health organizations.[14]

Several American studies relating income level to morbidity from disease have been reported. One of the most extensive epidemiological studies was done by Pell and D'Alonzo on men employed by the DuPont Company.[15] The major finding was the consistently low frequency of various chronic disease entities among men in the upper-income levels; that is, among men holding such positions as officials, executives, managers, research scientists, attorneys, and engineers. It was postulated that the lower disease rates among these men were associated with such factors as ability to adapt to stresses and pressures, education, past and present environment, health habits, mode of living, and possibly the degree and quality of medical surveillance they received. The diseases studied were myocardial infarction, cerebrovascular disease, hypertension, obesity, diabetes mellitus, and cancer.

As income and economic levels increase and economic productivity advances, the work week will continue to shorten. With a 32 hour work week free time may become tiresome to the individual. The implications for mental health are numerous. How to use this time advantageously will be an educational challenge. Recreational competency will become even more important, causing philosopher and educator alike to think carefully on the words of Alfred North Whitehead, that no civilization has ever learned to survive with a large amount of leisure.

As the economy, coupled with the charity of man, permits more education and opportunity for the poor, their health status can only improve. Social workers, teachers, and medical personnel, working through neighborhood health centers, are achieving concrete health gains for the people. In both Boston and Providence, the effects of placing a comprehensive health center in the middle of a low-income public housing development have been amazing. Hospital admissions decreased by 50 to 75 per cent. Even the length of stay in a hospital was only one-fifth of what it was before. This is significant evidence that the poor do value their health, providing it can be brought to their attention in a relevant way.

THE HEALTH OF THE CITIZENRY

There is a good deal of evidence to indicate that despite the great improvements in human well-being, and the gradual movement from superstition and ignorance to a somewhat scientific viewpoint regarding health, it is still not possible to say with certainty that optimum well-being today has become an accomplishment. In fact, man may never quite arrive at such an ideal state as long as his civilization becomes more complex and he must depend on techniques and knowledges from the health sciences in order to survive. But, he can be proud of what he *has* accomplished.

The death and illness rates from infectious diseases have been declining for years. Infections from all sources have been dramatically reduced. Although it is higher for non-whites, the infant mortality rate dropped significantly for both whites and non-whites over the last quarter century. A hundred years ago, over a fourth of the newborns died before age 5. Three fourths of the babies born today can expect to reach the age of 62, and one-fourth can expect to reach age 84.

---

[14]See Nicholas M. Griffin, "Health Manpower: Trends and Issues," *Journal of School Health*, 44:310–313, June 1974.

[15]Sidney Pell and C. A. D'Alonzo, "Chronic Disease Morbidity and Income Level," *American Journal of Public Health*, 60:116–129, January, 1970.

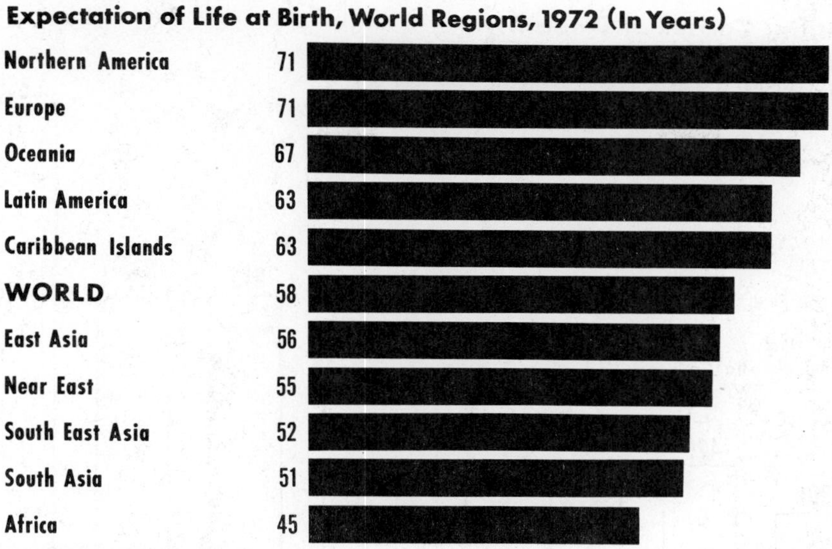

Expectation of Life at Birth, World Regions, 1972 (In Years)

Region	Years
Northern America	71
Europe	71
Oceania	67
Latin America	63
Caribbean Islands	63
WORLD	58
East Asia	56
Near East	55
South East Asia	52
South Asia	51
Africa	45

Source: Estimates from Bureau of the Census, "World Population: 1973, Recent Demographic Estimates for the Countries and Regions of the World," May 1974, pp. 5-11.

Figure 1-3   International longevity. (Courtesy of Metropolitan Life Insurance Company, *Statistical Bulletin*, May, 1974)

High living standards and medical science have increased longevity during recent years. In fact, the life expectancy at birth for the resident population of the United States increased to an all time high in 1974. The average length of life for the total population rose from 71.3 years in 1973 to 71.9 years in 1974—a gain of 12.7 years since 1929–31, when the average was about 59 years. Both sexes shared equally in the upswing. Expected lifetime rose to 68.1 years for the newborn male and to 75.8 years for the female. The favorable outlook reflected primarily a decline in deaths attributed to ischemic heart disease and other cardiovascular–renal diseases, as well as declines in fatalities from motor vehicle accidents and from pneumonia and influenza. The recent international trends in longevity in selected countries are shown in Figure 1–3. It is obvious that despite mean increases in the lifespan the maximum lifespan has remained unchanged at around 100 years. It is not likely, however, that the mean or maximum life expectancy figures will increase by any great amount in the years ahead. Current thinking suggests that the most disease-oriented biomedical research and anti-aging agents can do is to add perhaps 15 years to the mean life expectancy figures.

CURRENT HEALTH PROBLEMS

Although periodic medical examinations, early treatment, low cost vaccines, and superb hospital care have made a real impact on disease and disability, there are still a variety of both unsolved and solvable health problems. Through continued action in medical science and education it should be possible to substantially reduce conspicuous health problems such as the following.

Heart Disease

The cardiovascular diseases far outrank all other causes of death. Although mortality from heart disease has declined in the United States, it is by far the leading cause of

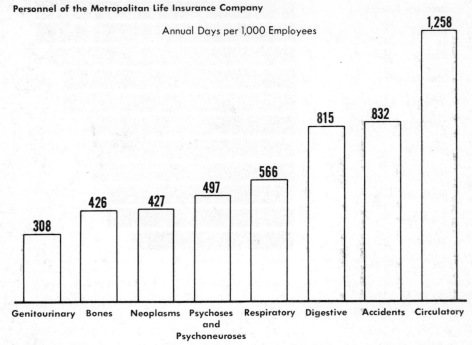

Figure 1–4   Leading causes of disability. (Courtesy of Metropolitan Life Insurance Company, *Statistical Bulletin*)

death, accounting for 38 per cent of all deaths in the nation. Almost 300,000 women suffered heart attacks in 1975. Any reduction in statistics appears to be related to the slow decline in cigarette smoking by men, a trend away from eating saturated fats which are high in artery-clogging cholesterol, and increased detection of hypertension. It should be noted that a great number of man-working days are lost by tens of thousands of people suffering from cardiac and other disabilities — people who have not yet contributed to mortality statistics, but are measurably unproductive, burdensome, and grossly unhappy (see Figure 1–4).

The public as a whole is short on knowledge in this area. A vast number of studies have shown a strong relationship between coronary heart disease and personal habits of physical activity, diet and obesity, cigarette smoking, and the extent of psychological stress. Coronary attacks come two to three times as often and are more severe in people who lead relatively inactive lives. In the well-known Framingham Heart Study, the "least active" men had more than three times the risk of having a heart attack than did the "most active" males. High-level physical activity confers protection against severe manifestations of coronary disease by stimulating the development of collateral circulation when the coronary blood flow is impaired. It also helps prevent overweight with attendant benefits of lower cholesterol levels, lower blood pressure, and reduced cardiac work load.

Considerable support for maintaining desirable body weight through proper eating and physical activity as an effective means of controlling blood cholesterol level comes from the Tecumseh, Michigan, community and a number of other studies. Interestingly, artery linings gather accumulations even in childhood. Blood cholesterol tests in more than 2000 normal children over a two-year period indicated that from 10 to 35 per cent of the children had an excess of cholesterol, and these levels were found to increase with age. Physicians caring for adolescents were advised to test blood cholesterol levels regularly and to help parents to plan diets when necessary.[16] Keeping physically active over the years seems to relate not only to serum lipid levels, but to the total glandular system. Thus the whole stress syndrome as it relates to the heart and other diseases needs study by young people. What Hans Selye wrote over two decades ago relative to human stress, emotional stability and disease is fundamental health education.[17]

Hypertension or high blood pressure is present in 15 to 20 per cent of the adult population. Some 24 million people are subject to stroke, heart disease, and kidney disease (see Figure 1–5). In fact, hypertension more than triples the risk. The significant point is that it can be readily discovered, treated, and kept under control. For many individuals control is difficult because of emotional interactions between a variety of socioeconomic stresses so common in modern life. In this respect, those prone to coronary heart disease belong to *behavior pattern type A*—characterized by personality traits such as aggressiveness, ambition, drive, competitiveness, and a profound sense of time urgency. Mannerisms and movements are rapid. Speech is usually forceful, fast, and often explosive and accompanied by sudden gestures such as fist-clenching and taut facial grimaces. These are the people who drive themselves to "get things done," they appear to be existing habitually under pressure of time. The type A person not only exhibits underlying

[16]Glenn Friedman and Stanley J. Goldberg, "Normal Serum Cholesterol Values," *Journal of the American Medical Association*, 225:610, August, 1973.

[17]Hans Selye, *The Stress of Life*, New York: McGraw-Hill Book Company, 1953.

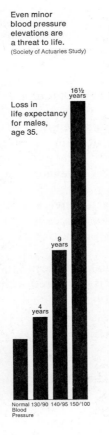

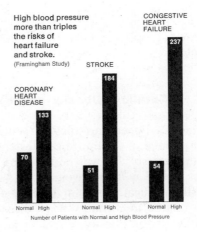

Figure 1–5 Normal and high blood pressure.

coronary arteriosclerosis, but he probably had hypertension in his early years. (Adolescent hypertension has been found in New York City high school students.) Thus, ongoing research is seeking the somewhat sophisticated relationship between the central nervous system and associated environmental stresses, and the role in the pathogenesis of coronary heart disease. These findings will in turn be compared with social class and racial differences in blood pressure. Blacks, for example, have higher average diastolic and systolic readings and a higher prevalence of hypertension than white males and females, and for all age groups.[18]

Not to be overlooked is the strong relationship between tobacco smoking and cardiovascular disease. The greater the cigarette consumption the greater the risk. The increase in the rise in fatal heart attacks among women is attributed to heavy cigarette smoking. Such smoking may cut a woman's life span as much as 19 years.[19] Active "intervention" programs to persuade men and women to reduce their smoking, cholesterol, and blood pressure are under way in a number of clinical centers of the National Heart and Lung Institute. These involve apparently healthy subjects who appear to be high risk individuals. The Framingham study's findings indicate that men with one of these risk factors have a 1.9 higher incidence of coronary heart disease than men with none of the factors. With two factors present the incidence is 3.4 times higher; with all three factors present, the incidence is 10.6 times higher.[20]

A rather large number of heart attacks occur without the awareness of the victim. It takes a routine health examination at a later time to show evidence of heart damage that had not been discovered earlier. Most of these recur, and half of the recurrences tend to be fatal. The real message here is one of knowledge and prevention. The late Paul Dudley White, cardiologist extraordinary, drives home a pedological point worth remembering:

> "We can and should pick out the potential candidates for heart attack as teenagers. This is where the school health education program comes in. What we do for someone in his 40's and 50's is much less important than what we do for him as a teenager. We know enough now to begin to educate the public how to prevent arteriosclerosis as a major cause of death."[21]

Nutrition, Obesity and Hypokinetic Disease

When Vermont's famed cardiologist, Wilhelm Raab, returned to America after a visit to Russia he spoke of the future of Western civilization in terms of "the survival of the fittest over the fattest." He was bothered by the great number of human diseases and inadequacies associated with overweight, obesity, and a sedentary type of living which requires very little physical energy in order to prevail.

Very much related to coronary heart disease, degenerative arthritis, and a number of lesser difficulties is the obesity prevalent in the affluent society — where three out of five men in their fifties are overweight, and half of the women over 40 years of age are at least 10 per cent above their optimum weight.

The major etiological factors in obesity are food intake in excess of needs, and physical inactivity. When the physical activity of the obese is compared with that of the non-

[18]S. Leonard Syme, et al., "Social Class and Racial Differences in Blood Pressure," *American Journal of Public Health,* 64:619–621, June, 1974.

[19]Editorial, "Women Smokers and Sudden Death," *Journal of the American Medical Association,* 226:2012, May, 1973.

[20]Medical News, "Six Years and 12,000 Men: Some Answers to Heart Disease," *Journal of the American Medical Association,* 227:1243–1244, March, 1974.

[21]Quoted from *School Health Review,* 1:19, September, 1969.

obese (matched for age, socioeconomic background, and occupation) there is a clear indication that obese men and women are far less active. Overeating is only part of the picture. Jean Mayer, the Tufts University nutritionist, believes that exercise and diet are
not alternatives but rather complements. When comparing obese girls with girls of normal weight for caloric intake and activity, Mayer discovered that the obese girls were
eating three to four hundred calories fewer per day than the girls of normal weight.[22] The
activity of these girls was studied by filming them at play. The obese girls spent only
about one-third as much time in physical activity as did girls of normal weight. Obese
girls stood motionless 80 to 90 per cent of the time in volleyball games or during swimming periods, while the other girls were motionless half that amount of time in volleyball
and only 20 per cent of the time in swimming. Mayer concluded that inactivity is a more
significant causative factor than overeating in the development of obesity. Moreover,
such things as parental nagging increase the obese youngster's sense of guilt and insecurity, causing even further withdrawal from normal physical activity. The University of
Washington School of Medicine compared obese teenagers with controls and discovered
that parents of the obese encouraged and perpetuated dependency, and they were not
really uncomfortable with the adolescent's social isolation. In fact, they usually viewed
the weight problem as the sole responsibility of the teenager and the professional, and
resisted becoming involved.

Obese adolescent girls seem to be much more knowledgeable about weight problems
than they are about solutions. Canning and Mayer compared 225 obese female adolescents
and 213 controls and discovered an obsession on the part of the obese with their weight, to
such an extent that areas of personality, looks, and emotional overtones became involved
in the issue.[23] Interestingly, the girls were aware of the role of exercise but lacked the
first-hand knowledge to get started. Both health education and physical education could
make a contribution here. Corbin and Pletcher arrived at the same general conclusion in
their comprehensive study of children.[24] They added the dimension that the pronounced
inactivity characteristic of the obese adolescents seems to be a carry-over from the inactive childhood years.

A nutrition education, coupled with physical exercise and psychological support, can
be introduced in a public school system. All it takes is cooperation. Seltzer and Mayer accomplished this in the Newton School System (Massachusetts) and made a strong case
for health education as follows:[25]

> "In our judgment, the opportunity for greatest success in the control of obesity lies in
> tackling the problem in the pre-adult stage, in obese children and adolescents, when the
> habits of diet and physical activity are more tractable to modifications and are not yet as
> firmly established as in adult life. In addition we believe the scope of the obesity problem
> in youngsters is so extensive (12% to 20% of the preadult population), that reliance can-
> not be placed on the individual initiative of parents and children to obtain weight control
> therapy where needed ... And, significantly, the eventual serious health consequences of
> the persistence of obesity into middle adult years make early obesity a *national public
> health problem* of communities across the country. The public school system, therefore,
> affords the most suitable and logical focus for an attack on the problem of weight control
> in our excessively fat youngsters."

[22]Jean Mayer, "Obesity Control for Adolescents," *Roche Medical Image,* 9:32–34, February, 1967.
[23]Helen Canning and Jean Mayer, "Obesity: Analysis of Attitudes and Knowledges of Weight Control in
Girls, " *Research Quarterly,* 39:894–899, December, 1968.
[24]Charles B. Corbin and Philip Pletcher, Diet and Physical Activity Patterns of Obese and Nonobese Elementary School Children," *Research Quarterly,* 39:922–928, December, 1968.
[25]Carl C. Seltzer and Jean Mayer, "An Effective Weight Control Program in a Public School System,"
American Journal of Public Health, 60:679–689, April, 1970.

Secondary school children have much to learn about foods and nutrition that has a bearing on human welfare and productivity. Few individuals have an understanding of the relationship between malnutrition and proper intellectual development. Separating sense from nonsense about nutrition is no small teaching assignment, for Americans seem willing to believe almost anything about diet. They seem to expect a certain magic from almost every kind of food. And to a certain extent some foods do indeed seem magical, especially when they are extrolled by writers and lecturers whose pronouncements are given unquestionable acceptance such as Linda Clark, Carleton Fredericks, Adelle Davis, and J. I. Rodale. With little nutrition education, it is difficult for youth to evaluate vegetarianism, Ohsawa's *Zen Macrobiotics,* Ehret's *Mucousless Diet Healing System,* and *Back to Eden,* by Kloss. The desperately overweight individual sees value in the Stillman Diet—a carbohydrate-restricted diet rich in protein and animal fat that calls for drinking at least eight glasses of water a day—resulting in a cholesterol consumption of more than twice the amount in the average American diet.[26]

Sifting truth from falsehood in the nutrition area is made difficult because of the varied ecological and political ideologies of youth. As individualism flourishes, eating philosophies become fragmented and adolescents embrace nonstandard eating patterns involving "health," "natural," and "organic" diets. In other circles changing life styles have caused people to seek convenience and nutritional impact. Thus, ready-to-eat cereals with milk enjoy wide consumption.

The diseases and inadequacies resulting from underactivity not only relate adversely to weight control, the cholesterol build-up, and circulatory disorders; they also have a bearing on other hypokinetic diseases such as undue muscle tension and low-back pain.[27] Psychiatrists employ exercise to relieve muscle tension. Exercise also aids in adaptation to the stress syndrome, with deep implications for mental health. It improves functional efficiency at any age and is a great aid to geriatricians, as it helps measurably to curtail both insomnia and fatigue in older citizens. However, while millions of individuals walk, ride bicycles, swim and jog, about 45 per cent of all adults do no engage in physical activity for the purpose of healthful exercise. Moreover, despite the activity of the President's Council on Physical Fitness and Sports, large numbers of adults report that they have not seen or heard information about the importance of physical fitness.

Lack of simple physical activity affects women as much as it does men. They suffer, often needlessly, from menstrual discomfort, backaches, and general fatigue due in part to inadequate muscle tone. In fact, large numbers of American women are not strong enough to stand the strains of pregnancy. As Evalyn Gendel of the University of Kansas Medical School points out, many girls and women are simply not prepared for the task of pregnancy when the time comes. They are not obese; they have a common history of inactivity from early childhood—little or no physical education, no bicycling, little dancing, and little walking or bowling. And they are completely unaware of the beneficial relationship of good abdominal tone and regular exercise in reducing menstrual pain.

Cancer

In the early 1900's there was practically no cure for cancer. By the 1930's the five-year survival rate was about one person in five. Ten years later it was one in four. Today it is about one in three. There are a million and a half living Americans who, five years

---

[26]Harvard Medical School findings reported in Rickman, F., et al., "Changes in Serum Cholesterol During the Stillman Diet," *Journal of the American Medical Association,* 228:54–58, April, 1974.

[27]See particularly Hans Kraus and Wilhelm Raab, *Hypokinetic Disease,* Springfield, Ill.: Charles C Thomas, 1961.

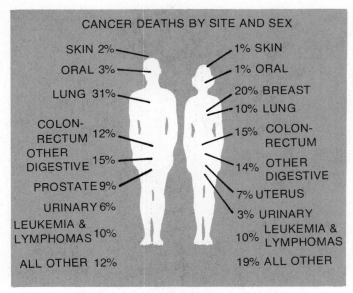

Figure 1-6   Cancer deaths by site and sex.

after diagnosis, show no evidence of the disease. This is real progress when 200,000 persons are saved each year.

However, cancer is still the number two killer with approximately 370,000 deaths in 1976.

Cancer of the breast is still the most frequently reported cancer among women, with 89,000 newly discovered cases in 1975 and 33,000 deaths. Cancer of the uterus figures, however, have improved measurably—from 28,000 deaths a year to 16,000. Most of these cancers occur in the cervix or neck of the uterus, and the Papanicolaou smear test for cancer is credited with the almost 50 per cent improvement in death rates. It has been suggested by cancer specialists that if every adult female would submit to this painless pelvic examination once a year, cancer of the uterus could be completely eliminated by early detection. Yet, almost 50 per cent of all women over 20 years of age have never been examined for cervical cancer. How to get the message across is the old question. The same public information question pertains to cancer of the colon and rectum, which is relatively easy to cure if discovered in time. It kills 48,000 people a year. The problem, as Holleb points out, is that people are still afraid of examinations, which are time-consuming processes, and they have little knowledge of how all kinds of cancer cases are being helped.[28]

Fifty years ago lung cancer was a rare disease, but it is now the most common cause of death from cancer among men and an increasingly common cause of death from cancer among women. Lung cancer occurs 5 times more frequently among men than among women; however, the incidence rate is rising rapidly among women and has increased ten-fold since 1964. After age 65, cancer risks for women are almost equal to that for men. The great problem continues to be pollutants in the respiratory system. The Nashville Air Pollution Study, as well as other pollution research, indicates that when extensive community-wide aerometric measurements are made and compared with the health status of the population there is a positive association between polluted air

---

[28]Arthur I. Holleb, "Using the Cancer Cures We Have Now," *Today's Health*, 48–49, April, 1970.

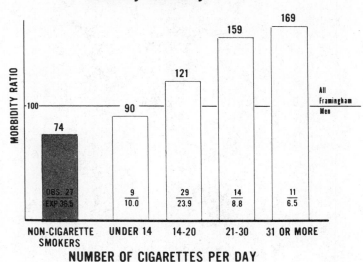

Figure 1–7   Cigarette smoking and coronary mortality. Coronary heart-disease risk increased with the *number* of cigarettes smoked daily. (Framingham Heart Study Report, U.S. Public Health Service, Pub. No. 1515, 1966)

and respiratory, gastric, and prostatic cancer. Mortality rates in high pollution zones were more than twice those in the lowest zones.[29]

Between the United States Public Health Service and the American Cancer Society, the topic of lung cancer and related diseases has been researched in more ways than almost any other disease known to mankind. Moreover, every major health group in the world has condemned cigarette smoking because of its direct relationship to cancer and emphysema in the respiratory system. Its relationship to coronary mortality is shown in Figure 1–7.

An impartial word about smoking is in order. It is related to a number of diseases besides cancer and coronary insufficiency. Risk of death from emphysema is six times greater for smokers than for non-smokers. This progressive respiratory disease causes 20,000 deaths a year. Smokers have more chronic bronchitis and hardening of the aorta. They also have more gingivitis, loss of bone surrounding the teeth, and other forms of periodontal disease. And of course they do not live as long as non-smokers. American Heart Association and American Cancer Society statistics show clearly that heavy smokers, on the average, lose about one minute of life for every minute they smoke. In fact, the death rate from lung cancer for men who are heavy smokers (more than 2 packs a day) is over 200 per 100,000, which is 15 to 20 times greater than that for men who do not smoke.

More young people smoke now than ever before.[30] By 1974 the proportion of teenage girls who smoked almost equalled, for the first time, the percentage of boys who smoked. Today, about 16 per cent of boys and an equal percentage of girls are smokers. There is still a link between smoking while pregnant and stillbirths, deaths among newborns, and lower birth weight of babies.

---

[29]Warren Winkelstein, Jr., and S. Kantor, "Air Pollution and Prostatic Cancer," *American Journal of Public Health,* 59:1134–1138, July, 1969.

[30]See result of an elaborate study by Saul R. Kelson, et al., "The Growing Epidemic: A Survey of Smoking Habits and Attitudes Among Students in Grades 7 Through 12, *American Journal of Public Health,* 65:923–938, September, 1975.

The no smoking movement in defense of clean air and the rights of nonsmokers should have an impact on those youths who are considering smoking. Outlawing smoking in public establishments to *protect* the majority puts smokers on the defensive. It also causes many smokers, who wish that they did not smoke anyway, to become reasonable about curtailing their habit.

The problem for the educator is to understand the underlying reasons for smoking behavior. Adolescents smoke because their parents do, and because they want to keep up with their peers. Their reasons for smoking cigarettes are the same as for smoking marijuana, taking "speed," and using other drugs, all of which present social and health problems. Frustrated kids want to experiment and sometimes rebel against an adult world. They need help, for they are happier, more self-confident, and more success-oriented when they don't smoke.

Dental Problems

Statistics in the area of dental health continue decade after decade to be almost beyond any real control. They seem to be as much a part of civilization as poetry and the arts. Yet, aberrations in dental health are closely related to numerous factors affecting human growth and well-being. Despite years of "school talk" relative to teeth, the same old factors are with us—poor diet, poor oral hygiene, and failure to receive prompt and adequate dental care.

It is interesting to note that the prevalence of men and women without natural teeth and the number of decayed, missing, and filled teeth are inversely related to rising levels of education and family income. Children in poverty areas all too often do not receive dental care. The result is that by the time they are 35 to 40 years of age, 70 per cent will need bridges or dentures to replace lost teeth.

There is an educational problem here. For one thing, severe dental caries are associated with poor academic achievement and a high absence rate. Also, they are highly related to how well a community is informed about the benefits of fluoridated water. Far too many people remain misinformed in this area despite the long-standing acknowledgement that fluoridation of the drinking water reduces tooth decay up to 70 per cent and cuts dental care costs per child to one half of what it is in non-fluoridated communities.

Fluorides not only reduce the hazards of malocclusion; they also contribute to stronger bones—less osteoporosis in older folks and therefore less likelihood of bone fracture due to an accidental fall. There appears to be a striking difference between high- and low-fluoride areas in the number of calcified body parts. In one study both men and women in a high fluoride area had 40 per cent fewer calcified aortas than men and women in low fluoride areas.[31]

Seldom, when teeth are discussed, is reference made to the adverse role of cigarette smoking. Yet, periodontal disease and ensuing tooth loss is considerably higher in smokers of both sexes. In fact, findings on some 10,000 patients at the Roswell Park Memorial Institute indicated that smokers have about twice the chance of experiencing periodontoclasia as do non-smokers.[32]

---

[31]Research reported by F. J. Stare. See *American Journal of Public Health,* 60:792, April, 1970.
[32]Harold Solomon, et al., "Cigarette Smoking and Periodontal Diseases," *Journal of the American Dental Association,* 77:1081–1084, November, 1968.

Mental Health

The magnitude of the problem of mental disorders is much greater than is revealed in presently available data. There is a difficulty in getting reports on the milder personality disorders. While the more severe forms of emotional disturbance, psychoses, are more readily detected and classified, the milder psychoneurotic conditions exhibit greater variability between patients in symptoms and signs, and greater differences between physicians in diagnostic judgment.

Despite the fact that half the hospital beds in the country are occupied by the mentally ill, a great number of people in poor mental health are simply at large in the community; an increasing number are being helped as outpatients, but many more are not being helped at all. Some 18 million Americans suffer mental disturbances and handicaps which to varying degrees limit their ability to carry on major life functions. Large numbers of people are depressed, and depression is the most untreated of all major diseases, despite the fact that in most cases it is relatively easy to handle.[33] Moreover, less than 5 per cent of the 20 million people a year that need help receive it at psychiatric treatment facilities.

A Senate committee has estimated that 10 per cent of public school children are emotionally disturbed and in need of psychiatric guidance. Moreover, there are few communities in this country which provide an acceptable standard of services for its mentally ill children. This is compounded by the projected estimates of children and youth who will require treatment in the future—a projection of a 164 per cent increase in the groups under 15 years of age. It follows, therefore, that learning to see oneself as a totality during the formative school years is a significant experience which all school children should share. In fact, learning to "know oneself" and communicate values is the only sound antidote to the wide variety of mental disorders and depressions, and the many instances of alcoholism, suicide, and downright irritable and sour personalities.

Poor mental health is manifested in many ways, including the 22,000 suicide deaths which occur each year. Moreover, for everyone who commits suicide there are 10 others who make an attempt and fail. About every minute someone either kills himself or tries to kill himself with conscious intent. Expert help and reassurance is needed at such times of suicidal crisis—a time when the pressures of life seem so intolerable to some people that suicide is considered. When studies are made of characteristics predisposing to suicide, it is generally found that anxiety and despair are in the forefront.

Unhappy secondary school and college students rank high among suicides today. They lack a dimension; they can't face defeat in familial, social and academic circles. Research has shown that a number of self-inflicted injuries and poisonings not ascribed to accidental circumstances were considered as suicides. Relatively few "accidental" poisoning cases involving adolescents brought to poison control centers are accidental. Most are suicide attempts. In an Omaha study of poisoning, 70 per cent turned out to be suicide gestures, and 26 per cent of the subjects had made previous suicide attempts.[34] In a high percentage of these cases, there was too much parental control and unreasonably high expectations. The automobile is also an almost ideal instrument for self-destruction. There is evidence to show that many people involved in single-car accidents may be trying to tell something, but no one is listening. They are unhappy and not well

---

[33]Nathan S. Kline, "Antidepressant Medications," *Journal of the American Medical Association,* 227:1158–60, March, 1974.

[34]Matilda S. McIntire and Carole R. Angle, "Psychological 'Biopsy' in Self-Poisoning of Children and Adolescents," *American Journal of Diseases of Children,* July, 1973.

adjusted; they have a greater number of highway accidents than people in good mental health.

Related to the general topic of mental health and suicide is the subject of death. It is not easy to discuss freely in most educational circles, yet it relates directly to the ultimate meaning of life and the values well-adjusted men and women live by. Leviton makes an admirable case for the study of man's ability to cope with his own imminent death and the death of others as a valid area of concern for health educators.[35] It deserves attention.

Accidents

If reasonable people know the truth about a problem, the truth in some way should help them solve the problem. This has certainly occurred to some degree as people everywhere have learned to live safely. Yet accidents continue to be the fourth leading cause of death for adults, and number one for children between the ages of 5 and 14 years.

More than 10,000 pedestrians die from traffic accidents every year, and about 20 per cent of these deaths are elementary and secondary school-age students. There are approximately 5 million injuries occurring each year about the home, 30,000 of which are fatal. An increase in home canning has brought on more food poisoning, chiefly botulism. Another 9000 people die each year from drowning despite widespread programs of swimming and water safety instruction; several thousand more succumb from participation in sports and recreation—a figure that has increased in recent years almost 8 per cent, due primarily to the sharp rise in leisure time sports and recreation throughout the western world; firearm accidents claim about 2800 lives, not counting suicides and homicides. Firearms injuries alone are well over the 100,000 mark each year; and bicycle accidents add up to an annual loss of over 800 lives and cause 150,000 disabling injuries.

The biggest contributor to accident statistics is the motor vehicle. Approximately 60,500 motor vehicle fatalities and 1.9 million disabling injuries occurred in 1973. One year later there was an 18 per cent drop in the number of persons killed in highway traffic accidents—a figure widely attributed to a mandatory reduction in driving speed associated with the national movement to conserve energy. This is partly due to the increasing number of people driving automobiles. When the motor vehicle hazard is appraised in several different ways, it appears that the safety record of the United States compares on the whole rather well with most other countries. However, there is considerable room for improvement, particularly when it comes to drinking and driving. Alcohol abuse by persons under 18 is increasing and adults frequently set poor examples. Few high school students drink at home, and in a National Highway Traffic Administration study half of them indicated that they had driven at least once or twice while intoxicated. The same government agency calls attention to the hazards of motorcycle driving, noting 3500 deaths in 1974 and a cycle death rate of 17 per 100 million miles of travel as compared to the 4.5 rate per 100 million miles for automobile travel.

Automobile research relative to accidents and safety practices indicates that factors of attitude, personality, and adjustment are of greater importance in safe driving than sensory defects, reaction time, and psychomotor skills. This means that education for safe driving has much to offer. How else can the gap between safety belt installation and

---

[35] Dan Leviton, "The Need for Education on Death and Suicide," *Journal of School Health,* 39:270–274, April, 1969.

safety belt *use* be closed? The belts are only used about 30 per cent of the time. There could be a saving of 10,000 lives a year instead of the 3000 now saved. And the use of shoulder straps could reduce deaths to almost zero at speeds under 60 miles an hour. Hopefully, there will develop a greater degree of cooperation between manufacturers and consumers. In any case, formal safety education has as much to offer as do legislation and product design.

The coupling of the two is important, especially when one considers that 400,000 people a year are burned or injured through fires alone. According to the Department of Health and Welfare figures there are an estimated 3000 to 5000 deaths annually from flammable wearing apparel, and from 150,000 to 200,000 burns each year from these materials. The following hospital intensive care unit report is not uncommon:

> In one isolation room a 78 year old Somerville woman lay swathed in blood-soaked bandages from head to toe, "like a mummy," her son said. Modern electronic devices and a maze of tubes were keeping her alive. She had already received 103 units of O-positive blood.
> Nine days earlier, about 11:30 p.m., her flannel nightgown had been ignited by an electric hotplate as she made a cup of coffee. Confused, she fled to the street a flaming torch—and by the time someone had called the fire department more than 80 per cent of her body had been covered with third degree burns. Only the back of her head was untouched by the flames.

Environmental Pollution

It has already been pointed out that any study of man's community must consider the total environment—an ecological view. Pollution is only one variable having to do with human ecology, but it is significant enough to have become the concern of business, government, public health, politics and education in several subject matter fields.

Americans generate a staggering amount of solid waste—150 million tons per year of rubbish, garbage, newspapers, beer cans, broken glass, plastic bottles, meat bones, grass cuttings, old mattresses, junked cars, and hundreds of other throwaway items. Someone has calculated that if New York City's domestic garbage was heaped in Yankee Stadium, it would make a mile-high mountain within a year.

Pollution is also the problem of the inner city with its overcrowding and burdensome demand for housing, employment, education, and recreation. The more crowded the city, the greater the atmospheric pollution, waste removal problems, crime, unresolved poverty, youth troubles, dehumanized individuals with family and neighborhood difficulties, and a variety of health disorders, from very specific diseases to vague unhappiness.

One asks, how do we encourage individuals to do something about the environmental problems? What does it mean to say that 20 billion dollars is the estimated cost of the havoc wrought annually by pollutants? The U.S. Environmental Protection Agency estimates 4000 deaths and 4 million sick days each year are attributed to automobile air pollution. A high percentage of this comes from exhaust systems and will not kill healthy individuals during a limited exposure. But it does cause faulty time judgments, headaches, and visual impairment problems. With additional exposure comes reduced ability to engage in physically active work, nausea, dizziness, and eventually convulsions and unconsciousness.

A minimum of 4000 cases of water-borne illnesses occur yearly in America. According to the Department of Health, Education and Welfare about 8 million people are served impure water through community water systems. And the ocean, with its vast amount of water, is too fragile to absorb sludge waste forever. In fact, says oceanographer

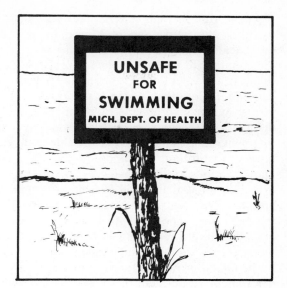

Figure 1-8   What does it take to engage our jaded attention?

Jacques Cousteau, the ocean is more than a weather-regulating system and source of food. It functions to absorb vast quantities of carbon dioxide and releases a major part of the oxygen one breathes.[36]

Lead and vinyl chloride poisoning, thermal pollution, and overexposure to radioactivity are significant environmental concerns. So is noise pollution, which fosters irritability and seriously threatens mental health. Yet, it is not the scientist making discoveries that affect health and general well-being who must make the value judgments and ultimate decisions. It is an individual and community decision. Human values and ecological considerations frequently collide in the political arena; health and welfare interests compete with other interests and a stalemate results. Fundamental to resolving the issues is an informed public that will support appropriate measures for its own survival. The role of the health educator, therefore, is especially important in helping to identify and remedy pollution problems, and offset the frequently heard doomsday philosophy that western civilization is on the way out—suffering irreversibly from suffocation, overbreeding, poisoning, and pollution.[37]

Alcohol and Drug Abuse

The dramatic increase in the use of alcohol and other drugs in the population, and particularly among youth at all socioeconomic levels, is of such magnitude that practically everyone agrees that there is a need for personalized education—one that is concerned with the psychological and sociological aspects of the motivation for using drugs.

As teenagers drink and ingest various mind-altering substances the theme again and again is one of disenchantment and alienation, particularly in the area of values. Youngsters are struck with a sense of futility about the basic institutions of their society,

---

[36]Jacques Cousteau, "The Perils and Potentials of a Watery Planet," *Saturday Review/World,* August 24, 1974, p. 41.

[37]For more details concerning environmental impact see Charles A. Bucher, Einar A. Olsen and Carl E. Willgoose, *Foundations of Health,* 2nd edition, Englewood Cliffs, N.J.: Prentice-Hall, Inc., 1976, pp. 292–326.

so they criticize their parents and challenge their teachers and clergy to relate to the world as the young see it. Moreover, it is a frequently distorted world with enough complications to test the fiber of the most informed and dedicated health teachers.

Immediate health problems are associated with the abuse of drugs. Some of these relate to the liver and the brain, but because the metabolism of drugs in the body is so complex many other systemic reactions occur. These include damage to genetic mechanisms, epilepsy, problems of pregnancy, the impairment of learning capacities, pelvic disorders in the female, birth defects, psychotic reactions leading to mental confusion, disorientation, hallucinations, suicide and violence, and social degradation leading to crime, prostitution, and unproductive lives. Moreover, there is no evidence that these manifestations are decreasing.

Alcohol statistics will continue to blemish the advances of civilization as mortality and morbidity figures rise due to excessive drinking. Twelve million people have drinking problems. Independent of dietary deficiencies, many have liver damage, phosphate depletion, and a reduction in bone density, leading to higher risk of fracture. Alcoholic women who are pregnant frequently bring on a "fetal alcohol syndrome" characterized by postnatal growth deficiency in length, weight, head circumference, and intelligence. With about 72 per cent of the population over age 15 consuming alcoholic beverages, it is apparent that mental health difficulties will continue to lead to more alcoholism. The National Institute of Mental Health reports that alcohol related health problems account for 26 per cent of all admissions to state and county mental hospitals. Fortunately, the majority of people who drink are not adversely affected by the custom. It is the minority—an increasing minority—that causes the problems.

A government study of 10,000 junior and senior high school students has shown that as many as 92 per cent have used alcohol at least once—with 7 per cent becoming intoxicated four times a year in the seventh grade and rising to 36 per cent by the 12th grade.[38] Among teenagers in Toronto the use of alcohol "at least once in a six month period" increased from 46 per cent in 1968 to 73 per cent in 1974.[39] In the San Mateo County, California, study the figures for "alcohol use during the past year" increased as follows:[40]

Year	Per Cent
1968	65
1969	73
1970	74
1971	77
1972	81
1973	85
1974	86

There is a possibility that a ceiling of alcohol use by youth is being approached, particularly by older teenage males.

Marijuana use among teenagers is reported in the vicinity of 34 per cent. It enjoys an increasing popularity which gives no evidence of disappearing. A few cigarettes (joints)

[38]Morris Chafetz, "Teenage Drinking Rising Sharply," *American Medical News,* July 22, 1974.
[39]R. M. Smart and D. Tefer, *"Changes In Drug Use in Toronto High School Students,* Toronto, Ontario. Addiction Research Foundation, 1974.
[40]Grace M. Barnes, "A Perspective On Drinking Among Teenagers with Special Reference to New York State Studies," *Journal of School Health,* 45:386–390, September, 1975.

present no hazard, but heavier use involves the active ingredient tetrahydrocannabinol (THC) with lipophilic brain tissues and with the production of DNA. When the DNA production process is slowed, the virus- and bacteria-fighting white blood cells become less efficient and less numerous.

Heroin use in America began a decline in the early 1970's, chiefly because of availability. By 1974, however, there was a sharp upturn in use due primarily to the "brown heroin" (brown because of impurities) brought to the country from Mexico. This caused the Drug Enforcement Administration to increase its budget to almost one half billion dollars. Infants born to narcotic-dependent mothers are often themselves physically dependent on heroin, and exhibit withdrawal symptons when deprived of the drugs.

As already indicated, young people use drugs for a number of social reasons, but experimentation was found to be the single most important motive in a Portland, Oregon, study of public high school students.[41] Here 12 hypotheses were tested concerning the motivations for use of barbiturates, hallucinogens, cocaine, sedatives, inhalants, amphetamines, and marijuana.

Almost everyone concedes that there is a serious drug problem in this country, but a logical discussion of its possible remedies is exceedingly difficult because of strong emotions about almost every one of its aspects. This is because this complex health concern is intricately tied in with the way modern people go about the business of living. Tranquilizers are used abundantly as one means of coping with stress. Is this drug abuse? Do physicians use drugs too freely and fail to control the refilling of prescriptions or employ too strong a drug when a simpler one would do? When the illicit use of drugs is discussed realistically it involves the people who demand an antibiotic everytime they catch a cold. Dana Farnsworth of Harvard University focuses on the difficulty:[42]

> . . . when we talk about the drug problem, we are talking about a people problem. We are talking about a tendency to substitute an instant evasion of our problems for a sound approach to their solution. This places a great burden on all of us . . . we have to show them [youth] that the only way to approach drugs of all types is to make them our servants rather than our master.

The physical and mental health teaching implications in this area are greater, perhaps, than any other. Humankind has come to look to drugs — both new and old — to bring about much needed temporary serenity. However, as values become disoriented and drugs are abused, something is lost in the process. How does one learn that chemical comforters, used increasingly as a substitute for coping with the challenges of living by means of personality resources, will lead eventually to less ability to cope with family responsibilities, financial worries, job situations, death, fear, and other stressful situations?

Human Sexuality

One of the foremost shortcomings having a bearing on health and happiness has to do with the widespread lack of knowledge and understanding of human sex and sexuality. It has been stated well that "sex is not something you do; it is something you are," and until this viewpoint prevails there will continue to be a variety of sex-related problems.

---

[41]Morris Weitman, et al. "Survey of Adolescent Drug Use," *American Journal of Public Health,* 64:417–421, May, 1974.
[42]Dana L. Farnsworth, "Drug Use for Pleasure: A Complex Social Problem," *Journal of School Health, 43*:153–158, March, 1973.

Venereal disease continues to be a blight on the land. It is primarily a teenage disease, striking the 15 to 19 year old group very hard. Ten years ago it was believed to be diminishing because of the increased availability of antibiotics, chiefly penicillin. Effective treatment should have led to its disappearance, but it has increased measurably since 1962. Moreover, the actual case rates are undoubtedly higher than those reported because physicians still fail to report a large number of venereal infections.

Primary and secondary syphilis started to drop during the late sixties. By 1970, however, the rate was heading up again to over 10 cases per 100,000 persons. By 1975 the incidence of syphilis had risen an incredible rate of 108 per cent in a 15 year period.[43] The gonorrhea toll, significantly, continues to rise every year, and in 1969 a staggering 494,227 cases were reported—a 14 per cent increase over the previous year—and involved 246 persons per 100,000 population. By 1974 there were over 900,000 such cases, but it was estimated that there were actually well over 3 million infections treated in the United States alone, and many more that were not treated. Worldwide figures indicate that approximately 150 million people were treated in a recent year. Such an uncontrolled state of disease (pandemic) is occurring throughout the civilized world except in Mainland China. About 75 per cent of females show no symptoms of the disease, and even men can carry the gonoccocal infection without symptoms—another reason why the disease is hard to control. Moreover, one of five women infected with gonorrhea develops pelvic inflammatory disease, and in a recent year 122,000 women experienced pelvic surgery because of it. Venereal disease is always greatest in the cities, where people are in close contact. New York, Miami, Chicago, and Detroit have very high rates. Venereal disease has now become the most prevalent reportable communicable disease in the nation and by the most conservative estimates, is clearly out of control. Almost every scientist writing on the topic has called for stepped-up education programs. This is particularly impressive when it is noted that ignorance is a significant factor. In New York City, where syphilis among teenage boys doubled in an eight-year period, a study showed that 32 per cent did not know that it could be cured, and 60 per cent did not know that venereal disease is transmitted through sexual intercourse.

Unknown to youth are the bacterial and viral diseases infecting the female vaginal tract. A leukorrhea infection caused by Trichomonas, a parasitic protozoan that produces a white-green watery and frothy discharge, is frequently mistaken by youths for the more common venereal diseases. The same can be said for the disagreeable odor and curd-like discharge of moniliasis (Monilia). Vaginal irritations and warts also present problems. The moist, alkaline climate of the vaginal tract created, in part, by the pill has made it easier for these infections to become seated. Ten years ago the herpes virus Type 2 was a rare infection; today it is exploding throughout the population with probably one half million cases being treated per year.[44] This painful genital herpes may be attributed in part to an increased practice of oral/genital sex. Preliminary research indicates that women suffering from herpes Type 2 infections are eight times more likely to develop cervical cancer than are those free of the disease.

Americans have grown increasingly tolerant of premarital sex, but the level of understanding among young people about pregnancies, contraception, abortion and boy-girl sex roles has not risen accordingly. Dynamic sociopolitical issues such as abortion, with 950,000 operations a year, continue to be neglected in school discussions—treated no differently than dozens of other marriage-family issues that miss the "teachable moment." Each year the illegitimacy rate is higher than the previous year despite the wide-

---

[43]Nicholas J. Fiumara, "Specifics for Syphilis", *Drug Therapy*, February, 1975.
[44]Genell Subak-Sharpe, "The Venereal Disease of the New Morality." *Today's Health,* March, 1975, p. 42.

spread use of effective contraceptives and an ever increasing opportunity to obtain a legal abortion. This clearly indicates a need for thorough sex education programs in large population areas so that attitudes toward sexuality can be thoroughly explored.

Schools are gradually facing the responsibility of teaching in the area of sex and family living education, but much remains to be done. Comprehensive programs for pregnant teenagers exist today by the hundreds in a number of the larger cities. The best sex education, coming too late, frequently takes place here, while other young people crave information and explanations. They seek standards to live by, and they want to talk about it. They know that parents are of little help and they are not about to change. They know that sex sells everything from automobiles to toothpaste and is on display everywhere, both in and out of the arts. It is used and abused in the culture, yet it is entwined practically, romantically and mysteriously with the all-encompassing subject of love. Where can it lead one? Where should it lead one? These are the questions for which youth seeks answers.

Sickle Cell Anemia

When a particular altered type of hemoglobin is present in red blood cells the inherited disease of sickle cell anemia is present. What causes it, who gets it, and how is it recognized are the kinds of questions that should be asked by a larger part of the public than now does so. Blood tests must be made and carriers advised about situations which might cause a moderate lack of oxygen, and ultimately result in death from infections, heart or kidney failure, or other vital organ damage. Since about 2 of 25 American blacks carry the sickle cell trait, an educational campaign to discover cases early is a part of the health education message.

Consumer Protection

The American public, bright as it is in numerous ways, can be a most gullible, superstitious, and misinformed composite of individuals when it comes to the consumption of health and health-related items. As much as two billion dollars is spent annually on falsely promoted, worthless, and frequently dangerous services, machines, and products.

Some 300 million dollars is spent annually on nonprescription products that claim to relieve cold symptoms, and another 70 million dollars is spent each year by promoters to extol the virtues of one brand over another. Arthritis is made to order for the quacks as they prescribe copper bracelets, honey and vinegar, colon irrigation and a variety of other fake "cures." The get-well schemes stimulate the hopes of those afflicted with cancer, obesity, impotence and general malaise—often the poor and, more than often, the elderly poor.

In the Gaines study, students right out of high school were sampled to determine their health misconceptions.[45] The misconceptions were classified into twelve consumer health content areas. The highest percentage of correct answers for any area was only 64.4 per cent. The lowest, 12.375 per cent, was in the legal area, where some 91 per cent of the students erroneously believed that "government public health agencies have the

[45]Josephine Gaines, "Some Possible Psychological Dynamics of Consumer Health Misconceptions," *Journal of School Health, 38*:489–493, October, 1968.

authority to enact legislation." Also, 100 per cent of the students did not believe that "much false and misleading information about nutrition can be published and freely circulated without fear of legal punishment or penalty."

The Gaines study also showed that 42 per cent believed that "health articles in popular magazines are always checked for their scientific and medical accuracy before they are published." The author goes on to say:

> "Other types of erroneous beliefs associated with current advertising included the need for special iron preparations, that osteoarthritis results from acid and poisons in the blood, that many diseases are caused by persistent acidosis and that daily bowel movements are essential to good health. The individuals tested tended to believe that electric vibrators and isometric exercises are effective means of weight reduction. One hundred per cent were of the opinion that increased consumption of proteins improves athletic performance. It seems apparent that many individuals do believe most of what is presented to them via the media — in written form, on radio and TV. It appears that the insinuations and messages of advertising have been effective. People have an uncritical and fantastic faith in the published word."

Many people seem to want to live, if not forever, at least an extra twenty-five or fifty years fat-free, pain-free, pimple-free, with unwrinkled skin, their own hair, sweet-smelling breath, and the energy of a young gazelle. Because of this, they'll swallow half-truths with truths and listen to the tub-thumpers and pitchmen who pursue and harass them from all sides. And if they suffer from infirmities associated with cancer, arthritis, or some disorder with unrelenting pain and misery, they'll ignore competent medical attention and squander family funds in order to support the charlatans and quacks dispensing the fads and fallacies.

An estimated ten million Americans spend a half-billion dollars a year on nutritional quackery alone. The greatest danger comes when sick people abandon accepted treatments to experiment with food fads or treat themselves with worthless dietary pills. Moreover, thousands of people do not know that scientific evidence *does not* support the popular premise that modern foods are nutritionally inadequate. Self-medication is always a questionable practice. Because aspirin will reduce fever and help relieve pain, there are people who use it erroneously for everything else that bothers them. Along with a wide variety of products for self-medication are the harmless but worthless kind. More tragic than the financial loss is the continued suffering and deaths in some cases, and the destroying of confidence in authentic agencies, services, and products.

An informed, thinking public is important in controlling medical quackery, misinformation, and fraudulent practices. Unfortunately, a surprisingly large number of people do not realize that there is a difference between a doctor holding an M.D. degree and a practitioner of dubious arts who may call himself "doctor." These same people fall easily for the "secret formula," the quick cure, the impressive testimonials and the often present argument that medical men are afraid of the competition.

Watchdogs in the private sector, such as *Consumer Reports,* offer a superb service. The relatively new role of the Federal Trade Commission in regulating advertising is also significant, but it has been condemned by many in business because it is cutting into the freedom afforded by the government's heretofore laissez-faire policy. Others applaud the FTC, realizing that decades of half-truths and outright lies in advertising have undermined the public's confidence in advertising.

Problems of the Aging

The time to prepare for old age is when you are young. This is the time to learn the value of regular physical, mental, and creative activities. The secret of life in retirement is to be interested in what is taking place—to be a participant in some small way. Yet thousands of oldsters simply vegetate year after year—bored by a lack of physical and mental stimulation to a point of chronic fatigue and low spirits.

It is not how long one lives but how well he lives that is important. There is no need for a person over sixty-five years of age to submit to the all too common sedentary existence of watching the passing scene and believing that a stiff, flabby, groaning, weak, tired, breathless body is quite normal. The average senior high school student has had enough background to discuss the ramifications of age in a meaningful way, and to discuss the Joe Lee philosophy that "we don't cease to play because we grow old; we grow old because we cease to play."

AN EDUCATION FOR HEALTH

It should be clear by now that the need for health teaching in the schools is anything but superficial. It is a deep topic of such magnitude that it affects every facet of life in the society. Significantly, a greater number of the problems, diseases, and inadequacies of adult mankind do not suddenly appear; rather, they come about gradually, having been established during the early school years. This is to say that obesity, coronary thromboses, ulcers, backaches, gastrointestinal pains, hypertension, chronic fatigue, and the neurotic and psychotic behaviors related to feelings of anxiety, apprehension, fear, worry, hatred, and jealousy are all tied ultimately to a *pattern of living*. It is this pattern of living which is favorably influenced when values are formed early in life.

The most stupendous of man's inventions, wrote Joseph Wood Krutch, ". . . was not the wheel, or the wedge, or the lever, but the values by which he has lived."[46] The true worth of an education, therefore, is found in how it affects values, judgments, and commitments. In terms of health, it has been known for some time that people who understand themselves make better patients when ill and recover sooner. They have what Maslow characterizes as an "appreciation of the body" which leads to an extension of the whole personality. This is the "healthy, self-actualizing person."[47] This is the individual who knows what to do and is moved to a state of doing it. He is not indifferent to the health consequences of his own acts. He is sensitive to the delicateness and dearness of life. He is profoundly aware of the potentialities of a fully awakened human being. Finally, he sees a relationship between the well-being of the individual and the healthy development of the society itself.

QUESTIONS FOR DISCUSSION

1. The question has been raised as to whether a society can meet the several pollution challenges without giving up anything. What are your thoughts about this? Is it possible that ecological expedience will require a kind of totalitarianism which will limit the freedom most people enjoy today?

2. Saul Kelson (see Selected References) writes about the increase in smoking among girls and women. What is the association here with health education practices in the community as well as secondary schools?

---

[46]Joseph Wood Krutch, *The Measure of Man,* New York: Bobbs-Merrill Co., Inc., 1954, p. 172.
[47]Abraham B. Maslow, *Toward A Psychology of Being,* Princeton, N.J.: D. Van Nostrand Co., Inc., 1962.

3. To what extent does the ecological philosophy of Rene Dubos influence your own attitudes towards well-being? Is man an ecological dominant at the center of things, or is he a part in the "flow" of life?

4. Elaborate on the multidimensional nature of health and health education by responding to the question: why is the subject of health education frequently difficult to grasp?

5. Just how serious is the threat to education of a changing national economy? Will school health services and teaching be affected? Will health manpower and hospital care problems be affected?

SUGGESTED ACTIVITIES

1. It was Prometheus, the "forethinker," that fire-breathing titan, who sought a "heroic" civilization in which the unyielding spirit of humankind could be expressed. Could this be the ultimate state of health? Examine the literature pertaining to definitions and philosophies of health and comment on your findings in terms of your own feelings.

2. Our planet could become unfit for human habitation if man continues blithely to ravage his delicately balanced environment. There are some signs that he is trying to veer off this collision course with doom. Ask several businessmen and college faculty members if they think man will be able to change direction far enough, and soon enough.

3. In an effort to see how widespread comprehensive health planning is today, visit a local hospital administrator or public health figure and solicit his opinions.

4. Health education is becoming stronger. It may relate to the statement of Alfred North Whitehead that we should teach about "life in all of its manifestations." How do school board members feel about this, especially when money is in short supply in many places? Speak to one or two school board members and share your findings with classmates.

5. Study the list of nine *Imperatives in Education* set forth by the American Association of School Administrators. Discuss ways in which health education can contribute to the fulfillment of these points and help meet the needs of the times.

SELECTED REFERENCES

Ager, Joel W., et al. "Vasectomy: Who Gets One and Why?" *American Journal of Public Health*, 64:680–684, July, 1974.

Bucher, Charles A., Einar A. Olsen, and Carl E. Willgoose, *Foundations of Health*. 2nd edition, Englewood Cliffs, N.J.: Prentice Hall, Inc., 1976.

Bates, David V. "Screening Smokers for Emphysema," *Medical World News*, November 23, 1973.

Browning, Charles H. "Suicide, Firearms, and Public Health," *American Journal of Public Health*, 64:313–319, April, 1974.

Consumer Union Editors. *The Medicine Show*, Orangeburg, N. Y.: Consumer Reports, 1974.

Ehrlich, Paul. "Eco-catastrophe," *Ramparts*, September, 1969.

Frankle, Reva and F. K. Heussentamin. "Food Zealotry and Youth," *American Journal of Public Health*, 64:11–16, January, 1974.

Gentry, Atron A., et al., *Urban Education: The Hope Factor*, Philadelphia: W. B. Saunders Co., 1972.

Glyer, John. "Diet Healing: A Case Study in the Sociology of Health," *Journal of Nutrition Education*, 4(4):163–166, Fall, 1972.

Hanlon, John. *Public Health: Administration and Practices*, 6th ed., St. Louis: C. V. Mosby Co., 1975.

Horn, Jack. "Bored to Sickness," *Psychology Today*, 9:92–94, November, 1975.

Kelson, Saul, R., et al. "The Growing Epidemic: A Survey of Smoking Habits and Attitudes Among Students in Grades 7 through 12." *American Journal of Public Health*, 15:923–938, September, 1975.

Lewin, Robert. "Starved Brains: New Research on Hunger's Damage," *Psychology Today, 9*:29–34, September, 1975.

Mayer, Jean. *A Diet for Living,* New York: McKay, 1975.

Moody, Howard. "Demythologizing Medicine: Redefining Health Care," *Christianity and Crisis, 35*:219–224, September, 1975.

Morehouse, Lawrence E. and Leonard Gross. *Total Fitness in Thirty Minutes a Week,* New York: Simon and Schuster, 1975.

Navarro, Vincent. "From Public Health to Health of the Public," *American Journal of Public Health, 64*:534–537, June, 1974.

Price, Weston A. *Nutrition and Physical Degeneration: A Comparison of Primitive and Modern Diets and Their Effects,* New York: Hoeber-Harper, 1942.

Rathbone, Frank S. and E. T. Rathbone. *Health and the Nature of Man,* New York: McGraw-Hill Co., 1971.

Rosenfeld, Albert. "Medicine's Mighty Molecules," *Saturday Review/World,* December 14, 1974, p. 50.

St. Pierre, Richard, and Carrie Lee Warren. "Smoking and Obesity: The Behavioral Ramifications," *Journal of School Health, 45*:406–409, September, 1975.

Stare, Frederick J. and Johanna Dwyer. "An Eye to the Future: Health Eating for Teenagers," *Journal of School Health, 39*:595–599, November, 1969.

Washington, Vivian E. "Baltimore's School Program for Teenage Mother," *School Health Review, 4*:7–9, May-June, 1973.

Willgoose, Carl E. "Education for Health," *The Instructor,* October, 1969.

Chapter 2

The Secondary School Health Program

"...you cannot separate the seamless coat of learning."

Alfred North Whitehead

As part of a larger society, junior and senior high schools suffer from the attendant economic perplexities, population shifts, and other problems. These schools do not exist in a vacuum and should have realistic programs. Recently, the Education Development Center working with five commissions explored the question of reforming secondary education and discovered that most adolescents spend a considerable amount of time in school corridors and classrooms, and that the schools too often served a custodial and protective function, isolating young people from the society they are about to enter.[1] Barriers, instead of bridges, between youth and the rest of society are erected. Moreover, the size of the school has worked against making daily education attractive, and schools are often caught between doing too much and doing too little. While the schools cannot solve all their difficulties, it was the feeling of the five commissions that it would help to reduce barriers between adolescents and the larger society by (1) generating work experiences and other community-related opportunities, (2) creating smaller schools, and (3) diversifying teacher roles so that subject areas are seen with all their overlapping contents and manifestations.

Beyond an element of doubt, Whitehead was right in his advice to educators to examine the multi-dimensional nature of all learning. The secondary schools are beginning to do this—particularly as they have felt the impact of alcohol, drugs, tobacco and sexual problems. Moreover, difficulties in national and world politics, starvation, pollution, abortion, and other community-wide concerns have been so profoundly related to the physical and mental well-being of large numbers of young people that health education now appears to have a continuous claim on educational priorities.

DEFINING THE ENDS

Education is a process of changing behavior toward certain preconceived goals. The emphasis is on the *process*. It is not haphazard; it is orderly and planned. In keeping

---

[1] Peggy Dulany and David F. Quattrone, "Reforming Secondary Education," *EDC News,* Newton, Mass.: Education Development Center, 1975.

30

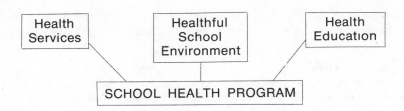

with the Latin root *educere,* it seeks to "lead forth" or "draw out" the latent or potential qualities in a person. In addition, education considers the whole man as he strives to fulfill some far-reaching purpose. Every subject matter area must ultimately do the same.

The *school health program* represents the combined effort of all school and community forces bearing upon the health of the school population. These forces are coordinated by school personnel and are channeled into three traditional divisions: health services, healthful school environment, and health education.

Health services comprise the many procedures used to determine the health status of the student, to enlist his cooperation in health protection and maintenance, and to work with parents to correct defects and to prevent illness.

Healthful school environment refers to the total school setting—a wholesome location, a healthful school day, and the existence of teacher-pupil relationships that are safe, sanitary, and favorable to the optimum development of everyone.

Health education is the instructional program—the organization of learning experiences. It is a subject matter area. More specifically, it is defined as *the sum of one's experiences which favorably influence health attitudes and practices.* It is an applied science that relates research findings to the lives of people by narrowing the gap between what is known and what is practiced. It is both a process and a program concerned with human values and behavior that are openly and subtly associated with such items as ecology and environmental well-being, nutrition and growth, mood-modifying substances, consumer health, sexuality, and the comprehensive treatment of major health problems of young people and adults. In a larger sense, the health education mission, according to Burt, is to assist the individual in the "acquisition and understanding of the knowledge required to select a life style that is actualizing, healthy, and happiness-promoting."[2] Moreover, it seeks understandings through a broad, multidimensional approach which frequently overlaps many other school subject areas.

The health effort will always be a multidisciplinary endeavor, for it is a study of what Whitehead describes as "life in all of its manifestations." Moreover, it cannot be approached in an isolated fashion. It requires direct attention in the classroom and the lunchroom as much as it does in the health office. This is because the topic of health is both subtle and dramatic, both obvious and hidden, and means many things to many people. Someone has said that "health is a crown on the well man's head that only the sick can see." From the Anglo-Saxon root, it means "hale," "sound," "whole," and is not simply an ideal state achieved through complete elimination of disease. What it is in reality is a *modus vivendi* enabling man to achieve a rewarding existence while he copes with an imperfect world.

The task of secondary education is to somehow infuse the means of health education with the values exposed in defining the ends. In the years ahead, health education

---

[2]John J. Burt, "Rational Selection of Life Style Components," *School Health Review,* 5:4–9, March-April, 1974.

must help students graduate from facts to feelings and from feelings to values. Goodlad makes this humanistic point very clear in writing about educational programs in 1980:

> The most important task for our schools during the next few years—and for many generations to come—is their daily practice and demonstration of those qualities of compassion, sensitivity, sound judgment, flexibility, adaptability, humanity, self-renewal—and many more that we have long claimed to be seeking in the human products of education.[3]

Early writers on education—Spencer, Comenius, Rousseau, and others—were just as enthusiastic about values and determining the ends for healthful living as are some of the more recent educators. This is fully documented in several lists of educational aims and objectives that have been periodically prepared over the decades. Most of these goals were set forth in broad philosophical categories such as "life and health," "optimum organic health," "healthful living," "to live most and to serve best," and "self-realization." This was helpful in pointing to educational requirements, but it left the reader the task of relating the health objective to the needs of the times.

---

[3]John I. Goodlad in *Designing Education for the Future, No. 2* by Edgar L. Morphet and Charles O. Ryan, New York: Citation Press, 1967, p. 47.

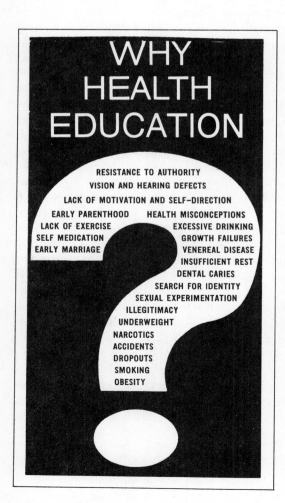

Figure 2–1 Why health education? (Courtesy of the American Medical Association)

No matter how the times change, they call for an individual who is dynamically healthy, able to satisfy his own needs and to contribute his share to the welfare of society. *The long-range goal of the health educator,* therefore, is to prepare persons with the wherewithal to struggle toward the imperatives because they possess:

1. Optimum organic health and the vitality to meet emergencies.
2. Mental well-being to meet the stresses of modern life.
3. Adaptability to and social awareness of the requirements of group living.
4. Attitudes and values leading to optimum health behavior, and
5. Moral and ethical qualities contributing to life in a democratic society.

HISTORICAL PERSPECTIVE

> If you have built castles in the air, your work need not be lost; that is where they should be. Now put the foundations under them.
>
> — *Thoreau*

To a large extent much of the early school health work was only a weak beginning. Few schools actually accomplished anything significant. It was indeed a case of building "castles in the air." However, in 1842 Horace Mann, editor of the Massachusetts *Common School Journal,* began to write about the need for "knowledge of laws of structure, growth, development, and health of the body" as essential to intellectual and moral behavior. This was a new twist, for it meant that educators and humanists, and not just the biologists and dispensers of medicine, were studying health. It was a slow move from a period when scientists were looking at the living organism in terms of the material bases of life and organismic functions to an era of dealing with the experiences of whole men and women responding in all their complexity to the stimuli and challenges of their total environment.

This slow-to-start shift in viewpoint regarding the health function of the school gradually began to be noticed. Late in his life William Alcott, named by James F. Rogers as the "father of health education," wrote a health book for schoolchildren and stressed both health services and health instruction.[4] By 1890 every state in the country had a law requiring instruction in the area of alcohol and narcotics. Much of this legislation was engineered by temperance societies unhappy over the increases in the use of alcohol and drugs.

By 1894 the Boston schools were starting regular medical examinations of schoolchildren. Chicago, New York, and Philadelphia followed. In 1909 the Metropolitan Life Insurance Company opened its health and welfare division to reduce preventable diseases and premature death through enlightenment of schoolchildren and the general public. Since that time this voluntary health agency has established an admirable record of having distributed about 21 billion pamphlets on health and safety and 15 billion health messages through the media carrying information on such timely topics as alcoholism, venereal disease, amphetamine abuse, and obesity.

The New York City Health Department established a bureau of health education in 1914. Although its main concern was public health, it had a favorable influence on school health practices in the city. Because of the work of official and voluntary health groups, numerous schools taught hygiene courses consisting chiefly of anatomy and

---

[4]For a full coverage of this early period see Richard K. Means, *A History of Health Education in the United States,* Philadelphia: Lea & Febiger, 1962, Chapters 2 and 4. See also the writings of Means under Selected References at the end of this chapter.

physiology. Interest was further generated for health teaching at this time by the efforts of the National Tuberculosis Association (1916) and the newly formed American Child Hygiene Association (1918). Perhaps the biggest boost to school health education came in 1924 with the publication of *Health Education* by the Joint Committee on Health Problems in Education of the National Education Association and the American Medical Association, the oldest NEA committee in existence, established in 1911.

In 1922 Clair E. Turner, working with Mary Spencer in Malden, Massachusetts, set up a school health demonstration project which extended over a two year period.[5] An experimental group of children was compared with a control group relative to growth, health status, and health practices as a result of formal health instruction. The demonstration was widely publicized and caused a number of school personnel to explore the area of health teaching more seriously.

About 1911, nurses were hired in schools to help control communicable diseases. Later it was decided that they could be useful as first aiders—perhaps to lessen the liability of the schools. In the 30's and 40's the follow-up of defects was considered to be the chief concern of the nurse. Slowly her role developed into one of education and she evolved from the nurse to the nurse-teacher category.

Over the years the School Health Section of the American Public Health Association, the American School Health Association, and the American Alliance for Health, Physical Education and Recreation have done a great deal to promote the total school health program throughout the nation. This support, added to the activities of the World Health Organization, state education departments, and professional education agencies, has brought the topic of the health of schoolchildren into almost every community. Sensing this increased concern for health instruction, the Joint Committee of the National School Boards Association and the American Association of School Administrators in 1968 recommended a comprehensive program of health education in grades K through 12 to meet the health needs, interests, and problems of the school-age group and prepare them for their role as future citizens.

THE UNIFIED APPROACH AND PRESENT TRENDS

Perhaps the most significant part of the recommendations of the Joint Committee of the National School Boards Association and the American Association of School Administrators was the unmistakably clear call for a *comprehensive* school health program:

> Such a comprehensive approach should be supported by groups interested in a single health area because it assures an orderly and progressive consideration of the separate topics in the context of total health and, hence, offers more effective student exposure through the grades. It avoids "band wagon" approaches, crash programs, and piecemeal efforts focused on one or a few topics that happen to be enjoying popularity or extensive press coverage at a particular time—an approach which on the basis of past experience has proved to be largely ineffective.

In 1969 the School Health Division of the American Association for Health, Physical Education and Recreation set forth a position paper stressing the need for a unified approach to health teaching. They too were aware of how easy it is to fragment health education into a number of unrelated parts. It was their recommendation, therefore, that the health instruction program be organized and scheduled to reflect proper scope and

---

[5]Clair E. Turner, "Malden Studies in Health Education and Growth," *American Journal of Public Health,* 18:1217–1230, 1928.

sequence through the years K—12, on a continuing basis; it should also emerge from curriculum development activities involving both school personnel and individuals from the voluntary and official health agencies.

Further support for the comprehensive school health program came early in 1970 from the National Congress of Parents and Teachers. This highly effective group also called for a specified time allotment, qualified teachers, an adequate budget, and a well-planned program of health instruction with appropriate progression.

By 1973 the American Academy of Pediatrics supported a proposition for a unified and comprehensive program of health instruction, one appropriate to the age and maturity of the pupils, and one that "should set high standards with requirements as exacting as those in any other area of instruction."[6] This, coupled in the same year with the report of the President's Committee on Health Education, helped bring out the need for good programs and pointed to the fact that even where programs do exist, there is fragmentation, a lack of planning, sequence, and evaluation, and a lack of commitment of time, money, administrative support, and legal sanction. In late 1974 the American Public Health Association's position paper on school health was welcomed; it went beyond comprehensive planning to stress the need for a better teaching-learning environment.[7] By late 1975 several comprehensive school health education bills were before Congress in a concerted effort to get programs started throughout the country with solid government support. One outcome was the establishment of the Bureau of Health Education as a part of the Center for Disease Control under the authority of the Secretary of Health, Education and Welfare. Its function is to "provide leadership to a comprehensive national health education program for the prevention of disease, disability, premature death, and undesirable and unnecessary health problems."

In comparing the school health practices of several decades ago with those of the present, it is noticeable that a number of improvements have been made. Some noteworthy examples are summarized in Table 2–1.

A significant trend is the upgrading of legislation pertaining to school health and health education. This has occurred in a number of states, both large and small. An excellent example is the *Revisions of the Commissioner's Regulations on Health Education* for the State of New York, which became law in 1969 and was implemented in the fall of 1970:

> Health (and safety) education in the secondary schools. The secondary school curriculum shall include health (and safety) education as a constant for all pupils. In addition to continued health guidance in the junior high school grades, provision shall also be made for (approved health and safety teaching either as part of a broad science program or as) a separate one-half year course. In addition to continued health guidance in the senior high school, provision shall also be made for an approved one-half year unit course (or its equivalent). Health (and safety) education shall be required for all pupils in the junior and senior high school grades and shall be taught by teachers (with approved preparation) *holding a certificate to teach health.* A member of each faculty with approved preparation shall be designated as health coordinator, in order that the entire faculty may cooperate in realizing the potential health-teaching values of the school program.

A final trend, which is barely in evidence, is the increasing attention being given to research in health instruction and health services. Numerous professionals in health education are today attempting to open boundless new horizons to human experience through research into methodology, aids, and behaviors. School health personnel con-

---

[6]Committee on School Health, "Health Education," *Pediatrics,* 52:458–459, September, 1973.
[7]School Health Section Position Paper, *Education for Health in the School Community Setting,* American Public Health Association, October 23, 1974.

TABLE 2-1 School Health Then and Now

PRESENT TRENDS	PAST PRACTICES
1. The function of the school health services department is concerned with every health-related factor in the school and community—medical, dental, psychological, and environmental.	1. Health services activities were generally limited to the giving of physical examinations and minor nursing duties.
2. Medical examinations of secondary school pupils are thorough and are given about every three years by either the family physician or the school physician. The follow-up of findings is a significant activity.	2. Medical examinations were given hastily on an annual basis, and with very poor organization for following up needy cases.
3. Teachers, nurses, physicians, and parents serve on health councils designed to determine individual pupil weaknesses and provide health guidance.	3. There was very little effort made for teachers, parents, and medical personnel to solve health problems.
4. Teachers are better prepared to teach with a multidisciplinary and ecological approach to health education, and a willingness to go beyond the classroom for a continual in-service education.	4. No special ability was required to teach "health and hygiene"; sometimes taught by the physical education instructor as a rainy day program.
5. Concepts, competencies, and behaviors are stressed rather than bits and pieces of knowledge. At examination time facts are recalled by students as a means of supporting major concepts.	5. Health facts were dispensed rather formally and related essentially to the particulars of anatomy and physiology.
6. School nurses with a health education background act as resource personnel for classroom teachers, and assist with program planning.	6. The school nurse remained pretty much in the health services office—more as a clerk first-aider than an educator.
7. Self-appraisals, in which students evaluate their own health practices, are carried out and followed up with informal discussion groups.	7. Students seldom related the health topics to themselves in a personal way, especially through any wide discussion and appraisal.

duct surveys and search for causes. Ultimately, every secondary school graduate should be able to determine his own course of action through a well-founded process of inquiry and decision-making. Local research projects, preferably involving students, have a significant role to play in educating for health.

It might appear from the above "trends" that everything is indeed rosy and beautiful today in health education practice. Talks with teachers and administrators, coupled with personal observations, will pretty much convince one that a great deal remains to be accomplished. There is still a need for more coordinators of health instruction, more detailed curriculum guides, less student indifference, better facilities, and teaching aids, increased parental support for programs and follow-up for children in need of health services, vitally interested teachers with a humanistic approach to teaching, sufficient time for in-depth instruction, and flexible scheduling of health classes to permit wider discussion of prime issues.

TABLE 2-1   School Health Then and Now (Continued)

PRESENT TRENDS	PAST PRACTICES
8. Health textbooks and other teaching aids are designed to guide discussion, provoke ideas, and suggest pupil activities leading to understanding and decision-making.	8. Textbooks tended to be straight health facts calling for more memorization activity than understanding and personal application.
9. Formal health education classes, which provide for a more in-depth treatment of topics and are more effective than integrated and correlated classes, are increasingly being taught in both small towns and large cities.	9. Health instruction, often haphazardly arranged, was frequently made a small part of such subjects as biology, science, home economics, physical education, and social studies.
10. Health education supervisors and consultants are employed to assist teachers in planning and teaching.	10. Supervisors were sometimes looked upon as quite unnecessary since they would do little actual classroom teaching themselves.
11. Health education receives near-equal or equal consideration with other subject areas in the curriculum.	11. Health education, if taught at all, was considered an "extra" or "fringe topic" in the school.
12. Standardized tests from reputable testing services are used to determine level of pupil knowledge and the extent to which it may be applied.	12. Knowledge tests, when employed at all, were used to measure knowledge of health facts only.
13. Attention is given to the mental and physical health of the teacher, since it frequently sets the tone of the classroom.	13. The health of the teacher was incidental to learning.
14. Curriculum development, with appropriate scope and sequence, is an almost common practice in alert communities, and leads to the construction of teacher guides and detailed courses of study.	14. The health "curriculum" was often carried in the head of one person, and not put down on paper with the help of school and community personnel.

ADMINISTRATIVE GUIDELINES

In an attempt to get away from "crash" programs and move toward solving some of the shortcomings related to health education, the California Association of School Administrators, the California School Boards Association, and the California Medical Association endorsed a set of administrative guidelines for health education in the California secondary schools.[8] These guidelines were developed specifically to assist school boards and administrators in the critical review of their programs. They are an admirable contribution to the field, for they spell out in clear-cut fashion just what is expected in order to have an adequate secondary school program of health education.

---

[8]Copies are available from the California Association of School Administrators.

Guidelines

Programs

1. Health education should be identified as a separate subject in the school curriculum.
2. School districts have an obligation to make provisions for health education as an integral part of general education.
3. Health education should be a planned sequential program in grades kindergarten through twelve; crash programs emphasizing special health topics should be avoided.
4. Adequate time and resources for health education should be provided.
5. Districts should be encouraged to explore innovative organizational patterns for instruction such as flexible scheduling in order to provide for effective health education.
6. Districts should also offer pre-school and adult health education programs, **if not otherwise available.**

Curriculum

1. Curriculum development should focus on student achievement of desired behavioral objectives.
2. Relevant health concepts should be included at the most appropriate developmental levels of children and youth.
3. Health education should be responsive to the needs of students and the demands of society, and should reflect current scientific knowledge.
4. The curriculum should focus on the positive aspects of health.
5. Students and the community should be involved in curriculum development to insure the inclusion of instruction based on health needs, interests and problems.
6. Districts should be encouraged to explore innovative and creative instructional methods which actively involve students in the achievement of established behavioral objectives such as small discussion groups, independent study and team teaching.

Time

1. Health education should receive equal consideration with other subject areas in the curriculum.
2. Adequate time should be provided to achieve the established behavioral goals and program objectives.
3. Specific time allotment should be given to the treatment of health education in depth as well as recognizing it as an inherent portion of several other disciplines.
4. Time allotment will vary depending on individual and community needs.

Teachers

1. Health education in schools should be taught by an adequately prepared teacher with a demonstrated interest and aptitude in health education. Wherever possible, the teacher should have a specific preparation in health education, preferably a major or minor.
2. Desirable teacher qualities should include: ability to interact meaningfully and honestly with students, to act capably as a resource for students, and to be sensitive to individual differences and needs.
3. Districts should provide continuing programs of in-service teacher preparation in health education that should also reflect current scientific information.

Coordination

1. Responsibility for the development, coordination and implementation of health education in the school district should be assigned to a specific person.
2. Districts should be encouraged to seek and utilize consultant services from county school offices, from medical and other sources.

Community

1. School districts should be responsive to and involve the community in planning, developing and implementing programs in a variety of ways, including the establishment of and/or the participation in school-community health councils.
2. Districts should never assume permanent acceptance of health education by the community but should constantly assess and revise the program in accordance with changing needs and attitudes.
3. Districts should enlist the help and support of community leaders.
4. Available community resources should be utilized to augment and enrich the instructional program.

Financing and Facilities

1. Sufficient financial support should be provided to insure adequate facilities, personnel and instructional materials to achieve the established objectives.
2. School districts should seek resources which may be available from a wide variety of community agencies and organizations.

Evaluation

The program should be periodically evaluated in terms of effectiveness based on realistic and measurable criteria.

Pupils, teachers, parents and others should be involved in the evaluation of the program at regular intervals in terms of relevance to pupils.

RELATIONSHIP OF HEALTH SERVICES TO HEALTH INSTRUCTION

The effectiveness of the health instruction program depends in part on the kind of relationships that exist between a number of school functions and personnel. Obviously, there should be a close bond of feeling and communication between the physician, nurse, and others in the health services department and the health instructor. There are opportunities to tie in classroom happenings with health services activities. When, for example, medical examinations are given to appraise health status, and when screening examinations are conducted for height-weight-growth, teeth, hearing, seeing, and so forth, there is an excellent opportunity to involve junior high school students (who are especially aware of their appearance and rapid growth changes) in classroom discussion. A significant function of school health services is to help prevent and control disease. Another is to provide emergency service for injury or sudden sickness. These functions require a fair amount of attention to the total school environment—everything from the quality of specific facilities to the health of the teacher. From a teaching viewpoint it is just as important to know about hazardous buildings, grounds, and equipment as it is to know about the number of decayed or missing teeth among members of the freshman class. Defective stair rails, broken sidewalks, obstructed exits, slippery floors and unsanitary lunchroom facilities are frequently being brought to the attention of health services personnel.

In some schools the school nurse is the only member of the health professions on the staff. She is a health specialist whose nursing skills are combined with a background in health and education. She acts as a consultant and helps plan and conduct health services as a positive learning experience which enhances formal health instruction. In some schools she teaches one or more classes. More and more she is being asked to participate in the design of the curriculum—a particularly significant activity in view of her traditional liaison with medicine, the home, and the community. In addition, her status is being upgraded in many schools. She is being freed from the band-aid-clerical image which she formerly projected in order to help teachers become skillful observers and sources of information about health problems.

The demand for fully trained nurse-teachers is growing, particularly as it becomes evident that the nurse is in the best position to tie together all parts of the school health program. Teachers require some prodding in order to take advantage of the numerous classroom opportunities both to observe and to instruct boys and girls along health lines. An active nurse gets around. In his study of school nurse services in several large cities, Jenne found a significant correlation between increased nurse-school contacts and the numbers of health observations made by teachers.[9]

Another concern is research. Research carried on by health services has practical use in the instruction program. Big cities and a number of smaller towns study their school population in several ways. Evidence relative to health practices is frequently on hand from group surveys, interviews, and case studies that may be used to make a health topic "real" in almost any location. What, for instance, do students know about school

---

[9]Frank H. Jenne, "Variations in Nursing Service Characteristics and Teachers' Health Observation Practices," *Journal of School Health,* 60:248–251, May, 1970.

absences? How meaningful are these kinds of statistics? The Delaware School Health Study, for example, discovered that high absence is associated with having low grades, being over age for one's grade, having low socio-economic status, coming from a broken home, and attending an urban school. Think of the several ways this information can be used in the classroom to make environmental or community health a vital topic.

In a number of states, particularly Colorado, California, and Wisconsin, the state medical societies have been very active in working with local health services personnel to improve health instruction in the schools. In Wisconsin, sex education, drug education, physical education, and the certification of teachers for health was given a big boost by medical personnel vitally interested in school health. Another example of how local medical associations have worked through school health services to make a contribution to health education is found in the activities of the Los Angeles City Unified School District. Here, the cooperation with the Los Angeles County Medical Association has been noteworthy in improving health education programs at all teaching levels. Additional noteworthy examples may be found in Seattle and San Diego.

The need for greater cooperation between health services personnel and health teachers is evident. Such activity stands to make local health problems real to students and provide incentives for prevention. Preventing disease, accidents, and injury is a social issue in which school and community groups ultimately have to work together, perhaps under the leadership of the health instructor or school nurse, where there is no health coordinator. In this respect, there is agreement that the role of the school nurse is to exert leadership in a school health interdisciplinary team.[10]

SCHOOL HEALTH POLICIES

A logical means of adding impetus and respectability to school health programs is to prepare separate statements or written affirmations outlining definite policies. They may be combined into a general procedures manual reserved for school health. Whatever form is selected should reflect the following points:

1. Existing policies should be known to students, school personnel, parents and community groups, and should provide the basis for decisions until it is deemed necessary to change or discontinue a policy.

2. Clear policies should govern certain specified areas of school health such as health instruction with its concern for course content, requirements, time allotment, evaluation and selection of resource materials and text books; also covered should be health services, healthful environment, health of school personnel, first aid and emergency care, control of communicable disease, qualifications of health education teachers, provisions for pupils with special needs, health administrative functions, and the school lunch program.

OTHER SCHOOL SUBJECTS AND HEALTH INSTRUCTION

The school health program would be incomplete if opportunities to tie in such subjects as home economics, science, physical education, social studies and English with the formal teaching of health were overlooked. Such opportunities are more apt to be planned for when a health consultant or health supervisor has been employed. This kind

---

[10]Shu-Pi C. Chen, "Role Relationships in a School Health Interdisciplinary Team," *Journal of School Health,* 45:172–176, March, 1975.

of person is a leader, a coordinator of all loose ends that can be brought together to form an optimum health program. Teachers and other health personnel work under this person's direction, and meaningful activities are arranged through clever integration and correlation of learning. (See information on methods in Chapter 10).

The day has long since passed when school health was limited to the health class. Every facet of instruction now bears on the health topic. Nowhere is this better illustrated than in the area of English when the teacher assigns such reading material as *Catcher in the Rye* and evokes a discussion which relates to learnings gathered in sex and family living education. Another example is the physiological nature of physical fitness (work capacity) and how it relates to coronary heart disease; it is of concern to health teachers and physical education instructors alike. The economics of our social system as it pertains directly to the health needs of the poor, race problems, the population explosion, and consumer welfare is another example of an area vital to the social sciences as well as to health education. There are many examples of these kinds of associations. They need more attention than they get. This is perhaps the chief reason why some health education programs are so barren and unrelated to the world in which students live. Moreover, the students are the first to say so, especially if they are asked.

There is always danger that because of the multidimensional nature of health instruction it could become lost in the educational shuffle and be a kind of "all things to all people" course without formal description. *Health education must remain identifiable and visible as a subject area capable of standing on its own.* It can do this and still embrace such flexible teaching concepts as open classrooms, humanistic education, minicourses, and alternative schools that are designed as a *way* to reach the affective and action domains.[11]

SCHOOL AND COMMUNITY HEALTH PLANNING

As indicated previously, there are numerous official and voluntary health organizations in the country today that are anxious to be of assistance in the school health program. Such groups are especially valuable at a time when the school is in the process of revising a course of study or preparing new curriculum materials. Those agencies having to do with child health, vital statistics, nutrition, accident prevention, fire protection, consumer health, drug abuse, alcoholism, cancer, heart, mental health, air and water pollution, respiratory disorders, and the several other degenerative diseases of mankind all have a real interest in assisting school health specialists and teachers to be more effective. Not to call on them regularly for help is to have tunnel vision, and to miss an excellent opportunity to improve school relations with the public.

By bringing representatives of all health-related agencies in a community together at the school, it is possible to achieve a balance in influence. That is, no one group will be quite so apt to unduly affect the program. It has happened in a number of instances that one or two well organized health agencies that distribute a large number of appropriate teaching aids have been able to dominate the curriculum emphasis—particularly if their field relates to the so-called "hot" topics of alcohol, drugs, tobacco, or mental health. Needless to say, the planners of the comprehensive curriculum keep this in mind as they strive to use the expertise of all community groups, and seek to achieve balance in the contributions from all contributors (See Figure 2–2.)

The comprehensive approach in any community looks at a wide range of health edu-

---

[11] For more on this viewpoint see Carl E. Willgoose, "Saving the Curriculum in Health Education," *Journal of School Health*, 43:189–191, March, 1973.

cation possibilities and relationships between the schools and non-school agencies. Planning brings together a variety of people, whose activities might otherwise be fragmented, to work on such things as school curriculum, a team approach to patient education in a hospital, an outreach education program by a home care agency, counseling of employees in an industry, neighborhood group discussions by a civic organization, parent effectiveness training, or mounting a consumer awareness campaign about a specific health problem.

In Ventura County, California, a consolidated comprehensive health planning group placed top priority on public health education, with a strong role for the secondary schools, after obtaining a variety of ideas from throughout the county. The survey unearthed a lack of public understanding about available health services, drug abuse, venereal disease, and nutrition, and a concern for health manpower shortages, environmental hazards and health-related social forces in the community. Certainly, there are a variety of significant links that pertain to health status, resources, and actions. As Figure 2–3 indicates, these links begin with people who wish to become involved.

The need to *collaborate* is real. It affords ordinary people a voice in the schools, reduces feelings of powerlessness resulting from unresponsive bureaucracies, and vastly improves the way schools utilize community resources to enrich programs. Moreover, community perceptions of local health problems are an adequate reflection of health problems which affect, or will affect, young people. Several surveys of what community respondents have perceived as their health problems have been helpful for health council discussions and secondary school health projects. Rank order listings of health problems

---

Resolution No. 5

adopted by
Joint Committee on Health Problems in Education
National Education Association - American Medical Association
February 13-16, 1971

Coordination of School-Community Health Programs

Whereas,   The component parts of the health program for
                schools frequently are fragmented, and

Whereas,   The overall school health program is ineffective if
                there is no organizational structure to coordinate
                the component parts of a school health program with
                all phases of the school system, and

Whereas,   The solution of major child and youth health issues
                requires the concerted action by the entire com-
                munity, including schools, therefore be it

Resolved,   That the component parts of a health program in a school
                system be coordinated by an advisory school health coun-
                cil consisting of representatives of the administration,
                instructional staff, students, parents, employees, and
                the health disciplines, and be it further

Resolved,   That local medical and dental societies, advisory school
                health councils, other educational related organizations,
                and all health related agencies be encouraged to work
                together through a Community Health Council or Comprehensive
                Health Planning Council to coordinate efforts in solving
                health issues in schools and communities.

Figure 2–2 Support for school-community cooperation.

DYNAMIC LINKAGES IN HEALTH EDUCATION

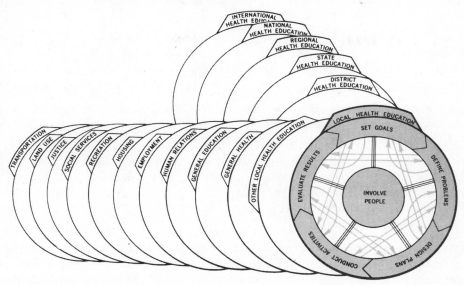

Figure 2–3 Comprehensive health planning begins with involved people. (Courtesy of Health Education Report, Ojai, California)

by community respondents often tie in fairly closely with the listings of social agencies and voluntary health agencies. Both groups frequently agree when surveyed that the schools could contribute to the solution of local health problems. There is some support for this viewpoint when one reviews the nationwide effort to promote the community-based drug prevention programs with youth expressing their ideas constructively in community life. Certainly, the varied community groups can no longer afford to remain as isolated entities prescribing remedial procedures for youth with medically related and academic problems. More extensive interdisciplinary involvement is necessary. In the U.S.S.R. prevention receives great emphasis. Physicians and the public work together; frequently, a family member is a "health volunteer" and is a community-school contact person. Physicians are expected to devote one hour daily to health education as a way of preventing disease and promoting health. The major purpose is to create active community participation.

QUESTIONS FOR DISCUSSION

1. Historically, the health education movement has received its greatest boost from small groups of individuals and organizations interested in human well-being. Presently, there is considerable legislative activity at state and federal levels to move health education into the mainstream of education. What are the factors that will contribute to the success of this effort?

2. In recent years secondary education has undergone a number of changes, including a movement from formality to flexibility. What has been the effect on health education programs?

3. In meeting the needs of certain young people, the alternative schools show considerable promise. What are the factors that put additional demands on health education teachers?

4. One of the liabilities of modern education, according to Norman Cousins, is that it has contributed to a compartmentalization of knowledge, and that what is needed today is an understanding of the interrelationships within the entire province of knowledge. Do you agree or disagree with this viewpoint? How do you see it relating to school health?

5. To what extent is it possible for high school students to actually carry on their own health research, either individually or as a part of a small group? What are the obstacles? Suggest ways of overcoming the obstacles.

6. It is possible that there needs to be a whole new approach to the teaching of health to secondary school students? Are they not more mature, perhaps more worldly, than they used to be a decade ago? Are they able to handle more indepth material, projects, tasks, and so on? Back up what you think by referring to the current literature pertaining to health instruction.

7. Do problems with alcohol, sex, and drugs on the college campus relate in any specific way to the lack of a high school health instruction experience? The answer to this question will be difficult to obtain, so discuss it rather thoroughly with others before you attempt an answer.

8. In reviewing the recommendations of several conferences having to do with the health of children and youth, it is quite common to find recommendations made for extended health services, a higher quality of health care, and a plea for more health manpower in the United States. Frequently missing is a recommendation for more formal health teaching. Why does this occur? Is it a case of forgetting the obvious, or a sign of lack of faith in what education can provide?

SUGGESTED ACTIVITIES

1. Over 100 years ago Spencer asked, "What knowledge is of most worth?" Ask one or two school administrators if they would be willing to convene a mixed group of secondary school teachers in order to discuss the Spencerian question in the light of a 1980 existence in the world as a whole. Note their comments whether or not they support the idea.

2. Review the list of nine *Imperatives in Education* prepared by the American Association of School Administrators (see *Selected References*). Enumerate several ways in which health education can contribute to the fulfillment of these items and help meet the needs of the times.

3. Interview several teachers of health education at either the junior or senior high school level. See if you can discover what they believe to be the most significant trends in health teaching today. Also, determine whether these teachers see any trends in the operation of the health services section.

4. Find out what kind of research is carried on by a large city health services department. Cleveland has for years been very thorough in surveying tooth decay and relating it to a number of school variables. How are the research findings used? Are those who teach health involved in any way?

5. Responding to the need for total community action on the drug use and abuse prob-

lems, numerous examples of cooperative effort are to be found. Investigate the means employed by a local town or city to be effective in the drug area. See if you can find out how the school health program at both health services and health teaching levels became involved in striving toward a solution to this particular health problem.

6. Form a small team of investigators to look into the duties of school nurses in a local area. Check several school systems to see if the nurse is primarily a kind of clerk-first aider or more of an educator. If possible, also interview some teachers who work with the nurse, and talk briefly with the school principal.

SELECTED REFERENCES

American Association of School Administrators. *Imperatives in Education,* Washington, D.C.: American Association of School Administrators, 1966.

Anderson, C. L. *School Health Practice,* 6th edition, St. Louis: The C. V. Mosby Co., 1976.

Bryan, Doris. *School Nursing in Transition,* St. Louis: The C. V. Mosby Co., 1975.

Cahn, Lorynne and Robert Peterson. "Education and Mental Health: A Need for Interdisciplinary Involvement," *Journal of School Health,* 43:218–222, April, 1973.

Creswell, William H. and Thomas M. Janeway. "A Comprehensive Health Education Program for Illinois Schools," *Journal of School Health,* 44:336–339, June, 1974.

Cunico, John A. and William H. Boothe. "Duluth's School Health Education Project: The Multiagency Approach," *Journal of School Health,* 43:11–15, January, 1974.

Dolfman, Michael L. "Toward Operational Definitions of Health," *Journal of School Health,* 45:200–210, April, 1974.

Eurich, Alvin C. *High School 1980: The Shape of the Future in American Secondary Education,* New York: Pitman, 1970.

Joint Committee on Health Problems in Education of the NEA/AMA. *Health Education,* 6th edition, Washington, D.C.: American Alliance for Health, Physical Education and Recreation, 1975.

Means, Richard K. *Historical Perspectives on School Health.* Thorofare, N.J.: Charles B. Slack, Inc., 1975.

Means, Richard K. "Can the Schools Teach Personal Responsibility for Health?" *Journal of School Health,* 43:171–175, March, 1973.

Newman, Ian M. and Cyrus Mayshark. "Health Education Planning and Community Perceptions of Local Health Problems," *Journal of School Health,* 43:458–460, September, 1973.

Oberteuffer, Delbert, Orvis A. Harrelson, and Marion B. Pollock. *School Health Education,* 5th edition, New York: Harper and Row, 1972, Chapter 2.

Schaller, Warren and Alma Nemir. *The School Health Program,* 4th edition, Philadelphia: W. B. Saunders Co., 1975.

Schiffers, Justus J. "The Health Educator: Neither Fish, nor Flesh, Nor Good Red Herring," *Journal of American College Health Association,* 22:265–270, April, 1974.

Willgoose, Carl E. "Providing for Change: New Directions," in Read, Donald A. (ed.). *New Directions in Health Education,* New York: Macmillan Co., 1971, pp. 1–17.

Chapter 3

The Student And Health Instruction

> The old, with their wisdom and earth bound experience, are necessary correctives to the warring fantasy, untested idealism, and despair of youth. But the intensity, idealism, and despair of youth are equally needed correctives to the pragmatism, cynicism, and pallor of age.
>
> *—John Silber*

> . . . each of us one time or another, can ride a white horse, can have rings on our fingers and bells on our toes, and if we can keep our senses open to the scents, sounds, and sights all around us, we shall have music wherever we go.
>
> *—Sean O'Casey*

> If you treat an individual as he is, he will remain as he is, but if you treat him as if he were what he ought to be and could be, he will become what he ought to be and could be.
>
> *—Goethe*

The college president, the Irish playwright, and the German philosopher have spoken above. It should be clear from them that youth are being accepted for themselves, for what they are and can be—idealists, visionaries with their "senses open" and awaiting an opportunity to discover the "scents, sounds, and sights" of the times.

The "teachable moment" is ever-present, because youth are willing to suffer through the best and worst of times and to take heart from the "spring of hope" and "winter of despair" as they reach for a fully human and genuine life style. In short, they frequently reflect the spirit of O'Casey, Teddy Roosevelt, and Dietrich Bonhoeffer as they seek teachers of authenticity who possess both vision and courage and who merge understanding and action.

WHO ARE THE STUDENTS OF THE TIME?

Are secondary school students causing civil war in their inner city and suburban schools?[1] A Senate subcommittee, using data from an 18-month study of 757 school districts, reported that vandalism alone in American public schools is costing taxpayers over one half billion dollars a year—as much as the cost of textbooks. Assaults on teachers increased 77 per cent over a 3-year period. At the same time the number of weapons

---

[1] John P. DeCecco and Arlene R. Richards, "Civil War by the High Schools," *Psychology Today*, November, 1975.

confiscated increased by 55 per cent. Does this mean that anger and conflict are taking an educational toll?

Are junior and senior high school students properly characterized as desperate? Are they spoiled brats, arrogant and disruptive, and intolerant rebels? In general, are they discourteous to parents and teachers, insensitive to the things for which America stands, anti-establishment, anti-police, anti-church, and "cop-outs" who are running away from the world in which they live? Is it true that most of them are so sophisticated beyond their years that it is difficult to reach them?

The answer to these questions is a resounding no. Although students come from diverse elementary school–neighborhood backgrounds that are fairly likely to cause friction at the secondary level, one must bear in mind that the vast majority of today's youth are quite normal in terms of what they tolerate and accept in the way of change. Given a chance, they will negotiate conflicts between themselves and teachers in the school setting. They have an impatient idealism that leads to change, and they want to talk about it in the light of society's health and welfare problems. They have learned that education is not just *for* life. It *is* life—here and now. The current high rate of secondary school disruptions suggests that the school has become a microcosm of the conflicts in the larger society around it. Poverty, pollution, disease, and inadequate health care cause youth to become "activists"—to become involved and thereby partially satisfy the impulse to grow, to reach out, to touch stars, to live freely, and to let their minds loose along unexplored corridors. Some believe they can attain their sweetest experiences by destroying hard-won structures, or using speed and other drugs; but most rise above these temptations. They are willing to find fault, discover facts and call them by their right names, engage in controversy, and try to understand.

In studying the motivations of youth for alcohol consumption, the Department of

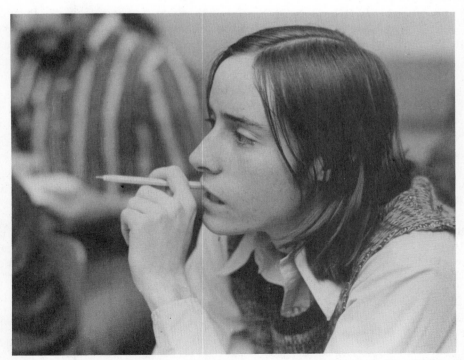

Figure 3–1 Inquiring youth—keen and attentive and not atypical. (Courtesy of Joe Di Dio, National Education Association Publishing.)

Health, Education and Welfare found that drinking students were not "far out," drop-outs, alienated, or underachieving types; on the contrary, they represented all levels of scholastic achievement and aspiration. They were somewhat liberal and permissive and felt that their social environment was overly restrictive and authoritarian in its attitudes toward young people. Moreover, they were heavily motivated by peer pressure and a feeling that they must escape with their friends to socialize. This is not a strange finding; when confidence in school personnel or parents is weak, students seek help with personal–social–emotional problems from a school-age friend.[2] Teenagers may be more effective teachers of their peers than adults. Programs in San Diego and San Francisco begun by youth themselves have proved highly effective in drug education and have reduced drug abuse among youthful participants beyond most expectations.[3] The message here is that adolescents are ready to identify with persons and issues. Erik Erikson said as much in *Dimensions of a New Identity*.[4] It is up to the educator to discover some means for the identification outlet. To do otherwise is to encourage more "safe" environments within the peer group, and risk losing student approval and respect.

Many youths have a deep feeling of helplessness because they see so many things that need to be set right in a "dehumanized," "materialistic," and "chemical" society. Moreover, they feel powerless to effect change, without realizing that they are not the first to have felt this way. If some are angry and frustrated and light fires and throw stones — for personal relief or exploitation — and make unjust accusations, it is unworthy of them. Most will work patiently to improve the inconsistencies of the society, and refuse to succumb to either cynicism or hopelessness.

The unhappiness and emotional abandonment found in some youths relates to the fact that there is today no clear-cut level when adulthood begins — so boys and girls assume adult roles early. They copy adults. They are trained for adulthood by exclusion from adulthood. What kind of example do they follow? Like the oldsters they see, they drink heavily, date steady, pet, speed in automobiles, smoke up a storm, use mood modifiers — and *act* like adults.[5]

As Piaget has indicated, the adolescent develops a new way of viewing his world by becoming somewhat absorbed in himself. Frequently, he or she becomes so involved in individual thought processes that reality becomes secondary to possibility with the ideal as a focus. This sometimes creates problems in which the individual becomes isolated by this egocentric thought and may not be sensitive to people nearby and to some of the realities of daily life. Such inner thought has a bearing on self-concept, or self-image. As a person feels about himself, so will he act. If he *feels* clumsy and inept, he will not move with grace, regardless of muscular and neurological condition. If he *feels* stupid or deprived of enlightenment he will present a non-comprehending face to the world. Unfortunately, it is all too often the school system, as Benjamin Bloom pointed out a decade ago, that reduces the aspirations of both students and teachers, and weakens the ego and self-concept of a sizable group of students. The difference between then and now is that students felt trapped in school 10 years ago, but they were less articulate and more afraid to express it then. Schools may have become more bureaucratic, with dry facts, dull lectures, recitations that do not permit students to think, and teachers who carefully steer them away from controversy. Most teachers are so used to schools like this that they seldom think what it means for pupils to spend day in and day out with their bosses

---

[2]Jean L. Perry, "Counselor Preferences of Female High School Students in the State of Illinois," *Research Quarterly*, 46:184–190, May, 1975.

[3]A. Gartner et al., *Children Teach Children: Learning by Teaching*, New York: Harper and Row, 1971.

[4]Erik Erikson, *Dimensions of a New Identity*, New York: W. W. Norton and Co., 1974, p. 124.

[5]The teenager today lives in a very confusing world. Half the adults are telling him to find himself, while the other half tell him to get lost.

telling them: sit down, keep quiet, speak up, hurry up, you can't do that without permission, I'm your friend, don't talk back to *me*, you should have gone to the bathroom before, you can't go now, your hair is too long, mind your own business . . . .

Not to acknowledge the plight of youth is to be hostile. Their plight is ours. Certainly it is not strange that in their blindness and confusion, denied explanations, they should experiment. They will admit being at times misdirected and ignorant, but are they asking too much when they seek a helping hand? Or is it too much when they want to be free, but not alone; loved, but not smothered; presented with expectations and limits, but not locked into someone else's manipulation?

In study after study the prime reasons teenagers drop out of school are marriage or pregnancy, and a lack of interest. Even then there is a searching for the meaning of things. It is not always a joyous time, for sometimes one searches, and there is little meaning to find. Yet, the struggle goes on for things of ultimate worth among affluent and minority groups alike.

Again, who are the students of the times? They are the ones that marry early in the teens (50 per cent), and most of the girls are pregnant at the time. Their interests give rise to their great mobility; they get around in cars so much that the car has become the standard projection of ego and virility. They own an estimated 20 per cent of all cars, and, of course, a good many family cars are driven, if not owned, by teens. They reflect the affluent society many of them live in—food, clothing, and housing. The nation's 26 million teenagers seek independence and get hung up on superficialities and fads. Their impulse purchases include 27 per cent of the cosmetics sold in the United States, 50 per cent of all records, 20 million radios, a million television sets, 24 per cent of all wristwatches, and 30 per cent of all low priced cameras. In short, youth is great for business.

Finally, to fully understand the adolescent one must realize that he or she lives in an intense present; "now" is so real that both past and future seem pallid by comparison. Everything that is important in life lies either in the immediate life situation or in the rather close future. For health instruction to be profitable, therefore, it must get close to the students' personal value system of the moment. Youth must experience events, says Joseph Conrad in *Lord Jim,* that " . . . reveal the inner worth of man; the edge of his temper, the fibre of his stuff; the quality of his resistance; the secret truth of his pretenses not only to himself but to others." This is the philosophy that must prevail today and be advanced through the art of teaching.

DETERMINING YOUTH NEEDS

Youths need an opportunity to think, explore, and feel the forces for optimum health. They need to receive from the secondary school what the culture embraces and society wants them to have. Their individual needs pertaining to interpersonal relations, self-development, and values must also be met. This means that pupils must be studied and taught in terms of age-level characteristics, health and safety practices in specific situations, local community health problems, the findings from medical examinations and screening tests, major interests, and current peer group concerns.

The Junior High School Student

This is an active period in the lives of boys and girls—a period for exploring and trying new things. The young people have not yet started to suffer very much from pseudomaturity and over-sophistication. Yet every time they move toward becoming young adults, there is another forgetful move when they fall back toward childhood be-haviors. In short, they frequently vacillate in responsibility from a position of strength to one of weakness, depending on individual mood and circumstances.

The physical, mental, and social characteristics of boys and girls tend to be similar, but there is in reality considerable variability. There is a balance, however, between the immature students at one end of the continuum and the more mature students at the other end, with the great mass of students falling somewhere in the middle.

1. Physical Characteristics and Needs. Growth is rapid and uneven; arms and legs grow rapidly. The lateral body form types (mesomorphs) mature earlier than the linear type (ectomorphs). Muscular development is rapid and frequently results in rela-tively poor coordination and the appearance of awkwardness. Health examinations and screening tests should be given routinely. In some cases acne may appear, causing an in-terest in skin conditions and the use of cosmetics. In this period there appears to be an unlimited source of energy, sometimes accompanied by great exuberance and boister-ousness. There is a need for a discussion of physical capacity, human energy, chronic fa-tigue, sleep, and instruction on how to relax. *Boys* have voice changes and pubic hair at about 13.5 years of age; sexual maturity and nocturnal emissions reached in most cases. Need to understand what these growth characteristics mean now and in the future. *Girls* are about 1½ years ahead of boys in maturation. Height increases rapidly. Secondary sex characteristics develop. Menstrual cycle irregular. Concern great for personal ap-pearance. Need chance to discuss growth variations and talk about one's figure and gen-eral appearance.

2. Mental-Social Development. Desire for independence from "old-fashioned" adults and school authorities. Great loyalty to group leaders. Need and want friends, and to measure themselves with friends through class projects, contests, and achievements. In-terest in impressing the opposite sex. Reality begins to hold sway over imagination. Ex-perimentation sometimes strong. Need for mental health, smoking, and drug education. Self-appraisal needed via a number of unrelated activities. A desire for clothes, movies, and parties. Need opportunity to develop social poise and confidence. Need to under-stand why health education is important now. *Boys* sometimes self-conscious about physical inadequacies; frequently think that physical prowess is all-important. Need sympathetic guidance from parents, teachers, and other adults. *Girls* need acceptance by peers. Need to know how to groom themselves and appear proper to peers. Need coeducational experiences to accompany interest in boys, dating, and dancing. As consumers, both sexes need consumer health understandings.

The Senior High School Student

Growth and maturation should be viewed as a continually evolving period through grades 7 to 12. Junior high school characteristics, therefore, will be seen among many upper grade students. In fact, most of the characteristics will change only by degree. For example, peer group association and interest in the opposite sex become more intense, and in a number of ways more mature—more responsible and of greater consequence.

1. Physical Characteristics and Needs. Musculature continues to grow among the boys; for girls there is some tapering off. Maturation in height and weight is almost complete, but there are some sex differences in timing of physical growth. Students rela-tively free from infections; reasonably healthy. Both sexes have a good appetite, but girls tend to restrict food intake. Need interesting nutrition discussions relating to use of food, food fads, and weight control. *Boys* catch up to girls in physical growth, improve in motor coordination and strength. Need to relate in school and out-of-school activities to food, exercise, rest, and medical advice. Strong sex drive which needs to be understood and related to responsible actions while dating. *Girls* tend to increase in weight as basal metabolism slowly decreases. Poise, grace, and grooming pronounced. Sexual maturity reached by senior year. Adult drives are strong. Need to understand own feelings and physical drives of boys.

2. *Mental-Social Development.* Tendency to be intensely emotional and complex. Need to see value in accepting both success and failure. Need to appreciate some limitations during early years of life. Both sexes more predictable, more cheerful, friendly, and out-going than in earlier grades. Status gained essentially through social activities. Highly critical of adults and sometimes even their peers. Dating is common; going steady is also quite common with social activities extending beyond home and school. Need to explore the intricacies of romantic love, marriage, and family relationships. Need opportunities to work with peers for common goals, to appreciate need for some rules for living, and the way to release tensions. *Boys* have mild to strong female interests. Need to understand sexual mores in the culture and their own limitations. *Girls* have a strong interest in boys, a narrowing interest in physical activities, and a strong interest in personal appearance and personal worth. Need is great to discover why they feel as they do and how to adjust to a busy world of persons and things.

STUDENT HEALTH INTERESTS AND MOTIVATIONS

A fair amount of research has been done in an effort to discover the real health concerns of youth and the underlying reasons for their prominence. This has been accomplished through surveys, checklists, and questionnaires for the most part. However, there are less objective methods of ascertaining pupil health interests that have value, such as observing their actions in and about the school community; listening as they talk together; appraising their stories; studying their paintings, drawings, and crafts; noticing their choices of foods, clothing, cosmetics, and reading material; and discussing them with their parents and former teachers.

Carefully interviewing students themselves can prove quite profitable in determining how adolescents view their health needs and problems. Brunswick, working with 12 to 17 year old students, spent an average of two and one-half hours per interview and found that youths were able to provide detailed information about their own feelings and perceptions regarding health matters. Their greatest concerns had to do with exercise, eating, smoking, and sleeping; they were also aware of problems having to do with alcohol, drugs, and the general condition of teeth.[6] In the same study, white youngsters appeared to take their health for granted while Spanish-speaking and Negro youngsters gave evidence of placing greater value on the importance of good health. This occurs frequently among minority groups. They appear to have considerable feeling for the mental and physical deprivations of individuals and groups.

The young person lives in a culture in which sex, alcohol, and drugs are being related to nearly every facet of living. Consequently, only a rare teenager fails to think about the SAD topics, and how they relate to the process of growing up. For example, several studies in recent years have indicated that students are eager to learn about alcohol, and they want objective and scientific data about intoxicants so that they can make their own decisions on whether or not to drink. Even more significant, in terms of what pupils can contribute regarding health teaching, was that too often parents emphasized only the evil nature of alcohol. Too often health was taught with a quickly detected bias or a one-sided approach to a controversial subject.

---

[6]Ann F. Brunswick, "Health Needs of Adolescents: How the Adolescent Sees Them." *American Journal of Public Health,* 59:1730–1745, September, 1969.

For several decades, Kilander measured and appraised the health interests of groups of students. He compiled information on numerous topics and in considerable detail. He discovered that adolescents are generally interested and aware of a good many items pertaining to nutrition, consumer health, misconceptions, superstitions, and venereal disease. His work on sex interests throws light on the kind of things that should be taught in secondary schools. Employing vocabulary checklists, questionnaires, and other interest-oriented means, he found that young people were extremely interested in dating customs and behavior, understanding the opposite sex, adult attitudes towards sex and dating, controlling the sex drive, sexual stimulation and sexual intercourse, reproduction, conception, contraception, pregnancy, and childbirth.[7] Moreover, Kilander's work on myths about sex and superstitions in general is a good indication of how far "off base" young people can be in the sex-related areas of health instruction.

One of the most enlightening studies of the health interests, concerns, and problems of young people was conducted by the Connecticut State Board of Education and involved over 5000 students.[8] In the course of the research it became apparent that the major health areas were common to all students regardless of whether they lived in rural, suburban, inner city, or high socioeconomic environments. Information pertaining to student interests was gathered in an unstructured manner by employing such questions as "What do you wish to know about your body?" or "What do you think the school should teach your younger brothers and sisters about health?" Free discussions and anonymous writing from whole class and small group meetings were reported by teachers who noted at the end of each day all observations and discussions seen or heard relative to health.

From this unique study comes the pupil-held viewpoint that health should be taught in every grade as a regular and required subject. The students thought that the following health areas should be taught in the secondary schools:

Sex Education
Drugs, Drinking, Smoking
Physical Development
Food, Nutrition, Diet
Personal Hygiene
Diseases
First Aid and Safety
Understanding Self and Others
Community Health
Grooming
Health Maintenance
Family Life
Birth Control and Birth Defects

More specifically, secondary school boys and girls were saying in their own words that they wanted information on the following:[9] "how to keep oneself healthy; eating properly, exercising, controlling weight, getting enough rest, and the like"; "changes taking place in both boys and girls"; "making oneself attractive to the opposite sex (dress, hair, makeup, skin care); on making a good appearance"; "safe driving"; "to understand and communicate with...parents"; "learn about differences among people (racially,

---

[7]H. Frederick Kilander, *Sex Education in the Schools,* New York: Macmillan Co., 1970, pp. 90, 137, 157.
[8]Ruth Byler, Gertrude Lewis, and Ruth Totman, *Teach Us What We Want to Know,* Hartford, Connecticut: Connecticut State Board of Education, 1969.
[9]See *Teach Us What We Want to Know,* pp. 154–157.

economically, the retarded, the mentally ill, etc.), something of the causes of differences, and should cultivate an attitude of tolerance and helpfulness"; "the major study of sexual development, relations, and behavior should be placed in grades 7 and 8, to prevent experimentation and illegitimacy due to ignorance"; "discussion of the choice of friends, of dating and 'going steady' . . . the dangers of venereal disease . . . pregnancy and birth control in grade 7, and again in grade 12 in a course on preparation for marriage"; "seniors should learn about genetics and birth, and birth abnormalities and their causes"; "learn to face life and its problems . . . there is so much to learn about the mind and how it works"; "alcohol and harmful drugs . . . major emphasis in grade 7 or 8 . . . the whole truth as to why people use them, what the results are, what the serious hazards are, how to avoid using them, and how excessive users can be helped"; "education about smoking

---

POLL REVEALS STUDENTS DRUG USE

According to a drug survey conducted during the week of March 2–6, nearly ⅓ of Brookline High students have tried marijuana. The survey, which was administered in random English classes, covered a variety of questions concerning drugs, and was answered by 380 students or about 16 per cent of the student body. The results of the poll are as follows:

1. Have you ever smoked marijuana?

Yes...............................32%
No 68%

Those students who answered "yes" to question 1 were asked several related questions.

a. Where have you smoked marijuana?
48 per cent stated that they had smoked at a friend's house. "Everywhere", "at home", "at parties", and "outside" were other popular answers.

b. How often do you smoke marijuana?
Have Quit.................................... 19%
A Few Times 14%
Infrequently (1 to 3 times per month)............ 27%
When Available 7%
No Comment 6%
One student said that he smoked marijuana between classes. Several others smoke "at least once a day".

c. Have you ever done any other drugs?
Yes...............................50%
No 48%
No Comment 2%

Those who answered "yes" to the preceding question (16 per cent of the total responses) were asked to list the drugs they had tried. Here are their answers:

L.S.D.. 40%
Heroin 6%
Speed (methedrine) 50%
Opium...................................... 18%
Hashish 55%
Others (Pills, Cocaine, etc.)............. 68%

It was on this question that several students let loose their hostile feelings toward drugs. One student listed "acid, speed, and downs" and added admonishingly, "(acid and speed kill your memory)". Another student who had taken "smack, speed, and acid" scrawled "I

HATE THEM" at the top of the survey, and "DRUGS ARE A SUPREME BUMMER" at the bottom.

What affects your use of drugs the most?

This question elicited varied responses. A majority of students attributed their drug taking either to the influence of their friends or to their minds. One student called his drug taking a result of the "chicken dilemma". Other answers included parents, curiosity, and schoolwork. One student explained, "My instability and fears hassle me until I get depressed, so I do dope as a release." The variety of responses to this item made statistical analysis impossible.

To explore the relationship between marijuana and cigarette smoking, the following question was asked of all students. The results were then broken down according to whether or not the student had tried marijuana.

2. Do You Smoke Cigarettes Regularly?
Marijuana   yes 45%
    Users   no... 55%
Non-Marijuana   yes 15%
    Users   no... 85%
Total (all students)   Yes 25%
                No 75%

Finally, all students were asked the following question:

3. Do you think the school should have any role in the apprehension of drug users? Explain.
a. Marijuana Users
School should have a role in apprehension...17%
School should have a role in rehabilitation...15%
School should have no role in apprehension...58%
No comment 10%

b. Non-Marijuana Users
School should have role in apprehension ... 33%
School should have role in rehabilitation......18%
School should have no role in apprehension...35%
No comment 14%

Figure 3–2 Poll reveals student drug use. (Brookline, Massachusetts High School Survey)

should begin in the fifth grade . . . teaching about these things later won't do any good because after grade nine they won't listen."

A significant outcome of the Connecticut study is that in addition to being a resource for health teaching, it has served as an example for a number of Connecticut schools that have developed their own local surveys. This has been helpful to school boards calling for documentation and to other school personnel having to do with guidance and services to youth.

THE LOCAL SURVEY

Almost any school system can sample the health interests and behaviors of youth. This is to say that they can go *beyond* a mere compendium of knowledge and discover the real concerns of boys and girls. Students themselves have prepared questionnaires about smoking, alcohol, mental health, sex education, and consumer health. They have questioned each other on how they feel about pornographic literature appearing on the shelves of their own community bookstores. They have studied local safety hazards and shown more than a passing interest. They have constructed and used clever survey instruments for finding out about food products, food prices, and food fads. They have also measured their own level of health misinformation and misconceptions.

Health classes in Brookline, Massachusetts, high schools were made more meaningful following a local inquiry (see Figure 3–2):

A number of junior and senior high school teachers of health courses have found the Dating Problems Checklist distributed by Family Life Publications (Durham, North Carolina) helpful in assessing the dating interests of young people. This is a 125-item listing of problems and concerns having to do with dating that, when completed, affords the teacher information pertaining to strong areas of student interest. Several local schools have accomplished the same end by having a student committee prepare direct questions for boys and girls to answer. Such checklists or questions are almost instantly successful in bringing forth an effective response from class members. Perhaps the least complicated way to take note of student interests is to ask several questions or list several sub-topics under each of the major health areas. The student would be asked to read each item carefully and put an X mark in the square out to the right of the page to signify degree of interest. Josephine Gaines has found a procedure that is very helpful for both pupil and teacher in assessing knowledge and interest. As shown in the following example, the student is asked to show *how much* knowledge and interest he has in the health item by responding rather carefully as follows:[10]

Under *Knowledge:*
None	You have no knowledge at all about the particular topic.
Little	You know what it is, but your knowledge is very limited and you feel you could know much more about the topic.
Some	You know something about the topic, but would find it helpful to have more information on this topic.
Adequate	You feel that your knowledge on this topic is extensive enough to meet your present health education needs.

Under *Interest:*
None	You have no interest at all in this topic.
Little	You have a limited amount of interest in this topic and would probably prefer studying another topic.
Considerable	You have considerable interest in this topic and would like to learn more about the subject.
Great	You have a great deal of interest and curiosity about this topic and would like to thoroughly explore the subject.

---

[10]Adapted from *Student Self-Appraisal Inventory of Interest and Estimated Knowledge in Major Health Areas* by Josephine Gaines, University of Washington.

	KNOWLEDGE				INTEREST			
	None	Little	Some	Adequate	None	Little	Considerable	Great
A. BASIC HEALTH CONCEPTS								
1. Defining and interpreting health................								
2. Relationship of health to effective living......								
3. Major factors influencing health................								
4. Individual health needs								
5. Characteristics of the healthy individual......								
6. Health in contemporary society.................								
B. NUTRITION AND DIET								
7. Essential nutrients................................								
8. Functions of food in the body.................								
9. Planning a healthful diet								
10. Food fads and fallacies............................								
11. Overweight and underweight.....................								
12. Physiological aspects of digestion..............								
13. Food deficiency diseases								
C. CONSUMER HEALTH								
14. Fraudulent practices and quackery								
15. Legal protection for the consumer								
16. Organizations and agencies protecting the consumer								
17. Criteria for selecting health products								
18. Qualifications and licensure of health personnel								
19. Criteria in selecting health services............								
20. Health and accident insurance policies								
21. Evaluating health information								
22. Dangers of self-diagnosis and treatment.....								
23. Health services available to the consumer...								

The *Health Problems Inventory For High School Students* developed by Phyllis O'Daniels has been used in Kentucky to assess the extent of problems common to high school boys and girls. It is available from Professor O'Daniels at the University of Kentucky in Lexington, Kentucky. Using the Inventory, it was discovered that health instructors are not really aware of the students' perceptions of health problems; and teaching can be improved when instruction is focused on these problems.

Working together to focus more clearly on family health problems, O'Rourke and Olsen at the University of Illinois sampled attitudes of adolescent students by appraising degrees of feelings on contrasting statements. Students expressed their feelings in simple Likert scale fashion, as illustrated by questions 75 to 79:*

75. *Divorce is a reflection of poor mate selection.*
A Strongly Agree   **B** Agree   **C** Undecided   **D** Disagree   **E** Strongly Disagree
76. *Divorce is immoral.*
A Strongly Agree   **B** Agree   **C** Undecided   **D** Disagree   **E** Strongly Disagree
77. *Family unity is the key to lowering the divorce rate in the United States.*
A Strongly Agree   **B** Agree   **C** Undecided   **D** Disagree   **E** Strongly Disagree
78. *Divorce is better than living with someone you do not love.*
A Strongly Agree   **B** Agree   **C** Undecided   **D** Disagree   **E** Strongly Disagree
79. *Divorce destroys society.*
A Strongly Agree   **B** Agree   **C** Undecided   **D** Disagree   **E** Strongly Disagree

* Used by permission of Thomas W. O'Rourke, University of Illinois, Champaign, Ill.

With respect to divorce, the majority of males and females felt that divorce is a better alternative than living with someone you do not love. A majority supported the family unit as important, and more than two-thirds of the youths disagreed with the concept that divorce will destroy society. In most of the sex and family health areas there was homogeneity of responses among males and females.[11] Mutual interest in human sexuality problems is strong most everywhere with youth. This was borne out in the 1975 studies, *What Arkansas Teenagers Have Asked About Sex.*[12]

Another source of health-related information has to do with the kinds of music being played and listened to by local youth. What are they hearing? What are the words saying to them? What is it telling the instructor? In their article, "Are You Listening to the Lyrics," Dezelsky and Toohey present a most convincing argument for why teachers should keep up to date on what their charges are following in the way of popular music.[13] It is probable that many young people are spending more time listening to music with their friends than they are at almost any other comparable activity. They may say that they are not listening to the words—only the beat—but they really do hear what is being said. In fact, they cannot help being influenced by the words, for music has always been a means of expressing ideas and experiences and recording feelings.

It is clear from an examination of the music young people spend hours listening to that it is by far the most open expression of sexuality, mental health, happiness, rebellion, and commentary on the social scene in existence today. For example, most people would

---

[11] For additional details involving earlier studies, see John A. Conley and Thomas W. O'Rourke, "Attitudes of College Students Toward Selected Issues in Human Sexuality," *Journal of School Health,* 43:286–292, May, 1973.

[12] Copies available from Arkansas Family Planning Council, P.O. Box 5149, Little Rock, Arkansas 72205.

[13] Thomas Dezelsky and J. V. Toohey, "Are You Listening to the Lyrics?" *Journal of School Health,* 60:40–42, January, 1970.

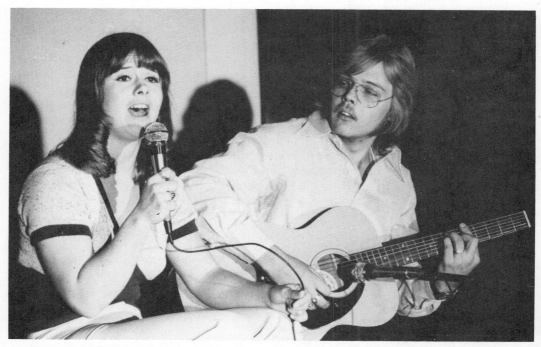

Figure 3–3 Student interests. What do they sing about? (Courtesy of Alcohol Safety Action Project, Phoenix, Arizona)

agree that John Denver's musical plea, "Please Daddy, Don't Get Drunk This Christmas," is real enough to relate to. So is his song, "Rhymes and Reasons:"[14]

> So you speak to me of sadness and the coming of the winter,
>   Fear that is within you now that seems to never end.
> And the dreams that have escaped you and the hope that you've forgotten
>   And you tell me that you need me now, and you want to be my friend,
> And you wonder where we're going, where's the rhyme and where's the reason . . . .

With the quick turnover in popular songs, such lyrics as the ones above may be outdated, but they serve as an example of what to look for in youth music.

THE STUDENT AND HIS KNOWLEDGE

Ever since the 1929 Carnegie report on the student and his knowledge, educators have never ceased to be amazed at what students of any age seem not to know.

The School Health Education Study discovered numerous gaps in knowledges and understandings pertaining to healthful living. It was an extensive study involving 529,656 elementary school students and 311,176 secondary school students in thirty-eight states.[15] Large, medium, and small school systems were studied. Health behavior questionnaires were submitted to the students in the sixth, ninth, and twelfth grades in order to secure information which would reflect the accumulation of health experience in the years prior to graduation. There were found to be serious misconceptions about health at all grade levels. Sixth graders scored poorly in safety education, and only one in five brushed his teeth or rinsed his mouth regularly after eating. In grade nine the average student could answer about two-thirds of the test questions correctly, with girls scoring higher than the boys. As might be expected, knowledge and attitude about health were better than health practices. In this same grade the weakest areas were consumer health, habit-forming substances, fatigue, sleep, and rest. Ninth graders generally accepted as being true health advertisements seen in print or heard on radio and television. Approximately half the ninth graders could not identify the recommended method for brushing the teeth. The high school seniors, although fairly well informed about drugs and mental health, showed weaknesses in the areas of nutrition, community health, chronic diseases, and the health of the consumer. It should be added that in a number of school systems some of these shortcomings may have been improved, because of the recent nationwide attention being given to mood modifiers, mental well-being, and personal adjustment.

In this same study it was found that hundreds of schools omitted certain health areas. Discussions pertaining to health careers and international health were treated poorly in some districts and better in others, but the study of research developments in health and medical science were noticeably missing throughout the school years.

Several state departments of education have surveyed the level of pupil knowledge prior to introducing stepped-up programs of health instruction. When Maine was experimenting with high school instruction in health it was conceded that if a pupil attained a reasonably good score on the Kilander Health Knowledge Test he would be excused from taking the health education course. Interestingly enough, only a rare student or two actually was excused from the course of instruction, for even the bright students pos-

---

[14]From *"Rhymes and Reasons"* by John Denver. © Copyright 1969 Cherry Lane Music Co. Used by permission—all rights reserved.
[15]Elena M. Sliepcevich, *School Health Education Study: A Summary Report*, Washington, D.C., 1964.

sessed numerous bits of misinformation pertaining to health practices and products; and when they *do know* what to do, they don't always do it. This, of course, comes as no surprise, for it was found in the Rhode Island School Health Education Study that the reason responses to health practices were poor was that pupils were not translating into everyday behavior the health understandings supposedly taught in their health education classes.[16] Moreover, these inadequacies were not related to economic status or intelligence. It was felt that the values held by the home, the neighborhood, and the peer group may play a real part. In any case, the percentage of high schools in Rhode Island listing required courses in health education is considerably higher than the national average. This may be due to the fact that 85 per cent of Rhode Island systems are in urban districts with large high schools, whereas much of the United States is made up of systems primarily located in small school districts.

In concluding this section on the student and his knowledge, it seems appropriate to point out that what the average adult citizen knows about health is a reflection of the public school system. This was made especially clear when CBS conducted a televised national health test covering a wide range of subject matter related to health knowledge and health behaviors of the viewers. The results provoked considerable concern among both public health and school health personnel, because the scores revealed that the American public is weak in health knowledge. For example, the great majority of the thousands tested didn't know their blood type, thought that venereal disease was spread through unclean toilets, believed that 20/20 vision assures freedom from eye trouble, and that a physician takes the blood pressure to measure the heart beat. They also believed that the chief cause of overweight is a glandular disorder, that milk should not be drunk immediately after eating citrus fruits, and that too much alcohol is dangerous because it overstimulates the brain. In short, adopting routine measures to determine what people — including students — know about health seems to be a most appropriate activity in which to engage prior to any large scale program of health education.

THE ENVIRONMENTAL SETTING

It would be a mistake to terminate a discussion of the peculiarities and interests of students without somehow relating them to the physical and emotional factors in the school environment. Obviously, health is best taught when the school environment is itself a healthful one.

Overcrowded classrooms, poor lighting, inadequate ventilation, unsatisfactory janitorial services, immovable desks and chairs, unattractive walls, and poor acoustics may be found in a number of schools today despite the increased attention given to the improvement of physical factors influencing education. In the heavily populated areas noise and congestion alone account for reduced classroom efficiency. Moreover, as the number of pupils packed into a building increases, the individual feeling of "being lost in a crowd" occurs more often. No one has really studied the effect of this kind of depersonalization or dehumanization on motivation and the involved process of intellectual development. A depersonalized setting is a health hazard. Rollo May says that, for the person involved, it is worse than physical pain.

The human or emotional factor is an especially important part of the environmental setting. Pupils learn better when they are happy with each other and with the teacher. Individual human factors such as idiosyncrasies, attitudes, prejudices, likes and dislikes, and the health status of the teacher at the moment have much to do with successful

---

[16]The Rhode Island Department of Education, *The Rhode Island School Health Study,* Providence, Rhode Island, 1969.

learning. It is interesting to note that a number of surveys have indicated that the physical and mental condition of teachers is frequently less than adequate. There is evidence that a good many are ill in one way or another. Unfortunately, only a few teachers in any school system are kept from teaching because of poor health. Research is needed to show more clearly the relationship between classroom-student efficiency and teacher health defects and illness. The grouchy teacher is a liability from the beginning. Moreover, teaching is a vigorous occupation requiring proper health conservation through attention to diet, rest, exercise, dental care and time for relaxation and enrichment away from the classroom. The teacher who understands this viewpoint will have the vigor and zest for working with young people, as well as mental health of sufficient balance to gain the respect of otherwise indifferent students.

HEALTH EDUCATION FOR THE UNDERPRIVILEGED STUDENT

There is a direct relationship between low socioeconomic status and poor health. The United States National Health Survey showed that low income families had a morbidity rate of 30 per cent. In contrast, a person in an income bracket only a few thousand dollars higher had a 7 per cent chance of morbidity limiting his activity. Also, students suffering from cultural and social deprivation have more school failures and health problems.

It is not uncommon to find studies showing that the less advantaged, the minority student, and other underprivileged need health education. They frequently value the importance of good health in their lives more than other youngsters. To effect needed improvements, however, it will be necessary to combine the efforts of health services and health instruction in a carefully designed program. An all-out approach has been made in the schools of Denver, Colorado, to do something about these problems — by helping students cope with themselves in learning to change and sometimes by changing their environment.[17]

In his Richmond, Virginia, study of inner city and outer city health needs, McCarthy discovered that inner city teachers regard such items as tooth care and disease prevention as far more important than do teachers in the outer city.[18] Therefore, making toothpowder, studying garbage and rubbish removal regulations, and learning how to take a sponge bath when bathing facilities are not available are practical curriculum items.

James Coleman and his colleagues recommend extensive involvement in community-based learning. Health projects and problems to solve outside the restrictive atmosphere of the school frequently represent real learning, carrying more impact than the "artificial" learning of the classroom.[19] Alternative schools with diverse health programs also have much to offer, chiefly because they provide choices and frequently permit individual students an active voice in how the program functions. Health education for the underprivileged must focus more on the student and less on the subject matter. The teacher must know more about the student — his thoughts, values, emotions, family life, and problems. Discussions seem to make these students feel especially good; lectures should be kept to a minimum.

[17]See report by Zoe VonEnde, "Denver Doesn't Quit on Problem Students," *American Education*, 6:18–22, June, 1970.

[18]Donald W. McCarthy, "Health Topics for Inner and Outer City Children," *School Health Review*, 1:27, April, 1970.

[19]James S. Coleman, *Transition to Adulthood*, Chicago: University of Chicago Press, 1974.

QUESTIONS FOR DISCUSSION

1. Philip Phenix, among others, has pointed out that there are several ways of knowing. (See his *Realms of Meaning* in Selected References.) Is it possible, therefore, that the diversity of students and types of learning suggests that we shall never find the ideal teacher, method, or climate for learning?

2. Over a half century ago, Oswald Spengler astounded the philosophical world by writing in *The Decline of the West* that the curtain is falling on Western civilization, that it is in the final stage, and that the route of decline is clearly visible. He reasoned that all societies eventually reach the top of their expectations, and from there they can only go down and slowly disintegrate. As you observe the health statistics and the health scene in general in America, do you see any evidence which might contribute to the validity of Spengler's viewpoint?

3. Which of Abraham Maslow's five levels of human needs seems to apply most to the topic of health education? Can man's level of "need satisfaction" be reached through health instruction?

4. Today student-held values appear more important than ever before. It is practically impossible to break through to the action realm with students without somehow relating to these values. How might this be accomplished in the area of health education?

5. Peer groups' interests and behaviors measurably influence the teaching process. This is especially true when one considers the kinds of health items purchased by teenagers. In teaching a series of lessons on consumer health, how might you take advantage of peer group interests?

6. Why is it that pupils frequently fail to translate into everyday behavior the health information taught in their health education classes? In the Rhode Island School Health Study it was felt that the values held by the home, neighborhood, and peer group were being overlooked in the teaching process. What are your comments?

7. Students who are culturally deprived and generally underprivileged need the kind of health education that appears to be immediately useful—a very practical kind of education. How can health be taught to meet this need?

SUGGESTED ACTIVITIES

1. Today's youth wants to identify with models for living in whom they can trust. They, like their heroes, are impatient with those who appear to base their authority simply on convention or tradition—no matter how sacrosanct the convention might be. What bearing does this attitude have on health teaching? Give some thought to this question and discuss it with classmates. A review of the Bonhoeffer biography by Bethge (see Selected References) may help, especially if this account of personal involvement in the plight of people is related to the diseases and disorders of individuals in the seventies.

2. Visit a busy eighth or ninth grade class of boys and girls, preferably one engaged in a health education lesson. From your observation formulate a list of individual and/or group characteristics and relate these to the level of interest in the particular health lesson. Compare your findings with those of your classmates. Where are they the same? Where do they differ?

3. Choose a half dozen recordings of music currently being heard by young people. Sit down with a friend or two and carefully listen to the words. What appears to be the "message"? Comment on whether you think there are implications here for health teaching.

4. Gather a small group of secondary school boys and girls together in an informal, non-school setting. Move from a general discussion of societal problems to the more specific health problems. Observe the level of youth interest in such items as weight reduction, pollution, mental disorders, and drug addiction. Eventually, raise the question as to whether these kinds of health topics can be properly taught in a school setting. Record your answers. Later, compare your answers with those of your classmates. What are the findings? Are there two or three significant conclusions that can be drawn from this experience? How may they be helpful to teachers?

5. Review some of the basic works in the area of motivation and interests. Texts having to do with general psychology and the psychology of learning should be helpful. What are the two or three essential points to consider when teaching a specific topic such as health? In short, what is the practical application of research pertaining to human interests and motivations?

SELECTED REFERENCES

Allen, Dwight W., and Jeffrey C. Hecht. *Controversies in Education*, Philadelphia: W. B. Saunders Co., 1975, Section seven.

Bethge, Eberhard. *Dietrich Bonhoeffer: Man of Vision, Man of Courage*, New York: Harper and Row, 1970.

Chafetz, Morris E. "Problems of Reaching Youth," *Journal of School Health*, 43:40–45, January, 1973.

Coleman, James S. *The Adolescent Society*, New York: Basic Books, 1965.

Coleman, James S. "The Children Have Outgrown the Schools," *National Elementary Principal*, October, 1972.

Coleman, James S. *Transition to Adulthood*, Chicago: University of Chicago Press, 1974.

Dillon, Stephen V. "Schools with Failure and Alienation," *Journal of School Health*, 45:324–326, June, 1975.

Farnsworth, Dana L. "Mental and Emotional Disturbances of the Secondary School-Age Student," *Journal of School Health*, 45:221–226, April, 1975.

Frankle, Reva T. and F. K. Heussentamm. "Food Zealotry and Youth," *American Journal of Public Health*, 64:11–18, January, 1974.

Hechinger, Fred M. "The All-New 'Law and Order' Classroom," *Saturday Review/World*, April 3, 1975.

Hentoff, Margot. "The Ungreening of Our Children," *Newsweek*, May 12, 1975.

Keniston, K. *Youth and Dissent: The Rise of a New Opposition*, New York: Harcourt, Brace, Jovanovich, 1971.

Maslow, Abraham H. *Motivation and Personality*, New York: Harper and Row, 1954.

Miller, John P. *Humanizing The Classroom*, New York: Praeger Publishers, 1976. Chapter 3.

Phenix, Philip. *Realms of Meaning: A Philosophy of the Curriculum*, New York: McGraw-Hill, 1964.

Schwartz, Audrey J. *The Schools and Socialization*, New York: Harper and Row, 1975. Chapters 2 and 6.

Willgoose, Carl E. *Health Education in the Elementary School*, 4th edition, Philadelphia: W. B. Saunders Co., 1974. Chapter 4.

Chapter 4

Planning and Implementing the Health Curriculum

The best laid schemes o' mice and men
Gang aft a-gley;
An lea'e us nought but grief and pain,
For promis'd joy.

—Robert Burns

All too often the best laid plans of men fail to work out as set forth. The "promised joy" that Burns speaks of is frequently lost by the wayside because the planning has been unrealistic or too far beyond the practical reach of the originator.

In an age when health education has yet to be fully understood and warmly received in hundreds of communities, it would be quite easy to make the error of overextending oneself in setting up an all-inclusive program designed to meet every health need from kindergarten to the adult level. A *reasonable* plan for each community should be the near-at-hand objective. Begin gradually, run pilot programs, solicit comments, evaluate results, and then with this background of experience the health effort can safely be extended.

Through advanced planning all health topics may be arranged in proper focus to achieve an "orchestration of many powers." "Harmony," said the Greeks, "is the music of the gods." Failure to seek a balanced and full health curriculum is to shortchange the student and mislead him so that he fails to appreciate the subtle particulars of the healthful life in a nuclear age. Furthermore, he may miss what Nobel laureate Jacques Monod considers vital—recognition of the distinction between objective knowledge and the realm of values.

PART I—CURRICULUM DEVELOPMENT
THE CURRICULUM DEFINED

The word curriculum is derived from the Latin word *currere,* which means "to run." It was earlier associated with race courses and the running of races. However, the more common definitions of a curriculum describe it as "a work schedule," or "any particular body of courses." The derived word seems to suggest an orderly plan and progression.

The employment of the word curriculum in the language of the American public school is as an all-inclusive term referring to the total program of the school. Thus, all of the academic programs, plus the extraclass activities, such as glee club, student council, band, clubs, and intramural and interscholastic athletics, are included. So integrated is

62

the total curriculum today that one speaks of "co-curricular" activities instead of the older term "extracurricular."

In discussing curriculum development in any subject matter area it is important to appreciate where the curriculum stands in relation to other educational influences.

```
┌─────────────────────────────────────┐
│                                     │
│      Philosophy of Life             │
│      Philosophy of Education        │
│      Aims and Objectives            │
│                                     │
│      ┌──────────────┐               │
│      │ Curriculum   │               │
│      └──────────────┘               │
│                                     │
│      Teaching Methods               │
│      Teaching Materials             │
│      Evaluation                     │
│                                     │
└─────────────────────────────────────┘
```

It is true that the curriculum, as a body of experiences, commands a central position. The degree to which it is implemented, however, depends on how highly motivated school personnel are to achieve their predetermined objectives, and upon the strength of the instructional methods, instructional materials, and evaluation techniques. In short, the most ideally planned curriculum may fail to be effective because of these other factors.

VARIETIES OF SECONDARY SCHOOL CURRICULA

In recent years the school curriculum has been widely studied, not only in the isolated subject areas but in terms of the total package—the ultimate influence of a secondary education on how one lives with himself and with other people in a society. Nevertheless, there is a dissatisfaction of both junior and senior high school students with curricula that fail to relate learning to real-life problems. The disaffection continues despite a wave of curriculum reform attempting to respond to this demand. Where before it was enough to leave the confines of the classroom and examine pond water to expose the mysteries of the ecosystem, now students are asked to *apply* such knowledge to solve pollution problems or to debate questions of environmental planning.

Goodlad, after an extensive study of curriculum change, stresses the fact that a curriculum should be built around unifying principles rather than specific bits and pieces of information.[1] He also observes that there are three recurring cycles of curriculum development: a concern for subject matter, a concern for the learner's total educational diet, and a concern for the individual as a human being. A look at these approaches is in order.

The *separate subject* or *subject matter curriculum* is the traditional approach to learning. The focus is on the academic subject rather than on the whole curriculum. It is a discipline-centered curriculum in which health is taught as a separate entity in the school. Frequently, there is little effort made to relate one school subject to another. For example, health is taught without reference to science, home economics, or physical education. There needs to be a strong emphasis upon problem-solving and learning how to handle new situations through a multidisciplinary approach to education. This is particularly true when it comes to health instruction. There is evidence that health is taught best

[1]John I. Goodlad, *School Curriculum and the Individual,* New York: Blaisdell Publishing Co., 1967.

in a specific setting as a subject by itself, especially when compared with the various "integrated" and "correlated" experiences of the past where it has really been lost in the shuffle. By taking a fresh approach, however, it is possible to recognize the multidimensional nature of health and set up a separate subject curriculum that is purposely constructed to relate to other academic fields in the particular school.

The *total curriculum* is something like the *broad fields curriculum* in which subject matter areas are grouped together. For example, spelling, oral communication, writing, reading, and grammar fall under the broad topic of language arts. Health has been included under the over-all heading of science. It has also been part of the umbrella of health, safety, and physical education. Relationships between several subjects are sometimes learned in this manner. However, health education has frequently suffered when combined with a biological science, because the zoological and botanical requirements in science demand a large share of the time assigned to the subject. Also, when health education is bracketed with physical education it often gets treated as an "also ran" topic or a rainy day activity. Health education can stand on its own two feet and still relate to the total curriculum. Moreover, when asked, most separate subject matter teachers would prefer to have health education taught as a separate subject; they already have more than enough material to cover in their own areas. The dilemma will continue as one compares the virtues of the total curriculum with the subject-matter curriculum, for the great explosion in knowledge demands a need for breadth, while the ability to deal forcefully with one aspect of the knowledge explosion demands depth. In the *activity curriculum* and *emerging curriculum* there is an emphasis on creativity through the planning of both students and teachers.

Alternative Programs

A more recent curriculum that provides choices in education is alternative programs. These may be part of an existing school or an alternative school. To a large extent content and courses are chosen by the students. Smaller units of study are made available with program differentiation. The *mini-course curriculum* fits this plan quite well. Here, short term courses appeal to students who might otherwise not be motivated.[2]

In the health area schools can provide "sanctuaries" from the typical school setting, where students have a chance to focus on their own concerns and problems, work out alternate ways to handle them, and receive the support they need to implement the alternatives. For example, in drug prevention programs in New York, California, and elsewhere goal-oriented rap sessions, frequently led by the students themselves, have been quite effective. It is these "positive alternatives," which have to be worked out and implemented, that make this type of curriculum difficult to operate. Yet, based on the theory that many secondary school drug abusers are simply bored with the typical school, one Lower East Side school center in New York City has had considerable success in weaning drug users from their habits through yoga. There are other ways to reach non-chemical "highs," such as following the lead of the Black Panthers by emphasizing various political and economic actions as an alternative to drug abuse.

The alternative curriculum must generate more than recreational programs of arts, crafts, and sports. The critical question is whether a "positive alternatives" program contributes to the development of a life style or simply fills up some loose hours. Alan

---

[2]See Allan A. Glatthorn, *Alternatives in Education: Schools and Programs,* New York: Dodd, Mead and Company, 1975, Chapter 5.

Cohen and others have established extensive lists of activities that permit matching alternatives to specific drug behaviors. These cover a wide range of experiences—from physical-sensory items such as dance training and massage, to emotional awareness, exercises, psycho dramas, photography, creative fantasy, non-partisan lobbying for environmental health projects, social service involvement, workshops on values and morality, self-reliance training, and "Outward Bound" survival training. Here, affective education is married to effective personal action. Even in traditional schools the provision for alternative health education paths could lead to responsible decision making.

Humanistic Education

Goodlad's thinking centered on a *humanistic curriculum* that functions in the area of human interests, feelings, and values. Perhaps more than a program it is a method or way of teaching—a warm technique grounded on the principle of respect for the individual personality. It focuses on what kind of persons students should be, rather than strictly upon what they know about processes, items, and other things. A number of affective procedures are offspring of the humanistic or human potential movement. Weinstein and Fantini have shown how students can observe their inner selves with a minimum of defensiveness and obstructive self-judging and see real values in situations related to numerous subject areas, especially in social issues and mental well-being.[3]

Multicultural Health Education

America is not a melting pot but a multicultural society. The concept of the melting pot never really worked well; it rejected as "unmeltable" many ethnic groups, including native Americans, blacks, Spanish-speaking individuals, and Orientals. There was an assumption that those who wished to be absorbed by the mostly Anglo-Saxon melting pot had to surrender their own cultural heritage. Today, with the acceptance of the culturally pluralistic nature of society, what is taught in the educational system must take into account a wide range of individuals, groups, and life styles.

Health education can be multicultural if it is oriented toward the enrichment of youth through preservation of cultural diversities in such areas as food choice and preparation, drinking practices, family mores, ethnic attitudes toward death and dying, and practices relating to a positive state of emotional well-being. This concept has the advantage of holding the student's interest, as well as developing stronger school and family bonds. Moreover, in a search for an improved motivation, the multicultural concept can be extended to class structure, as British educator Denis Lawton has suggested, noting that working class people have a different culture and, therefore, need a different kind of education.[4]

ERA OF MAJOR CURRICULUM STUDIES

It has become almost fashionable to prepare and rework educational programs from the point of view of both the total school and individual subjects. However, in many

---

[3]Gerald Weinstein and Mario Fantini, *Toward Humanistic Education: A Curriculum of Affect,* New York: Praeger Press, 1970.

[4]Denis Lawton, *Class, Culture and the Curriculum,* Boston: Routledge and Kegan Paul, 1975.

cases the exploration and curriculum planning have been shallow. There seems to be only a slight relationship between success as measured in the classroom and subsequent demonstration of those virtues inherent in most educational aims. Knowledge test scores leading to high marks in a health education class are virtually useless as predictors of health leadership, creativity, inventiveness, health citizenship in the community, family happiness, and a healthful way of life.

A large number of state and local efforts are being made today to restructure the curriculum and improve education in the United States and Canada. Curriculum reform is designed chiefly to update the content of instruction, but it must do more than this. It must provide structured approaches to otherwise unmanageable accumulations of knowledge.

Over the years from 1959 to 1967 the high school physics program was overhauled by the Physical Science Study Committee (PSSC). During the same period, and at a cost of several million dollars, the Biological Sciences Curriculum Study (BSCS) upgraded biology. The National Science Foundation funded several years of research and experimentation by the School Mathematics Study Group (SMSG) in an effort to plan and implement a first-class mathematics curriculum. Other subject matter areas have struggled to create a better program. Over 40 major curriculum projects were initiated in the social studies area in the last several years.

Most of the new patterns of curriculum planning have attempted to better recognize individual student differences; encourage flexible grouping; and plan for the use of certain instructional personnel from outside the school. Instead of swinging from an emphasis on breadth to an emphasis on depth, as was done in past cycles, there is an effort being made to balance the two. There is also a trend that is particularly helpful for health education. This is the organizing of parts of the curriculum, such as study of alcohol and drug problems, around current problems of young people or pressing problems of the generation. In previous eras these approaches have been considered of doubtful value.

In the past decade several state-sponsored and big-city curriculum projects have resulted in new guides and courses of study for a number of teaching fields. The Educational Research Council of Greater Cleveland is one example of a city organization that thoroughly studied ways to provide a better curriculum in all subjects and at all grade levels—a major undertaking of significance to other areas of the country. It influenced health teaching far beyond the Cleveland city limits. Finally, with the establishment of the Center for the Study of Instruction at the National Education Association in Washington, D.C., it was possible to encourage and help all subject matter personnel upgrade their special programs.

HEALTH CURRICULUM STUDIES

Short term and hastily conducted investigations pertaining to health education programs were generally the rule up until 1961, when the Samuel Bronfman Foundation sponsored the School Health Education Study (SHES).[5] Information was gathered from large, medium, and small school systems about the accumulation of health experiences and understandings. Health specialists and teachers were brought together to prepare sample experimental curriculum materials based on a concept approach. Subsequently, these materials were appraised in try-out centers in Alhambra, California; Evanston, Illinois; Tacoma, Washington; and Great Neck–Garden City, New York.

---

[5]Elena M. Sliepcevich, *School Health Education Study: A Summary Report,* Washington, D.C.: SHES, 1964. See also Richard K. Means, "The School Health Education Study: A Pattern in Curriculum Development," *Journal of School Health,* 36:1–11, January, 1966.

The development and publication of SHES curriculum materials began in 1966 when the project came under the control of the Minnesota Mining and Manufacturing Company (3M). The basic publication for teachers, *Health Education: A Conceptual Approach to Curriculum Design, Grades Kindergarten Through Twelve,* appeared in 1967 and set up a framework for the health education curriculum that had both depth and flexibility. Three concepts representing the unifying threads of the curriculum were developed:

> *Growing and developing:* a dynamic life process in which the individual is in some ways like all other individuals, in some ways like some other individuals, and in some ways like no other individuals.
> *Interacting:* an ongoing process in which the individual is affected by and in turn affects certain biological, social, psychological, economic, cultural, and physical forces in the environment.
> *Decision making:* a process, unique to man, of consciously deciding to take an action, or of choosing one alternative rather than another.[6]

These three concepts are considered *key* concepts and are related specifically to ten curriculum concepts developed by the study:

1. Growth and development influence and are influenced by the structure and functioning of the individual.
2. Growing and developing follow a predictable sequence, yet are unique for each individual.
3. Protection and promotion of health is an individual, community, and international responsibility.
4. The potential for hazards and accidents exists, whatever the environment.
5. There are reciprocal relationships involving man, disease, and environment.
6. The family serves to perpetuate man and to fulfill certain health needs.
7. Personal health practices are affected by a complexity of forces, often conflicting.
8. Utilization of health information, products, and services is guided by values and perceptions.
9. Use of substances that modify mood and behavior arises from a variety of motivations.
10. Food selection and eating patterns are determined by physical, social, mental, economic, and cultural factors.

These curriculum concepts reflect the scope of health education, and because they relate to thinking and acting in a comprehensive way, they are viewed by SHES as especially valuable in that phase of program planning that is concerned with appropriate repetition and the integration of ideas.

Under each of the ten curriculum concepts there were developed a number of sub-concepts. These are set up to bear upon physical, mental, and social dimensions so that the individual can react and make decisions in respect to his total surroundings — surroundings which cause him to view himself in terms of physical status, mental well-being, and social awareness.

From the sub-concepts were developed the long range goals, which ". . . reflect what is expected of the student after experiencing the total health education program based on the conceptual approach."[7] These goals were formulated in three domains and were based in part on the pioneering work of Bloom and Krathwohl.[8]

---

[6] School Health Education Study, *Health Education: A Conceptual Approach to Curriculum Design,* St. Paul, Minnesota: 3M Education Press, 1967, p. 20.

[7] Ibid, p. 26.

[8] Benjamin S. Bloom, ed., *Taxonomy of Educational Objectives, Handbook I: Cognitive Domain,* New York: David McKay Co., Inc., 1956. See also David K. Krathwohl et al., *Taxonomy of Educational Objectives, Handbook II: Affective Domain,* New York: David McKay Co., Inc., 1964.

The final effort in the School Health Education Study was to create behavioral objectives (progessions and sequences) for each of the ten concepts. These were set up as four levels of progression rather than by the more traditional grade level approach. This was done to provide for individual and administrative variations and to ensure a degree of flexibility. The SHES program has been used directly by a number of school systems, for it is a curriculum package complete with instruction materials and follow-up information. It has also been used as a guide in the preparation of health education programs. In this respect it is most helpful in getting local curriculum committee personnel to relate local philosophy and objectives to the practical aspects of content and teaching progressions.

Another excellent health curriculum study was carried out by the Curriculum Commission of the School Health Education Division (AAHPER) in 1967.[9] It contains concepts and supporting data relating to some of the major health problems facing youth in the decade of the seventies. National organizations concerned with these health problems and outstanding health authorities assisted the members of the Curriculum Commission in this work. Significantly, the publication was prepared to help teachers in developing curriculum and teaching guides.

In recent years, several state departments of education have conducted their own health curriculum studies. In addition to throwing light on the shortcomings of secondary school students, the studies have resulted in the preparation of curriculum guides which set forth program suggestions and even complete programs. Noteworthy studies and programs have been accomplished in such states as Pennsylvania, Illinois, Florida, Oregon, Colorado, New York, Rhode Island, Massachusetts, Maine, and California. By way of example, the Pennsylvania program for total school health, *Conceptual Guidelines for School Health Programs in Pennsylvania,* is a superb publication complete with appendices and practical ideas for program activities.[10] Equally impressive is the New York State Education Department's study of the health curriculum.[11] This publication, *Suggested Guidelines for the Development of Courses of Study in Health Education for Junior and Senior High Schools,* is of particular value to secondly school teachers. (See pp. 81 to 82.)

New curriculum studies leading to more effective health courses are on the horizon. The Decision Making Model of the Educational Research Council of America examines motivating forces and relates these to personal standards and practices prior to beginning learning activities.[12] The Risk-Taking Curriculum of Shirreffs' is another example in which the curriculum is approached differently.[13] Here, the integration of subject matter

---

[9]Health Education Division, *Health Concepts: Guide for Health Instruction,* Report of Curriculum Commission, Washington, D.C.: American Association for Health, Physical Education and Recreation, 1967.

[10]Pennsylvania Department of Education, *Conceptual Guidelines for School Health Programs in Pennsylvania,* Harrisburg: Pennsylvania Department of Education, 1970.

[11]New York State Education Department, *Suggested Guidelines for the Development of Courses of Study in Health Education for Junior and Senior High Schools,* Albany: The State Education Department, 1970.

[12]Lester V. Smith, "A Decision Making Model," *School Health Review,* January-February, 1974.

[13]Janet Shirreffs, "A Risk-Taking Curriculum," *School Health Review,* July-August, 1973.

TABLE 4–1 Long Range Goals

COGNITIVE DOMAIN	AFFECTIVE DOMAIN	ACTION DOMAIN

Understanding
Comprehending
Realizing
(Knowledge, intellectual
  abilities, skills)
	Awareness
	Appreciation
	Consciousness
	(Interests, attitudes,
	  values)
		Improving
		Modifying
		Developing
		(Application of
		  knowledge and
		  attitudes)

is stressed by focusing on behavior that actually threatens the life or well-being of the individual. Self-destruction as a psychological entity is woven into the course of study.

School Health Education Curriculum Project (SHECP)

A relatively recent core curriculum in health education (SHECP) was designed by the national clearinghouse for smoking and health of the Department of Health, Education and Welfare. As a central theme a different body system is utilized at each grade level (five, six, and seven); the program is anatomically and physiologically based. A multiplicity of learning experiences is used along with multi-media aids appropriate to learning. Teachers involved in the project participate in a two-week workshop designed to acquaint them with the same learning experiences that their students will have. Although this carefully structured curriculum has been tried from Berkeley to Boston, its effectiveness is under continuous study at six regional training centers throughout the country. It appears, however, that this curriculum has a positive influence on health knowledge and attitudes.

CONCEPTS IN CURRICULUM DEVELOPMENT

Before getting into curriculum construction, it seems appropriate to take a look at *concepts* and *competencies*—terms often employed to denote learning outcomes. They are much alike, but they are different. The concept is a point of view or idea held about something, whereas a competency is a solid ability or proficiency. Both are needed in health education. *Ultimate health behavior starts with one or more health concepts and culminates in a skillful and appropriate action—a health competency.*

The concept approach to program planning is sound, for it is based on the premise that a concept is a relatively meaningful and complete idea in the mind of the student that he can perceive according to his experience. Concepts are built from a number of related sensations, precepts, and images. They range from ideas about very elemental things to high-level abstractions.

TABLE 4–2   *Examples of Concepts*

Accidents:	Man interacts with people, things, and events in his environment. That which occurs but was unplanned is an accident; the result may be desirable or undesirable.
Dental Health:	The dental needs of the community must be recognized and studied for methods of prevention and correction. There are various methods of financing dental care.
Smoking:	Smoking seems to be related to a range of diverse psychological behaviors which may be set off by different personal needs.

A concept is actually a *personal* understanding, feeling, or interpretation of something to which an individual has been exposed. Therefore, concepts cannot be taught as such; but teaching can be directed *toward* concepts. Setting up a curriculum in terms of student concepts appears to be far superior to the more traditional listing of specific objectives, goals, and outcomes of the past. For one thing, these ends tend to be more teacher-oriented than pupil-oriented. Morever, they encourage the objectivation of factual information, which is too often unrelated to larger generalizations. For too long, hundreds of health facts have been tossed around without the student seeing them as a part of the whole—a part of *his* life. This is one reason why the School Health Education Study people stressed the need to conceptualize learning in all health areas—not only in terms of the individual student and his personal feeling, but of his family and community at large.

If, as Gagne and others have pointed out, concept learning requires the student to make a response to a number of stimuli that may differ from each other, then the curriculum of study must provide several avenues for personal exploration.[14] Curriculum builders must see concepts "...as the skeleton of sweeping ideas the understanding of which permits the learner to reach Gagne's most complicated varieties of learning, principle learning, and problem solving."[15]

There are a number of examples one might use to show how concepts are brought into play in curriculum planning. In most instances it takes a fair amount of time to identify and formulate appropriately worded concepts for a particular educational level. By way of illustration, the Curriculum Commission of the School Health Education Division (AAHPER) tried to think in terms of conceptualizations that should be held by reasonably mature individuals. In the mental health area, for instance, several concepts suitable for senior high school students are as follows:

Human behavior tends to be ordered and patterned.

Behavior is complex.

Behavior is characterized by adaptability.

Interpersonal relationships are enhanced through an understanding of the factors underlying behavior, including behavior of self and others.

---

[14]Eight varieties of learning are discussed by R. M. Gagne, *The Conditions of Learning,* New York: Holt, Rinehart, Winston, Inc., 1965, p. 32.

[15]Cyrus Mayshark and Leslie W. Irwin, *Health Education in Secondary Schools,* 2nd edition, St. Louis: C. V. Mosby Co., 1968, p. 162.

NUTRITION

CONCEPT	JUNIOR HIGH	SENIOR HIGH
Nutrition is important in the everyday functioning of an individual.*	**Grade Level Concept:** Nutritional practices contribute to the development of diseases and disorders.	The level of nutrition of people affects their health, which in turn affects the productivity of their country.
	Objective: Describes chronic diseases and disorders which may be associated with nutritional practices.	Summarizes effects of nutrition upon the productivity of the individual and society.
	Content: (1) obesity; (2) underweight; (3) diabetes; (4) cardiovascular disease; (5) acne; (6) allergies; (7) central nervous system disorders; (8) vitamin deficiency diseases; (9) dental disorders.	(1) life expectancy; (2) growth and development; (3) endurance required to work; (4) nation's productivity.

CONSUMER HEALTH (Grades 7, 8 and 9)

OUTLINE OF CONTENT	MAJOR UNDERSTANDINGS AND FUNDAMENTAL CONCEPTS	SUGGESTED TEACHING AIDS AND LEARNING ACTIVITIES	SUPPLEMENTARY INFORMATION FOR TEACHERS
I. Quackery and Quacks 　A. Definitions 　　1. Health Quackery	Health quackery prevents consumers from engaging in sound health practices and deprives them of adequate health protection.	———	———

Extensive research in the behavioral sciences has provided a basis for determining possible causes of certain behavior patterns.

In the California Public Schools framework for health instruction there is an overall concept for each major health area. This is followed by a grade level concept. This in turn is followed by examples of objectives and teaching content. By way of illustration, the Nutrition area might look as shown in the diagram above.[16]

In the New York curriculum materials, the State Education Department has kept concepts practical by tying them closely with the content outline, the learning activities, and teaching suggestions. An example of a consumer health concept suitable for grades 7, 8, and 9 is as follows: (See diagram below.)

Generally speaking, a local committee charged with preparing a health curriculum should think in terms of overall aims and goals for a particular major health area. When the discussion is concluded, it should boil down to a carefully worded and all-encompassing generalization—a major concept for the area. Once this has been accomplished, a sizable listing of related concepts can be written. Later these will be assigned according to beginning, intermediate, and advanced instructional levels or to specific grade levels in the junior and senior high schools.

Helping students to conceptualize health material has given way in recent years to use of behavioral objectives and competency-based activity. This may be due in part to findings which indicate that the concept approach to learning is not sufficient to produce a substantial number of changes in student-reported health behavior patterns.[17]

Behavioral Objectives

Since behavioral objectives are stated in precise fashion and describe a behavior, they are obviously student objectives, as opposed to the objectives of an institution or a society. They represent something that can be achieved and readily measured. They are written in terms of actions rather than thoughts and feelings. Action words associated with the verb *to do,* such as the following, generally preface the stated objectives:

analyzes	relates	plans
identifies	improves	produces
evaluates	modifies	designs
describes	performs	judges
gives	makes	formulates
applies	distinguishes	writes

[16]State of California, *Framework for Health Instruction in California Public Schools,* Sacramento: The California State Board of Education, 1970.

[17]Robert E. Allen and Owen J. Holyoak, "Evaluation of the Conceptual Approach to Teaching Health Education: A Second Look," *Journal of School Health,* 43:293–296, May, 1973.

In the following example note the difference between the writing of a traditional objective, a concept, and a behavioral objective; note especially the weight placed on the first behavioral objective word *(performs):*

> *Example*
> *Traditional objective:*   To understand that the first aid practice for asphyxiation due to drowning or electric shock is artificial respiration.
> *Concept:*   Artificial respiration is employed as a first aid measure for asphyxiation from drowning or electric shock.
> *Behavioral objective:*   Performs artificial respiration as a first aid procedure for asphyxiation from drowning or electric shock.

A number of state and city health curriculum guides combine grade level concepts and behavioral objectives as a part of each major health unit. Behavioral objectives were also developed for each of the 10 fundamental concepts in the School Health Education Study.[18] The Maryland State Education Department has available an excellent chart in which conceptual and sub-conceptual statements preface clearly stated behavioral objectives in all the major health areas, grades 6 to 8 and 9 to 12. Human external and internal environments are separated for purposes of study and the objectives have both depth and breadth. Note the extent of activity called for in the following examples:[19]

> Given a description of an interaction which occurs between man and natural conditions and which has a detrimental influence on health, the learner will be able to develop a plan for coping with the problems and for reversing the negative aspects of the interaction.
> Given a description of the relationship of a local, state, national, or international community with a natural condition, the learner will be able to develop a plan for utilizing and protecting the natural condition in a healthful manner which requires the cooperation of the communities involved.

In these examples the behavioral objective is carried through to the action domain by having the student develop a plan. If this provision is not made the objective will be no different from those that have been written for decades on a purely teacher-oriented level. Other examples of in-depth objectives calling for student involvement may be found in *You, Behavioral Objectives and Nutrition Education* from the National Dairy Council, and in the Appendix of this book.

For some time Arthur W. Combs, a perceptual psychologist of considerable reputation, has been unhappy with the emphasis on behavior objectives. He considers the behavioral objective approach to be somewhat limited to a symptomatic approach to behavior change.[20] How one sees himself and acts at the moment is a symptom of what is taking place inside the individual. In short, a person behaves in keeping with his perceptions of his world. Combs warns that one should concentrate attention, therefore, on the *origins of the behavior* rather than the actions at the end of the process. However, in the planning stages of education it still appears possible and appropriate to live with Combs' concern by first determining the kinds of health behavior worthy of goal identification, and then establish the ways and means of getting at perceptions, beliefs, hopes, desires, and values. In short, focusing on behavioral objectives has value only if they are viewed as one part of the teaching process. In this respect, the objectives are of limited

---

[18]Available in wall chart form from Minnesota Mining and Manufacturing Company, Box 1300, St. Paul, Minn. 55101

[19]Adapted from *Health Education: A Curricular Approach to Optimum Health*, Division of Instruction, Maryland State Department of Education.

[20]Arthur W. Combs, *Educational Accountability: Beyond Behavioral Objectives*, Washington, D.C.: Association for Supervision and Curriculum Development, 1972.

value unless they are a part of an evaluation feed-back process which describes student attainment in light of stated goals. A prime reason for the limited use of behavioral objectives is the great amount of energy that must be expended by a school faculty to describe and measure outcomes sought in the various subject areas.

Competency-Based Programs

The assumption behind competency-based instruction (CBI) is that specific skills, knowledge, and behavior can be identified in each major health area. In this respect, it is essential that performance criteria be explicitly stated in behavioral objective form, describing the components of a competency area. Competencies are defined and stated in advance of instruction. The criteria for evaluation are also designed and made public to all participants, i.e., students, teachers, and parents. There is a progression in competencies that the learner must follow. As proficiency is demonstrated the learner moves ahead—and the responsibility of this learning lies with the student.

Obviously there are many activities employed to put across a health topic, especially when the student is to work essentially on his own competencies. Learning modules take the form of mini-courses which are helpful; so are mini-lessons in which certain key parts of a health area are stressed in connection with other activities, such as reading, observing, and appraising the circumstances. The teacher is free to be a resource person, to observe, and to check, among other things, with a student's peers about his or her advancement in competencies. It has been said that CBI is more of a method than a program.[21]

DEVELOPING THE HEALTH CURRICULUM

There has to be order in developing a curriculum. This is especially true when one realizes that the knowledge explosion has provided far more health information than can ever be included at any grade level and for any one topic. The selection of content under these topics has to be screened carefully. As the Harvard Report pointed out a quarter century ago, "Selection is the essence of teaching.... Since the problem of choice can under no circumstances be avoided, the problem becomes what, rather than how much, to teach...."[22]

In determining *what* to teach, it has already been pointed out that student interests, student needs, and the health problems of the society and local community provide considerable information. In addition, it is helpful to review successful programs in other localities, and to study recently developed curriculum guides and courses of study gathered from several sources. In this connection, most state departments of education have either a health education consultant or someone assigned to the area who will make certain publications available at the local level. Moreover, several states have a health advisory committee that works to develop curriculum items, health needs research, and other health-related items of immediate use in the schools and colleges.

---

[21]Thomas L. Good, et al., *Teachers Make a Difference,* New York: Holt, Rinehart and Winston, 1975, pp. 34–37.

[22]Report of Harvard Committee, *General Education in a Free Society,* Cambridge, Massachusetts: Harvard University Press, 1948, p. 63.

ELEMENTS THAT AFFECT PLANNING FOR HEALTH EDUCATION

Health Needs	Societal Needs
Health Knowledge	Significant Curriculum Trends
Health Attitudes	State and Local Courses of Study
Health Behavior	Organization of Total School Curriculum
Health Status	Organization of Health Curriculum
Health Interests	Time Allotments
Characteristics of Growth and Development	Scheduling of Classes
Individual Variations in Physical and	Health Education Research
Social Capacities	Health of Teachers

STUDENT

State Education Department	School Environment
Secondary School Education Objectives	Adequate Facilities
Health Education Objectives	Qualified Health Education Staff
School Department Policies,	Special Resources Personnel
School Committee, School Objectives	Available Teaching Materials and Supplies
Governmental and Private Bulletins	Parents and Community

There are a great many elements that have a significant bearing on health curriculum building. They are best accounted for by structuring them about the student as follows: (See table above.)

Despite the profusion of factors having to do with curriculum construction, and the inherent difficulty of trying to juggle all of these so that they can have a beneficial bearing during the planning stages, there are nevertheless hundreds of local committees that have created admirable programs that are functioning well today. One reason for this is the attention given to the organization of people for curriculum development.

THE CURRICULUM COORDINATING COMMITTEE

The working organization for a health curriculum production is the curriculum coordinating committee (see Figure 4–1). Because of the multidimensional nature of health, this committee requires a breadth of experience and "feel" for the needs and problems of secondary school youth.

The committee should not be large—five or six people are enough to act as coordinators of the efforts of several sub-groups of junior and senior high school teachers. Sub-groups should consist of teachers of health and related health topics such as science, biology, home economics, and social studies. An interested parent, an administrator, and a student or two usually rounds out the sub-group so that a variety of viewpoints and experience are represented. In the larger communities, personnel from the more active voluntary health agencies and the local health department are invited to be a part of and to make contributions to the sub-groups. Significantly, the multiagency approach does much to improve curriculum development and the implementation processes. In fact, in the Duluth School Health Education Project, the comprehensive health program was given a real boost by local committees interested in upgrading the curriculum.[23]

The sub-groups break themselves down into feeder groups. A sub-group of a dozen or 15 workers might break down into feeder groups of two or three people. It is the

---

[23]For details concerning input see John A. Cunico and William H. Boothe, "Duluth's School Health Education Project: The Multiagency Approach." *Journal of School Health,* 44:11–15, January, 1974.

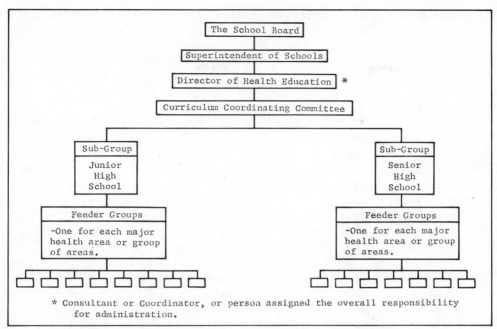

Figure 4–1   Organization for curriculum development in Health Education.

feeder groups that prepare the initial materials, frequently in rough form. A particular feeder group works up health concepts, objectives, content, learning activities, teaching materials, and evaluation suggestions for a major health area or for a grouping of health topics. Feeder groups can get help from a number of sources. They review materials, guides, research, and so on, and may bring in resource personnel from the community. Their efforts, however, are always related to what other feeder groups are doing and are coordinated through meetings of their sub-group. In short, the sub-group is a well-informed group of people who are working directly on parts of the health curriculum.

It is the job of the Curriculum Coordinating Committee, frequently under the chairmanship of the Director of Health Education, to work closely with the sub-groups so that there is proper progression from junior high to senior high health instruction. More specifically, the task of the Curriculum Coordinating Committee is to:

1. Set the stage for curriculum discussion. Expressions of dissatisfaction with the present curriculum require exploring. A number of school personnel can contribute information here—sometimes through a simple survey questionnaire. Parents, students, and community health workers also have valuable viewpoints to consider.
2. Meet with the junior and senior high school principals and eventually with the school board in order to clarify necessary administrative procedures.
   a. Obtain released time for health education teachers or other personnel to attend professional meetings and visit out-of-town school systems, and to report back the new ideas and practices elsewhere.
   b. Arrange for some teachers to attend summer institutes and in-service workshops in order to be better prepared to work with sequences, learning experiences, and so forth.
   c. Consider budget provisions for curriculum materials, final copy, and possibly the employment of an outside curriculum consultant.
3. Establish appropriate procedures underlying the organization of the curriculum at both levels and the construction of the curriculum guide.

4. Formulate satisfactory work schedules so that working together in sub-groups and feeder group activity will be a challenge.
5. Arrange stages of work both within and between the sub-groups.
6. Appoint personnel to the subgroups and oversee the assignments to feeder groups.
7. Review junior and senior high school sub-group preparations for completeness, sequences, and general smoothness of flow.
8. Arrange for the writing and publication of the curriculum guides.

The task of preparing a thoroughly effective secondary school health instruction program is not one that can be done in a hurry. More than a few meetings are needed to iron out all the possibilities involved in writing appropriate level concepts, spelling out content, reviewing and suggesting learning experiences, seeking pertinent teaching aids, and formulating some kind of evaluation procedure. The Los Angeles County School initiated Project Quest with three years of time given to planning and operating a health instruction program. That much time was needed in order to involve teachers, students, parents, physicians, and health specialists and get feed-back from the developed programs and begin to make changes in guides and appraisal techniques.

How does one know whether the committee is following acceptable curriculum development practices? How can a local curriculum coordinating committee be certain it is doing all that it should in developing a subject matter area? An excellent way is to review the detailed checklist on curriculum development procedures set forth by the National Study of Secondary School Evaluation in its *Evaluative Criteria* publication.[24] In addition, Figure 4–2 summarizes some of the essential items to be considered when a new program is being prepared or an old one revised. If most of the 20 "concerns" can be embraced and given a "yes" or "no" answer, the effort to develop a sound health education curriculum will be productive.

CONSTRUCTING THE CURRICULUM GUIDE

The libraries of most teacher preparation institutions carry examples of local curriculum guides in health education. They generally include manuals from large cities, small towns, suburban regions, and rural areas. It is a good idea to carefully examine several recent guides or courses of study.

A curriculum guide in one community may depict a full program—actually a complete course of study for the secondary school teacher's use. Everything is there in the way of procedures, suggestions, resources, and concrete examples. In another community, however, the guide may be no more than an outline of essential topics and their rough placement within the grade levels concerned. Because of these differences in depth, it is common practice to use the terms "curriculum guide" and "course of study" synonymously. Experience indicates that teachers welcome help, and that they will render a better instructional program if they have something more than a skeleton outline from which to work.

If a guide is going to be helpful to the classroom teacher, and especially the increasing number of new teachers assigned to health instruction, it must elaborate on each major health area. Therefore, dental health, drug education, or anything else must be clearly conceptualized and the behavior idealized for each teaching level, and followed by examples of content, learning experiences, teaching suggestions, resource materials,

---

[24]National Study of Secondary School Evaluation, *Evaluative Criteria,* 4th edition, Washington, D.C.: NSSSE, 1969, p. 41. Copies may be obtained from the Study at 1785 Massachusetts Avenue, N.W., Washington, D.C. 20036. This 356 page book is set up so that health education and every other subject matter area can be thoroughly evaluated by a local school system.

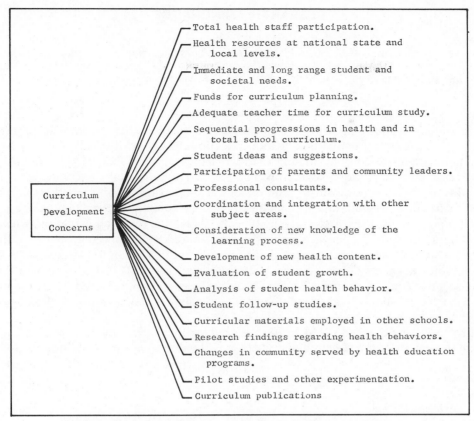

Total health staff participation.

Health resources at national state and local levels.

Immediate and long range student and societal needs.

Funds for curriculum planning.

Adequate teacher time for curriculum study.

Sequential progressions in health and in total school curriculum.

Student ideas and suggestions.

Participation of parents and community leaders.

Professional consultants.

Coordination and integration with other subject areas.

Consideration of new knowledge of the learning process.

Development of new health content.

Evaluation of student growth.

Analysis of student health behavior.

Student follow-up studies.

Curricular materials employed in other schools.

Research findings regarding health behaviors.

Changes in community served by health education programs.

Pilot studies and other experimentation.

Curriculum publications

Curriculum Development Concerns

Figure 4–2   Summary of essential curriculum development concerns.

and evaluation procedures. To put this in the right setting, most curriculum guides start off with the school's position on health philosophy, principles, and goals; this is frequently coupled with comments pertaining to student needs and the learning process.

Very often the junior high school guide is constructed separately from that of the senior high school. This provides two neat packages and keeps the size of the manual under control. If health education is taught every year, grades 7 to 12, then each manual will be rather heavy with details for each grade level. However, if health is taught only once in the junior high school and once in the senior high school it probably would be desirable to print both programs in the one curriculum guide. The minimum contents of a guide are outlined as follows:

I. Introduction
II. Philosophy of Health Education
   Health Education Defined
   Why Health Education?
   Health Education in Education
III. Health Education Program
   Objectives
   General Objectives
   Objectives for junior high school
   (or senior high)
IV. Instructional Methods in
   Health Education
   How To Use This Guide
   Conceptual Learning in Health
   Education
V. Health Teaching Areas

Grade Seven ⎫   ⎧ Level I
Grade Eight ⎬ or ⎨ Level II
Grade Nine ⎭   ⎩ Level III
Each Major Health Area
   (for each grade or level)
   Fundamental Concept
   Grade Level objectives or
      competencies
   Content
   Suggested Learning Activities
   Resource Aids and Materials
   Evaluation Suggestions
   Selected References
      For Students
      For Instructor
VI. Evaluation in Health Education
VII. References

RESEARCH AND CHANGE

". . . in personal affairs, as in history, change is a constant. The ignorant sometimes learn; the poor become rich; the powerless, influential. It is a test of life. . . to come to terms with change; neither to hide from it, nor to waste too much time in protest."

—*John J. Putnam*

In surveying the total school curriculum, it is apparent that no one subject area is more concerned with research than health education. Every medical advance and educational innovation related to health and welfare is pertinent to some part of the health education presentation. There are numerous implications of individual value judgments, anxieties, life styles, and the ever-present ecological dimension. This is one reason why a health instruction program must remain flexible and accommodate frequent changes.

Although medical research is ancient, health education research is relatively new. It has its limitations. Yet, if most health research is carefully interpreted, there is often a way in which it can be implemented, at least in part. Research workers may offer prescriptions, even very good ones, but research itself, says Sir Ronald Gould, "cannot be prescriptive, only descriptive." Thus, both the research worker and the research user must face the question of value and consider curriculum changes in terms of philosophy and goals.

Professional periodicals which are more educational than medical, and frequently present health education research and ideas of real value to teachers, include the following:

American Journal of Public Health
Childhood Education
Consumer Reports
Family Health (formerly *Today's Health*)
International Journal of Health Education
Journal of School Health
Safety Education
Health Education (AAHPER)
School Safety
Science
Scientific American
Statistical Bulletin of Metropolitan Life Insurance Co.
Research Quarterly (AAHPER)

There is considerable value in regularly reviewing health and health education research. It will not always be immediately useful in terms of content and teaching method, but many times it will start the reader thinking about new ways to meet an old health problem. Consider for the moment the following research titles from recent issues of the *Journal of School Health*. How might each article influence curriculum reform?

"The Use of Selected Value-Clarifying Strategies in Health Education" (Osman).
"A Perspective on Drinking Among Teenagers with Special Reference to New York State Studies" (Barnes).
"Mental Health Benefits of Small Group Experiences in the Affective Domain" (Garner).
"The Feasibility of Establishing a Breakfast Program in the Middle Class Secondary School" (Stewart).
"Behavior Modification Techniques in the School Setting" (Snow).
"An Analysis of the Perceptions of High School Principals in Public and Catholic Schools Relative to the Importance of Sex Education in the Curriculum" (Read).

"A Pilot Program Using Videotapes as a Health Education Medium with Students in Grades Six to Nine" (Zimmerli, Weppner, Lalor, and Rabinowitz).

At first glance, it might appear that only one or two of these research studies would have any bearing on program development. Yet, upon investigation, it will be discovered that each article makes a worthwhile contribution to health education — in terms of either content, teaching emphasis, or methodology. The need to read health education research publications, therefore, is an ever-present need, the neglect of which frequently leads to routine, dry, outdated, and non-stimulating courses that turn 10 students off for every one they turn on.

PART II—ORGANIZING FOR HEALTH TEACHING

Perhaps more than anyone else, Alfred North Whitehead championed the theory that student experiences have their origin in the activities of the *whole* organism. The theory of organism is expressed more clearly when Whitehead says that ". . . you cannot separate the seamless coat of learning."[25] All learnings have a connection with other learnings. This is especially true in the health field and is an excellent reason why stress is placed on organizing health teaching activities in terms of a unified or comprehensive health program. Important as they are, special courses in drug education, sex education, tobacco smoking, nutrition, or mental health belong as major health topics in a comprehensive health education course. Moreover, most school systems cannot afford the time for special topic concentration at the expense of other health topics. Properly organized, all health topics can be expected to receive adequate attention when they are parts of a long-range program.

THE MAJOR HEALTH TOPICS

There are a number of ways to arrive at a list of major health topics. Perhaps the most practical way is to take a look at the listings of local schools, state departments of education, and other health interested organizations. By scrutinizing these health curriculum topics it is possible to observe variations in emphasis and the manner in which some topics are grouped together.

Determining which is a major health topic and which is minor will have to be a local decision. Depending on how divisions are made there are probably 12 or 13 topics, each worthy of concentrated planning and graduated programming for grades 7 to 12. The author has worked with these topics for a number of years:

- Physical Activity, Sleep, Rest and Relaxation
- Nutrition and Growth
- Dental Health
- Body Structure and Operation (including the senses and skin)
- Prevention and Control of Disease
- Safety and First Aid
- Mental Health
- Sex and Family Living Education
- Environmental and Community Health
- Alcohol, Drugs and Tobacco
- Consumer Health
- World Health
- Health Careers

---

[25] Alfred North Whitehead, *Science and Philosophy*, New York: Philosophical Library, 1946.

In planning for grades 7 to 9, 10 to 12, the Pennsylvania Department of Education set up the following major health topics with full elaboration for classroom activities:[26]

Alcohol	Heredity and Environment
Anatomy	Human Sexuality
Community Health	Mental Health
Consumer Health	Nutrition
Dental Health	Physical Fitness
Disease Control	Physiology
Drugs and Narcotics	Safety
Family Relationships	Smoking
Health Careers	

In the Pennsylvania breakdown the topics of Anatomy, Physiology, and Heredity receive special attention, and Family Relationships and Human Sexuality appear as two major areas of emphasis.

In attempting to arrive at major health areas of value in the development of appraisal instruments for health knowledge and application, the Educational Testing Service came up with eleven areas as follows:[27]

Consumer Health	Growth and Development
Quackery	Physical
Delivery of Health Care	Emotional
Health Economics	Social
Patient-Doctor Relationship	Special Concerns
Community Health	Nutrition
Environmental Problems	Food Utilization
Health Organizations	Food Fads
International Health	Weight Control
Organizations	Food Processing
Major Problems	Mental Health
Diseases and Disorders	Personality Development
Prevention and Control	Escape Mechanism
Communicable	Psychosomatic Relationships
Non-Communicable	Mental Illness
Personal Health Care	Human Relationships
Oral Health	Drug Use and Abuse
Special Senses	Alcohol
Physical Activity	Tobacco
Sleep, Rest, Relaxation	Other Drugs
Skin Care	Drug Respect
Sex Education	Safety and First Aid
Family Planning	Accident Prevention
Psycho-sexual Development	Injury Prevention and Control
Physical Development	

The ETS breakdown of topics is helpful because it shows the subtopics and indicates how certain topics are grouped.

In the Oregon plan, Family Living is considered to be a part of the larger domain of Mental Health. This arrangement is also encompassed in both the New York and Mas-

---

[26]Pennsylvania Department of Education, *Conceptual Guidelines for School Health Programs in Pennsylvania,* Harrisburg: Pennsylvania Department of Education, 1970, p. 16.

[27]A project sponsored by the School Health Division of AAHPER, researched and developed by Educational Testing Service, Princeton, New Jersey. The health tests are designed to measure health knowledge, application, analysis, and evaluation.

sachusetts groupings. The Massachusetts Health Education Curriculum was developed over a two year period by an extensive Health Education Advisory Committee. Four areas of program emphasis were set forth as follows:

Area I *Physical Health*
    Body Structure and Function
    Cleanliness and Appearance
    Dental Health
    Fitness and Body Dynamics
    Nutrition
    Diseases and Disorders
    Sensory Perception
    Sleep, Rest, Relaxation

Area II *Mental and Social Health*
    Drugs, Alcohol and Tobacco
    Emotional Development
    Sexuality and Family Life

Area III *Consumer and Environmental Health*
    Ecology
    Health Careers
    Community and World Health
    Consumer Health

Area IV *Safe Living*
    First Aid and Emergencies
    Safety and Accident Prevention

Perhaps the most thoroughly researched health education curriculum was developed in New York State and set up for grade levels in five strands (see Figure 4–3). Each of the five strands is designed to simplify the teaching of substrands as much as possible for the teacher who "(1) has little formal background in the area; (2) has some background but needs updating or; (3) has sufficient technical knowledge but desires some broad guidelines for teaching the areas."[28] The New York State strands and substrands break down by secondary instructional level as follows:

Strand and Substrand	Grade 7–9	Level 10–12	Strand and Substrand	Grade 7–9	Level 10–12
I. Physical Health			IV. Environmental and Community Health		
Health Status	X		Environmental and Public Health	X	X
Nutrition	X	X	World Health	X	X
Sensory Perception	X		Ecology and Epidemiology of Health	X	X
Dental Health	X		Consumer Health	X	X
Disease Prevention and Control	X	X	V. Education for Survival		
II. Sociological Health Problems			Safety	X	
Smoking and Health	X	X	First Aid and Survival Education	X	X
Alcohol Education	X	X			
Drugs and Narcotic Education	X	X			
III. Mental Health					
Personality Development	X	X			
Sexuality	X	X			
Family Life Education	X	X			

[28]The State Education Department, *Suggested Guidelines for the Development of Courses of Study in Health Education for Junior and Senior High Schools*, Albany, New York: The State Education Department, 1970.

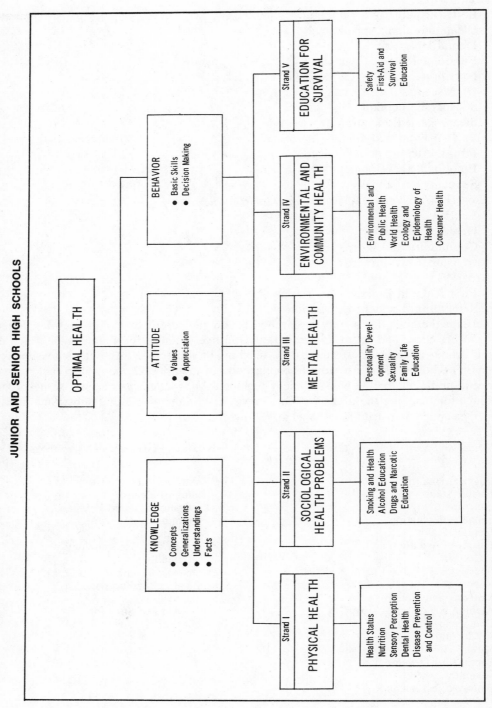

Figure 4–3 The three dimensions of optimal health expressed in five strands. (Courtesy of New York Education Department)

Educational consultants working in the State of California, 75 per cent of whom were classroom teachers, developed and evaluated a framework for health instruction which consists of an overview, major concepts, grade level concepts, suggested behavioral objectives, and suggested examples of content for each of the content areas.[29] Although the framework is subject to change, the content areas are reproduced here for scrutiny. More specific grade level concepts are included in the basic publication.

California Content Areas

1. Consumer health
2. Mental-emotional health
3. Drug use and misuse
4. Family health
5. Oral health, vision, hearing

6. Nutrition
7. Exercise, rest, posture
8. Diseases and disorders
9. Environmental health hazards
10. Community health resources

DETERMINATION OF SCOPE AND SEQUENCE

It may seem like a short distance from major health topics, strands, areas, and groups to grade level objectives, scope, and sequences. In a concentrated curriculum study it would take quite a while to check out and establish grade level scope for each junior and senior high school grade.

The word "scope" refers to the breadth of the health education curriculum — *what* should be taught at all levels. Scope varies according to the student and societal requirements of the moment. Sequence refers to the *when* of the curriculum — the grade placement of the health education experiences. Sequence defines the curriculum vertically, whereas scope defines it horizontally.

In determining scope, first review the *total* health education program, from kindergarten to grade 12. This view of all the health content in perspective gives the planner an opportunity to envision a complete program of health experiences in the life of a school child, prior to breaking it down into primary, intermediate, junior, and senior high school divisions. Scope is reviewed periodically by laying out all content in broad categories of instruction. This traditional approach, however, was discarded in Project Quest of the Los Angeles County Schools in favor of a course of study organized around students' health goals — in other words, it was learner centered. The emphasis was on student health behavior rather than knowledge. The scope, therefore, was to measure how well students (1) cared for their bodies; (2) developed mature personalities; (3) built satisfying human relationships; (4) assumed responsible health roles in their communities; and (5) coped with contemporary health problems.

In the Connecticut study of pupil interests and concerns, it was decided that the scope of any health education program must relate directly to student appeal: "Don't teach us what you want to teach; teach us what we want to know."[30] The scope of the program in grades 7, 8, and 9, therefore, would have to do with puberty, sexual concerns, self-concept, adolescent diseases, and *individual* problems associated with alcohol, drugs, and smoking. In grades 10, 11, and 12, sexual problems continued, but the emphasis in the areas of alcohol, drugs, and smoking was on *social* issues.

---

[29]State of California, *Framework for Health Instruction in California Public Schools,* Sacramento, California: State Department of Education, 1970.

[30]Ruth Byler, Gertrude Lewis, and Ruth Totman, *Teach Us What We Want to Know,* Hartford, Connecticut: The Connecticut State Board of Education, 1969, p. 170.

Suggested Scope and Sequence

B = Basic Content Development
H = Heaviest Concentration
C = Continuing Emphasis
R = Reinforcement of Content

	7–9	10–12	13
Alcohol	H	H	C
Anatomy	H	R	—
Community Health	H	C	R
Consumer Health	H	H	C
Dental Health	C	R	—
Disease Control	H	H	C
Drugs and Narcotics	H	H	C
Family Relationships	H	H	C
Health Careers	B	H	C
Heredity and Environment	H	C	R
Human Sexuality	H	H	C
Mental Health	H	H	C
Nutrition	H	C	R
Physical Fitness	H	H	C
Physiology	H	C	R
Safety	H	C	—
Smoking	H	C	C

Proper sequence, along with the right amount of emphasis, is what makes health education vital. For too long health topics have been taught at random in a number of grades as a kind of "do-gooder" activity. This, coupled with highly repetitive material, made health classes very unpopular, especially among the bright, eager-to-learn students. Because of this the Pennsylvania guidelines call for scope and sequence by degree; that is, suggested periods of greatest concentration:[31]

Barrett followed the Pennsylvania suggestion of identifying "periods of greatest concentration" for secondary school programs and developed his scope chart accordingly:[32]

---

[31]Pennsylvania Department of Education, *Conceptual Guidelines for School Health Programs*, op. cit., p. 16.
[32]Morris Barrett, *Health Education Guide: A Design for Teaching*, 2nd edition, Philadelphia: Lea and Febiger, Co., 1974, p. 6.

TOPIC	GRADES 7 TO 9	10 TO 12
Aging Process	C	H
Anatomy and Physiology	C	H
Dental Health	C	C
Nutrition	H	C
Physical Fitness	H	H
Heredity and Genetics	H	C
Human Sexuality	H	H
Mental Health	H	H
Family Relationships	H	H
Alcohol	H	H
Smoking	H	C
Drugs and Narcotics	H	H
Human Ecology	C	H
Consumer Health	H	C
Safety	H	C
Disease Control	H	H

H = Heaviest concentration
C = Continuing emphasis

Publishers of health textbooks for junior and senior high school consumption frequently make available a scope and sequence chart with a rationale for following it. In this respect Laidlow Brothers has a very detailed chart setting forth 11 health area strands. Scott, Foresman and Co. also makes available a chart with an appropriate breakdown of topics in sequence. These charts display reasonable validity as they reflect the experiences of reputable authors.

There is really only one adequate way for the teacher to appreciate the sequential development of health topics, and that is to carefully examine curriculum guides and courses of study. Progressions within an area are spelled out along with appropriate content, materials, and teaching ideas in far more detail than can be set forth on these pages. Guidelines vary, of course, but the efforts of the New York State Education Department are worth some additional attention. They are especially clear in getting at scope and sequence so that the average teacher of health has something immediately useful.[33]

The strands and substrands of the New York course of study have already been mentioned. (See Figure 4–3.) To clarify scope, there are broad guidelines for each of the five strands. Objectives are also set forth for each strand so that the health instructor knows what he is after. This is followed by an outline of content.

Consumer Health, for example, is a part of Strand IV, *Environmental and Community Health.*

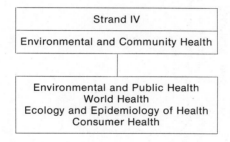

In order to get a "feel" for intermediate grade and secondary school grade areas of concentration, the following units of work are set up to show relationships under the Consumer Health topic.

---

[33]The State Education Department, *Suggested Guidelines for the Development of Courses of Study in Health Education for Junior and Senior High School,* op. cit.

CONSUMER HEALTH (Grades 4–12)		
INTERMEDIATE GRADES	**JUNIOR HIGH SCHOOL**	**SENIOR HIGH SCHOOL**
I. The Health Consumer	I. Quackery and Quacks	I. Influences on Consumer Behavior
II. Ethical Advertising and Protection	II. Consumer Protection	II. Contemporary Quackery and Pseudoscientific Practice
III. Undesirable Promotional and Advertising Techniques	III. Consumer Motivation	III. Health Personnel and Medical Care

OUTLINE OF CONTENT	MAJOR UNDERSTANDINGS AND FUNDAMENTAL CONCEPTS	SUGGESTED TEACHING AIDS AND LEARNING ACTIVITIES	SUPPLEMENTARY INFORMATION FOR TEACHERS
I. Quackery and Quacks A. Definitions 1. Health quackery	Health quackery prevents consumers from engaging in sound health practices and deprives them of adequate health protection.	Keep a running list of vocabulary words for each major area in this unit. Review from time to time with flash cards.	*Health quackery* embraces all of those practices engaged in for economic gain or out of distorted belief, which lead the individual from intelligent health practices or deprive him of adequate health protection.
2. Health quack	Health quacks are those who make false claims to medical knowledge, or who make fraudulent claims of treatment or cure.		The quack may be a physician, a practitioner of a healing cult, or he may claim no medical education whatsoever. The vast majority of quacks are dishonest and their motive is to make money at the expense of unwary customers. However, a few of these individuals are sincere in believing they have health panacea. *Sincerity,* however, is *not* a test of truth. It is impossible to distinguish a health quack from a legitimate health practitioner by appearance alone.
B. Recognizing the quack	There are definite characteristics by which an informed public may recognize the health quack.	Prepare a bulletin board to highlight those traits that identify a health quack.	Health quackery may not be characterized by all of these characteristics. Usually, more than one of the following traits can be identified.

1. Secret formulas or devices	Reputable physicians share their ideas, findings, and other pertinent information with the rest of the scientific community.	Quacks often claim not only an absolute cure, but a quick and permanent cure. Many times they claim that their cure is known only to themselves and may bear the quack's own name or that of a fictitious research foundation.
2. Guarantee of cure	Unlike reliable practitioners, the quack promises sure and quick cures.	Reputable medical practitioners characteristically refrain from promising cures, although they may express optimism in their prognosis.
3. Use of advertisements and case histories	A doctor's reputation becomes well known by his professional qualifications and it is unnecessary for him to advertise for clients as do many medical frauds.	It is not uncommon for reputable medical personnel, new to a community, to announce that they are establishing a professional practice. The quack, however, routinely advertises to encourage new business. Often, case histories (real or imagined) are used in these advertisements.
4. Testimonials	The reliability of testimonials is often doubtful and the health consumer should realize that fraudulent practitioners often use testimonials to increase sales.	Locate testimonials in magazines. With opaque projector project these on a wall, and discuss how they are lacking in scientific validity. Testimonials are statements made by real or imagined people, attesting to the success of a quack's treatment. Those providing testimonials may be relatives or friends of the quack or, as in many instances, fictitious people. Sometimes, those making the testimonial are paid quite handsomely.

(Outline continued on following page)

OUTLINE OF CONTENT	MAJOR UNDERSTANDINGS AND FUNDAMENTAL CONCEPTS	SUGGESTED TEACHING AIDS AND LEARNING ACTIVITIES	SUPPLEMENTARY INFORMATION FOR TEACHERS
			Reliable health practitioners become known because of their professional competency and do not have to rely on such questionable promotional practices as testimonials.
5. Clamor for medical investigation and recognition	Legally any promoter of a drug must undertake the responsibility of proving its safety and effectiveness prior to interstate shipment. Many quacks turn this responsibility around in their promotion to the public.		Many who testify in support of a quack's treatment have only the quack's word that they were afflicted with a particular disease which had "disappeared."
6. Claims of persecution by medical men who are afraid of competition	When the health fraud is exposed by his professional colleagues, he may react by claiming that he is being persecuted by them.	Invite a qualified person from the community to visit the class to talk on quacks, faddists, and cults.	The American Medical Association's Department of Investigation and state and county medical societies check on practices in medical quackery.
7. Claims that conventional forms of therapy will cause more harm than good	Quacks may ridicule conventional forms of diagnosis and/or treatment and substitute a technique or device known only to themselves.	Plan a skit that will illustrate the different characteristics of the health quack. Students should be able to identify these traits.	Frequently, quacks claim that drugs, surgery, and X-ray treatment will do more harm than good. They may discourage a client from seeking consultation with competent medical counsel. The resultant delay in diagnosis and treatment may have serious consequences for the client.

The *Content* outlines for *Consumer Health* are as follows:

Grades 7, 8, 9

I. Quackery and Quacks
  A. Definitions
    1. Health Quackery
    2. Health Quack
  B. Recognizing the quack
    1. Secret formula or devices
    2. Guarantee of cure
    3. Use of advertisements and case histories
    4. Testimonials
    5. Clamor for medical investigation and recognition
    6. Claims of persecution by medical men who are afraid of competition
    7. Claims that conventional forms of therapy will cause more harm than good
  C. Quack modalities
    1. Nostrums
    2. Mechanical devices
    3. Secret regimens
  D. Common quack approaches
    1. House-to-house peddling
    2. Health lectures
    3. Mail order gimmicks
    4. Books and literature
    5. "Health" practitioners
  E. The hazards of quackery
    1. Discourages one from seeing a competent physician
    2. Human suffering and loss of life
    3. Useless expenditure of money
    4. Self-propagating nature of quackery
  F. Why do people consult medical frauds?
    1. Fear
    2. Persons ill with incurable or poorly understood illnesses
    3. Lack of information
    4. The antimedical personality
    5. Modern health trends
  G. Highlights in the history of quackery
    1. Quackery in Colonial America
    2. Contemporary case studies

II. Consumer Protection
  A. Early efforts
  B. 20th century legislation
    1. Food and Drug Act of 1906
    2. Federal Food, Drug and Cosmetic Act of 1938
    3. Other significant legislation
      a. July 6, 1945 (certification of safety and efficacy of penicillin)
      b. Durham-Humphrey Amendment, October 26, 1951
      c. October 10, 1962 (Kefauver-Harris Drug Amendments)
  C. Federal organizations
    1. Food and Drug Administration
    2. Federal Trade Commission
      a. safeguards the free-enterprise system
      b. false advertising
    3. Post office department
      a. tries to protect the public from mail fraud
      b. controls obscenity in the mail
  D. Professional Groups
    1. American Medical, Dental, Dietetic, and Hospital Associations
    2. State and local professional societies
  E. Voluntary health agencies
    1. American Cancer Society
    2. Arthritis Foundation, Inc.
  F. Commercial groups
    1. Consumer's Research
    2. Consumers Union, Inc.
    3. Magazine Testing and Rating Services
      a. *Good Housekeeping*
      b. *Parents' Magazine*
      c. *Changing Times*

III. Consumer Motivation
  A. Motives
  B. Role of motives (incentives) in consumer behavior
  C. Classification of Motives
    1. Rational motives
    2. Emotional motives

D. Consumer purchasing patterns
  1. Products people buy
  2. When people buy
  3. Fashion and fads
E. The teen-age consumer
  1. Buying power
  2. Influence on family buying patterns
  3. From dependent childhood to independent adulthood
Suggested References
  Books
  Pamphlets
  Periodicals
  Films
  Transparencies

Grades 10, 11, 12

I. Influence on Consumer Behavior
  A. Psychological considerations
    1. Persuasion
      a. people enjoy buying
      b. rational and irrational consumer motives
    2. The use of symbols
      a. symbols defined
      b. function of symbols
        (1) to reinforce selfimage
        (2) to reflect sexuality
        (3) to symbolize age
        (4) to symbolize social participation
    3. Motivational mechanisms
      a. aggression
      b. ambivalence
      c. anxiety
      d. autonomy
      e. compensation
      f. fantasy
  B. Other influences on consumer behavior
    1. Ignorance and gullibility
      a. ignorance
      b. gullibility
    2. Promotional techniques
    3. Social pressure
  C. Advertising and Selling Approaches
    1. Low-pressure selling
    2. High-pressure selling
    3. Positive approaches
    4. Analysis of advertisements
    5. Creative Code of the American Association of Advertising

D. Health Information
  1. Unreliable sources
    a. superstitions
    b. ignorance or prejudice
    c. customs
    d. expoundings of the quack
    e. commercialized health information
  2. Reliable sources of health information
  3. Criteria for evaluation of health information

II. Contemporary Quackery and Pseudoscientific Practice
  A. Cancer and arthritis quackery
    1. Cancer
      a. quack techniques
        (1) poultices and pastes
        (2) sprays
        (3) gadgets
        (4) internal remedies
        (5) diet
      b. Mexican centers for cancer cures
      c. I.A.C.V.F. (International Association of Cancer Victims and Friends)
      d. patrons of the cancer quack
        (1) neurotics
        (2) former cancer patients
        (3) patients in early stages of cancer
        (4) incurable cancer patients
    2. Arthritis and rheumatism quackery
      a. review of concepts
      b. quack remedies
        (1) devices
        (2) uranium mines
        (3) mineral spas and baths
        (4) drugs
        (5) curative foods
        (6) liniments
  B. Pseudoscientific practices
    1. Physiological basis
      a. homeopathy
      b. naturopathy
    2. Psychologically based
      a. hypothesis
      b. psycho-quacks
      c. others

III. Health Personnel and Medical Care
  A. Physicians and dentists
    1. General practitioner
    2. Medical specialist
      a. board qualified specialist
      b. diplomate
      c. types of medical specialists
    3. Dental specialists (not covered in 4, 5, 6)
      a. endodontist
      b. oral pathologist
      c. oral surgeon
      d. prosthodontist
    4. Selecting a Physician or Dentist
      a. criteria
      b. procedures
  B. Paramedical specialties
  C. Other health personnel
  D. Medical care
    1. Trends
      a. physician-patient ratio
      b. method of payment
    2. Medical care plans
      a. voluntary health insurance programs
        (1) Blue Cross-Blue Shield
        (2) types of voluntary health protection available
          —loss of income protection
          —hospital expense protection
          —surgical expense
          —regular medical expense
          —major medical expense
        (3) HIP (Health Insurance Plan)
      b. criteria for selecting a plan
      c. compulsory or government medical care programs

        (1) Medicare
          —basic plan
          —voluntary plan
        (2) Medicaid
        (3) New York State's Medicaid
    3. Medical care facilities
      a. hospitals
      b. hospital systems
        (1) Government hospitals
        (2) non-government hospitals
          —voluntary community hospitals
          —proprietary hospitals
          —nursing homes
  E. The Consumer and the Drug Industry
    1. Ethical drug companies
    2. Cost of drugs
      a. advertising
      b. generic versus brand name drugs
      c. geographic influence
      d. type of purchase
      e. research and drug cost
    3. New drugs
      a. patents for new drugs
      b. trademarks
      c. drug testing

Appendix A. Critical Analysis of Advertisements
Appendix B. Selected Internal Nostrums
Appendix C. Paramedical Personnel
Appendix D. Other Health Personnel
Books
Pamphlets
Periodicals
Films
Transparencies

At this point the teacher of consumer health knows its limitations as a part of Strand IV, Environmental and Community Health. Now, by looking over the separate consumer health manuals for junior high and senior high, the content may be studied in greater detail, and in terms of fundamental concepts, suggested teaching aids, and learning activities. This is nicely organized in the manuals in the following style.[34]

[34]Taken from the beginning of the material on Consumer Health for Grades 7, 8, and 9, *Strand IV Environmental and Community Health,* Albany, New York: The State Education Department, 1970, pp. 1–3.

CYCLE PLANNING

Repetition is not all bad. Repeating information in order to firmly root certain concepts is good. It need not be done *ad nauseam* several years in a row, particularly if the repetitive health topic is organized on an every other year or three year cycle. The cycle selected may vary slightly for each major health topic. All topics should probably be introduced to the junior high school student early in the seventh or eighth grades according to emerging interests or needs. The following year, or on the next occasion when health education is taught, certain areas may be dropped so that greater time can be allotted to critical or priority areas. Such a practice is beneficial to the instructor also, for it permits a more complete development of content material, teaching methods, and evaluations.

While it will be desirable in some instances to omit a major health area altogether in a certain year, there are a number of schools that will want to briefly review areas not treated in depth in a particular year. This might result in a cycle breakdown such as in Table 4–3, which provides for a seventh grade exposure of nine "emphasis" topics, and reduces in number over the remaining years from seven to five topics per year.

SCHEDULING AND TIME ALLOTMENT

Scheduling is essentially an administrative procedure. A "perfect" health education program on paper is successful chiefly because of the manner in which it is implemented—proper teaching methods and adequate scheduling. In the modern school, several questions arise:

1. What are the state health education requirements?
2. How much total time is set aside for health education in the particular secondary school?
3. Is the time block to be the same length each period the classes meet?
4. Is health education scheduled daily, or once or twice a week?
5. Is the schedule flexible enough to vary the length of a class period in keeping with the nature of the lesson?
6. Does the schedule accommodate team teaching, mini-lessons, mini-courses, and flexibility for innovative programs?

TABLE 4–3   Cycle of Topics by Grade

MAJOR HEALTH TOPICS	7	8	9	10	11	12
Physical Activity, Sleep, Rest and Relaxation	X	R	X	R	X	R
Nutrition and Growth	R	X	R	X	R	X
Dental Health	R	X				
Body Structure and Function	X	R	X	X		
Prevention and Control of Disease	X	X	R	X	R	X
Safety and First Aid	X	R	X	R	X	R
Mental Health	X	X	R	X	R	X
Sex & Family Living Education	X	R	X	R	X	R
Environmental & Community Health	R	X	R	X	R	X
Alcohol, Drugs & Tobacco	X	X	X	R	X	R
Consumer Health / Health Quackery	X	R	X	X	R	X
World Health	R	X	R	X	R	X
Health Careers	X	R	X	R	X	

X = Emphasis year
R = Review year

Scheduling is a task that takes the school administrator most of the summer months to complete, even with the help of computers. Scheduling is relatively easy if health education is an elective, and difficult when it is required of everyone in the school. In addition to being based on the number and kinds of students, it must consider the number of teaching staff available and the adequacy of classrooms, laboratories, and library materials.

The time allotted to a comprehensive coverage in health education should be a minimum of a half-year course each year, grades 7 through 12. A more acceptable plan is a full-year course in which the class meets on a daily basis. This puts the course on a status level with math, English, science, and social studies. It permits continuity of thought by students with less need for daily reviews, encourages the employment of trained health education teachers, and makes the program worthy of academic credit toward secondary school graduation. Such regularity of instruction makes it possible for the teacher to make a thorough preparation, use outside resource people, and (perhaps most of all) continue in-depth discussions from one day to another. Moreover, there is time to appraise student health behavior and to advance some integrative and correlative teaching with other subjects. Integration or correlation *alone* is not very effective. Too often health objectives are loosely planned for in science, home economics, or social studies. Research indicates that the formal regular health course is the most effective in terms of student knowledges and understandings. In addition, health education, when taught as a separate course over a full year, will generally be accepted for college entrance credit.

Bensley makes a plea for a concentration of health teaching in three grades—fourth, seventh, and eleventh. It is his observation, from working with youth over a number of years, that these three periods are where health teaching can be most effective.[35] If concentrated here many of the objectives may be achieved in the limited time allotted, he maintains. Bensley reasons that this task will be accomplished in better fashion with short-term courses—a variety of micro-courses with attractive titles. Waltham High School in Massachusetts and Lewisberg Area High School in Pennsylvania have had excellent student acceptance of short-term electives within the program. The secret, in part, is to use attractive course titles such as: "You Are What You Eat," "Sexuality and You," "Death and Dying," and "Suicide in the Seventies."

A less effective means of scheduling health education involves blocks of time alternated with physical education. In one system this takes the form of two conventional class periods per week of physical education and one of health education. Thus, in the course of the school year there are 36 to 40 periods of health instruction in secondary school. This is far better than much of the incidental health instruction that goes on in the country at large, but it means that the class meets only once per week and some time is wasted reviewing material at every meeting. To alleviate this weekly lapse of time, some schools have set aside 40 class periods in a row for health education. On a daily schedule this would require eight weeks of concentrated work. In the previous example of three periods per week of health education and physical education, all three periods would go to health and require about thirteen weeks of exposure. Frequently, this causes the physical education personnel to take a dim view of the arrangement, because their programs cease for the thirteen weeks. These kinds of difficulties will continue to arise until health education is taught as a separate subject and not linked so closely with physical education that it has to be watered down because of the time element.

---

[35]Loren B. Bensley, Jr., "Five Cures for Dull Health Curriculums," *School Health Review*, July-August, 1973.

THE ON-GOING CURRICULUM

Health education programs will not remain static in a day when curriculum revision is so well understood. Teachers of health, therefore, will be revising curricula several times a decade. They will have to be careful not to put every "new" idea or method into the program without first appraising results with students. Change for change's sake means very little. Move slowly, plan thoroughly and prove all things.

PART III—IMPLEMENTING THE HEALTH CURRICULUM

Well over a decade ago Arthur Koestler wrote that the modern individual is an "urban barbarian" that lives isolated in his artificial environment with little comprehension of the forces which make it work.[36] If, indeed, the environment *is* artificial and Koestler is right, then the task of implementing vital health education programs is a formidable one. Reality indicates that many people are dreamers; fewer are successful planners, and fewer still are able to implement. Thus, in health education circles and elsewhere, there is a significant challenge to maneuver health content and learning activities so that students comprehend essential dynamics and consequences in the affairs of people.

The word "implementation" comes from the Latin *implere,* meaning to fill up or finish. It is associated with such words as accomplish, fulfill, carry out, and complete. In health education, therefore, it relates to putting the health plans in action, the selection of learning activities, the varieties of student experiences, teaching techniques, resources and aids, and evaluation practices.

BALANCE, BREADTH AND DEPTH

To begin with, it is not likely that a health topic can be fully implemented if it is not taken apart and put back together again in a setting that relates to physical, mental, and social ramifications. Learning activities employed in instruction need both breadth and depth. The pupil needs a broad and varied health experience. There is a need to "taste" health relationships in many areas—personal, community-wide, and even economic. One asks, how comprehensive can a program of health education be when many teachers have one or two "pet activities" they like to stress? Or, consider the school that pushes the "hot" topics (sex education, alcohol, and drugs) at the expense of some less popular but nevertheless worthwhile topics. Only a broad and varied health program will appeal to all students. It is particularly important that the junior high school student investigate and react to all of the major health topics even if the class time assigned is limited. This is the age level at which it is time to learn in detail that optimal health contributes measurably to the full use of human resources. "Harmony," said the Greeks, "is the music of the gods." Putting all of the health topics into proper focus, therefore, is to achieve an "orchestration of many powers." Concepts and competencies derived from this approach will carry over into the senior high school health curriculum and provide the student with a wider health dimension, insuring against any narrowness that may exist when certain health topics are studied in greater depth.

---

[36] Arthur Koestler, *Act of Creation,* New York: Macmillan Co., 1964.

The need for program balance is always present, not only to insure continued pupil interest, but to be certain that the essential health concepts are covered. This is not at all easy to accomplish in an era when medical science is daily spewing forth great amounts of new knowledge about health and disease. Yet, there is not time in any health area to cover everything from the new to the old. As previously indicated, selection is the important task in teaching. The sheer number of health items — facts, stories, experiences — defeats any effort to make a selection in haste. Learning activities, therefore, must be selected that *combine* the values of several activities into a common concept. This practice, of course, must relate to such things as the sequence of health education activities both within a school year and over a span of several years. It will also consider what is significant enough to be selected for repetition. Repetition to advance recall and retention is good, but health education in the past has harbored the reputation of reviewing health items to an *ad nauseam* stage, with the result that more students were turned off than were turned on in the course of the school year.

Where there is a serious question about the proper selection of health teaching content, a review of existing curriculum guides may be helpful. Experimental efforts are also helpful. Pilot studies involving a small number of pupils frequently provide answers to the questions of time allocation, meaningful sequences, over-repetitious activities, and what students prefer or dislike.

CHOOSING THE MAJOR HEALTH TOPICS

There are a number of listings of the major health topics appearing in state and local curriculum guides. Generally, these lists include all or most of the following 14 topics — each of which is of sufficient importance to warrant a separate chapter where it can be fully presented and discussed in terms of what and how to teach:

1. Physical Activity, Sleep, Rest and Relaxation
2. Nutrition and Growth
3. Dental Health
4. Body Structure and Operation (Including Special Senses and Skin Care)
5. Prevention and Control of Disease
6. Mental Health (Including Death Education)
7. Consumer Health
8. World Health
9. Health Careers
10. Alcohol and Drugs
11. Smoking Education
12. Sex and Family Living Education
13. Safety Education
14. Environmental Health

Although there is little agreement on where the emphasis should be placed, there is common agreement on how the major health topics may be grouped (New York, *Strands*; Massachusetts, *Areas*). Thus, in the next four chapters, the 14 major health topics are grouped accordingly — to put into practice the principle of combining several related areas that share common concepts:

Area I *Physical Health*

1. Physical Activity, Sleep, Rest and Relaxation
2. Nutrition and Growth
3. Dental Health
4. Body Structure and Operation (Including Special Senses and Skin Care)
5. Prevention and Control of Disease

Area II *Mental Health*
    6. Mental Health (Including Death Education)
    7. Alcohol and Drugs
    8. Smoking Education
    9. Sex and Family Living Education
Area III *Environmental and Consumer Health*
    10. Environmental Health
    11. Consumer Health
    12. World Health
    13. Health Careers
Area IV *Safety Education*
    14. Safety Education

Each major health topic in Chapters 5, 6, 7, and 8 is presented in terms of four areas of information for the teacher:

Comments concerning instruction.

Behavioral objectives for junior high school and senior high school students.

Essential topics to be included at each level.

Suggested activities for each secondary school level.

The *Behavioral objectives* should be considered as samples of what might be developed at the local level. They are reasonably appropriate for the grade level. However, it is always desirable that concepts or objectives be developed by teachers themselves; the objectives set forth here may serve as a guide. Teachers will go on from here, in many cases, to develop their own more specific objectives. After examining the list of *Essential topics,* they should construct their outline of content for the particular area under study. The sample of *Suggested activities* for learning has been tried in various parts of the country and found useful. However, it is well known that an instructional activity may work well in one school and be less than satisfactory in another—being governed in part by local surroundings and teacher expertise. Moreover, activities suggested for the junior and senior high school years are not "perfect" for these years. Although they are approximately suited to the particular age period, they may work well enough a grade above or a grade below. In any case each teacher will have to decide which of the learning experiences set forth seem suitable for the health class of the moment.

In using the suggested material, bear in mind that the instruction will be more effective when related to improved teaching methods, appropriate teaching materials, and evaluation techniques. *Chapter 11 should be carefully examined as each major health topic is studied, for the sources of materials here are considerable (films, filmstrips, pamphlets, posters, charts, age-level stories, and others).*

Finally, if the suggested learning activities really do contribute to pupil conceptualization and feelings, then there should be signs of behavior change in each of the major health areas. In short, the learning activities will have been proved to be consequential—viewed by the student as worth the effort, and by the teacher as of decision-making quality. This will result, among other things, in the student taking better care of the body, developing a more mature personality, building close human relationships, coping with contemporary health problems, and assuming responsible health roles in the community.

QUESTIONS FOR DISCUSSION

1. A careful look at the wording of traditional objectives, concepts, and behavioral objectives indicates considerable similarity. If one fails to teach for decision-making

action, the previously stated goals mean very little. This is one reason why the relevance of utilizing behavioral objectives has been a source of debate since 1918. What is the background here? (See Ebel's research in Selected References).

2. If curriculum is an outgrowth of one's philosophy of health education, how do you account for the fact that more than a few programs of health education appear to be just "thrown together"?

3. Joseph Wood Krutch has written that the school curriculum should provide greater opportunity for social intercourse that would foster mental health. Comment on how this can be planned for in the secondary school.

4. What are the several advantages and disadvantages in preparing curriculum materials over a short time period?

5. Teachers frequently complain that they have very little time to do research, think about it, and then modify their health teaching programs accordingly. If this is reasonably true, how can we expect to capitalize on current school research to any great extent? Your comments will be more meaningful if you discuss this topic with a teacher or two.

6. There is a similarity in the Massachusetts and New York State "areas" and "strands" arrangements for health education topics. How does this kind of grouping appeal to you? Explain the answer.

7. How can teachers get away from needless repetition in health education? What is your opinion of cycle plans? Are concepts better than objectives for developing non-repetitive teaching materials?

8. What are some of the arrangements for scheduling and allotting time for health education in junior and senior high schools in your locality? Comment on the effectiveness of these programs.

SUGGESTED ACTIVITIES

1. Examine a number of curriculum guides in secondary school health education. Usually these can be found in the college library. Note some of the ways they differ and some of the ways in which they are similar. See especially guides from the states of California, Pennsylvania, Oregon, and New York.

2. In the last several years curriculum changes have been more widespread and intensive than at any time in the history of American schools. One should ask whether these changes in curriculum are really significant. Do children learn better in the new programs than they did in the old? Have curriculum modifications been made because it is popular to do so? Suggest several means of finding out how valuable changes have been in a school.

3. Evaluate a chosen school system in terms of how it approaches the topic of curriculum development in health education. Consider the organization for planning, the offerings, direction of learning, and outcomes. To help you structure your appraisal, look over section four of *Evaluative Criteria for the Evaluation of Secondary Schools*, 4th ed., Washington, D. C.: National Study of Secondary School Evaluation, 1969.

4. Look over the health curriculum materials used in a particular secondary school. *How* are they used to put across certain content? Are students only mildly involved,

and if so is it due to poor motivation or to the weakness of the materials? For example, does displaying "before" and "after" plaster of Paris models of maloccluded teeth *affect* the class in any noticeable way — or is this about as effective as a filmstrip on the topic? Also, comment on the difficulty of doing a good evaluation here.

5. Examine the writings of Robert F. Mager (see Selected References) and comment on how he would avoid "pitfalls" and "barnacles" in establishing instructional objectives. Indicate whether Mager varies substantially in his views from other curriculum specialists.

6. Select a major health topic and experiment with diagramming a structure to show how one moves from objectives, through planned content and implementation to student decision-making.

7. Contact the health education consultant (or person assigned to the health area) in your state department of education. Find out what curriculum materials are available to teachers who are charged with upgrading the health education program or developing a course of study in grades kindergarten through 12. If possible, compare the services provided by several states.

8. Look through three recent years of research articles reported in such publications as *Journal of School Health* and *American Journal of Public Health*. List the several titles that appear to influence health teaching methods. Make another listing of those that appear to have a bearing on curriculum content in the secondary schools. Formulate a statement on the practical value of such articles.

SELECTED REFERENCES

Allen, Robert E., and Owen J. Holyoak. "Evaluating the Conceptual Approach to Teaching Health Education," *Journal of School Health,* 42:118–119, February, 1972.

Barrett, Morris. *Health Education Guide,* 2nd edition, Philadelphia: Lea and Febiger, 1974.

Bremer, John. "The Learning Society," in Dwight W. Allen and Jeffrey C. Hecht, editors, *Controversies in Education,* Philadelphia: W. B. Saunders Co., 1974, p. 125.

Bruess, Clinton E., and Thomas J. Fisher. *Selected Readings in Health,* New York: Macmillan Co., 1970.

Burns, Richard W. "Behavioral Objectives for Competency-Based Education," *Educational Technology,* November, 1972, pp. 22–25.

Caramanica, Virginia P. "Evaluation of Effects of Performance-Based Teacher Education on the Health, Knowledge and Attitudes of Fifth Grade Students." *Journal of School Health,* 44:449–454, October, 1974.

Conroy, William G. "The Synthesized Behavioral Objective," *Educational Technology,* October, 1973.

Ebel, A. L. "Behavioral Objectives: A Close Look," *Phi Delta Kappan,* 52:171–173, November, 1970.

Eisner, Elliot W., and Elizabeth Vallance. *Conflicting Conceptions of Curriculum,* Berkeley, California: McCutchan Publishing Corporation, 1975.

Freischlag, Jerry. "Competency Based Instruction," *Journal of Health, Physical Education and Recreation,* 45:29–32, January, 1974.

Krutch, Joseph Wood. "A Humanistic Approach," *Phi Delta Kappan,* 52:376–378, March, 1970.

Lasch, Henry A. "A Study of Health Policies In Public School Administration," *Journal of School Health,* 46:204–207, April, 1976.

Leigh, Terrence M. "Will the Real Health Education Please Stand Up," *School Health Review,* March/April, 1974, p. 10.

Lynch, L. Riddick. "The Conceptual Approach to Teaching Health Education," *Journal of School Health,* 43:130–135, February, 1973.

Mager, Robert F. *Goal Analysis,* Belmont, California: Fearon Publishers, 1972.

Mager, Robert F. *Preparing Instructional Objectives,* Belmont, California: Fearon Publishers, 1975.

Oberteuffer, Delbert, Orvis A. Harrelson, and Marion B. Pollack. *School Health Education,* 5th edition, New York: Harper and Row, 1972, Chapters 2 and 4.

Reid, William A., and Decker F. Walker. *Case Studies in Curriculum Change,* Boston: Routledge and Kegan Paul, 1975.

Unruh, Glenys. *Responsive Curriculum Development,* Berkeley, California: McCutchan Publishing Corporation, 1975.

Van Til, William. *Curriculum: Quest for Relevance,* Boston: Houghton Mifflin Co., 1971.

Willgoose, Carl E. "Sequential K-12 Courses Replace Old Style 'Health,'" *Nation's Schools,* 85:78–79, March, 1970.

Chapter 5

Area I — Physical Health

Components:
1. Physical Activity, Sleep, Rest, and Relaxation
2. Nutrition and Growth
3. Dental Health
4. Body Structure and Operation (Including Special Senses and Skin Care)
5. Prevention and Control of Disease

Somewhere early in the study of human development and well-being there is a need to examine carefully the physical structure and to develop an appreciation for the physical components of cells and specialized organs that work together to produce an extremely efficient motor mechanism—a mechanism that functions properly when food, activity, rest, and disease elements are under control. It is from this human movement or physical base that the mental, environmental, and intellectual ingredients of individual health can better be examined.

1. PHYSICAL ACTIVITY, SLEEP, REST, AND RELAXATION

The role of physical activity and the benefits of sleep and relaxation are significant in the prevention of disease and human inefficiency. However, in a great many schools this kind of information is almost entirely omitted from health education classes. Neither is it discussed in physical education classes. This is one of the reasons that there is a real need for youngsters to understand early what physical education is and what it means to the individual in his personal and community life. Junior high school boys and girls both need to talk over the practical aspects of "physical fitness," "high energy levels," "work capacity," and "pep," and relate such terms to their personal stamina to run, jump, climb, swim, throw, dance, hike, and perform other play-work activities. By combining the discussion of human movement with the recuperative forces of sleep and rest, the common forms of chronic fatigue, listlessness, boredom, tenseness, poor posture, and lack of stamina for athletic performance or anything else are more apt to be made meaningful.

With the amount of leisure that is becoming available for most individuals, it is proper to learn that recreation can be both stimulating and relaxing and is in fact "an attitude of mind" contributing not only to physical well-being but to the advancement of mental health. The intricacies of psychological stress and patterns of sleep, especially as they pertain to the culture of the moment, will be of interest to the older adolescent who is mature enough to consider the sensitivities and fragilities of the human being, and ponder their value in his emerging style of living.

This particular health topic lends itself very well to a discussion of such degenerative difficulties as low back pain, coronary disease, and obesity. If the first two topics were taught here, they wouldn't have to be taught in detail under the topic of *Body Structure and Function*. Information about obesity, however, should probably come up here and again under the *Nutrition* topic. Teenage girls, frequently more than the boys, are quite willing to talk about self-improvement programs to reduce their overweight through proper diet and exercise. There is one major difficulty, however, that needs to be cleared up in class. This is the general indifference to fitness of the average nonathletic woman. A tired, cross companion or friend is no joy to anyone. In fact, says Dr. Evalyn S. Gendel of the Kansas State Department of Health, the least physically active women have far and away the most complaints of menstrual difficulty, fatigue, digestive disorders, and headache! These same women have high heart rates in work tests and a high incidence of backache complaints. One must conclude that conditioning for life "work loads" should become as important as the conditioning usually insisted upon for athletes.

Childhood obesity has to be worked on at a pre-adult level, which means that obese teenagers must become involved beyond the academic level. In addition to nutrition sessions and an increase in physical movement, there has to be an acceptable atmosphere in which to interact with peers, develop some new social skills (such as speaking with confidence), and improve the self-image. Health instruction in such instances becomes very involved—combining the best of the classroom with individual health counseling.

The need for understanding in the broad area of human movement is considerable. Although recent surveys conducted by the President's Council on Physical Fitness and Sports show that 55 per cent of American adults exercise (18 million ride bicycles, and 44 million walk for their motor activity), there are millions of people who lead very quiet, sedentary existences. About half the people surveyed take exercise for reasons of health and recreation, and 9 of 10 favor school physical education programs. In this respect, the better programs are tying motor skills instruction and conditioning activities to health teaching. Exercise physiology concepts are being learned and applied. In East Hartford, Connecticut, for example, Edward Meyers has instituted a program that emphasizes the body systems before, during, and after exercise and training.[1] In the laboratory the senior high students test muscle strength, muscle endurance, and cardiovascular endurance; they experiment with pulse rate and blood pressure, body density, lean body weight, and percentage of fat. Program evaluations have been quite favorable. Similar types of health instruction have been very well received in the Orangeview Junior High School of Anaheim, California, and the San Antonio and Fort Worth areas of Texas. In Fort Worth, Kenneth Cooper and other investigators from the Institute for Aerobics Research worked with secondary school physical education students and discovered that cardiovascular endurance training and classroom instruction together could yield an improvement in the fitness of the students—a concrete behavioral manifestation.[2]

---

[1] Edward J. Meyers, "Exercise Physiology in Secondary School," *Journal of Health, Physical Education and Recreation,* 46:30–31, January, 1975.

[2] Kenneth H. Cooper, et al., "An Aerobics Conditioning Program for the Fort Worth, Texas, School District," *Research Quarterly,* 46:345–350, October, 1975.

Attention also should be given to sleep deprivation. In his work with adolescents, Holland determined that the performance of a selected number of arduous and long-term tasks was measurably worsened by the loss of a single night's sleep.[3] Senior high school students find the experimental study of human fatigue interesting because it can be related to so many everyday work and play activities as well as to emotional stability.

Behavioral Objectives

(*Junior High Level*)

Plans a balanced program of physical activity and rest which contributes to general fitness.

Demonstrates how vigorous physical activity increases the efficiency of the cardio-vascular and respiratory systems.

Explains how daily activities and environmental factors influence energy expenditure and sleep.

Lists the several kinds of recreational activities which supplement and complement other daily activities and influence rest and relaxation.

Takes rest, recreation, and exercise in order to contribute to physical, emotional, and social needs.

Shows how periodic physical examinations and planning of daily activities, including hobbies, help make effective healthful living possible.

Diagrams the relationship of every part of the body to the well-being of the entire body.

Describes how rest and sleep are needed to enable the body to repair itself, to remove fatigue products, and to enable muscles to relax and replenish their store of fuel.

Essential Topics

Physical fitness defined
Body dynamics and human movement
Functional efficiency and exercise
Chronic fatigue
Sleep and rest
Relaxation
Leisure-time activities
Periodic health examinations
School-community factors influencing energy expenditure
Rest and mental health

Behavioral Objectives

(*Senior High Level*)

Explains why the proper time to acquire sound practices to be used in the mainte-nance of physical fitness is during the adolescent period.

Relates own experiences of physical activity as valuable in helping to cope with the stress, tension, and mental strain sometimes experienced in daily living.

Takes a physical fitness test that has been developed to show how well a person

---

[3]George J. Holland, "Effects of Limited Sleep Deprivation on Performance of Selected Motor Tasks," *The Research Quarterly*, 39:265–294, May, 1968.

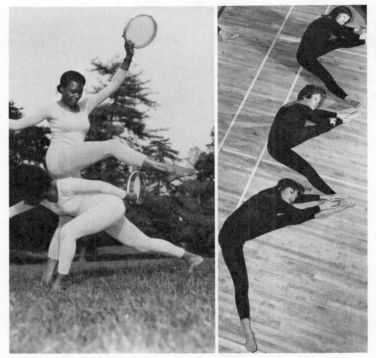

Figure 5–1   Dancing for fitness and relaxation. (Courtesy of Dorothy P. Stanley)

performs physical tasks and how well individuals are prepared for emergencies as well as for daily work, study, and play.

Illustrates how sedentary practices of modern living reduce the effectiveness of body functions.

Analyzes why recreation is a fundamental human need essential to the well-being and fitness of everyone, and why it contributes to mental health by helping to provide a balanced program of living.

Explains individual tolerances in the requirements for sleep which relate to overall living practices and temperament.

Describes the differences between those social forces that encourage activity rather than sleep, and those factors that encourage sedentary rather than active use of time.

Essential Topics

Degenerative disease and physical condition
Role of activity in preventive medicine
Psychological stress
Recreation and mental health
Sedentary living
Rest-activity styles of living
Sleep patterns and variations
"Jogging," swimming, bicycling, and other repetitive activities
Human efficiency research

Suggested Activites

(Junior High Level)

1. Obtain the physical fitness test scores from the physical education department for individual class members. Discuss what specifically is being measured and what the

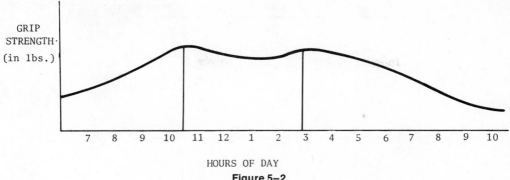

HOURS OF DAY

Figure 5–2

significance of these things is. If scores are not available, organize the class to administer the Youth Fitness Test of the AAHPER.[4]

2. Have several boys and girls measure their grip strength with a hand dynamometer (manuometer). Record the results, in pounds, every hour of the day for a full day. Plot the results on graph paper to establish a curve. Note the direction of the curve as fatigue sets in between meals and toward the end of the day. A somewhat typical diurnal curve is shown in Figure 5–2.[5]

3. Set up a panel discussion on the topic *Fitness For What?* Encourage class participation following panel member presentations.

4. Invite one of the school coaches to speak on the relationship between physical performance and training practices—with specific reference to nutrition, sleep and rest, mental attitudes, and exercise.

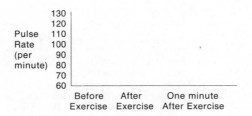

5. Demonstrate the immediate effect of exercise on the heart, circulation, and respiration. Measure the pulse rate before and after exercise. Note the change in the respiration rate.

6. Perform a three-minute step test:
   a. Take the pulse rate for 30 seconds and multiply by 2.
   b. Step up and down on a steady chair for three minutes, to a count of "step up—step down; step up—step down."
   c. Take the pulse rate again for 30 seconds and multiply by 2.
   d. One minute later repeat the pulse measurement.
   e. Plot the curve.
   f. Compare individual curves. Note great increase in pulse beat in some individuals and slow return after one minute to the before-exercise rate.

---

[4]Test procedures may be found in a number of references and in the *Youth Fitness Test Manual* (rev.) of the American Alliance for Health, Physical Education and Recreation, Washington, D.C.

[5]For more details and findings from previous research see Chapter 7 and pages 129–131 in Carl E. Willgoose, *Evaluation in Health Education and Physical Education,* New York: McGraw-Hill Book Co., 1961.

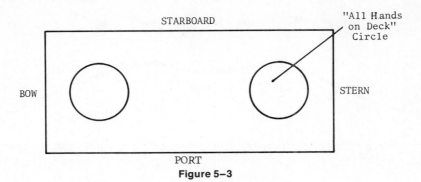

Figure 5–3

7. Discuss the practice of relaxing just before meals. Stress a pleasant mealtime as an aid to digestion.

8. Appraise the posture of several pupils. Use a Polaroid camera to photograph a student against a wall so that vertical and horizontal alignment can be observed.

9. Play a vigorous game such as *Shipwreck:*

    a. Consider the gymnasium floor to be the deck of a large sailing ship. See Figure 5–3.

    b. Assign one end of the gym as the *Bow* and the other as the *Stern.*

    c. Assign one wall or sideline of the gym as *Starboard* and the other side as *Port.*

    d. To begin the game, all class members stand in the center of the playing area (the deck of the ship).

    e. When the following commands are given, assume positions as *indicated immediately:*

COMMAND	ACT
"All hands on deck"	Run and put both hands in one of the deck circles.
"Port"	Run to Port side of ship.
"Starboard"	Run to Starboard side of ship.
"Boom coming over"	Flatten out on stomach on floor, hands out front.
"Bow"	Run to Bow of ship.
"Stern"	Run to Stern of ship.
"Man overboard"	Quickly pair up with another boy or girl in a horse and rider position. Either person can be the horse or rider.
"Freeze"	Don't move at all!

    f. As fast as a command is given, move to the proper position.

    g. The last person to move to a proper position on command is automatically eliminated. Continue until everyone is so tired that they begin to make errors. Eventually all players but one will be eliminated.

    h. Following the game ask these questions:

        (1) Was the game vigorous enough to challenge your physical condition? If you played it often enough would it build physical condition?

        (2) Was it fun to play? Was it too fatiguing to be fun?

10. On the bulletin board, display pictures of the kinds of recreational activities which tend to be (a) restful and relaxing, (b) social, and (c) vigorous.

11. Go over the make-up of a periodic medical examination and relate this to functional efficiency and emotional well-being. Emphasize that prime responsibility lies with the individual. Use school examination forms to make topic real.

Suggested Activities

(Senior High Level)

1. Research and report on the criteria to be used in determining how much daily exercise one should experience; consider (a) age, (b) results of medical examinations, (c) general reaction to and recovery from physical activity, (d) daily work and play routine, and (e) relaxation and rest practices.

2. Run a survey in the community to ascertain the frequency and kinds of exercise that adults undertake. What are the popular activities? Who belongs to health clubs and similar organizations promoting motor activity? Are women as active as men (they were more so in one survey carried out by the President's Council on Physical Fitness and Sports)?

3. Research and report on the training activities used to develop cardiorespiratory efficiency—circuit training, interval training, and the overload principle.

4. Assign a small committee of students to read Nathaniel Kleitman's *Sleep and Wakefulness* (University of Chicago Press, 1963.) Report on some of the fascinating studies to the class at a later date.

5. Study human fatigue through personal involvement. Employ a combination of walking and running a mile in the fastest time possible. Have class members describe how they feel when they finish. Concentrate on "gut feelings" in the *affective* domain. Write such one or two word descriptions as these on the board for discussion:

exhausted	tight
sleepy	breathless
fatigued	heartbeat
exhilarated	tired back
aching legs	happy feeling

6. Investigate the activities of the President's Council on Fitness and Sports. Materials may be obtained from the Council at the White House, Washington, D.C. 20202.

7. Evaluate the effectiveness of certain recreational activities in maintaining optimum levels of fitness: swimming, walking, jogging, cycling, mountain climbing, bowling, volleyball, and other games and sports.

8. Examine a weight reduction program as prescribed by a local physician. Refer to safety in lowering body weight, the role of diet, and the particulars relative to exercise. Note the effect of cholesterol in bringing on cardiovascular disease.

9. Discuss the manifestations of psychological stress (worry, anxiety, apprehension, anger, jealousy, hatred, and so on) and relate them to chronic fatigue, joint pain, ulcers, gastrointestinal upsets, and other physical symptoms. Show the role of rest and sleep in helping to offset undue stress and tension.

10. Define recreation in terms of re-creation, rejuvenation, relaxation, and divergence from the routines of living in a pressure-type culture. Also, consider the population pressures, noise, confusion, and city-type stresses leading to poor mental health.

11. Ask a group of girls to set forth a number of objections to exercise and some of the myths associated with the topic when related to female participation. This could be a very interesting topic. Do girls get bulky muscles from physical activity? Do girls require as much sleep as boys of the same age? Should girls take physical activity during the menstrual period? Are highly active girls always looked upon as tomboys? Are views about girls' physical activities changing?

12. Chart the physical, emotional, and environmental conditions that influence fatigue. Look at industry, at schools, and at the home. Don't overlook the effects of boredom, motivation, and aspiration level.

2. NUTRITION AND GROWTH

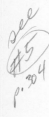

(Nutrition education should be one of the most involved and personal studies in the school curriculum.) If worldwide conditions and the possibility of an ecological catastrophe of mass starvation within 50 years mean anything, then the study of deprived peoples, food technology, and the newer topics of sea farming and jungle cultivation should be investigated and responded to by all youth. Moreover, as the CBS television documentary "Hunger in America" pointed out, there are gross nutritional problems in the American population that relate to the social–political–economic confines which entrap a large segment of society. Malnutrition causes a loss of 30 billion dollars a year as a result of poorer health, and exceeds the cost of other major health problems such as drug abuse and alcoholism.

As a multidimensional topic nutrition education requires a multidimensional approach—one that relates food to feelings and aspirations, to human efficiency, and to the multicultural and pluralistic practices of people. (The school's task) is considerably broader than identifying vitamins and minerals. It (calls for a serious look at obesity and

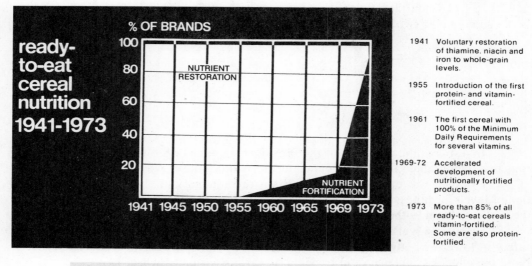

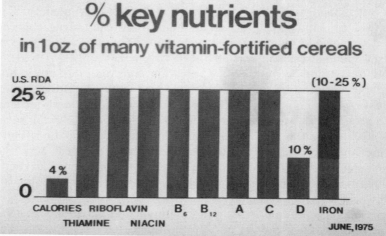

Figure 5–4   Nutritional enhancement of breakfast cereals. (Courtesy of Cereal Institute, Inc.)

the related factors of food intake, exercise, life style, food preferences, heredity, glandular and body malfunctions, and psychological and social problems. It calls for a look at nutritional values of all foods, because there are changes from year to year. There are also changes in food selection practices too.) For example, in a 5-year period, ready-to-eat cereals and toaster products increased 11.7 and 19.6 per cent, respectively, while eggs and meat dropped off 14.5 and 17.3 per cent, respectively.[6] Also, about 13 per cent of the United States population select no breakfast at home and about 5 per cent choose coffee only. Since the consumption of cereals has gone up, it is fortunate that they have been fortified with added nutrients to the point where many provide 25 per cent of the United States recommended daily allowance (RDA) for at least seven vitamins, prior to the addition of milk (see Figure 5–4).

Complicating the topic of nutrition education are the longstanding parental admonitions to "eat this food and not eat that," which frequently leave young people rebellious, as the enormous popularity of nonnutritional snacks proves. Yet, the topic *can* be made vital. The elementary school is the place to begin. (By the junior high school period one can concentrate on nutrition and link it to interest-centered topics such as growth and personal appearance.) Begin with cell structure and move from there to energy requirements for daily activities. Discuss human growth as it relates to factors such as height, weight, skeletal and dental development, and maturation; relate these factors to food requirements so that the four basic food groups can be translated into the activities of the day. Variations here are interesting. For example, people of different ages have different requirements. A seventh grader requires more Vitamin D than men and most women over the age of 19. And for proper efficiency, a grandparent in a family requires more Vitamin A for an aging skin and weakening vision than each of the children at the meal table. How do we know this? What role does the Food and Nutrition Board of the National Research Council play? How are the recommended daily allowances figured by this council? How do unusual amounts of physical activity at any age raise the food requirements above those recommended? How does illness raise the requirements?

(For the early secondary school student, the science of nutrition can be made practical through a study of home meals, restaurant menus, and the school lunch program. Food from each of the food groups can be incorporated into a hearty meal.) Meals can be planned around the following one-third. Recommended Daily Dietary Allowances pertaining to a Type A lunch (National School Lunch Program Regulations established by Congress in 1946):

- ½ pint of fluid whole milk served as a beverage.
- 2 oz. (edible portion as served) of lean meat, poultry, fish; or 2 oz. of cheese; or one egg; or ½ cup of cooked dry beans or peas; or 4 tablespoons of peanut butter; or an equivalent of any combination of these foods.
- ¾ cup of two or more vegetables or fruits, or both. A serving of full strength vegetable or fruit juice may be counted as not more than one-third of this requirement.
- 1 slice of whole-grain or enriched bread; or a serving of other bread such as cornbread, biscuits, rolls, muffins, made with whole-grained or enriched meal or flour.
- 2 teaspoons of butter or fortified margarine.

Slightly larger amounts are suggested for senior high students. Also recommended is a food rich in Vitamin C each day, and a food rich in Vitamin A twice a week.

As Dr. Frederick J. Stare of Harvard University has said, one can think of nutrition in terms of meat, potatoes and carrots, or he can think of it in terms of vitamins, minerals, and amino acids. It really makes very little difference how nutrition is thought of, as

---

[6]Market Research Corporation of America, *Fourth National Household Menu Census,* Chicago, Illinois, 1975.

Iron
   Men = 10 milligrams   Women = 12 to 15 milligrams

Boys and Girls	7 mg	8 mg.	10 mg.	12 mg	15 mg
	Age 1–3	4–6	7–9	10–12	13–19

Calcium
   Men = 800 milligrams   Women = 800 to 1500 milligrams

Boys and Girls	1000 mg	1200 mg	1400 mg
	Age 1–9	10–12	13–19

long as the pertinent information is translated into appropriate eating behavior. Students need to work with the nutrition charts of the National Research Council and work with grams and milligrams—which are just as easy to work with as pounds and ounces. The chart, for example, indicates a need for 85 grams of protein in the daily diet of a 13 to 15 year old boy. By turning to a list of foods containing protein, the student can discover several ways of eating a total of 85 grams of protein.

Here is one way:

serving of beef	= 30 g.
3 cups of milk	= 27 g.
1 egg	= 6 g.
peanut butter sandwich	= 8 g.
2 hot dogs	= 14 g.

How many ways can *you* add up 85 grams of protein? Which way seems the most expensive? The least expensive?

There should be an opportunity to observe that as age increases, so do the requirements for essential foods.

Although scientific meal planning is frequently a senior high school activity, some experience should be gained during the earlier years. Checking the nutritive value of foods can be fun, especially as one compares a juicy hamburger with a slice of custard pie. A meal planning work form can be constructed. Somehow, meal planning has to relate directly to meals eaten at home and at school. For example, studies of breakfasts eaten by secondary school pupils are still showing that either students haven't heard of the Iowa Breakfast Study research or they don't believe it. Perhaps some believe it but it

Protein

FOOD	QUANTITY	GRAMS
Beef	3½ oz.	30
Veal	3½ oz.	33
Pork	3½ oz.	28
Frankfurters	2	14
Eggs	1	6
Milk	1 cup	9
Dried beans	¾ cup	11
Peanut butter	1 tblsp.	4

doesn't cause them to change their practices. This was brought out vividly by Harris in his study of high school students:[7]

- Only 12 per cent of the girls and 14 per cent of the boys ate breakfasts that adequately met their nutritional requirements.
- Boys ate slightly better breakfasts than girls.
- The addition of milk or citrus fruit or both would have improved the nutritional quality of the breakfasts.
- Over 50 per cent of the students said they were hungry between 10:00 A.M. and 11:00 A.M.
- Reasons given for not eating an adequate breakfast were not getting up in time to develop an appetite and insufficient time to eat leisurely.

Especially fine reading for secondary school students are the nutrition book choices of Jean Mayer, former professor of nutrition at the Harvard School of Public Health:

Live High on Low Fat by Sylvia Rosenthal (Lippincott)

Diet for a Small Planet by Frances Moore Lappe (Ballantine)

How to Eat Well and Stay Well The Mediterranean Way by Ancel and Margaret Keys (Doubleday)

Panic In The Pantry by Elizabeth Whelan and Frederick J. Stare (Atheneum)

The Mirage of Safety by Beatrice Trum Hunter (Scribners)

Keeping Food Safe by Hassell Bradley and Carole Sundberg (Doubleday)

Dictionary of Protein by Barbara Kraus (Harper Magazine Press)

Fiber In Foods by Barbara Kraus (Signet)

People and Plows Against Hunger by Herbert Black (Marlborough House)

By Bread Alone by Lester Brown and Erik Eckholm (Praeger)

This Hungry World by Ray Vickers (Scribners)

The Conquest of Famine by W. R. Aykroyd (Readers Digest Press)

Food In History by Reay Tannahill (Stein and Day)

A Diet For Living by Jean Mayer (McKay)

Behavioral Objectives

(Junior High Level)

Diagrams how the body requires food energy and nutrients to carry on its vital functions, to build new cells for growth and repair, and to supply energy for physical activity.

Describes how a state of dynamic balance exists with regard to intake and outgo of food energy and nutrients by the body.

Observes that people vary considerably in their requirements for food. Body size, rate of growth, heredity, physical activity, and individual metabolic rates all affect caloric needs.

Explains how lack of sufficient nutrients can lead to nutritional deficiency diseases.

Notices that individuals who are growing fast during adolescence show the effect of an inadequate food supply more quickly than others.

Identifies obesity in individuals and notes that it may affect appearance, self-confidence, life expectancy, and one's relationships with others.

Distinguishes among people that while almost everyone follows the same general pattern of growth and development, there is a wide range of variation within the normal growth pattern; potential for growth is fixed by heredity and modified by environment.

---

[7] William H. Harris, "A Survey of Breakfasts Eaten by High School Students," *Journal of School Health,* 40:323–325, June, 1970.

Observes that pleasant surroundings and friends and good manners affect the enjoyment of food.

Explains how skeletal age can be measured by a physician, dental age by a dentist, and sexual age by noting the appearance of secondary sex characteristics.

Writes about how body build cannot be changed, but fatness may be changed by eating and exercise patterns.

Investigates how the processing of foods and the control of commercial preparations helps protect the consumer.

Lists ways in which food quacks and food faddists can endanger the health of their followers.

Essential Topics

Cellular growth and repair	Growth variations
Dynamic energy	Digestion and assimilation
Nutritional deficiencies	Mealtime surroundings
Food requirements	Morphological age
Caloric needs	Weight control
Basic four variations	Food processing
Growth spurts	Nutritional fads and myths

Behavioral Objectives

(Senior High Level)

Formulates a statement supporting the concept that a nation's productivity ultimately depends on a significant amount of human endurance to work; this applies both in America and in the developing nations of the world.

Discusses the fact that nutrition is important before and during pregnancy, to both mother and baby.

Explains how proper nourishment and favorable emotional experiences for the infant may be provided with either breast or bottle feeding.

Demonstrates how widespread malnutrition in the developing nations of the world interacts with disease and other factors to produce reduced life expectancies and poor health for many people; this is not helped by a world population that is growing in geometric fashion.

Reasons that personal, community, and worldwide nutritional health needs may be met by regulating caloric intake and activity, choosing balanced meals, and improving food production and processing.

Analyzes the way in which the homemaker prepares foods and how this influences the quality of nutrition of family members.

Essential Topics

Human productivity—mental and physical dimensions
Weight control and degenerative disease
Prenatal and early childhood nutrition
Nutrition and emotional health
Malnutrition in the United States
Malnutrition in developing nations
Food production and processing
Family health and food preparation
Cultural considerations: myths, superstitions, varieties of meals
Medical quackery

FOOD MEASURE	PRO-TEIN GM.	IRON GM.	CAL-CIUM GM.	VIT. A. I.U.	THIA-MINE MG.	RIBO-FLAVIN MG.	NIACIN MG.	ASCOR-BIC ACID (C)	CAL-ORIES
RECOMMENDED DAILY REQUIREMENTS*									
BREAKFAST									
LUNCH									
DINNER									

*Boy or girl, age 13 to 15.

Suggested Activities

(Junior High Level)

1. Since nationally recognized nutritionists such as Dr. Frederick Stare and Dr. Jean Mayer have "snapped, crackled, and popped" over widely publicized charges by engineer Robert Choate that most breakfast cereals are poor food, it would be most appropriate to study some of the more than 400 million cereal boxes appearing on the grocers' shelves. Just how nutritious are the cereals? And how much more so when milk is added? What about the value of a bowl of "Special K" or "Cream of Wheat"? Is the protein and iron percentage impressive or weak? Is drinking an "instant breakfast" a sound practice, or should one sit down to a bacon and eggs meal?

2. Adapt television's "Password" game to nutrition. The words to be suggested will depend upon the objective of the teacher. They may include any nutritional terms or be limited to foods, nutrients, body processes, nutritional recommendations, and so on. The class is divided into groups of five, including a moderator, two students to give clues and two to guess. Those giving clues receive a word from the moderator and try to lead the

TABLE 5–1   Carnation Instant Breakfast* Nutritional Analysis

	ONE ENVELOPE INSTANT BREAKFAST	ONE ENVELOPE WITH 8 FL. OZ. MILK
Protein	24.0%	17.5 gm. +
Carbohydrate	64.9%	35.4 gm.
Fat	0.65%	8.73 gm.
Calories	128	290
Vitamin A	26% MDR	35% MDR
Niacin	25% MDR	27% MDR
Vitamin B_1	20% MDR	30% MDR
Vitamin B_2	11% MDR	48% MDR
Vitamin B_4	.287 mg.	—
Vitamin B_{12}	.17 mg.	—
Vitamin C	93% MDR	100% MDR
Vitamin D	0% MDR	25% MDR
Iron	25% MDR	20% MDR
Copper	.194 mg.	—
Calcium	15% MDR	55% MDR
Phosphorus	18% MDR	49% MDR

MDR = Minimum Daily Requirements

*Carnation Company, Los Angeles, California 90036.

DAY	BREAKFAST FOOD	NO. OF CAL.	LUNCH FOOD	NO. OF CAL.	DINNER FOOD	NO. OF CAL.	SNACKS FOOD	NO. OF CAL.	TOTAL CALORIES FOR DAY

DATES_____ TO_____

_____ TOTAL CALORIES FOR WEEK

others to guess it by providing *one word* clues *related to nutrition*. A time limit is agreed upon and no references are used. Hang a simple sign before the game begins:

"PASSWORD"

3. Plan three meals for one day (see diagram above).
   a. Consult a food table for the necessary information on quantities and values. Write this information in the appropriate spaces of the Meal Planning Work Form.
   b. Total the figures in each column to see if the person has met the daily recommmended dietary allowances for an adequate diet.
4. Plan a five day food record in order to relate calories to activities.
   a. People vary in amount of calories used. A poor swimmer struggling through the water to move ahead and keep afloat may use up to 400 calories an hour, while a skillful swimmer of the same size who glides through the water, relaxing between strokes, may use only 250 calories an hour. It would make a difference how cold and rough the water is.
   b. Estimate the number of calories you use performing an activity.
      (1) Multiply your body weight by the number of calories used per pound per hour.
      (2) Multiply this figure by the fraction of an hour you actually spent on the activity.

Example:
   If you weigh 90 lbs. and play pingpong for 15 minutes you will be working at the rate of 225 calories per hour. Thus, in 15 minutes you will use about 56 calories.

   c. If you are a very active person, is it possible that you may eat more calories per day than other individuals, yet not be overweight? What are your comments?
5. Talk about the meaning of height and weight charts. How should they be used? Examine the Meredith Tables to note growth curves for each sex as girls grow rapidly

80 LB. GIRL CAL./HR.

Sleeping 3.2
Walking 120
Running 500
Swimming 320

*TABLE 5–2 Energy Expenditures for
Everyday Activities*

ACTIVITY	CALORIES PER POUND PER HOUR
Dressing and undressing	0.8
Household tasks (cleaning, dusting, sweeping, etc.)	1.2
Knitting	0.8
Playing piano...........................	0.9
Playing pingpong	2.5
Running	3.7
Sitting, eating, reading, sewing, etc............................	0.7
Sleeping or resting	0.4
Swimming	4.1
Typing	1.0
Walking slowly	1.1
Walking moderately (3 miles an hour)	1.4

from 10 to 15 and boys 12 to 17. (Height-weight charts for boys and girls can also be obtained free from Wheatena, Standard Milling Co., Kansas City, Missouri.)

6. Sketch the three extremes of body types (Sheldon's somatotypes) on the chalk board. Refer to genetic influences and body measurements. See Figure 5–5.

7. Set up a committee to interview fruit and vegetable merchants. What are the methods in judging the quality in fresh fruits and vegetables?

8. Examine the relationship between jogging and caloric expenditure. Review and comment on Table 5–3.

According to an Air Force Academy study, a 170 pound man running 1.45 miles in 8 minutes would burn up 175 calories. Running more slowly — 16 minutes for the distance — he would use 157 calories. A 120 pound man would expend fewer calories for the same exercise output; a 220 pound man would burn considerably more.[8] One study finding is that the speeder who tears up the track burns only a few more calories than the jogger who putters along at an easy pace. However, a faster running speed is better for heart tone and lung action than is leisurely trotting.

---

[8]Harger, B. S., et al., "The Caloric Cost of Running," *Journal of the American Medical Association,* 228:482–483, April, 1974.

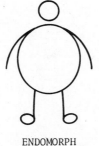 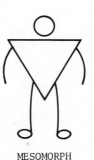 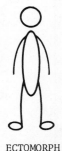

ENDOMORPH   MESOMORPH   ECTOMORPH

Figure 5–5   Sheldon Somatotypes.

TABLE 5–3 Caloric Values in Jogging

CALORIC VALUES FOR RUNNING 2.413 km. (1.45 mi.)

Weight kg.	(lbs.)	Calories/min.								
		8	9	10	11	12	13	14	15	16
54.5	(120)	125	124	121	120	119	117	116	114	112
59.0	(130)	135	133	132	130	128	126	125	123	121
63.6	(140)	145	143	141	139	138	136	134	132	130
68.1	(150)	155	153	151	149	147	145	143	141	139
72.6	(160)	165	163	161	159	156	154	152	150	148
77.2	(170)	175	173	170	168	166	164	161	159	157
81.7	(180)	185	182	180	178	175	173	171	168	166
86.3	(190)	195	192	190	187	185	182	180	177	175
90.8	(200)	205	202	199	197	194	192	189	186	184
95.3	(210)	215	212	209	206	204	201	198	195	193
99.9	(220)	225	222	219	216	213	210	207	204	202

9. Potassium helps maintain moisture in body cells and is required in muscle tissue. The potassium need is the greatest in girls between the ages 12 and 14 and in boys aged 14 to 16. It is found in oranges and in apples. Apples make up 10 per cent of all fresh produce sold. Look into where they come from, in the United States and locally, and find out what other food value they possess.

10. Prepare a short paper entitled, "Obesity is a disease of civilization."

11. Examine the 40-frame filmstrip, *Consumer Tips on Fresh Citrus* (Sunkist Growers, Inc.). Discuss the place of citrus fruits in the diet. Prepare a recipe using "tips" provided in the filmstrip.

12. Test for Carbohydrates.

Method:

1. Put corn syrup in a test tube.
2. Add one ounce of Benedicts' solution.
3. Heat, and wait for blue color to change to red-orange. This red-orange color is a positive indication that sugar is present.

Try the test with other foods. Put a small piece of food into a test tube, add about one ounce of Benedicts' solution, heat, and wait for color change. Some foods that contain sugar are oranges, cookies, and ripe bananas. Some foods that do not contain sugar are meat, cheese, and nuts.

Supplies	*Foods to Test*
Corn syrup	Cookies
Benedicts' solution	Potato
Dropper	Meat
Sterno can or bunsen burner	Cheese
8 test tubes	Orange
rack	Nut
2 test tube holders	Milk
paring knife	
matches	

13. Research the question: "What's in a Cranberry?" Can anyone name the 12 minerals? (See pamphlets available from Ocean Spray, Hanson, Massachusetts 02341.)

14. Give students a weekend assignment to "teach" someone something relating to nutrition and to write up the experience on a single page.

15. Class activity: List your 10 favorite foods.

1. Draw a circle around the food you could most easily do without for one year.
2. Mark a plus (+) next to each food that is high in nutrients.
3. Put a dash (−) in front of those foods high in calories and low in nutrients.
4. Put a star (*) in front of those foods low in calories.
5. Put a (#) in front of those foods you eat too much of and/or too often.
6. Put a five (5) in front of those foods that would *not* have been on your list 5 years ago.
7. Put an (x) in front of "junk" foods or empty calorie foods.
   a. What did the "Ten Foods" exercise reveal to you about your food selection?
   b. Are all of the food groups represented? In balanced amounts?
   c. What, if anything, do you plan to do as a result of this exercise?

16. Investigate changes in eating habits during the twentieth century. Are the changes sound?

17. Value Ranking

Ranking gets at priorities. Priorities reveal values. Value discussions often bring out inconsistencies, faulty reasoning, misinformation, or new information. Ask students to rank three or four items. The variations in answers create interesting discussion.[9]

1. Rank as most nutritious:

"Instant breakfast" with water
Salted peanuts
Pizza with pepperoni
Orange drink with a B-complex pill

---

[9]Adapted from a report by Jack D. Osman, "Teaching Nutrition With a Focus on Values," *Nutrition News,* 36:5–9, April, 1973.

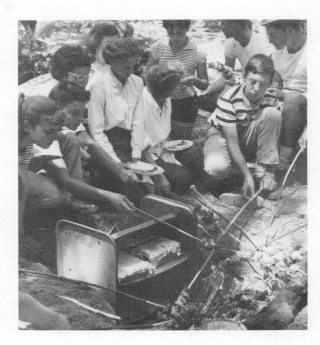

Figure 5–6 Junior high school outdoor cooking project.

2. Rank food with most calories first:
   Medium-sized baked potato
   Nine potato chips
   Extra large apple
   Ten celery stalks
3. Rank drink with most calories first:
   Beer, 8 oz.
   Whole milk, 8 oz.
   Skim milk, 8 oz.
   Cola drink, 8 oz.
4. Rank as most reliable source of weight control information:
   Dietitian
   Magazine ad
   Pharmacist

18. Gather and post newspaper clippings and advertisements about dieting, crash diets, fad diets, reducing pills, and food quackery. Refer also to "health foods."

19. Invite a physician to class to lead a discussion on weight control. Have an athletic coach contribute to the discussion by referring to weight loss and gain in the training of athletes.

20. With the help of the school dietitian and student committee, promote lunch room attractiveness through the use of pictures, table settings, flowers, and so forth.

21. Appoint groups of three students each to create nutrition crossword puzzles. Approximately 20 questions "down" and 20 questions "across" is adequate.

Suggested Activities

(Senior High Level)

1. Identify the word *psychosomatic,* and show relationships between mind and body, psychological stress and chronic fatigue (sub-energy levels), the inability to relax and underweight, and general mental health and eating practices. Have the class members contribute examples from their observation at home and in the community. Follow this with references and cases from the literature.

2. Discuss social customs and nutrition. Bring out the pro and con factors associated with the "coffee break," "snacking," "beer and television," "refreshing Coke," and so on.

3. Investigate the topic of malnutrition among schoolchildren. Divide the class into several small groups, each with a task to perform as follows:

Group I   Nutrition and Mental Retardation
Group II   Causes of Malnutrition
Group III   Signs of Malnutrition
Group IV   Pictures and Stories of the Malnourished
Group V   Rehabilitation of the Malnourished

4. A malnourished individual may suffer from a number of subclinical conditions and not look or feel sick enough to visit a physician. Discuss how the following characteristics associated with malnutrition may come about, and how they are related to human efficiency:
   Easily fatigued
   Exhibits poor posture much of the time
   Restless and irritable

Frequent and prolonged infections

Sleep difficulties

Lack of ambition in school or elsewhere

Flabby musculature

Lack of appetite

Dry scaly scalp, hair, and skin

Sore mouth, tongue and gums

5. Distribute the pamphlet "If You Think Breakfast Is for the Birds... Think Again!" (free from Cereal Institute Inc.). Then engage the class in discussion of following questions:

Do you eat breakfast alone or with members of your family?

Do you fix your own breakfast?

What effect does a good breakfast have on *your* day?

What does eating breakfast have to do with weight control? See Figure 5–7.

6. Develop a "capsule" story of several key nutrients. Have students make charts in bar graph form to show, for example, the amount of protein in various protein-rich foods. (Especially helpful are the *Food Value Charts* available from the National Live Stock and Meat Board. They are also available in wall size and in color.)

7. Invite a local pediatrician to speak to the class on nutrition and early growth. Prior to the talk have each student review the recommended food requirements for pre-school children.

8. Post pictures showing starving children in various parts of the world. Then discuss the intricate relationships between food, local customs and politics.

9. Demonstrate and discuss the *color* in fruits and vegetables.

   a. Carotene (pro-vitamin A) depends on the amount of chlorophyll in leafy vegetables, where *green* leaves may contain 50 times as much as inner white leaves.

   b. High content of *red-yellow* (beta-carotene) in carrots yields 60 to 120 mcg./g. of vitamin A.

   c. *Yellow* corn contains vitamin A.

   d. Sweet potatoes' *yellow-orange* hue derives from beta-carotene, a precursor of vitamin A.

   e. *Flesh color* of cantaloupes contains pigment that is 95 per cent beta-carotene.

   f. *Bright red* tomato color is not an index of vitamin A, although the fruit is a good source of vitamin A.

10. Visit a "health food" store. Note the wide variety of bread products, bone meal preparations, and other food items that are available. Note especially the pamphlets, leaflets, and labels created to sell these "health foods" and make them seem more nutritious than those most people can purchase in their own grocery store.

11. Investigate nutrition labeling. Obtain the U.S. Government Printing Office publication *Nutrition Labeling—Tools For Its Use,* and the superb poster on labeling from the Cereal Institute, Inc., Chicago, Ill. 60603 (see Figure 5–8). Look over food labels with the following in mind:

> Nutrition information on food packages can help consumers
> — *become more aware of key nutrients required for good nutrition and health.*
> — *recognize the specific nutrients present in different foods.*
> — *compare the nutritive values and relative costs of different foods.*
> — *select foods throughout the day that in total will supply the recommended amounts of key nutrients.*

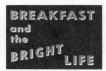

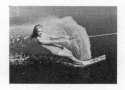

You feel better and work better...

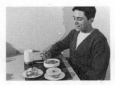

because you can get a good share of your daily protein, vitamins and minerals in the morning meal. Science has added even more nutrition to the natural food value of certain cereals.

At the same time, cereal with skim milk is low in fat—just 150 calories a serving . . .

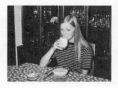

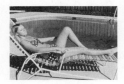

ideal for weight-watchers.

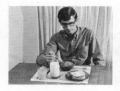

Whether you're working on a sensational figure or not . . .

everyone—young and old —can live longer, happier, healthier lives by choosing from a wide variety of foods, mostly low in fat, like those in the recommended breakfast.

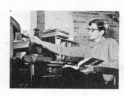

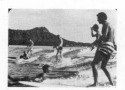

A basic breakfast helps cut down the yen for sweet or rich snacks and heavy evening meals— enemies of the trim figure and a carefree life.

Figure 5–7   Cuts from a dynamic film strip for high school use. (Courtesy of Cereal Institute, Inc.)

NUTRITION FACTS TO GUIDE YOUR FOOD CHOICES

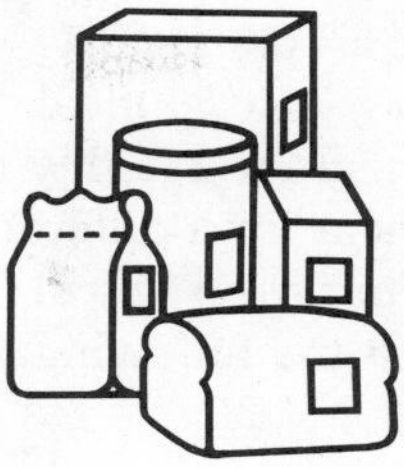

NUTRITION INFORMATION PER SERVING

SERVING SIZE: One ounce (1⅓ cup) Corn flakes alone and in combination with ½ cup vitamin D fortified whole milk.

SERVINGS PER CONTAINER: 12

	CORN FLAKES	
	1 oz.	with ½ cup whole milk
CALORIES	110	190
PROTEIN	2 gm	6 gm
CARBOHYDRATES	24 gm	30 gm
FAT	0 gm	4 gm

PERCENTAGE OF U.S. RECOMMENDED DAILY ALLOWANCE (U.S. RDA)

	CORN FLAKES	
	1 oz.	with ½ cup whole milk
PROTEIN	2	10
VITAMIN A	25	25
VITAMIN C	25	25
THIAMINE	25	25
RIBOFLAVIN	25	35
NIACIN	25	25
CALCIUM	*	15
IRON	10	10
VITAMIN D	10	25
VITAMIN B_6	25	25
FOLIC ACID	25	25
PHOSPHORUS	*	10
MAGNESIUM	*	4

*Contains less than 2 percent of the U.S. RDA of these nutrients.

The GOAL of Nutrition Labeling is to provide nutrient information in the same form on many foods.

Nutrition Labeling can help you:

■ become more aware of key nutrients needed for good nutrition and health.

■ recognize the specific nutrients present in individual foods.

■ compare the nutritive values and relative costs of different foods.

■ select foods for the whole day that *in total* will supply the recommended amounts of vital nutrients.

One example of Nutrition Labeling on cereals. Since cereals are usually eaten with milk, nutrition information is shown for the cereal alone and for a serving of the cereal with milk.

Figure 5–8 Nutrition labeling poster. (Courtesy of Cereal Institute, Inc.)

12. At the 1969 White House Conference on Food, Nutrition and Health it was recommended that more public service time on radio and television be devoted to nutrition. With this in mind, have a small group approach a popular disk jockey, sports figure, or entertainer to see how he might help in nutrition education.

13. Carefully examine the colorful booklet, "Recipes For Fat-Controlled Meals," available free from the Florida Department of Citrus, Lakeland, Fla. 33802. Discuss whether there are cultural, ethnic, or economic reasons why these recipes would not be used locally.

14. Divide the class into several small groups, each group to make up a day's meal plan for one of the following:

    a. meal for a teenage boy or girl

    b. low-cost meal

    c. low-calorie meal

    d. meal for a family of four, with a girl, 8, and a boy, 15, who carry their lunches

    e. meal for a different season

    f. "hurry-up" meal

15. Post the following for later discussion:

CHECKING FATS

Cholesterol is a substance that is manufactured by the body and that is also obtained from certain foods. Since it is used for the formation of hormones and vitamin D, it is essential for good health. However, a problem arises when there is too much cholesterol, because it then accumulates in the blood. Also, some of the excess may be deposited in the inner layers of the arteries and thus begin to interfere with the flow of blood—a process called *atherosclerosis*.

Problems that research has been studying—and today's answers:

1. Does the amount of cholesterol in the food affect the level of cholesterol in the blood? Yes.
2. Does the type of food fat (saturated or unsaturated) affect the level of cholesterol in the blood? Yes.
3. Can blood cholesterol levels be lowered? Yes.
4. Does lowering the level of blood cholesterol reduce the risk of heart attack? Yes.

---

16. Establish a committee to investigate *algae*.

ALGAE: GREEN FOOD FOR THOUGHT

Do algae—the pesky, microscopic plants which sometimes form a green haze on aquarium glass—hold the key to solution of our world food shortage? What a preposterious question! Or is it? Scientific research leads to some intriguing speculation along these lines.

For use inside space ships, a small plant was needed, one which was easy of culture and could be grown in the tank of a "green machine" called a photosynthetic gas exchanger. Chlorella, a species of algae, met all these requirements, and in addition, it grew so rapidly that a surplus of edible plant material was produced. In fact, the amount of Chlorella needed for a man's oxygen supply would also provide the exact amount of food he needed!

What does this "food" taste like? When processed into powder, Chlorella has a flavor somewhat like dried lima beans. It contains more than twice as much protein as steak, and has all essential vitamins except vitamin C.

Chlorella can be grown in outdoor ponds or in rooftop pools. The Arthur D. Little Co. of Cambridge, Mass., built a pilot plant for mass production, and engineers deduced that a full-sized plant, covering 100 acres, would yield 12,500 pounds of dry algae per day. Will such a facility ever be built?

---

17. Depict how the better food films can make nutrition interesting. For example, consider a list of titles such as the following:

Apples Away[10]
Food, Sunshine, and You[10]
Green Gold—Bananas[10]
Menu For An Astronaut[10]
Lights, Camera, Lettuce[10]
How Red Berry Saved White Man From Singing Blues[10]
Nutrition Sense and Nonsense[10]
The Real Talking, Singing Action Movie About Nutrition[11]
Let's Have a Porkecue[12]
Beef Says It Best[12]
You Can Reduce[12]

18. Examine nutritional aids in another language.[11]

In *French:*

> Les agrumes frais,
> sources de sante

In *Spanish:*

> Construya un Cuerpo mas
> Saludable con Citricos Frescos

19. As a class project, investigate the validity of the "inorganic foods" movement. This can be a significant project for mature students. In "organic" farming, all fertilizers are decomposed animal or vegetable matter, and no chemical sprays or fertilizers are used. Patrons of "organic" farms travel many miles to pay $1.50 a dozen for eggs and $2.50 a pound for ground beef. This is all part of a growing demand for "organic foods," the shorthand term for anything produced the old-fashioned "natural" way. Animals raised on organically managed land are permitted to roam freely and are untreated with antibiotics, hormones, pesticides, or irradiation. Even pasteurized milk is out. Only certified (raw) milk will suffice. With the exception of the pesticide consideration, there is no evidence to support these foods—but let the student researchers find this out.

> "ORGANIC FOODS"

> "NATURAL FOODS"

> ?

---

[10]Available from United Fresh Fruit and Vegetable Association, 1019 19th St. N.W., Washington, D.C. 20036.

[11]Available from Sunkist Growers, P.O. Box 7888, Valley Annex, Van Nuys, Calif. 91409. See also National Dairy Council materials in both English and Spanish.

[12]Available from National Live Stock and Meat Board, 36 S. Wabash, Chicago, Ill. 60603.

20. Obtain a number of copies of *Nutrition News* (National Dairy Council) free and *Nutrition Notes* free (United Fresh Fruit and Vegetable Association). Ask class members to report on something they have read that is new to them. How does it relate to their lives?

3. DENTAL HEALTH

(To the early adolescent it should be obvious that healthy teeth and gums are important to appearance, speech, and the enjoyment of living. Yet, the message is a difficult one to put across) throughout the world. Somehow, formally and informally, a greater degree of critical thinking must be applied to selecting products pertaining to dental health, choosing dental services, cleansing and eating practices, and the several other factors having a bearing on oral health.

(A large number of young people are not thoroughly convinced that the food they eat contributes in any significant manner to their tooth structure, so they eat what they want? For decades the English have done poorly with their eating and brushing. They have gone light on calcium-loaded dairy products and heavy on sugar (111 pounds per person per year), leading one British dentist to remark that "behind their mythologically stiff upper lips hang some of the sweetest and rottenest teeth in the world."

(Interestingly, economic deprivation and social deprivation correlate positively with poor dental health.) This has been shown in a number of studies, including the United States National Health Survey. (There are, nevertheless, numerous affluent families whose children lack essential dental care.) It is not surprising, therefore, that one survey conducted by a committee of the American School Health Association found that the biggest obstacle to good dental health was "need of parent education." Obviously, well informed parents can contribute more to the reduction of tooth decay than the feeble efforts of their offspring. One concrete way is to demand fluoridated drinking water. This action alone will reduce tooth decay up to 70 per cent when youngsters begin early. There is real work to do here, for after a quarter century only a little more than half the United States population is using fluoridated public water supplies. This addition of sodium fluoride to drinking water is a practice that holds high promise for the poor, who frequently lack proper home dental care, nutrition, and hygiene. Most objections are based on unscientific reports and political rather than scientific reasons. Education is needed to show that fluoridation is not socialized medicine or an example of unnecessary and unwarranted government action. The courts have consistently upheld fluoridation.

What can the secondary schools do that is better than what they have been doing? Why is it that even after dental health instruction, almost half of the students in the School Health Education Study did not know how to brush their teeth properly? In another study of first year high school students it was concluded that dental health facts may be learned after childhood, but that increasing knowledge does little to change preformed habits. Essentially the same thing was found in Kalamazoo, Michigan, where (oral health practices coincided poorly with students' knowledge.)[13] And in Tennessee, a high school evaluation of dental health education showed little positive relationship between dental health knowledge and attitude scores and periodontal findings.[14] From such studies as these (one gathers that too much attention has been given to the knowledge target rather than the behavioral target.) Schools have taught their lessons without working coopera-

---

[13]William C. Love, "An Assessment of the Knowledge and Practice of Oral Health by Selected School Children in Kalamazoo, Michigan," *Journal of Public Health Dentistry,* 28:153–166, Summer, 1968.

[14]Durwood R. Collier and Earl J. Williams, "The Evaluation of an Educational Program in Preventive Periodontics," *Journal of Tennessee State Dental Association,* 48:92–103, April, 1968.

tively with the family dentist and the home. There has been too much talk in the classroom.

After carefully reviewing a number of unsuccessful and successful programs of dental health education, Cohen and Lucye determined that known behavior-changing methods simply were not being practical. (They recommended a theoretical model for the classroom which limited lecturing, included numerous role playing activities, and personalized the subject.) For example, instead of telling the student to visit the dentist, the student was asked to make his own arrangements.[15]

In terms of material aids and current scientific research findings, the American Dental Association has the most extensive supplies for teachers. Their publications, exhibits and audiovisual materials are superb, for they have been tested in dental practice and in schools at various grade levels. Their current catalog of listings is available from 211 E. Chicago Ave., Chicago, Illinois 60611.

Studies continue to indicate that *tooth brushing experiences* in the school are worthwhile. In Torrance, California, Meier found the usual instruction methods inferior to supervised brushing practice. By employing the Bass brushing technique the formation of plaque did not occur (prevented by its daily disorganization). The Bass technique is being taught in many schools today. Here, toothbrushes with rounded bristles are used without toothpaste or powder. The bristles are pointed toward the teeth at a 45-degree angle and the brush is vibrated in place in a gentle, circular motion. About two teeth at a time are cleaned in this fashion.

Where teachers are trained, as in the Model Teacher-School Dental Hygiene Program of Texarkana, Texas, the reduction in plaque and improvement in oral hygiene skills is significant.[16] Here, the teachers had a teaching guide, films, and toothkeeper kits containing toothbrushes, plaque-disclosing tablets, dental floss, and hand mirrors.[17] Students were trained to recognize plaque and employ red disclosing tablets to note personal changes in the cleanliness of teeth. Darwin Dennison, in his several experiments concerning motivational models, has also found skills instruction to be more effective than cognitive and affective experiences alone.[18]

Perhaps a *variety* of experiences, exercises, and demonstrations which are *not purely* informational in nature, can be effective. Terhune believes so, and has set up several exercises or learning activities which relate directly to plaque production and sugar consumption over a three-day period[19] (see Suggested Activities, No. 1, p. 125).

Behavioral Objectives

(Junior High Level)
Explains that all over the world teeth are susceptible to decay by certain foods, but most people appear to be indifferent to its consequences.

---

[15]Lois K. Cohen and Helen Lucye, "A Position on School Dental Health Education," *Journal of School Health,* 40:361–365, September, 1970.

[16]Lawrence A. Friedman, "Impact of Teacher-Student Dental Health Education," *Journal of School Health,* 44:140–145, March, 1974.

[17]The Toothkeeper System is distributed by Health Education Division, Den-Tal-Ez Manufacturing Company, 1201 W.E. Diehl Ave., Des Moines, Iowa 50315.

[18]Darwin Dennison, "A Motivational Model to Modify Actual Health Behavior," *Journal of School Health,* 44:16–22, January, 1974.

[19]James A. Terhune, "Developing Positive Dental Health Practices," *Journal of School Health,* 6:23–28, January-February, 1975.

Documents the fact that appearance, speech, and economic success are related to sound teeth and gums.

Illustrates how proper dental practices will bring freedom from dental discomfort, reduce time and money spent on dental corrections, and improve well-being.

Describes how neglect of teeth may result in oral disorders which in turn may adversely affect other parts of the body.

Evaluates the literature on the use of fluorides as a very effective way of preventing tooth decay.

Practices individual safety measures which help prevent dental accidents.

Compares the number of people requiring treatment for malocclusion with those who do not, and acknowledges that this is partly due to the steadily increasing demand for orthodontic care by better educated people.

Practices persistent daily attention to dental care.

Identifies the specialized personnel who treat dental disorders.

Essential topics

Dental caries control

Abscesses and total health

Selecting dental products

Choice of foods with the emphasis on sugar content

Fluoridation—water supply

Fluoridation—topical application

Accidents to teeth

Personal attractiveness

Speech irregularities

Malocclusion

Individual dental practices—toothbrushing skills

Behavioral Objectives

(Senior High Level)

Surveys a group of individuals to discover that the prevention and correction of dental disease depends upon the motivation of individuals.

Explains how dental decay has plagued both civilized and uncivilized peoples since time began. Writes that only a few people in isolated areas of the world today are not affected by dental decay.

Identifies the variables in tooth decay and gives attention to tooth structure irregularities, alignment, dental plaque, mouth bacteria, acids, foods, saliva, gum disorders, cleansing practices, and emotional tension.

Explains that there is no evidence to support the claim that toothpaste or mouthwash can significantly reduce or destroy mouth bacteria.

Prepares an article stating that the most significant innovation in preventive dentistry is the fluoridation of the drinking water in the larger cities and towns, and fluoridization (topical applications) in rural communities where it is not practical to provide controlled fluoridation measures.

Contrasts the several methods of financing dental care.

Essential topics

Motivating dental care; parental and peer group influences

International dental needs

Public health activities in the larger community

Para-dental personnel

Professional care

Cancer of the mouth
Periodontal disease
Fluoridation research
Dental insurance
Gingivitis

Suggested Activities

(Junior High Level)
1. Record meal and snack activity, particularly in terms of sugar consumed. Show a relationship between meals and snacks and bacterial-plaque acid production by using red erythrosine dye disclosing tablets. Terhune employs a stain with Plak-Lite in order to show contrasting mouths.[20] Students examine their own teeth before and after the stain has been added.

2. Set up the fluoridation controversy for role playing—i.e., mayor, city council, proponents, opponents, etc. Debate the pro and con issues associated with the topic.

3. Post such words as the following for definition:

halitosis   periodontal disease
malocclusion   caries
gingivitis   discolored teeth
erosion   abrasion

4. Have a small committee report on career opportunities available in dentistry. Consider also the auxiliary fields such as dental hygienist, technician, research assistant, and manufacturer of dental supplies and equipment.

5. Prepare a game board on which students can move a marker (bean, corn, etc.) from space to space with the roll of a die. The spaces call for questions to be answered. Successful answers permit the student to stay on a space. Unsuccessful answers result in the student returning to where the marker rested prior to the roll of the die. (For an already prepared "Dentopoly" game see Engs et al., p. 87, in Selected References at the end of this chapter.)

6. Depict information about dental decay by line, bar, or pie graph. For example, have a pie graph show that less than 4 per cent of high school pupils are free of dental decay, or that by the age of 55 years, 1 in every 2 persons needs dentures.

7. Determine how many class members have had accidents injuring teeth. Follow this up with student suggestions as to how these accidents might have been prevented.

8. Look into the reasons for using x-ray film. A small group may visit a local dentist in order to get his views.

9. Borrow plaster molds from the dentist showing "before" and "after" cases of individual malocclusion. This is a highly effective way to show what braces can do to straighten teeth and make orthodontia a more pleasant experience.

10. Ask a football team player to report on and demonstrate the use of mouth pieces.

---

[20]Plak-Lites, which have a white light source and cause stained plaque to glow a brilliant yellow, may be obtained from International Pharmaceutical Corporation, 400 Valley Road, Warrington, Pa. 18976.

11. Consider dental costs by comparing expenses for treatment of minor caries as opposed to those for more involved work such as root canal procedures or a dental bridge. Contrast early and regular dental attention with neglectful situations where there is toothache, loss of teeth, drifting of teeth, and an appearance problem. Solicit student experiences.

12. Distribute back issues of such magazines as *Consumer Reports, Family Health,* and *Journal of the American Dental Association.* Record all references to teeth and dental issues. In this *guided discovery* activity have class members orally recall what they have found and of what significance it appears to be. Diet research provides new ideas. For example, a low-calcium diet hastens the loss of bone that supports teeth in the gums, leading to the possibility of periodontal disease as a first clinical sign of osteoporosis, a crippling disease of older adults characterized by a loss of calcium from skeletal bone and subsequent softening of the bone.

13. Distribute a number of dental instruments for class inspection. See how many students know what they are and what they are used for.

14. Collect toothbrush and dentifrice advertisements; study the claims made. Gather information to determine whether the claims are reasonable and accurate.

15. Have the class practice using dental floss. Distribute a 10-inch piece to each pupil. Have the class practice using the floss by moving it gently back and forth between the teeth.

Suggested Activities

(Senior High Level)
1. Report on the several specialties of dentistry, such as oral surgery, orthodontia, periodontia, prosthodontics, and oral pathology. This may be accomplished through committee study or by bringing specialists to class to discuss selected health careers.

2. Investigate dental care group insurance. Should it be a part of the Blue Shield plan everywhere? Will it cost the participant more or less money than the more traditional way of securing dental care? This can be a *problem solving* project in which several students or small groups of three each take a different approach.

3. Research the statement:

Debilitating childhood diseases or any disease causing a high fever for longer than 24 hours' duration can cause improper or poor calcification and lead to easily decayed teeth.

4. Survey the community, listing all the facilities for providing dental care. Elaborate on the findings by doing the following:
a. Determine the proportion of dentists to the general population of the community.
b. Find out how the community or county provides for people who cannot afford dental care.
c. Use survey facts as basis for a report for publication in school or local newspaper.
d. Consult with the county or state dental society to see what their comments about the findings of the survey are.

5. Use models to help show what happens when food is permitted to remain on the necks of the teeth, or becomes lodged between the gum margin and the neck of the tooth. This is an opportune time to demonstrate the effects of proper brushing on tissue tone and gingival health.

6. Show the film, *Dentistry Through the Age of Man,* available from the American

Dental Association. Raise several questions related to historical facts. Why, for example, have we not found a way to eliminate dental problems when the topic is so well known—and goes back to the era of Rhodesian man, estimated to have lived 250,000 years ago?

7. Have each student experiment with and describe his saliva flow—the amount of which influences natural mouth cleanliness. Sample foods such as the following: marshmallows, peanut butter and crackers, caramels, bread, nuts, potato chips, celery, apples, and carrots. Acid foods stimulate a free flow of saliva; sweets stimulate a low, thick flow which tends to adhere to the teeth. Citric acid found in hard candies is especially damaging if left on the teeth over a long period. Phosphoric acid from soft drinks is almost as severe, and lactic acid produced by mouth bacteria ranks next in destructiveness.

Tooth Destroying Acids

Citric (Hard Candies)
Phosphoric (Soft Drinks)
Lactic (Mouth Bacteria)
Acetic (Vinegar)
   —Ranking by U.S.P.H.S.

---

8. Experiment in order to evaluate the claim that a certain dentrifice "kills mouth bacteria." How much does toothbrushing reduce the number of lactobacillus bacteria (*Lactobacillus acidophilus*)?

a. Take a lactobacillus colony count.

b. Materials needed:
   1. Sterile saline solution
   2. Sterile test tubes
   3. Petri dishes
   4. Pipettes
   5. Agar medium (sterile)
   6. Incubator (or a warm place)

c. Procedure:
   1. Secure saliva sample or separate samples from persons with different caries susceptibility.
   2. Mix 1 ml. of saliva with 9 ml. saline solution.
   3. From the 1:10 mixture make other mixtures in the ratios of 1:100 and 1:1000. With pipettes, transfer 1 ml. of each dilution to the next 9 ml. of sterile saline.
   4. Transfer 0.1 ml. of each sample to an agar plate.
   5. Incubate agar plates at 37.5°C. for 2 or 3 days or put in a warm place.
   6. Compare number of colonies on each plate according to dilution.
   7. On plates containing 50 to 100 colonies, count the colonies and estimate the total number of *L. acidophilus* per milliliter of undiluted saliva.

d. Check the likelihood of decay:

Colonies of L.A. per ml. of saliva	Extent of Decay
Under 2000	Very little
2000 to 10,000	Moderate
Over 10,000	Extensive

---

9. Experiment in class with the amount and strength of acid formed by mouth bacteria by color testing.

a. Materials needed:
   1. Tooth picks

    2. Microscope and slides

    3. Methyl red indicator

    4. Sugar

b. Procedure:

    1. Remove material from around the necks of the teeth with a toothpick.

    2. Arrange the material in a ¼ inch doughnut-shaped circle on the slide.

    3. Place a few drops of 0.02 per cent aqueous methyl red (20 mg. soluble methyl red in 100 mg. of water) over and around the outer rim of the circle.

    4. Place a few grains of sugar inside the circle.

    5. The indicator will turn red if acid is formed. Rapidity of the color change indicates acid production and caries susceptibility.

c. Point out that it is known that people who are relatively immune to dental decay have saliva that is somewhat alkaline.

    10. Organize groups of students to assist health services personnel in their follow-up efforts to encourage dental care among a group of elementary school children (Youth-to-Youth activity).

    11. Use a student-prepared dental health quiz in interviewing several adults to see what ideas people have about modern dental health. The survey findings should be returned to the classroom for comment.

    12. Talk over the problem of oral cancer—where about 90 per cent of the over

How do you rate in oral hygiene?

(Score 10 for each correct answer. A score of 90 to 100 means you really know your stuff; 70 to 100 – – no reason why you shouldn't have a very attractive smile; 50 to 70 – – better take a good look at the answers; below 50 – – where were you all through elementary school?)

1. What is the main dental problem for teenagers?

    A. tooth decay ( )
    B. gum disease ( )
    C. crooked teeth ( )

2. Most people lose their teeth through decay.

    True ( )
    False ( )

3. Sugars and starches cause tooth decay by

    A. weakening the gums and letting infection in ( )
    B. forming acids which dissolve enamel ( )
    C. being deficient in vitamins and minerals ( )

4. Eating good food makes the enamel of your teeth stronger.

    True ( )
    False ( )

5. Tooth decay can be largely prevented by (select two):

    A. brushing teeth twice a day ( )
    B. cutting down on sugars and sweets ( )
    C. drinking more milk ( )
    D. having decayed teeth taken out ( )
    E. brushing teeth after every meal ( )
    F. chewing gum ( )

6. Your dentist can help you to protect your gums, if you visit him regularly, by

    A. frequent X-rays ( )
    B. removing tartar deposits and cleaning your teeth ( )
    C. checking your teeth for cavities ( )
    D. applying sodium fluoride to your teeth ( )

7. The best dentifrice is

    A. plain water ( )
    B. an ammoniated dentifrice ( )
    C. baking soda and salt ( )
    D. the least expensive ( )
    E. a stannous fluoride dentifrice ( )

8. If you can't brush your teeth after meals, the next best thing is to

    A. eat an apple ( )
    B. chew gum ( )
    C. rinse your mouth with water ( )
    D. use a toothpick ( )

9. The most important reason for maintaining good teeth

    A. to keep up bodily resistance to disease ( )
    B. for a good smile and a pleasant appearance ( )
    C. it costs less to maintain than to repair ( )
    D. oral hygiene is part of general cleanliness ( )
    E. for chewing food efficiently ( )
    F. for clearness in speaking ( )

Figure 5–9

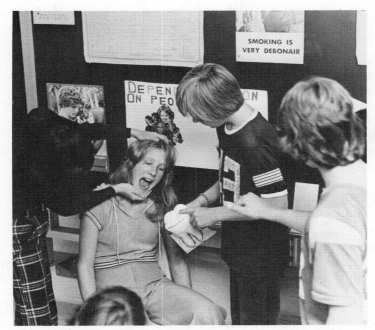

Figure 5–10   In dental health education, students examine the real thing along with the model. (Courtesy of Loren Bensley, Jr., and Brad Fleming, Central Michigan University)

35,000 cases a year are smokers. Smokers have four times greater risk of death from oral cancer than non-smokers and far more periodontal disease. In addition, they have more stained teeth, more bad breath, and a duller sense of taste and smell. (The American Dental Association puts out an excellent folded leaflet entitled *Smoking And Your Oral Health.*)

13.   Take the Canadian *Teenager's Tooth Test,* shown in Figure 5–9.[21]

Answers

1. A.   Tooth decay attacks 9 of 10 people and is most active during the teens. Gum disease is more serious among adults. See Figure 5–9.
2. True of people under 35. People over 35 suffer tooth loss through gum disease, though decay remains a problem throughout life.
3. B.   Bacteria feed on sugar in the mouth and acids are formed which dissolve the enamel.
4. False.   Enamel is fully formed by the age of 8. Teenagers cannot improve their teeth by good food, but they can harm them by eating too much sweet food.
5. B and E.   Cutting down on sugar consumption, and cutting down the time it stays in your mouth, are your best preventives against decay.
6. B.   Most cases of gingivitis result from local irritations, such as tartar formation, poor oral hygiene, etc.
7. E.   Teeth may benefit from some stannous fluoride dentrifices, but when and how you brush them is very important.
8. C.   Rinsing your mouth of food particles immediately after eating can cut down tooth decay.
9. E.   The chief purpose of teeth is to prepare food for digestion. The other reasons are important too.

---

[21]Distributed by the Department of National Health and Welfare, Ottawa, Canada.

4. BODY STRUCTURE AND OPERATION (INCLUDING SPECIAL SENSES AND SKIN CARE)

The purpose of this major topic is to present a picture of the basic structure of the human body and how it relates to function. Bones, connective tissue, musculature, and organic systems are viewed in terms of a total operation—the active, living organism as a superb example of balanced forces in operation. For some instructors this is a starting point in health teaching. For others it would appear to be unsatisfactory because one might run the risk of being too anatomical and physiological in instruction.

There will be a number of teachers who may wish to omit *Body Structure and Operation* altogether as a major health area and treat the respective body systems and their functions as they pertain to specific health problems. For example, the skeleto-muscular system would be set forth in some detail when body mechanics and physical activity were discussed; the function of the respiratory system would be studied along with smoking and respiratory difficulties; digestive functions would accompany nutrition education; a review of degenerative diseases would present an opportunity to look at the intricacies of the cardiovascular system; and the topic of mental health would call for a close look at the brain as the center of the nervous system responsible for behavior and conditioning.

Somewhere, however, attention should be given to the sense organs and senses. Some curriculum developers have scheduled this as a part of the nutrition topic (taste and smell functions) and mental health (seeing, hearing, and touching). Also, the subject of skin needs to be well covered. It could be discussed in several different places, for it relates to personal appearance, the sensory apparatus, heat regulatory mechanism, and the excretory system. In addition, it is frequently referred to under Consumer Health.

Experience indicates that for many boys and girls, their first formal health education course with a degree of depth and challenge comes when they enter the middle school or junior high school. Early in the course there appears to be an immediate need to take a look at the human being in terms of overall structure and its function. This is a time when an understanding of the multifunctional makeup of the body is needed in order to conceive the "whole person" idea and appreciate the fact that what affects individuals mentally and emotionally has a bearing on them physically, and vice versa. By noting the supportive and cooperative actions of all body systems, one begins to learn early the meaning of the words "balance in living," and understand that most of the difficulties of mankind have to do with a pattern of living practiced over the years.

If the body systems and organ functions have been well covered at the early secondary school level, there should be no need to schedule this area as a separate topic. It can be reviewed in other health areas. Moreover, there is a shortage of health teaching time in most high schools as certain major health topics demand in-depth attention not provided previously. For instance, in several high school health education programs the total emphasis is on five or six topics such as mental health, consumer health, alcohol, drugs, and tobacco, sex and family living education, and safe living.

Early in the junior high school, one should learn that the individual is a performer. Whether active in sports or engaged in earning a living, the individual is impelled to strive in all seasons, under many conditions which often involve severe stress. Fortunately, as growth continues through adolescence the individual develops defenses and learns to meet the demands of the environment. This is an excellent time to discuss fully the topic of individual growth—of height-weight concerns, skeletal development, maturation, chronological-physiological age, puberty, and self acceptance. It is a time to study height-weight charts distributed by reliable organizations such as insurance companies. The Meredith Tables are especially revealing. So is much of the material in the "Kit on Body Systems" put out by the Cleveland Health Museum.[22] Also, a number of films have been produced that introduce the student to the human body (see Chapter 12 for sources). The American Heart Association film, *About The Human Body,* was developed for this age level and looks at the major body functions from the point of view of a student being given a complete physical examination. The American Heart Association poster, "Your Heart and How It Works," is especially well done in terms of circulation mechanics.

(As a topic, the study of the skin can be made most interesting. Acne is by all odds the most common skin disease of the adolescent. The earlier it is treated, the less likely it is to result in the psychic scarring of personality and pitting and scarring of the skin. With an understanding of the pathogenesis of skin diseases, students can begin to appreciate a rational approach to skin care.) Medication, nutrition, cleansing practices, and emotional needs cover considerable ground and indicate the depth of study needed to enhance personal appearance, body image, and self-esteem. Feelings of acceptability, especially among adolescents, are associated with the appearance of the surface of the skin—so much so that with skin disease there is almost always an emotional impact.[23] The subject of climate and the skin (thermal homeostasis), sweating, hormonal and circulatory controls, heat loss, and heat safety can be covered quite successfully at this student age level.

Contributing further to the topic of appearance and total body functioning is the discussion of other sensory organs. Vision and hearing contribute greatly to physical and mental efficiency and need to be covered in depth. Over 100 million people in the United States wear eyeglasses. The topic is relevant to the age, especially when one considers the problems associated with such things as hearing impairment, contact lenses, safety glasses, plastic lenses, sunglasses, sports participation, reading and studying, and earning a living.

Behavioral Objectives*

(Junior High Level)

Tells how growth and development is a sequential yet unique process determined by the structure and function of the individual.

Describes how hormones secreted by endocrine glands have an effect on the physical growth and development of the whole body.

Confirms the fact that the normal function of the body is sometimes interrupted by disease, accidents and malformation.

Diagrams how a number of vision and hearing disorders can be treated and corrected, and how professional personnel are essential in this process.

Demonstrates how eyeglasses are worn to correct refractive errors; they do not cure the error.

Investigates the validity of the statement that the leading cause of loss of sight among adolescents is injury to one or both eyes.

Initiates and leads a discussion supporting the fact that hearing, like vision, is both a function of the structure and a learning center in the brain.

---

[22]Meredith Tables, American Medical Association, 535 N. Dearborn Street, Chicago, Illinois 60610; Cleveland Health Museum, 8911 Euclid Avenue, Cleveland, Ohio 44106.

[23]See two highly useful articles for the teacher: John A. Kennedy, "Treatment of Skin Diseases of the Adolescent," *Journal of School Health,* 40:7–10, January, 1970; and William W. Zeller, "Adolescent Attitudes and Cutaneous Health," *Journal of School Health,* 40:115–120, March, 1970.

*No behavioral objectives and learning activities are listed for the senior high level because this topic is considered to be appropriate only for the lower secondary grades.

Explains how the skin protects the body from the outside world, helps regulate body temperature, and provides sensations relative to touch, pain, warm, and cold.

Experiments with the senses of smell and taste, which are related and bring about enjoyment during the act of eating.

Essential Topics

Bones and connective tissue stability
Musculature for human movement
Placement of organs
Intra-organ dependency (balances)
Growth and maturation—genetic forces
Growth and maturation—environmental forces
Puberty as an "event"
Skin structure and function
Acne and other adolescent difficulties
Periodic eye and ear examinations
Eye and ear problems
Contact lenses, safety glasses, and sunglasses
Hearing aids, noise pollution, and deafness
Taste and smell sensations

Suggested Activities

(Junior High Level)

1. Dissect a frog or other animal to isolate organs and tissues. Note location of organs within body framework.

2. Examine the skeleton of a human being and note the places where muscles attach to bones. Using wide elastic bands, illustrate how a muscle contracts and moves the body parts.

3. Post a height-weight-age chart and discuss what it says and what this means to members of the class. Consider the extremes of body types in the light of individual genetic-familial influences. Consider also the environmental influences.

4. Invite a physical therapist to class to show how rehabilitation work is done. Illustrate how low back pain or some other body weakness can be helped.

5. Discuss movement—how it takes place from nervous system direction to muscle contraction and how all body functions occur because of muscle stimulation.

6. Display materials written in Braille. Investigate the Braille system.

7. Demonstrate how contact lenses stay in place. Ask for experiences about when they have not done so.

8. Examine the topic of perception. Compare it to seeing as a mechanical affair. Show that it is possible to improve one's perception. Place some common objects in a box (pin, paper clips, erasers, etc.). Require each student to look into the box for 30 seconds. Then ask:

How many paper clips did you see?

Was the pin opened?

Ask a question about something that did not exist in the box. Compare accuracies. From here proceed to a discussion of visual perception.

9. Diagram on a blackboard or wallboard how visual acuity works. Draw a sketch of the eyeball with light rays coming through the lens toward the retina. Illustrate myopia, hyperopia, and astigmatism situations and show how eyeglasses ground in a certain way are able to correct or improve vision.

Figure 5–11

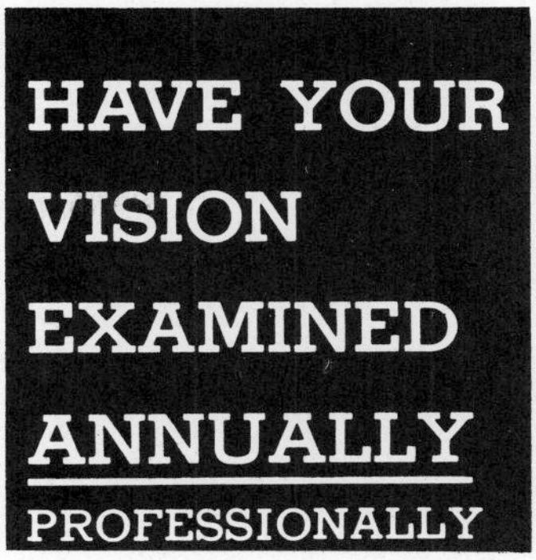

HAVE YOUR
VISION
EXAMINED
ANNUALLY
PROFESSIONALLY

10. Have the class establish a list of those things most likely to damage the eye causing partial or complete loss of sight.

11. Raise the sign in Figure 5–11 before the class. Then discuss its validity.

12. Form separate groups of two or three students to discuss and report on "vision in sports." The booklet, "You Can't Hit It... If You Can't See It," will be helpful. It is available from the American Optometric Association. So is the very informative student booklet, "Your Vision And How It Works."

13. Use the strategy of "brainstorming" to:
   a. Assist the students to appreciate the sense of sight. Placing a time limit of three minutes on the activity, direct the students to record on a sheet of paper "all the things we do that require eyesight," or "all the ways that we use our eyes in learning."
   b. Find out what students know and what they want to know about vision and the eye. (This class activity may be conducted in small groups or as an individual assignment.) Appoint a student recorder to list the ideas on the chalkboard under the following headings: *Already Know, Do not Know, Would Like to Know.* Announce to the students: "There are many things you probably know about the eyes and vision, especially after viewing the program. Let's see what you already know..."
   "...Now, what are some things you don't know or would like to know more about?"

14. Select a body system to study. Relate it to the individual student and the community. The function of the heart and circulatory system, for example, can be related to the saving of human life instead of being associated with tragedy and death. Invite a Red Cross speaker to class to talk about the blood center. Appropriate booklets on blood are available for the class reading shelf from the American National Red Cross.

15. Study acne by illustrating on a model of the skin how the oil glands become plugged, causing the sebum to exude onto the skin and bring about inflammatory pimples or cysts. Have the class find out how to care for the condition.

16. Illustrate the effect of wind on the surface temperature of the skin. For example, if the wind is blowing 20 miles per hour at 15° above zero, it will feel the same as 15° below zero. Initiate discussion by posting Table 5–4.

17. Obtain a *Coronary Care display* and set it up for individual game use in the classroom.[24] The purpose of the Guide to Coronary Care is to give an estimate (not a medical diagnosis) of a person's chances of suffering a heart attack or stroke. By learning to win at this game of coronary care, a person can learn to be a winner in the real game of health.

---

[24]Available from Spenco Medical Corporation, P. O. Box 8113, Waco, Texas 76710.

TABLE 5–4 *Wind Chill Table*

WHEN THER-MOMETER READS ↓	Calm	WHEN THE WIND BLOWS AT THE M.P.H. BELOW, YOUR BODY WILL REACT AS IF THE TEMPERATURE WERE:							
		5 mph	10 mph	15 mph	20 mph	25 mph	30 mph	35 mph	40 mph
+50	50	48	40	36	32	30	28	27	26
+40	40	37	28	22	18	16	13	11	10
+30	30	27	16	9	4	0	−2	−4	−6
+20	20	16	4	−5	−10	−15	−18	−20	−21
+10	10	6	−9	−18	−25	−29	−33	−35	−37
0	0	−5	−21	−36	−39	−44	−48	−49	−53
−10	−10	−15	−33	−45	−53	−59	−63	−67	−69
−20	−20	−26	−46	−58	−67	−74	−79	−82	−85
−30	−30	−36	−58	−72	−82	−88	−94	−98	−100
−40	−40	−47	−70	−88	−96	−104	−109	−113	−116
−50	−50	−57	−85	−99	−110	−118	−125	−129	−132
−60	−60	−68	−95	−112	−124	−133	−140	−145	−148

Coronary Care is played by moving numbers of rings from the 10 short poles to the center tall pole. Each ring represents one year of life. The short poles represent risk factors known to influence a person's chances of suffering a heart attack or stroke. The center pole stands for the total predicted years of life.

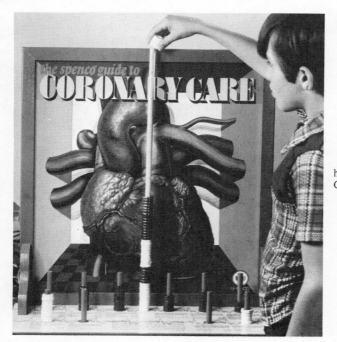

Figure 5–12 Education can prevent heart attacks. (Courtesy of Spenco Medical Corp.)

The coronary risk factors include sex, family history, diabetes, overweight, smoking, exercise, stress, personality type, high cholesterol, and high blood pressure. After studying each risk factor, a person selects his personal health habits and moves the rings from the short risk factor poles to the center longevity pole as directed. The number of unmoved rings lost because of poor health habits is a strikingly firm motivator for improved health care. (See Figure 5–12.)

5. PREVENTION AND CONTROL OF DISEASE

This is a rather broad health area, especially when considering that the term "disease" can be applied to just about every physical and mental ailment afflicting mankind. For this reason disease prevention should be discussed in a general way — in terms of contributing elements such as antibodies and immunity, chronic fatigue, infectious organisms, degenerative conditions, and defective organs. Moreover, the word disease should be conceptualized as dis-ease. Disease means a lack of ease. It can be due to high blood pressure, a cramp in the stomach, an unresponsive administration bureaucracy; it can be due to erratic transportation, and it can be due to a lack of jobs or civil rights. Students must examine these larger dimensions of dis-ease that are all about them today.

Disease should be seen as the great deterrent to the advance of a civilization. It should be viewed historically as well as in contemporary situations. Philosophers have observed that it seems always to be with us. Thoreau wrote, "There is hardly a lily pad afloat on the pond that hasn't been riddled by insects."

If cost were any indication of disease control, then America would be the healthiest nation in recorded history. No other country can match our 6.7 per cent expenditure for health care. Yet 14 nations do a better job of preventing infant deaths. The Scandinavian countries have the lowest rate, probably because about 90 per cent of pregnant women visit physicians during the first three months — a health practice that is not followed by a large number of American women. Twelve nations have a lower maternal mortality rate,

Infant Mortality
Fifteen Countries

RANK	COUNTRY	INFANT MORTALITY PER 1000 BIRTHS
1	Sweden	12.9
2	Netherlands	13.4
3	Finland	14.2
4	Norway	14.6
5	Japan	15.0
6	Denmark	15.8
7	Switzerland	17.5
8	New Zealand	18.0
9	Australia	18.3
10	Britain	18.8
11	France	20.6
12	East Germany	21.2
13	Canada	22.0
14	United States	22.1
15	West Germany	22.8

Source: U.N., U.S. Dept. of Health, Education and Welfare

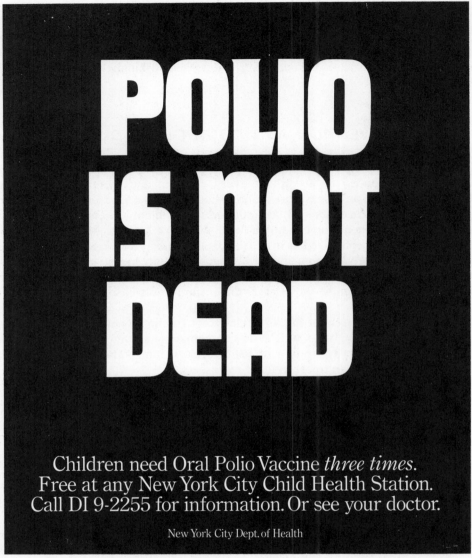

Figure 5–13 New York poster—an immunization message of concern.

and longevity rates for both men and women are higher in a dozen countries. Somehow personal living habits, coupled with inadequate health education, genetics, and the physical and social environment have combined with medical care deficiencies to produce American health inadequacies. Bacteria have been brought fairly well under control by antibiotics, but only a few virus-induced diseases can be prevented—polio, smallpox, influenza, measles, and yellow fever. Encephalitis and the common cold are still around, along with arthritis, hardening of the arteries, cancer, and coronary disease (see Figure 5–13).

The future, however, looks bright. The teacher can convey a positive outlook. Molecular biology, it is hoped, is the key that will unlock the remaining secrets of nature. Chemicals that are effective at the molecular level may influence genetic control and may prevent birth defects.

Early in the junior high school, the topic of immunization should be discussed, with practical examples coming from such diseases as smallpox, diphtheria, whooping cough, tetanus, polio, measles, German measles, influenza, mumps, and typhoid fever. Infections should be studied in the light of the infection triad—host, bacteria, and antibiotic. Eli Lilly Company distributes an excellent booklet entitled "The Triad of Infection," with clear color photographs of infected tissues.

In studying the communicable diseases, the effort will be more rewarding if the particulars can be translated into real situations, such as case studies or location studies in a community (see suggested activity on a waterborne disease, page 141). The same approach can be followed in studying the nature and prevention of coronary disease. Senior high school students are able to become involved in exciting projects such as the Columbus Study, where a community program was established to screen large numbers of individuals for risk factors.[25]

The topic of cancer is an appropriate area of instruction to illustrate the need for disease prevention. Although other degenerative diseases will be covered, cancer deserves full treatment at the secondary level. This is the time to go over breast cancer detection techniques and point out that one of every 15 women will develop breast cancer sometime in her life. The Betsi Breast Teaching Model[26] is an excellent aid on which to perfect self-examination skills (see Figure 5–14). Here, one can learn exactly what a "lump" feels like. Each breast in the model contains different lesions which provide a range of tactile characteristics. Prevention can be a real item, particularly in the case of cancer of the respiratory tract. The argument favoring periodic medical examinations and how this relates to early detection of cancer is important. The materials

---

[25]See the report by Martin D. Keller and staff, "A Study of the Primary Prevention of Coronary Heart Disease," *American Journal of Public Health*, 60:1466–1476, August, 1970.

[26]Available from OMNI Educational System, Ortho Pharmaceutical Corporation, Raritan, N.J. 08869. The company also distributes two very economical visual cassettes and viewers which can be used by the individual to learn breast self-examination skills and how a Pap smear test is taken to check for cervical cancer.

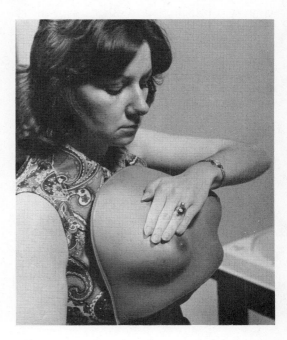

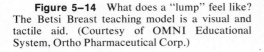

Figure 5–14 What does a "lump" feel like? The Betsi Breast teaching model is a visual and tactile aid. (Courtesy of OMNI Educational System, Ortho Pharmaceutical Corp.)

from the American Cancer Society are most helpful for teachers, particularly the booklet "Teaching About Cancer." The opportunity to tie this topic in with smoking, coronary disease variables, and environmental health (air pollution, etc.) should not be overlooked.

Behavioral Objectives

(Junior High Level)

Explains that it is easier and less expensive to prevent diseases than to cure them.

Illustrates how the degenerative, chronic, and constitutional diseases have taken a prominent role in affecting health all over the world.

Discovers that there has been an increase in the health and life expectancy of all age groups due to advances in medical sciences.

Relates how some diseases are caused by microorganisms such as bacteria, viruses, rickettsia, fungi, and protozoa.

Diagrams how the spread of disease is influenced by both the social conditions and the physical nature of the environment.

Creates a chart that depicts how disease is actually any condition which interferes with the proper functions of the individual; it may be either communicable or non-communicable in nature.

Defines the "lines of defense" which help protect the body against disease.

Checks own immunization record and acknowledges that immunization is an important protective measure against certain diseases; it may be acquired naturally by having had the disease, or artificially as a result of medically introduced substances.

Directs fellow students to public health facilities in the community where medical personnel are capable of treating and eradicating venereal disease.

Explains how degenerative or constitutional diseases (cancer, heart, and others) cannot be transmitted to others; they may be controlled by individuals, families, and the community.

Essential Topics

History and broad definition of disease (dis-ease)
Infectious disease
Degenerative disease
Immunization procedures and timetables
Cancer
High blood pressure
Arthritis
Coronary heart disease
Venereal disease
Bacterial disease (tuberculosis, strep)
Viral disease (colds, hepatitis)
Fungal disease (ringworm)
Protozoal disease (malaria)
Parasitic disease (worms)
Common cold—personal status, absenteeism, and economic consequences
Early detection practices
Case-finding

Behavioral Objectives

(Senior High Level)

Shows how chronic disorders such as diabetes, arthritis, cancer, and heart disease have similar general effects as well as unique effects on individuals and society.

Acknowledges that all tissue is vulnerable to cancerous growths.

Explains how varied and complex factors interrelate in the transmission and development of respiratory diseases such as colds, asthma, emphysema, lung cancer, pleurisy, and pneumonia.

States that through early diagnosis of some cancers it may be possible to obtain a complete cure and prolong health and longevity.

Tells others that the chief danger from a cold is that it leaves one susceptible to secondary infections such as pneumonia.

Discovers that although "cold shots" do not prevent the cold, they may reduce the severity, duration, and frequency of attacks.

Maintains that individuals have a responsibility to assist in community efforts for control and prevention of disease and disorders.

Illustrates how history demonstrates that diseases have affected the growth and development of a number of countries. Studies these situations to gain insight into future health practices.

Observes and describes mononucleosis as an infectious disease of unknown origin, with involvement of glandular tissues; it is prevalent during the spring and fall seasons.

Essential Topics

Cellular changes during some illnesses

Infectious hepatitis

Mononucleosis—implications for individual life style

Community controls of disease

Diagnostic techniques

Disease research

Cardiovascular problems

Heredity and disease

Insect control and anti-pollution

Travel restrictions

Quarantine

Venereal and vaginal diseases

Germ warfare—biological and societal implications

Public health and epidemiology

Suggested Activities

(Junior High Level)

1. Set up a family record of immunizations. Having accomplished this, open up a class discussion of the extent to which family members are properly immunized against disease. An excellent record in booklet form for class use is the "Family Health Record," distributed at 30 cents each by the American Medical Association.

2. Post a sign: *How Common Is The Common Cold?* Think of all the ideas employed to keep from getting a cold. (Eating onions, giving up kissing, standing on one's head, growing a beard to protect the throat, being sewn into long winter underwear, and refraining from bathing during the winter months are some methods that have been tried. Sir William Osler said that the cold sufferer should hang his hat on a

bedpost, get into the bed and drink whiskey until he saw two hats.) Public Affair Pamphlet No. 395, "Viruses, Colds, and Flu," is quite informative and is available from 381 Park Ave. South, New York, N.Y. 10016.

3. Trace the spread of venereal disease by constructing a Boy-Girl Infection Chart. Discuss these questions:

a. What do you think is the reason syphilis is increasing among teenagers and young adults?

b. Why is it that most cases do not get reported to public health officials despite the law requiring that this be done?

4. A half million students have had rheumatic fever. Spend time looking at the streptococcus bacillus as it invades the throat, the ear, and even the brain. Use the microscope. Illustrate by diagram the location of possible heart valve damage. What are the implications relative to prevention and living with a damaged heart.

5. Post recent news clippings about cholera in certain parts of the world. Why does this occur in countries where cleanliness and sanitary practice is not the rule? Correlate health conditions with the sociology of developing nations.

6. Show the film *Breathing Easy*.[27] Then ask the class to write a list of the kinds of health problems that were directly and indirectly referred to. Is there agreement, or are a variety of problems noted by class members?

7. Examine the class for dermatophytosis ("athlete's foot"). This may be accomplished with all class members seated along the wall of a classroom or gymnasium. Shoes and socks are removed. As the instructor walks along the line of students, each student spreads his toes. This activity can be employed to initiate a discussion of fungi and ringworm.

8. Invite a resource person from an organization such as the American Heart Association or the American Cancer Society to speak to the class about chronic diseases. Prepare individual questions to ask before the speaker comes to the class.

9. "Experience" a chronic disease by choosing to actually visit a patient with emphysema, diabetes, heart disease, cancer, and so on. Arrangements can be made to go to a hospital or rehabilitation center, or spend part of the day with a visiting public health or community nurse. Similar "experiences" can be accomplished with the emergency squad of the fire department, in a hospital emergency room, and so on.

10. Not long ago, the Los Angeles City schools were closed because of heavy air pollution. Relate polluted air (particularly from tobacco) to reduced respiratory efficiency and ultimate physical performance in such personal activities as athletics—particularly endurance events such as running, bicycling, and swimming (through decreased oxygen uptake and increased carbon monoxide).

Suggested Activities

(Senior High Level)

1. Look into the possibility of visiting a cancer clinic that is actively engaged in cancer treatment, to discuss approved methods of cancer treatment such as chemotherapy, radiation, and surgery. This must be a carefully organized project, but it can be accomplished in numerous communities.

2. Show the girls the films *Breast Cancer: Self Examination* and *Breast Exam For Teenagers,* available from the American Cancer Society as well as a number of state

---

[27]Available from the American Lung Association, 1740 Broadway, New York, N.Y. 10019.

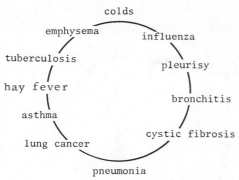

colds

emphysema   influenza

tuberculosis   pleurisy

hay fever   bronchitis

asthma   cystic fibrosis

lung cancer

pneumonia

Figure 5-15

departments of public health. At this time also distribute the American Cancer Society leaflet, "A Breast Check," which illustrates the "how to" examination.

3. Have the class work in small (3 or 4 person) committees and search for the common disease factors causing certain respiratory difficulties. (See Figure 5-15.)

4. Study the cell wall structure of bacteria in relation to antibiotic treatment. Investigate cell wall synthesis and how it is affected by the penicillins, vancomycin, and other antibiotics. The staphylococci are interesting bacteria to study. This project, if done by the students, will involve library research into the areas of medicine, biology, and biochemistry. Opportunity also exists here for some in-depth studies of disease.

5. Everybody has an opinion on the cold. Whoever named it the common cold knew what he was doing. Adults have an average of 3 colds a year; small children have 12. Ask the question: "Do you think cold tablets help?" In a 5-year study at the University of Minnesota, thousands of sniffling students were given pills—some of them sugar pills, others actual cold medicines. The students who received sugar pills got rid of their colds just as fast as the ones who took cold tablets. What is a possible explanation? With this question leave the class on their own to discover information about colds and unpredictable viruses.

6. Read the following brief summary of research having to do with a waterborne disease; then ask the class if a similar survey could be carried out by students in a local survey of a health problem:[28]

A geographically defined widespread outbreak of gastroenteritis was reported in the early spring of 1968 in western New York State.

A random sample survey of 622 subjects at risk revealed an illness attack rate of 30 per cent as compared to an attack rate of 8 per cent among 157 subjects residing nearby but with a different water supply. Symptoms of the illness were mainly abdominal pain, nausea, and diarrhea of 48 to 72 hours duration. There were no areas of clustering or absence of disease and all age groups were affected.

Water source for the affected area came from Lake Erie and was processed by a water treatment plant utilizing rapid sand filtration and sedimentation.

Specimens from multiple sources in the water supply and stools from ill subjects were all negative on bacteriologic, virologic, and chemical analysis.

Despite these negative results, the characteristics and distribution of this illness, as well as its relationship to the water treatment plant and its distribution lines, clearly pointed out the waterborne nature of this outbreak.

---

[28]Adapted from research by Harvey H. Borden, et al., "A Waterborne Outbreak of Gastroenteritis in Western New York State," *American Journal of Public Health,* 60:283-288, February, 1970.

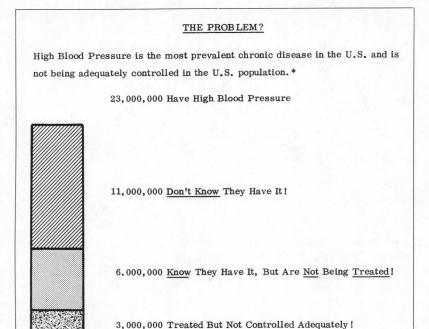

7. Like atherosclerosis, high blood pressure begins early in life. Most people do not understand this hypertension problem, nor do they realize that it affects them. Post the following chart from the National High Blood Pressure Education Program (National Institute of Health, Bethesda, Md. 20014). Let the class members size up the problem and describe what they might do about it.

8. The American Cancer Society strongly encourages teachers and students to telephone them for concrete help in learning about chronic disease. Appoint an individual to do this. Available for the teacher is the booklet, "Teacher, Please Call Us!" Also, the 3′ × 4′ wall chart guide on combating cancer, put out by Eli Lilly Company, is a superb addition to teaching aids.

9. Mononucleosis is a disease common in high school and college students. In its unusual forms it may appear as an acute infection of the liver, or as atypical pneumonia. Or it may appear as nothing at all—many people carry the disease around without even feeling sick. Why is this so? Leave the class with this question and see if they can discover an answer. Cap off the study by bringing into class two students who have had mononucleosis at some time, to discuss their symptoms and problems.

10. Look into the artificial kidneys and the use of dialysis machines. If possible, visit a clinic to see one of these prized pieces of apparatus in operation. Discuss the limitations of this treatment, as well as the "master chemist" function of the human kidney.

11. Study a food service operation, possibly a local eating establishment, for sanitary conditions. (See Figure 5–16.) Look into:
Food storage
Food preparation
Refrigeration
Disposal
Maintenance

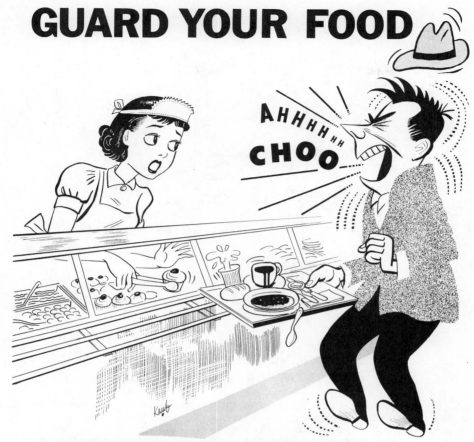

GUARD YOUR FOOD

PROTECT IT DURING STORAGE, PREPARATION, DISPLAY AND SERVICE

Figure 5–16 A poster for the classroom.

Animals, rodents, vermin
Food display and service
Handling eating utensils
Dishwashing
Paper service
Water supply and toilet
Lighting and ventilation

12. Examine plastic replicas of poison ivy, poison oak, and poison sumac in order to initiate study of poisonous plants. A fine plastic replica kit is available from Eli Lilly and Company without charge.

13. Study the operation of an artificial heart. Consider the problem of finding suitable materials for its construction, developing an implantable rechargeable power source, and devising an implantable control mechanism to meet shifting circulatory needs. (The American Heart Association film *The Heart—How It Works* should be used to introduce this assignment.) (See Figure 5–17.)

14. Look into the career of genetic counseling. What does the genetic counselor do? What kind of preparation is necessary for this profession? Use materials from The National Foundation, 800 Second Ave., New York, N.Y. 10017.

RELATION OF AUXILIARY VENTRICLE TO HEART AND AORTA

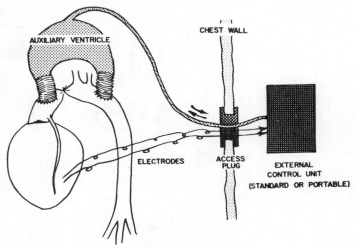

Figure 5–17

DIRECTIONS FOR RISKO (TABLE 5–5)

The purpose of this game is to give you an estimate of your chances of suffering heart attack.

The game is played by marking squares which —from left to right—represent an increase in your *risk factors.* These are medical conditions and habits associated with an increased danger of heart attack. Not all risk factors are measurable enough to be included in this game.

RULES: Study each risk factor and its row. Find the box applicable to you and circle the large number in it. For example, if you are 37, circle the number in the box labeled 31 to 40. After checking out all the rows, add the circled numbers. This total—your score—is an estimate of your risk. (See score tally below risk chart.)

HEREDITY: Count parents, grandparents, brothers, and sisters who have had heart attack and/or stroke.

TOBACCO SMOKING: If you inhale deeply and smoke a cigarette way down, add one to your classification. Do NOT subtract because you think you do not inhale or because you smoke only a half inch on a cigarette.

EXERCISE: Lower your score one point if you exercise regularly and frequently.

CHOLESTEROL OR SATURATED FAT INTAKE: A cholesterol blood level is best. If you can't get one from your doctor, then estimate honestly the percentage of solid fats you eat. These are usually of animal origin—lard, cream, butter, and beef and lamb fat. If you eat much of this, your cholesterol level probably will be high. The U.S. average, 40 percent, is too high for good health.

BLOOD PRESSURE: If you have no recent reading but have passed an insurance industrial examination, chances are you are 140 or less.

SEX: This line takes into account the fact that men have from 6 to 10 times more heart attacks than women of childbearing age.

Because of the difficulty in measuring them, the following risk factors are not included in the chart:

DIABETES: particularly when present for many years.

CHARACTER OR PERSONALITY and the STRESS under which you live.

VITAL CAPACITY: determined by measuring the amount of air you can take into your lungs in proportion to the size of your lungs. The less air you can breathe, the higher your risk.

ELECTROCARDIOGRAM: if certain abnormalities are present in the record of the electrical currents generated by your heart, you have a higher risk.

GOUT: is caused by a higher than normal amount of uric acid in the blood. Patients have an increased risk.

If you have a number of risk factors, for the sake of your health, ask your doctor to check your medical conditions and quit your risk-factor habits.

NOTE: The fact that various habits or conditions may be rated similarly in this test does not mean these are of equal risk. The reaction of individual human beings to risk factors—as to many other things—is so varied it is impossible to draw valid conclusions for any individual.

This scale has been developed only to highlight what the risk factors are and what can be done about them. It is not designed to be a medical diagnosis.

	1	2	3	4	6	8
AGE	10 to 20	21 to 30	31 to 40	41 to 50	51 to 60	61 and over
	1	2	3	4	6	7
HEREDITY	No known history of heart disease	1 relative with cardiovascular disease over 60	2 relatives with cardiovascular disease over 60	1 relative with cardiovascular disease under 60	2 relatives with cardiovascular disease under 60	3 relatives with cardiovascular disease under 60
	0	1	2	3	5	7
WEIGHT	More than 5 lbs. below standard weight	- 5 to + 5 lbs. standard weight	6-20 lbs. overweight	21-35 lbs. overweight	36-50 lbs. overweight	51 or more lbs. overweight
	0	1	2	4	6	10
TOBACCO SMOKING	Non-user	Cigar and/or pipe	10 cigarets or less a day	20 cigarets a day	30 cigarets a day	40 cigarets or more a day
	1	2	3	5	6	8
EXERCISE	Intensive occupational and recreational exertion	Moderate occupational and recreational exertion	Sedentary work and intense recreational exertion	Sedentary occupational and moderate recreational exertion	Sedentary work and light recreational exertion	Complete lack of all exercise
	1	2	3	4	5	7
CHOLESTEROL OR FAT % IN DIET	Cholesterol below 180 mg. Diet contains no animal or solid fats	Cholesterol 181-205 mg. Diet contains 10% animal or solid fats	Cholesterol 206-230 mg. Diet contains 20% animal or solid fats	Cholesterol 231-255 mg. Diet contains 30% animal or solid fats	Cholesterol 256-280 mg. Diet contains 40% animal or solid fats	Cholesterol 281 or more mg. Diet contains 50% or more animal or solid fats
	1	2	3	4	6	8
BLOOD PRESSURE	100 upper reading	120 upper reading	140 upper reading	160 upper reading	180 upper reading	200 or over upper reading
	1	2	3	5	6	7
SEX	Female under 40	Female 40-50	Female over 50	Male	Stocky male	Bald stocky male

If You Score:

6-11	Risk well below average
12-17	Risk below average
18-24	Risk generally average
25-31	Risk moderate
32-40	Risk at a dangerous level
41-62	Danger urgent. See your doctor now.

15. Display the 4′ × 4′ chart, "The Good Seed," distributed by Eli Lilly Company (no charge). This elaborate chart is a pictorial story explaining the search for microorganisms in the soil that may produce lifesaving antibiotics, and the manufacturing processes required to make them available to physicians. It is a complete story pertaining to screening, culture propagation, fermentation, filtration, isolation, purification, sterile transfer room, testing procedures, finishing, and distribution.

16. Carefully study Table 5–5 and the accompanying directions. This game of **RISKO** was developed by the Michigan Heart Association and can be of considerable

significance to high school students—not only in terms of their own lives, but the lives of family members and the peer group. Permit individuals to voluntarily score a parent or friend in an older age bracket.

QUESTIONS FOR DISCUSSION

1. To what extent is it true that publicity given to genuine medical advances has alerted the members of our society, arousing in them a feeling of impatience when confronting a difficult, chronic problem? Is this impatience justified? Is it not true that over the years medicine has proved its ability to find the cause and cure (or prevention) of many diseases?

2. Is there a *need to believe* something that is untrue, and therefore be out of the ordinary reach of education and persuasion? Are there people who align themselves against the "establishment" and frequently identify strongly with the "out" group—especially when they feel persecuted by an "in" group, such as the American Medical Association?

3. Have the medical and health professions been too lax in dealing with clearly unethical or shoddy practices of their members? Would a Ralph Nader or Common Cause investigation do more harm than good? Shouldn't reputable groups be able to influence their own people?

4. If, indeed,"selection is the essence of teaching," how does one determine just *what* to teach in such a broad area as Physical Health? In short, what determines the selection of more or less material and activities pertaining to nutrition as compared with physical activity, or disease control as compared with dental health?

5. To implement is to accomplish, to fulfill, to carry out what was conceived in the first place. Comment on the influence of content selection, educational methods, and teaching aids as implementation variables.

6. Terhune believes that it is most important to determine if students who have poor dietary and dental care habits are *willing* to modify their behavior. If you were teaching dental health what might you do at this crucial starting point?

7. If you agree that multicultural family practices are an important consideration in education, then how would you relate food to feelings and aspirations in a classroom discussion?

SUGGESTED ACTIVITIES

1. Visit a college or university library where there are professional education materials, and carefully examine several curriculum guides pertaining to junior and senior high school health education. Are purposes set up in terms of teacher goals? Concepts? Behavioral objectives? Competencies? Is there a rationale behind the terms used? Are provisions made for evaluating students in the Physical Health area? If not, try to develop some evaluation techniques (e.g., appraise how well students count calories and relate them to food intake, see how they score in a motor fitness test, record individual attitudes toward medical personnel and public health agencies responsible for various regulations pertaining to disease control).

2. Health departments through the country have been very successful in conducting rubella clinics. Because of intense educational campaigns, well over 90 per cent of tar-

get age groups in most communities were reached. Interview a local public health officer to hear a first hand account of a rubella program. Why should rebella protection work while it is so difficult for cigarette smoking and fluoridation campaigns to succeed in some places? Search the literature for possible answers.

3. Much has been written, particularly by Dr. Kenneth H. Cooper, about the value of aerobic conditioning programs for the general public. Look up some articles having to do with exercise physiology and compare aerobics with some other kind of physical exercise routine in terms of (1) weight control and (2) cardiorespiratory endurance.

4. How practical in the average high school is it to experiment with pulse rate, blood pressure, body density, body weight, and breathing rate? Survey several nearby secondary schools to ascertain the extent to which the above experimentation takes place.

5. Examine the health curriculum materials used in a particular secondary school. *How* are they used to put across certain content? Are students only mildly involved, and if so is it due to poor motivation or to the inherent weakness of materials? For example, does displaying "before" and "after" plaster of paris models of maloccluded teeth *move* the class in any noticeable way — or is this about as effective as a filmstrip on the topic? Also, comment on the difficulty of doing a good evaluation here.

6. Among other things, the movement to liberate women has helped to dispel the idea that girls should not exert themselves physically lest they somehow develop male-like muscles, disturb the menstrual cycle, and become overly aggressive. Survey (1) secondary school girls, (2) secondary school boys, and (3) a cross section of teachers to find out what they think about vigorous exercise for women. Pool your findings with other class members.

7. Study body composition and its relationship to weight control activities by doing skinfold measurements. Complete instructions and appropriate examples of data recording forms are described in the manual by Wayne E. Sinning on pages 46 to 50. (See Selected References at the end of this chapter.)

SELECTED REFERENCES

Albertini, Tullio, et al. "A Dental Health Education Program in the Open Classroom: Report of a Pilot Study," *Journal of School Health*, 43:566–571, November, 1973.

Allensworth, Diane, D. "Common Intestinal Parasitic Infections in the School-Age Population," *Journal of School Health*, 45:331–338, June, 1975.

Barrett, Morris. *Health Education Guide*. Second edition, Philadelphia: Lea and Febiger, 1975.

Cornacchia, Harold J. *Consumer Health*, St. Louis: C. V. Mosby Co., 1976. Chapters 10 and 11.

Dearth, Florean. *Dental Health Education*, Thorofare, N.J.: Charles B. Slack Co., 1975.

Edington, D. W., and Lee Cunningham. "More On Applied Physiology of Exercise," *Journal of Health, Physical Education and Recreation*, 45:18–20, February, 1974.

Engs, Ruth C., H. Eugene Barnes, and Molly Wantz. *Health Games Students Play: Creative Strategies for Health Education*, Dubuque, Iowa: Kendall-Hunt Publishing Co., 1975, Chapter 7, 8.

Maness William. "What Do You Really Know About Exercise?" *Today's Health*, 53:14–17, November, 1975.

McInnis, Mary E. *Essentials of Communicable Disease*, St. Louis: C. V. Mosby Co., 1975.

McWilliams, Margaret. *Nutrition for the Growing Years*, New York: John Wiley & Sons, Inc., 1975.

Oja, Pekka, et al. "Feasibility of An 18 Months' Physical Training Program for Middle-Aged Men and Its Effect on Physical Fitness," *American Journal of Public Health*, 64:459–460, May, 1974.

Read, Donald, A., and Walter H. Green. *Creative Teaching in Health*. Second edition, New York: Macmillan Co., 1975, Chapter 3.

Sinning, Wayne E. *Experiments and Demonstrations in Exercise Physiology*, Philadelphia: W. B. Saunders Co., 1975, pp. 35–40.

Swartz, Hillary, et al. "Differences in Mean Adolescent Blood Pressure by Age, Sex, Ethnic Origin, Obesity, and Familial Tendency," *Journal of School Health*, 45:71–75, February, 1975.

Zeller, William W. "Adolescent Attitudes and Cutaneous Health," *Journal of School Health*, 40:115–120, March, 1970.

Chapter 6

Area II—Mental Health

Components:
1. Mental Health (Including Death Education)
2. Alcohol and Drugs
3. Smoking Education
4. Sex and Family Living Education

Although each of the above major topics is clearcut and able to stand very well by itself, there is, nevertheless, a substantial degree of communality. There is a common bond which pertains to how one lives, aspires, and directs oneself. This is related to a mental outlook in which a level of self-concept and self-actualization is manifested. In more than a passing way, therefore, there is a mental health base that has much to do with alcoholism and drug abuse, with boy-girl relationships and human sexuality, and, frequently, the heavy use of tobacco. In short, alienated and unhappy youth frequently demonstrate the symptoms of poor mental health when they abuse and overindulge in the chemical world or display an irresponsible attitude and behavior toward sexual relationships. Peculiar to all four areas, and noticeably absent when problems arise, is the positive *humanistic dimension.*

Humanism is not a new concept. Humanistic education, in which teachers reach out to young people with warmth and empathy and are concerned with the affective domain, is not new either. But it is essential that it be viewed for what it is worth in each of the four areas, simply because young people have been turned off too many times during their developing years by some parents, some teachers, and the "establishment." Consequently, they do not become close enough to people who can help them gain appropriate health understanding and bolster their levels of self-esteem and self-acceptance.

Self-actualization is the primary goal of education, says Arthur Combs. This is because self-actualizing persons are (1) well informed, (2) possessed of positive self-concepts, (3) open to experience, and (4) possessed of deep feelings of identification with others. Involved here for the educator are mental health ramifications which are rooted in humanistic goals of education. Combs expresses his concern for *personal meaning* in education as follows:[1]

> Modern education must produce far more than persons with cognitive skills. It must produce *humane* individuals, persons who can be relied upon to pull their own weight in

---

[1]Arthur W. Combs, *Educational Accountability: Beyond Behavioral Objectives,* Washington, D.C.: Association for Supervision and Curriculum Development, 1972, p. 23.

148

our society, who can be counted upon to behave responsibly and cooperatively. We need good citizens, free of prejudice, concerned about their fellow citizens, loving, caring fathers and mothers, persons of goodwill whose values and purposes are positive-feeling persons with wants and desires likely to motivate them toward positive interactions. These are the things that make us human. Without them we are automatons, fair game for whatever crowd-swaying, stimulus-manipulating demagogue comes down the pike. The humane qualities are absolutely essential to our way of life—far more important, even, than the learning of reading, for example. We can live with a bad reader; a bigot is a danger to everyone.[1]

An excellent example of how the humanistic view is being applied is in Dade County, Florida, where the school program aims at providing students, parents, and other community members with skills for resolving abuses and other life problems before they reach crisis proportions. Based on the premise that abuse is a symptom of an individual's problem or problems, the program emphasizes personal development of students, interpersonal awareness, teacher-student interaction, the development of personal value systems, and individual decision-making skills. There are other major components including peer counseling for high school students, alternative activities outside school hours, and staff development programs to train teachers in affective education approaches. Significantly, the evaluation of this program after its first two years was positive, with pre- and post-testing and student survey reports clearly indicating increases in leadership skills, individual responsibility, self-concept, and teacher-student communications.

1. MENTAL HEALTH

One of the most significant contributions of the behavioral sciences today is the idea that one's feelings about self are the basic determinant in mental health. Because of the magnitude of the topic this entire book could easily be devoted to the mental health education concerns of youth.

The school has at least two especially significant tasks. First, it should help develop a mentally healthy person who perceives reality with minimal distortion and is able to communicate these perceptions effectively. Second, it should develop a proper level of self-esteem which contributes both to intellectual functioning and general health status. The task is difficult to accomplish because there are so many negative influences in society which serve as poor examples of adjustment among peers and parents alike.

Another disturbing factor is that there is an increasing number of secondary school age youngsters who are unhappy, disenchanted, and mentally ill to the point of considering suicide. Over 25,000 persons committed suicide in a recent year, and somewhere between a quarter and a half million attempted it. It has been shown that loneliness is in back of much of the despair and depression of young people. It is they who should ask the question: What is loneliness? How does it come about? In the Montgomery County (Maryland) crisis intervention program, teenagers themselves were part of the action. They exchanged information, planned services to adolescents, carried on discussion groups with mental health workers, gathered local statistics, and helped man the "hot line." These students *experienced* mental health needs at first hand. In the evaluation of "hot line" data, it was found that two and a half times as many girls called as did boys; one of four of the callers was 13 or 14 years old. The ages calling were broken down into percentages: 12 and under, 16%; 13 through 15, 40%; 16 through 18, 32%; and 19 and over, 12%. In a one week period the chief reasons for calls were, in order of frequency: boy/girl relationships, family conflict, just to "talk," drugs, pregnancy, and social inhibition. This led the adolescents and adults alike to conclude that young people need help,

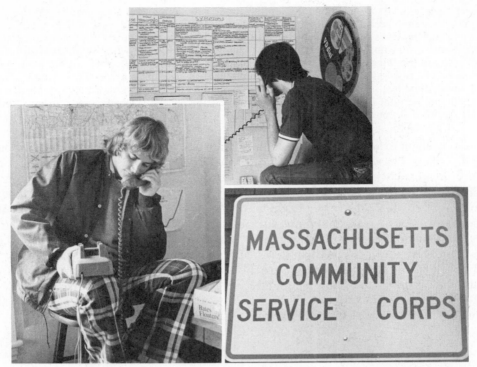

Figure 6–1   Student-initiated "Hotline." (Courtesy of Massachusetts Community Service Corps)

but they also need mental health resources in elementary and junior high schools. When resources are missing students can be motivated to initiate action. In Massachusetts a group of high school students simply established their own "Operation Venus," not only to help in the battle to eradicate venereal disease, but to solve social and psychological problems through an effective "hotline" arrangement. This small student operation later blossomed into the Massachusetts Community Service Corps (see Figure 6–1).

From an instructional viewpoint, what can be done with the rank and file junior-senior high school students to develop a proper attitude toward managing onself and one's environment? How do students see the topic as relevant? How can we teach the particulars and discuss the causes and effects without appearing to be misunderstood moralists?

It seems important to draw from the class members their acknowledged problems or concerns, no matter how minor they may appear. These can be volunteered at random or gathered through checklist tabulation. Not only will this approach get a number of topics out on the table, but it will serve to point up the fact that what one student believes to be *his* problem is frequently possessed by others. Such things such as acne pimples, voice irregularities, shyness, lack of confidence, and insecurity can be shared in a "misery loves company" manner. This normally will help bring about a classroom climate which seems appropriate for the instruction to follow. This is at least one good reason for formally structuring a unit or lessons specifically on mental health.

There have been a few studies reported that indicate a significant correlation between the problem-solving method of teaching and a more effective development of perceptions, emotions, and interpersonal relationships of students. Time is given to students to assess a problem, to collect data related to it, and then reach a solution on the basis of the data collection. Small group activity here helps boys and girls to understand and respect the viewpoints of their classmates. Gaining this respect early in the junior high years contributes to the process of maturation and self-discovery.)The teacher, however, must be able to foster group activity and be aware of a number of effective techniques. Society discourages intimacy between people, which makes the job that much more difficult for the teacher. The task is to assist students to:[2]

1. Develop an understanding of the physical basis of communication.

2. Make maximum use of cognitive and affective abilities to facilitate successful interaction with life situations.

3. Develop nonverbal as well as verbal communication skills.

4. Establish the universality of problems.

5. Experiment with alternative behaviors resulting in an enlarged view of their potential and competence.

6. Assess actual behavior as it deviates from conscious intentions.

7. Develop an awareness of the effects of their behavior on others.

8. Develop an acceptance of the constructive aspects of criticism that can direct behavior toward goal achievement.

9. Enhance self-esteem, decrease defensive reactions, and facilitate meaningful personal relationships.

10. Accept the attitudes and values of others.

11. Differentiate ways in which people satisfy their needs.

12. Listen to and empathize with others.

13. Affirm themselves in group situations.

14. Develop an appreciation for group cohesiveness in the decision making process.

---

[2]Adapted from Ronald A. Fusco and Michael J. Perlin, "Guidelines For Group Process," *School Health Review,* 5:37, July-August, 1974.

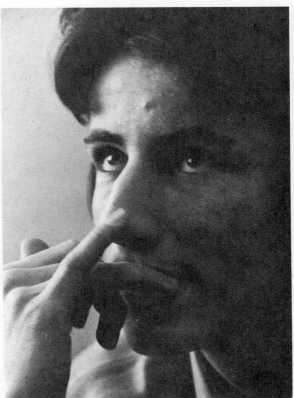

Figure 6–2 Just when so many other pressing problems have to be solved, these bumps, scars and pimples may make things worse, particularly with all the pressure from films and publicity which try to persuade you to be handsome at all costs. Acne may be as much a symptom as a cause of anxiety. Sex, scholastic achievement, attitude towards parents, trying to be an adult—all contribute to an adolescent's physical and mental state. (Courtesy of World Health Organization)

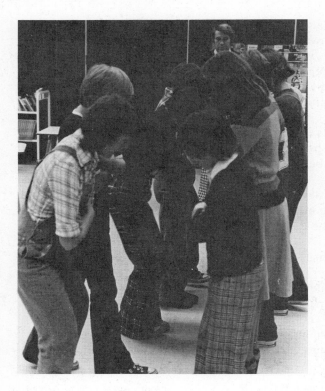

Figure 6–3 A non-verbal activity to demonstrate personal reactions to conflicts of individual freedoms. Note the teacher taking part in the activity. (Courtesy of Loren Bensley, Jr., and Brad Fleming, Central Michigan University)

The senior high school pupil may appear to have discovered himself; he is more organized, often more achieving, but frequently more anxious, more concerned about the larger world, and needs greatly to be understood. At this period the health teaching should be directed toward an identification with the larger community where he can think and act—something that both transcends the person and gives him a worth greater than any he might achieve alone. It is possible to shape an individual's sense of significance both by his communities and his position within them. Significance here refers to the value placed upon the person by key people in his environment. It complements how he views himself (self-esteem). Moreover, when older students work with others in the community, there occur certain preventive aspects of community mental health.[3] In short, there is some profit all around as students move out of the classroom and into their local environment to help solve problems, be of assistance to others, discover new things about others as well as themselves, and return to the classroom to share their experiences with class members. There is an opportunity to visit hobby shops and recreation centers, industries, mental institutions and prisons, and talk with social agency personnel directly concerned with delinquent youths.

Perhaps most of all, effective instruction in the mental health area will present learning situations where students begin to acknowledge more and more that the *Weltanschauung* ("world view") of each person begins with "me." For many this will be a newly-discovered reality. Too early they have heard and used the worlds "they," "he," "you," and "others," on all issues. They (we) speak of problems, "out there," of violence "out there," of poorly adjusted folks "out there" somewhere; and yet much of the "out there" is really close at hand and a part of their lives. Slowly there will grow an in-

---

[3]For an elaboration on this view see Donald C. Klein, "The Meaning of Community in a Preventive Mental Health Program," *American Journal of Public Health,* 59:2005–2012, November, 1969.

creasing consciousness that starts with the first person, with "I." With the determination of each "I" the world view will change and the individual pupil will begin to make his life more accountable to the highest purposes. Instead of pointing to the frailties and faults of society, each person will have a logic for his own decision-making, and this is the foundation of the corporate society.

Much has been written about ways of making the mental health topic more meaningful. In this respect value clarification techniques have much to offer—perhaps more here than in other health areas.

Although considerable information has been prepared both in support of and illustrating value clarification techniques, there is much evidence to indicate that many teachers do not engage in this dynamic process (for details see Chapter 9). As Dalis and Strasser point out, they discuss health issues and assign "thought" questions, but they do not begin at the "starting point of values modification or reinforcement."[4] A real awareness of self and of self with others must occur in relation to a particular health value if the stage is to be set for action. Certainly, an individual's values are modified only when he or she decides they should be changed.

Particularly useful in helping to implement value clarification techniques in the mental health area are materials from the Center for Humanities, Inc., 2 Holland Ave., White Plains, N.Y. 10603. Excellent guideline sheets are available for teachers to freely reproduce for class use. A number of particularly appropriate audio-visual programs may also be obtained from this organization.

Present day mental health education is deeply involved in *death education*. In fact, the area is so important that the Educational Resources Information Center (ERIC) now treats the subject as part of the health education curriculum.[5] Certainly, it is a fascinating topic to examine in a society which frequently attempts to avoid the particulars of aging and dying. An understanding of death is a preparation for living. The adolescent lives for the present, but frequently has real fears about death in the remote future. In coming to grips with the dying process a person may gain a deeper understanding of his own feelings and those of others. Numerous authors point out that death frequently presents a crisis state out of which coping with a new life style becomes difficult. Especially helpful for class use are these sources:

Leviton, Daniel, "A Course on Death Education and Suicide Prevention: Implication for Health Education," *Journal of the American College Health Association*, April, 1971, pp. 217–220.

Kubler-Ross, Elizabeth, *Questions and Answers on Death and Dying*, New York: Macmillan Co., 1974.

Alterkruse Berger, Carol and Alterkruse Berger, Patrick F., "Death on Demand," *Commonweal*, 52:585–589, December, 1975.

Feifel, H., "Perceptions of Death," *Annals of the New York Academy of Sciences*, December 19, 1969, pp. 669–677.

Berg, D. W., and G. W. Daugherty, "Teaching About Death," *Today's Education*, 62:47–51, March, 1973.

Toynbee, Arnold, et al., *Man's Concern With Death*, New York: McGraw-Hill, Inc., 1969.

---

[4]Gus T. Dalis and Ben B. Strassen, "The Starting Point for Values Clarification," *School Health Review*, 5:6–10, January/February, 1974. See also Sidney Simon, Leland W. Howe, and Howard Kirschenbaum, *Values Clarification: A Handbook of Practical Strategies for Students and Teachers*, New York: Hart Publishing Co., 1972.

[5]See the informative teaching publication by Loren B. Bensley, Jr., "Death Education as a Learning Experience," Washington, D.C.: ERIC Clearinghouse on Teacher Education, 1975. (1 Dupont Circle, Washington, D.C. 20036).

Green, B. R., and D. P. Irish (editors), *Death Education: Preparation for Living,* Cambridge, Mass.: Schenkman Publishing Co., 1971.

Crase, Dixie, R., and Crase, Darrell. "Live Issues Surrounding Death Education," *Journal of School Health,* 44:70–75, February, 1974.

In their treatment of the subject Crase and Crase are quick to point out that successful death education contributes considerably to optimum mental health if the instructor determines student interests and attitudes early in the course. There should also be an interdisciplinary approach involving medicine, law, insurance, psychology, sociology, and theology. Resource persons should be brought into the classroom, and comparisons of death practices made of various ethnic, cultural, and religious groups. Current death issues pertaining to such sociobiological concerns as abortion, suicide, and euthanasia would be included.

In establishing a unit of study on death education McMahon prefaces her work with high school students with a death questionnaire to spark interest and sample viewpoints.[6] Then she raises questions and sets up student activities covering the following units:

The Taboo of Death
Definitions of Death: Biological, Social, and Psychological
The Crisis of Man
Views on Death and Dying
Understanding the Dying Patient or Relative
The Funeral, Burial, and Bereavement: Psychological Implications
Understanding Suicide and Self-destructive Behavior

---

[6]Joan D. McMahon, "A Unit for Independent Study in Death Education," *Journal of School Health,* 43:27–34, October, 1973.

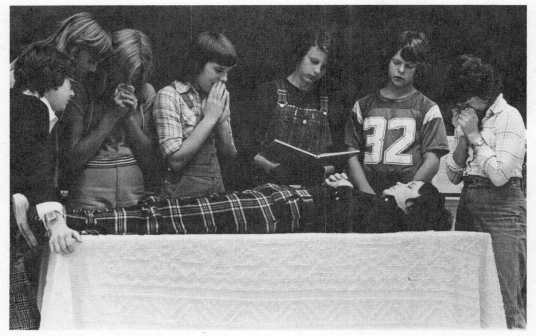

Figure 6–4   Death education through role play to better understand feelings. (Courtesy of Loren Bensley, Jr., and Brad Fleming, Central Michigan University)

Behavioral Objectives

(Junior High Level)

Demonstrates how sound mental health means being on "good terms with yourself," accepting others as they are, and meeting the demands of life as best you can.

Indicates that personality develops as a continuing process; there are ways to develop a worthy personality.

Shows a delicate balance between self-expression and self-control.

Explains that no one factor is responsible for one's mental health; heredity sets limits and environment determines levels of attainment.

Describes how environmental stress can cause physiological reactions which in turn may cause anxiety; a pleasant environment may bring about feelings of calm and tranquility.

Tells how growing up means facing and carrying through tasks without frequently finding excuses for failure.

Details how teenage popularity is based on many factors; peer pressures sometimes produce stress which individuals can learn to handle; self-respect is a prerequisite for receiving and giving respect to others.

Expresses emotions in an acceptable manner and they can be controlled; individuals with problems can be helped.

Outlines how people learn to cope with the changes and complexities of society; problems and frustrations are individual, yet all people of all societies deal with similar problems.

Explains how individuals must assume responsibility for their own health; almost everyone has the capacity for physical, mental and emotional growth.

Essential Topics

Personal values	Happiness
Heredity and environment	Teenage popularity
Success and attainment	Mental illness
Emotional outlets	Citizenship and mental health
Growth differences	Parental conflicts
Personality development	Leadership responsibilities
	Self-acceptance

Behavioral Objectives

(Senior High Level)

Describes the complexity of human behavior, and how personality is a composite of one's total being.

Demonstrates how socially useful work gives a person dignity; achievements and improved status add to the self-image.

Illustrates a variety of possible life plans with probable courses; identifies needs, abilities and problems that help one choose a possible life plan.

Explains in detail how mental illness is one of the major health problems of Western civilization; mentally ill individuals are being helped in a number of ways.

Names a number of common misconceptions and fallacies concerning mental illness.

Shows how the mentally mature person strives to accept worthiness of all people regardless of cultural, ethnic, or religious characteristics.

Sets forth several illustrations of psychological stress and how it produces physiological changes which may lead to chronic disease and disorders.

Names a number of challenging health careers directly and indirectly associated with the mental health area.

Organizes a play therapy session that might be used with institutionalized individuals.

Writes clearly about own feelings concerning death and dying attitudes and practices in the local community.

Essential Topics

Theories of personality	Status seekers versus true leaders
Goal-directed behavior	Achievement level and longevity
Adjustment patterns	Aging and mental health
Mental hospitals	Psychological stress
Sheltered workshops	Mental disorders
Community mental health centers	Emotional climate
Recreation and mental well being	Socioeconomic status
Mental health professionals	Alcoholism
Cultural determinants of behavior	Play therapy
Mental maturity	Death and dying

Suggested Activities

(Junior High Level)

1. Arrange to view the instructional television series, "Self Incorporated." It is designed to help early adolescents better deal with the problems of growing up; there are 15-minute programs where 11 to 13 year olds reflect on who they are, their normalcy, and where they are going. Workshop materials for classes are available from the Agency for Instructional Television, Box A, Bloomington, Indiana 47401.

2. Prepare a paper (or it could be a short talk) on "The Most Unforgettable Individual I Have Ever Known."

3. Initiate a discussion of basic human needs by writing on the board the needs as they are suggested by the students (love, security, acceptance, etc.). Follow this up with suggestions as to *how* these needs are met.

4. Illustrate through role playing appropriate and inappropriate expressions of the emotions. Properly worked out ahead of time, this can be a presentation that is both humorous and meaningful. It will take a degree of skill to illustrate rather well such examples as anxiety, fear, apprehension, worry, hatred, and jealousy.

5. Post the following quotation in large print where the class can readily observe it for two or three days. Then take a look at what pupils think it means:

> "Give me the power to change those things that should be changed; to leave unchanged those things that should not be changed; and the wisdom to know the difference."

Later, refer to the value of adaptability or the courage to "accept what cannot be changed."

6. Investigate the characteristics of a "group." Why do they hold together? Why is a peer-group something pretty special? How is the group strengthened by positive contributions of individual members? Do this by establishing a double circle of chairs, with *participants* in the inner circle discussing the issue, and *observers* on the outside listening only. Then reverse the participant-observer roles.

7. Employ the Value Continuum referred to by Simon, Howe, and Kirschenbaum to appraise feelings on controversial issues.[7] After students have checked their position on the pro-con scale, open the issue for discussion.

The Value Continuum

Pro / / / / / Con
View ⟋ ⟋ ⟋ ⟋ ⟋ View

8. Formulate a list of persons and organizations to which an individual may turn for help when problems arise. After this activity, it may be timely to invite a counselor, clergyman, social worker, or similar person to visit the classroom and tell of his work.

9. Arrange to complete a *Personal Coat of Arms* in Sidney Simon style.[8] This activity provides students with an opportunity for internal reflection. As students continue to work with value clarification activities, the following types of questions may arise: "Am I satisfied with my life and the goals I have set for myself? Are there changes I want to make in my life?" The personal coat of arms activity is a fun way for students to consider these questions.

Directions

Provide students with a full-page copy of the following coat of arms or let them draw their own:

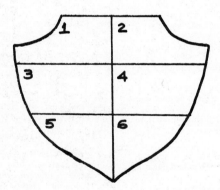

Pictures representing a student's answers to the following questions should be sketched in the appropriate areas of their coats of arms.

a. Draw a picture to represent one thing you do very well and one picture to represent something you are struggling to improve. This area will have two pictures.

b. Represent one value about which you have a deep commitment and would "never budge."

c. Draw the material possession most significant to you.

d. Draw two pictures in this area—one to represent your greatest achievement of the past year and the other to show your biggest setback, failure, or defeat.

e. Show what you would do with your life if you had one year to do whatever you wanted with guaranteed success.

f. What three descriptive words would you like people to write on your gravemarker.

---

[7]Sidney Simon, Leland Howe, and Howard Kirschenbaum, *Values Clarification: A Handbook of Practical Strategies for Teachers and Students,* New York: Hart Publishing Co., 1972.

[8]This particular activity was reported by Richard G. Schlaadt, "Implementing the Values Clarification Process," *School Health Review,* 5:10–13, January/February, 1974.

Emphasize that their drawings can be simple (stick figures, etc.) and need not have meaning to anyone but themselves. The coats of arms can be shared and discussed, if students choose to do so.

10. Express opinions on how junior high school age people can be helped when having troubles of a mental-emotional nature. A qualified specialist can help those who:

> persistently lie, cheat, steal
> take advantage of other students
> defy the teacher and school as a whole
> hold themselves away from the rest of the group
> seem excessively shy
> do an excessive amount of daydreaming
> work far below the level of their ability

11. Employ parts of the Center for Humanities material shown below. Several programs like this are available on request.

Am I Worthwhile? Identity and Self-Image

This program represents a new approach to the area of adolescent development. Relevant works of literature are combined with movie stills, photographs, graphics, as well as masterpieces of art, to give young people a broader perspective on their own lives. They are reassured that the struggles and difficulties of growing up are not unique to their generation alone. All people in all times and in all places have confronted similar problems. By discovering how others have solved these problems, adolescents can learn how to strengthen their own personalities and make their futures more purposeful and fulfilling.

The Program at a Glance . . .

Part I:

All human beings must examine themselves in order to determine who they are and what their worth is. Throughout life, this process of evaluation and discovery is repeated, but it is most notable during adolescence.

1. Our self-image is, in part, influenced by the image others have of us.
2. Young adults are often concerned with who they are and who they will be.
3. Our identity is defined by our emotions and goals.
4. By establishing independence and a sense of individuality we can shape our self-image.
5. It is only after an individual feels worthwhile, that he or she can reach out and help others.

Part II:

Everyone is capable of making a contribution to society; by recognizing the gifts of others, we enrich and heighten our own sense of self-esteem.

1. Individuals often feel cut off from society and unable to find people who accept them as they are.
2. Society often seems less interested in who a person really is than in his outside image.
3. Competition can isolate people from one another.
4. Love is a universal need; it is a unifying force in human relationships and essential in the development of self-awareness.
5. The dignity of all humans depends on their feeling useful in society and worthy of giving and receiving love.

Use this program when discussing:

Guidance:

1. The differences between how we see ourselves and how others see us (Marilyn Monroe).
2. The positive and negative aspects of conforming to peer and parental influence.
3. The importance of critical thinking in defining goals.
4. The establishment of meaningful human relationships.

5. The achievement of responsible independence and self-confidence.

English:

1. The identity crises expressed in literature (Arthur Cavanaugh's "Roseanne of Yesterday"; Edgar Friedenberg's *The Vanishing Adolescent;* John Knowles's *A Separate Peace).*
2. Individuality versus conformity (Paul Zindel's *The Pigman,* S. E. Hinton's *That Was Then, This is Now).*
3. Defining one's sense of worth within the framework of society (Charlotte Brontë's *Jane Eyre,* Hinton's *That Was Then, This Is Now).*
4. The expression of different forms of love (Carson McCullers' "The Ballad of the Sad Café"; Mary Stolz's *Wait For Me, Michael).*

Social Studies:

1. Culture as an influence on the development of self-image.
2. Peer influence in the search for one's identity.
3. The contribution to be made by each individual to society (Edward Everett Hale's "I Am One"; Nikki Giovanni's "Winter Poem").
4. The influence of the family in the development of self-worth (Margaret Mead's *Family).*

Humanities:

1. The expression of individuality through the arts.
2. The feeling of worth derived from helping others.
3. Alienation as a major theme in 20th-century art and literature.
4. The importance of human interaction.

Art

Includes works by Benton, Burchfield, Cézanne, Degas, Gauguin, Homer, Hopper, Hundertwasser, Matisse, Picasso, Renoir, Shahn, Toulouse-Lautrec, Van Gogh, Wyeth; plus cartoons; photographs by Ken Heyman and Dorothea Lange; and movie stills.

Music

Includes excerpts from Don McLean's "Crossroads," Pete Seeger's "Little Boxes Song," The Beatles' "Eleanor Rigby," and songs by Woody Guthrie.

A service of The Center for Humanities, Inc.

Two Holland Avenue/White Plains, New York 10603/(914) 946-0601

No. 601

12. Assign class members to a supplementary reading list in which they are to select some descriptions of emotions people have felt and the ways in which they expressed them. This is an attempt to help students understand their own emotions better. The class members should comment on the descriptions and note whether they have felt the same in similar situations.

13. Collect and post photographs, drawings, and pictures from newspapers and magazines that express emotions and attitudes. What effect might a particular facial expression have on different people in a variety of situations? Will an expression of emotion affect an individual one way and a mob another? What is "mob hysteria"? Continue to use the pictures to show how posture reveals attitudes and feelings.

14. Examine the issue of individual freedoms. Try an activity in which each student has a chance to complete the following form:

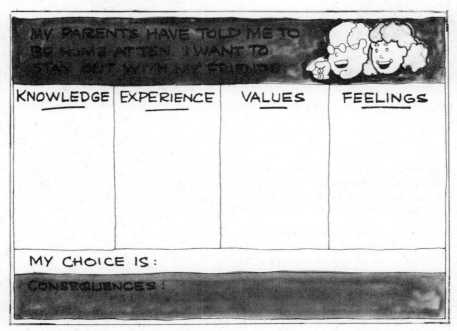

15. Make an assignment to watch one or two "family situation comedies" on television. Ask what roles were played by the father, mother, children. Were they real? How were recognition, security, and affection shown? When were there times of need for parental guidance?

16. Set up a group of students to implement the concept of "people helping people" by applying it to "children helping children." This is a project-oriented type of learning activity. What are the kinds of things that can be done? How do pupils *feel* about doing them?

17. Request a one sentence reaction to the poem *"Richard Cory"* by Edwin Arlington Robinson:

Whenever Richard Cory went downtown,
  We people on the pavement looked at him:
He was a gentleman from sole to crown,
  Clean favored, and imperially slim.

And he was always quietly arrayed,
  And he was always human when he talked;
But still he fluttered pulses when he said,
  "Good-morning," and he glittered when he walked.

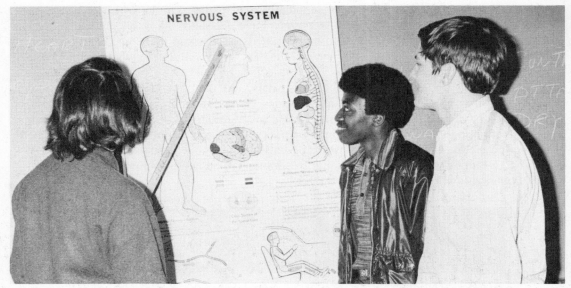

Figure 6–5   Examining the physical basis of mental health. (Courtesy of Norfolk, Virginia, Public Schools)

And he was rich—yes, richer than a king—
   And admirably schooled in every grace;
In fine, we thought that he was everything
   to make us wish that we were in his place.

So on we worked, and waited for the light,
   And went without the meat, and cursed the bread;
And Richard Cory, one calm summer night,
   Went home and put a bullet through his head.

18. Demonstrate states of mental health. Cut up individual pieces of paper with the words anger, hatred, jealousy, fear, worry, anxiety, and so on, written on each piece. Have class members draw a slip and act out the particular emotional state. For additional ideas see the superb book *Alternative Pursuits For America's 3rd Century*.[8a]

Suggested Activities

(Senior High Level)

1. Consider how personal participation in clubs, councils, and athletics enhances one's self-image. Discuss how certain recreational activities reduce tension and release energy, and contribute to a student's mental health. How does one school program complement another?

2. Success is a health item. Senior students should discuss its meaning. Introduce the idea that successful people live longer. This may come as a surprise, but high levels of achievement in the business world are related to longevity.[9]

[8a]Available free from the National Institute on Drug Abuse, 11400 Rockville Pike, Rockville, Maryland 20852.

[9]Jules V. Quint and Bianca R. Cody, "Preeminence and Mortality: Longevity of Prominent Men," *American Journal of Public Health*, 60:1118–1124, June, 1970.

3. Study the relationship between the extent of the work week, adequate rest and relaxation, and mental health. A Norwegian study reports that the 5-day work week is too long and that as workers get older they require longer vacation periods (it is fixed by law at four weeks). The research finding is that the short rest and relaxation period brings about a rush to use the leisure hours, which produces a stress situation like the rest of the week. What do class members observe in America?

4. Prepare and distribute copies of the following. Divide the class into groups of four people to discuss alternative ways of living.[10] What is the class feeling about "alternative pursuits"?

"ABOUT WHAT TO DO ON MONDAY MORNING"

"I went down to the Piraeus yesterday with Glaucon, Ariston's son, to pay my devotion to the goddess, and at the same time I wanted to see how they would manage the festival, since this was the first time they held it."

Thus starts one of the Western World's most significant books: Plato's *Republic.* As much as any other, and far more than most, it shaped civilization for the next two and one half millennia.

As Lin Yu Tang observed about it, the book "does not begin...with some such sentence as 'Human civilization, as seen through its successive stages of development, is a dynamic movement from heterogeneity,' or some equally incomprehensible rot."

Just: "I went down to the Piraeus..." and a world was changed.

In your search for alternative pursuits:
Don't be pompous.
Take a walk; look around.
See.
See again.
See beyond what is, to what could be.
Talk about it with someone else.
Take refreshment.
Walk.
Hang loose. Be open to its happening.
When it clicks, go!

---

5. Create a panel presentation to talk about the role of recreation in the maintenance of mental health. Inquire as to *how* hobbies contribute to personal creativity, self-assurance, and maturity.

— Is it true that in an increasingly impersonal society many people want most to use their hands on leather, metal, wood, glass, or clay?

— Will people work for less to be able to do their own thing and escape the treadmill?

— Will a person contribute more to the salvation of the world as a physicist than as a cobbler?

— What is the *full* meaning of the word "leisure"?

— What do "play," "amusement," "relaxation," "rejuvenation," and "diversion" have in common?

— Why is recreation referred to as "an attitude of mind"?[11]

---

[10]Adapted from *Alternative Pursuits for America's 3rd Century,* National Institute on Drug Abuse: Rockville, Maryland.

[11]See Carl E. Willgoose, "Recreation: An Attitude of Mind," *Education,* 81:42–44, September, 1960.

6. Visit a local industry in order to see the different kinds of tasks people perform in earning a living. Try to locate a production line operation where workers do essentially the same movements throughout the day. After returning to the classroom, discuss the relationship of such things as happiness on the job and pride in one's work to the maintenance of mental well-being.

> TALK
> HEALS

7. Post a "talk heals" sign at the front of the classroom. Show that psychotherapy, when all the technical language is stripped away, is this: talk heals. But it isn't just any kind of talk. It is talk sprung loose from the restraints of daily living; an uninhibited, free association of thoughts and ideas whose patterns reveal underlying emotional drives that cause psychic conflicts. Show further that it's the kind of talk that can only take place with a trained, understanding, non-judging person who wants to help.

How We Become Ourselves: The Shaping of Personality

The Program at a Glance . . .

Part I:

Each of us has a sense of our own personality. In understanding and accepting the many levels of personality and the various forces which shape it, we can learn to enjoy life's pleasures and deal with its trials.

1. Defining one's own personality is difficult since: our view of ourself is often different from the view others have of us; there are parts of our personality we are not aware of; and no personality is fixed.
2. There are three basic levels of the mind — id, ego, and superego.
3. There are two basic influences on the personality — heredity and environment.
4. In our social environment, our parents have the most influence on our personality; our relationship with them forms the basis for all later relationships.
5. Childhood and adolescence are times of great discovery and pain.
6. The greatest challenge in the formation of personality is in knowing and defining one's inner self, and learning to express one's inner wishes.

Part II:

Conflict is a central fact in human life, and dealing with it and anxiety is perhaps the most crucial task in our development; overcoming conflict enables us to live to our fullest potential.

1. Reaching intellectual and emotional maturity is difficult since we are influenced by many factors — both inside and outside.
2. Outside influences — parents, teachers, friends — and inside influences — memories, thoughts, feelings — are often in conflict.
3. Anxiety — the product of conflict — can both cause pain and impair judgment.
4. To protect ourselves from emotional conflict and anxiety, our minds use defense mechanisms.
5. The causes of personality problems seem most often to stem from child/parent relationships (William Branden, *Breaking Free*).
6. Insight into why we behave as we do and why we are what we are is a key element in mental health.

Use this program when discussing:

Psychology:

1. A study of the influences of heredity and environment on the individual.

2. The levels of personality — id, ego, superego — their functions, and their interrelationship.
3. A comparison of the basic elements in healthy and unhealthy relationships.
4. The functions of suppression and repression in the development of personality.
5. The positive and negative effects of the superego on personality.
6. A study of anxiety — various types and causes.
7. Personality disorders (neurosis, psychosis).

Guidance:

1. Basic human instincts and their relationship to thoughts and feelings.
2. The formation of emotional and physical bonds in human relationships.
3. The ability to examine alternatives and make realistic choices.
4. The formation of behavior patterns.
5. The need for personal expression and freedom.
6. The importance of self-acceptance.
7. Positive (sublimation) and negative (rationalization, denial, projection) defense mechanisms.

Humanities:

1. The influences of society in the shaping of personality.
2. The arts as an expression of self.
3. The roles of fantasy and dream in creative expression.

English:

1. The search for identity as a literary theme (*The Adventures of Huckleberry Finn*, Herman Wouk's "The Terrible Teens," Eve Merriam's "Thumbprints").
2. The conflict of motives as expressed in literature. (Elder Olson's "Directions to the Armorer," Buzz Aldrin's *Return to Earth*).

Social Studies:

1. The life and works of Sigmund Freud; his influence on modern psychology.
2. Conflicting social mores which complicate the process of growing up (sexual standards).

Art:

Includes works by William Blake, Bonnard, Cassatt, Chagall, M. C. Escher, Hopper, Lichtenstein, Matisse, Munch, Rockwell, Rodin, Shahn, Van Gogh, Grant Wood, Wyeth. Special sequences of drawings by William Steig and Saul Steinberg show the inner and outer conflicts we all must face.

A service of The Center for Humanities, Inc.

8. Assign projects dealing with the separate parts of the Center for Humanities material on page 162. Other programs like this are available on request.

9. Relate alcohol drinking to mental well-being. Initiate the topic by having a member of Alcoholics Anonymous come into the classroom for questioning. Treat statements that show misunderstandings:

"But I'm too young to be an alcoholic!"

"I only began to drink two years ago — nobody turns into an alcoholic *that fast*!"

"As long as I drink only beer I'll be O.K."

Show that alcohol in our drinking society is essentially a management problem and that Alcoholics Anonymous is a powerful force for improved mental health in almost every large community. For school use, see especially *Young People and AA,* distributed by AA, 468 Park Ave., South, New York, N.Y. 10016.

10. Research and list locations of excess noise in the community. Solicit expert medical and engineering opinion. Physically and psychologically, noise has been named the third pollution. Jets, jackhammers, sirens, food blenders, electronic music — all contribute to making the sound of our cities almost unbearable. Noise levels affect hearing, but the psychological effects are more subtle, and are centered on fear and annoyance. A noisy job or a noisy home fosters irritability, and mental health is seriously threatened.

11. In a three-year study of more than 5000 high school juniors and seniors in 11 schools in New York State, Morris Rosenberg of the National Institute of Mental Health discovered that the teenager with strong *self-esteem* is a remarkably productive citizen. He or she is likely to be a class officer, does well scholastically, enjoys competition, accepts responsibility, and is admired by classmates. Ask the students if the Rosenberg experience is in keeping with their own views of teenage performance.

12. Introduce the topic of death and dying by following McMahon's subunit:[12]

SUBUNIT A: THE TABOO OF DEATH

Behavioral Objective: The student will be able to freely discuss and come to terms with his own feeling concerning death.

Answer the following questions:

a. Why do language barriers exist on the subject of death and dying?

b. How do you perceive death?

c. What euphemisms can you think of to describe death and dying?

d. Do all persons have a negative attitude toward dying?

Activities: Interview a person about his feeling toward death.

Assessment Task: Either talk with someone about your ideas on death or tape record your ideas and replay them.

---

13. Divide the students into teams and permit each team to select a mental health problem to look into. Research over the last two decades indicates that team solutions of problems tend to be superior in many dimensions to individual solutions. Teams ask more questions and thus get more information. Also, they tend to summarize information and formulate more hypotheses leading to better solutions.

---

[12]Joan D. McMahon, "A Unit for Independent Study in Death Education," *School Health Review,* 4:27–34, July/August, 1973.

14. Examine aging and mental health. Request a comparison of older persons' views with young persons' views.

15. Review the research on violence—a topic which frequently fascinates high school students because they can relate to it. Discuss deliberate automobile "accidents" that may be caused by lack of emotional maturity and emotional control. Also, look into the theory that some persons may have a disturbed biologic base. Both animal and human research are revealing that aggression, rage, and other emotional extremes correspond to strong electrochemical activity in the brain. Genetic disorders, poorly developed central nervous systems, glandular secretions, brain diseases, and severe head injuries have been linked to aggressive actions.

An Old Woman Speaks[13]

"What is it to be a human being? Am I but a reflection cast into the lives of other persons? Does a tree falling in the forest make a sound if there are no ears to hear it? Is a person human when he has shrunk into the basic core of self and others have moved away like loose-hanging folds of skin?"

A Young Person Responds

"I see you, old woman. I see the *you*, not the old. In your eyes I read the story of the years, of the pain, the sweet delights, the tender pain. I see you *woman*, know your femininity, your graceful movements, your healing tenderness."

---

16. Investigate mental health films available as part of the Mental Health in the Classroom series from National Institute of Mental Health, 5600 Fishers Lane, Rockville, Md. 20852, and Human Relations Medical Center, 22 Clemons Square, Pound Ridge, N.Y. 10576. See also Chapter 10 of this text. The admirable films *Aspects of Behavior, The Sensory World,* and *Personality* are available from Boston University Film Service, 765 Commonwealth Avenue, Boston, Mass. 02215.

17. Encourage poster artwork in class, or purchase 14" × 22" posters from Spenco Medical Corporation (see list of sources in Chapter 10) which cover such amusing and debatable titles as:

"Alcohol, the All-American Cop-out"

"Stop Discrimination. Hate Everybody"

"There Is No Cure for Birth and Death, Save to Enjoy the Interval"

"A Man's Venom Poisons Himself More Than His Victim"

"Man Is Not the Creature of Circumstances—Circumstances Are the Creature of Man."

"Maybe Death Is Nature's Way of Telling Us to Slow Down"

"Humor Is the Only Thing that Stands Between Us and the Dark"

18. Expose the class to group problem solving through outdoor survival activities such as Outward Bound and Project Adventure (see *Adventure Curriculum,* Project Adventure, 775 Bay Rd., Hamilton, Mass. 01936). In group involvement activities everyone is concerned about the success of everyone else. In a sense everyone turns out a winner. Students put themselves in the hands of others and must trust them completely—a rare and exciting experience.

19. Engage the class in a Personality Spokes activity:[14]

a. Have each student pick a partner.

b. Each student is to draw three half dollar size circles: two at the top and one at the bottom of a piece of paper (see example). Next he is to draw spokes as if these circles

---

[13]Bert Kruger Smith, *Aging in America,* Boston: Beacon Press, 1973, p. 196.

[14]From Rosa Sullivan, "Personality Spokes," *Health Education* 6:36. January/February, 1975.

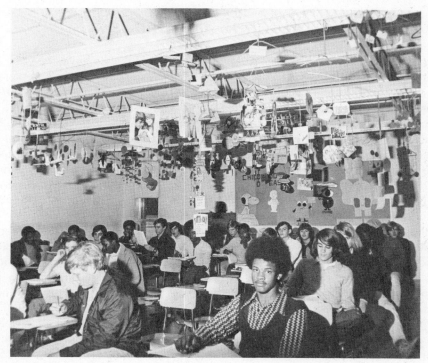

Figure 6–6   Mental health mobiles stimulate interest. (Courtesy of Norfolk, Virginia, Public Schools)

were wheels. One top circle has 10 spokes and is labeled personality assets. The other top circle has 5 spokes and is labeled faults. The bottom wheel has 5 spokes and is labeled ambitions.

c. Each student is to fill in the spokes accordingly, examine what they wrote and then draw lines from the assets to the ambitions these assets will help satisfy. Then the student is to draw lines from the faults to the ambitions that these faults will prevent from satisfying.

d. The students should then exchange and examine each other's papers.

e. Each student next explains to his partner why these assets and faults will help or hinder his ambitions. They also should talk about *how* important these ambitions are to them, and *why* they are so important.

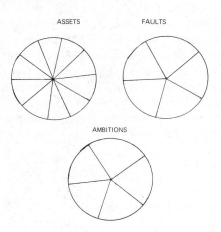

2. ALCOHOL AND DRUGS

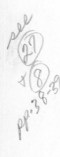

Ours is a drug-taking society where over 300 new chemicals have been produced in the last decade alone—for a variety of purposes—to restore health, lessen pain, induce calm, increase energy, create euphoria, and bring about sleep or alertness. Four million amphetamine pills are produced each year with very little medical need for any of them. They are abused because people believe in chemicals for everything—the sniffles, the mood, backache—which creates a frame of reference that says that all discomforts can be handled with a chemical cure. So tranquilizers and antihistamines are overused to a point where they can cause inattention, confusion, and drowsiness. When such drugs are used in combination with alcohol, the combined effect may be extremely hazardous, particularly in terms of automobile driving. Yet driving is necessary, and people of all ages drink without thinking.

Alcohol drinking has been socially acceptable for a long time. It is undeniably a family affair—affecting family stability, unity, values, mental and physical health, and pocketbooks. About 95 million Americans—over two thirds of the adult population—use alcoholic beverages without ill effects. However, there are some nine million persons who have become problem drinkers or alcoholics. The extent of the problem has been measured in a variety of ways. As many as 5 per cent of the employed population have drinking problems with a cost to the occupational sector of about 9.5 billion dollars per year. These costs are generally passed on to the consumer. Additional costs pertaining to personal and property damage bring the expense of problem drinking to 15 billion dollars a year. Other enormous items of economic and human welfare involve traffic fatalities, homicides, mental disorders, heart disease, cirrhosis of the liver, lowered resistance to infection, increased crime, untold thousands of unhappy marriages and broken homes, two million arrests annually for drunkenness, and incalculable costs in human suffering.

Back in 1971, the National Commission on Marihuana and Drug Abuse estimated that 24 million Americans had tried marijuana, with eight million using it regularly. Three years later the Drug Abuse Council in Washington, D.C., surveyed the country and found that 29 million Americans had tried marijuana, with 12 million of them using it regularly. Among teenagers, age 12 to 17, approximately 14 per cent indicated that they had tried marijuana and 5 per cent said they were current users.

As Ray earlier noted in his exhaustive study of drugs, society, and behavior, it would be expected that a very high percentage of the population uses one type of drug or another.[15] A look at the home drug cabinet will surprise many people with its stashed away agents to "cure" colds and other illnesses. The Stanford Research Institute discovered in one study that the average household had 30 different drugs. One of five was a prescription item, but the other four were over-the-counter drugs that could be purchased by anyone in any amount. Under these circumstances it is not surprising to find that a very high percentage of people have used a psychoactive drug—one that has a primary effect on the brain to alter mood and/or consciousness. From sleeping pills to tranquilizers, an army of individuals seek a way out of their immediate difficulties—and spread the word about how effective it is. Yet, barbiturate addiction with psychic depression is real. It even contributes to suicide; the familiar and unpleasant patterns of addiction and withdrawal are found with such tranquilizers as Librium and Valium, used by thousands of individuals.

---

[15]Oakley S. Ray, *Drugs, Society, and Human Behavior,* St. Louis: C. V. Mosby Co., 1972, Chapter 1.

YOUTH AND THE CHEMICAL SOCIETY

Drug abuse and narcotic addiction are a complex and difficult dilemma for which there is no simple solution. It is a health, legal, social, economic, and moral problem that will require a massive effort devoted to the discovery of new knowledge as well as the development of imaginative approaches to prevention.

With today's affluence, there is time and money to support drug excesses. Loss of goals and drives can be a by-product of affluence. Where leisure time hangs heavily and there are no viable goals, individuals become bored or alienated, and vulnerable to the temptations of using chemical substances for productive living. Unfortunately, youths are quite aware of these circumstances and question the relevance of social values and institutions. They recognize adult hypocrisy and want "out." Youngsters who feel helpless to accommodate to or change an unacceptable world, consciously choose to alter their own. For them, life is a "drag." It lacks meaning because there is no engagement; the future is unknown and probably horrible. For some, there seem to be no alternatives. Since you cannot alter the world, you alter your state of consciousness and perception, that is, experience the world through a "high."

In this age of hedonism and instant gratification, where one can "buy now and pay later," the youths listen to the advertising telling them how to get pepped up or toned down and seek chemical relief from normal tensions and stresses. Too often they become escape oriented. Like their older friends they want to smoke, chew, eat, drink, smell, or inject various chemicals to relieve the dailiness of their lives — to escape reality. As far as school is concerned, many students would drop out if there was something better to do; there too often prevails a passive acquiescence in boredom — incredibly mobile but profoundly unhappy students.

Lest this description of youth be applied too generally, it should be noted that not all youth fit the "unhappy" and "alienated" category. In fact Yankelovich, who does survey research for the government, finds that the youth are not becoming a nation of young junkies, and that drugs are losing their value as protest symbols, with a rising number of students rejecting them — or certainly using them less often than liquor.[16] However, there is widespread experimentation with drugs and with drugs in combination with alcohol. There is considerable variation in drug use. In studying the life styles and values of youth the Institute for Social Research at the University of Michigan discovered that 55 per cent of young people had tried illegal drugs by age 18 — a figure almost three times as high as in 1969. Use of marijuana had jumped from 19 per cent to 54 per cent, while the number using amphetamines had doubled and the number using barbiturates tripled. Lloyd Johnson, who carried out a United States Office of Education study also found that experimentation with illegal drugs was a common occurrence, with one third of those using each drug doing so no more than once or twice a year (see Table 6–1).[17]

Weitman also found that experimentation was the single most important motive contributing to the use of drugs in high schools.[18] Johnson's findings were that the amount of nonaddictive illegal drug use has been much less for youth than is frequently reported in the media, and the relationship between addictive drug use and such items as delinquency and poor academic performance is far less serious than commonly believed. Youth appear to be more interested, but more tolerant, of psychoactive drugs than in

[16]Daniel Yankelovich, "How Students Control Their Drug Crisis," *Psychology Today,* October, 1975, pp. 39–42. See also Yankelovich's book *The New Morality,* New York: McGraw-Hill Inc., 1974.

[17]Lloyd D. Johnson, "Drug Use During and After High School," *American Journal of Public Health* (Supplement), 64:29–35, December, 1974.

[18]Morris Weitman, et al., "Survey of Adolescent Drug Use," *American Journal of Public Health,* 64:417–422, May, 1974.

TABLE 6–1   Percentage of Self-reported Usage Rates during the High School Years and the Year Following

DRUG	DURING HIGH SCHOOL YEARS		YEAR AFTER HIGH SCHOOL	
	Any Use	Weekly Use	Any Use	Weekly Use
Marijuana or Hashish	21	6	34	10
Hallucinogens	7	1	11	1
Amphetamines	10	2	14	2
Barbiturates	6	1	9	1
Heroin	2	1	2	1
Alcoholic Beverages	81	33	89	44
Cigarettes	66	36*	68	41*

*The figures on cigarette use refer to daily rather than weekly use. (Courtesy of Dr. Lloyd D. Johnston, University of Michigan, Ann Arbor. From American Journal of Public Health, December, 1974.)

other years. Moreover, the vast number of students using drugs are not abusers, and are not likely to become so. They are not dropping out of school like earlier delinquents and the intellectually alienated. Their grades are about the same as nonusers. They employ drugs for the same reasons that social drinkers use alcohol.

There appears to be less alienation among youth today than five to 10 years ago. Drug experimentation and alcohol consumption is more likely to be part of the "in" thing to do, with individuals conforming in part to maintain peer approval. Most are reasonably normal and frequently superior teenagers. Many of them have humanitarian goals, aspirations, and creativity, and they cherish self-expression.

It may be a myth that stereotypes young drug-users in terms of alienation and emotional disturbances. Anthropologist Margaret Mead dismisses the idea that activist American youth is in any way alienated. She suggests in fact that young people today could be regarded as a new kind of world immigrant, acquiring and using experiences that their parents have not had, and at the same time not in possession of a historical sense.

Students do have values. First of all they are searching for meaning. This is why they joke half seriously about having an "identity crisis." They wonder what life means, where they are headed, and what really matters. Secondly, they embrace the cult of experience and seek immediate pleasure and satisfaction. From high school right into college they begin to fear that instead of becoming more open to themselves and to experience, they are becoming increasingly numbed and closed off from all that is exciting and beautiful. Both of these values are related to the use and abuse of drugs by students. Searching for meaning and experience is, unfortunately, part of the cultism and propaganda that surrounds drugs. Thus hallucinogens are consumed to produce a revelation of life's meaning, and amphetamines are ingested to intensify ordinary states of consciousness. As erroneous as the practice may be, it does take place—chiefly because no one has demonstrated to students that there are better and more lasting ways to experience the fullness, the depth, the variety and richness of life.

DELIBERATIONS ON THE CURRENT DRUG SCENE

The primary purpose of this chapter is to consider *what* and *how* to teach in the area of alcohol and drugs. It is not to spend a great amount of time describing today's youth and to quote lengthy statistics about the alarming state of affairs. Yet it is practically impossible to talk intelligently in terms of concepts and behaviors without an understanding of how students *feel* about their world and how extensive their problem has become.

Interestingly, most students do not know that any one of them could be potentially drug-dependent persons. They will tell you that it is the "other fellow" who is the troubled, isolated, alienated person for whom group drug usage provides a sense of community when he is unable to find himself by normal social means. Yet it has been shown that there are a number of young people from affluent homes and with higher than average intellectual ability who have quick tempers, little tolerance for frustration or postponement, and little tolerance for anxiety. They demand instant gratification and instant relief, and have found that drugs offer both of these.

It is acknowledged by many that this is an age when the expression "credibility gap" is associated all too often with many sources of information. It is par for the course to ask "when did you hear *that*?" or "who says so?" Usually, the degree to which certain facts are questioned is related to the past experiences of the questioner. Both the well-adjusted and poorly adjusted student, therefore, will find it easy on occasion to doubt much of what he hears from parents and teachers. Very often he will operate on the "I've got to be shown" or "prove it to me" basis. This makes formal education difficult at best, for the teacher is continually challenged to get the facts straight and present them without an obvious and overriding bias. This is hardly a new thought—only an amplification of a fundamental ingredient of good teaching. However, it does point up the fact that the alcohol and drug area is more difficult to teach than many other areas in the curriculum, and therefore requires a well versed and skilled teacher.

Posting an essential information chart in the classroom can be helpful (see Figure 6–7). It may be used to encourage the search for additional facts, particularly in the grey areas where there are questions not completely resolved.

THE MARIJUANA ENIGMA

A pertinent example of the unresolved question is the use of marijuana. Both inside and outside the classroom it continues to be a topic of conversation, from mild to heated discourse. This is to be expected if marijuana is indeed the "new social drug" affecting 12 million Americans, and showing its greatest increase in usage among middle-class adolescents and young adults. All of this is highly complicated by cultural, medical, and legal perspectives.[19]

In terms of secondary education, marijuana is directly related to the life styles of "turned on" youth. If there really is a generation gap, then marijuana enforces it. All too often the controversy is primarily *political* rather than *scientific*. "Grass" becomes a symbol for a number of positions and beliefs, in which those who use the drug are frequently labeled as "politically radical," "sexually loose," "unpatriotic," and a member of the "communist conspiracy." So the ideological argument continues with both sides invoking scientific findings which they believe support a position already taken. The school teacher, of all people, must show open-mindedness and permit an airing of opposite viewpoints in the controversy.

Information to be brought out includes the following:

1. In general, adolescents are introduced to marijuana by others in their peer group. There is little evidence to confirm the belief that "pushers" are needed to "turn on" a novice. His "friends" do it for him.

---

[19]Both instructor and student will profit from David E. Smith's *The New Social Drug,* Englewood Cliffs, N.J.: Prentice-Hall, Inc., 1970. The chapter by Eric Goode (p. 168), "Marijuana And The Politics of Reality," is especially good reading. See also the *Federal Source Book: Answers to the Most Frequently Asked Questions About Drug Abuse,* National Clearinghouse For Drug Abuse Information, 5454 Wisconsin Avenue, Chevy Chase, Maryland 20015.

Chart Listing Drugs, Medical Uses, Symptoms Produced and their Dependence Potentials

(Question marks indicate conflict of opinion)

Name	Slang name	Chemical or trade name	Source	Classification	Medical use	How taken	Usual Dose	Duration of effect	Effects sought	Long-term symptoms	Physical dependence potential	Mental dependence potential	Organic damage potential
Heroin	H., Horse, Scat, Junk, Smack, Scag, Stuff, Harry	Diacetyl-morphine	Semi-Synthetic (from Morphine)	Narcotic	Pain relief	Injected or Sniffed	Varies	4 hrs.	Euphoria, Prevent withdrawal discomfort	Addiction Constipation Loss of Appetite	Yes	Yes	No
Morphine	White stuff, M.	Morphine sulphate	Natural (from Opium)	Narcotic	Pain relief	Swallowed or Injected	15 Milligrams	6 hrs.	Euphoria, Prevent withdrawal discomfort	Addiction Constipation Loss of Appetite	Yes	Yes	No
Codeine	Schoolboy	Methylmorphine	Natural (from Opium), Semi-Synthetic (from Morphine)	Narcotic	Ease Pain and coughing	Swallowed	30 Milligrams	4 hrs.	Euphoria, Prevent withdrawal discomfort	Addiction Constipation Loss of Appetite	Yes	Yes	No
Methadone	Dolly	Dolophine Amidone	Synthetic	Narcotic	Pain relief	Swallowed or Injected	10 Milligrams	4–6 hrs.	Prevent withdrawal discomfort	Addiction Constipation Loss of Appetite	Yes	Yes	No
Cocaine	Corrine, Gold Dust, Coke, Bernice, Flake, Star Dust, Snow	Methylester of benzoylecgonine	Natural (from coca, NOT cacao)	Stimulant, Local Anesthesia	Local Anesthesia	Sniffed, Injected or Swallowed	Varies	Varies, Short	Excitation Talkativeness	Depression Convulsions	No	Yes	Yes?
Marijuana	Pot, Grass, Hashish, Tea, Gage, Reefers	Cannabis sativa	Natural	Relaxant, Euphoriant, In high doses Hallucinogen	None in U.S.	Smoked, Swallowed, or Sniffed	1–2 Cigarettes	4 hrs.	Relaxation, increased euphoria, Perceptions, Sociability	Usually None	No	Yes?	No
Barbiturates	Barbs, Blue Devils, Candy, Yellow Jackets, Phennies, Peanuts, Blue Heavens	Phenobarbital Nembutal, Seconal, Amytal	Synthetic	Sedative-hypnotic	Sedation, Relieve high blood pressure, epilepsy, hyperthyroidism	Swallowed or Injected	50–100 Milligrams	4 hrs.	Anxiety reduction, Euphoria	Addiction w/ severe withdrawal symptoms. Possible convulsions, toxic psychosis	Yes	Yes	Yes
Amphetamines	Bennies, Dexies, Speed, Wake-Ups, Lid Poppers, Hearts, Pep Pills	Benzedrine, Dexedrine, Desoxyn, Methamphetamine, Methedrine	Synthetic	Sympatho-mimetic	Relieve mild depression, control appetite and narcolepsy	Swallowed or Injected	2.5–5 Milligrams	1 hrs.	Alertness Activeness	Loss of Appetite Delusions Hallucinations Toxic psychosis	No?	Yes	Yes?
LSD	Acid, Sugar, Big D, Cubes, Trips	d-lysergic acid diethylamide	Semi-Synthetic (from ergot alkaloids)	Hallucinogen	Experimental study of mental function, alcoholism	Swallowed	100–500 Micrograms	10 hrs.	Insightful experiences, exhilaration, Distortion of senses	May intensify existing psychosis, panic reactions	No	No?	No?
DMT	AMT, Businessman's High	Dimethyl-triptamine	Synthetic	Hallucinogen	None	Injected	1–3 Milligram	Less than 1 hr.	Insightful experiences, exhilaration, Distortion of senses	?	No	No?	No?
Mescaline	Mesc.	3,4,5-trimethoxyphenethylamine	Natural (from Peyote)	Hallucinogen	None	Swallowed	350 Micrograms	12 hrs.	Insightful experiences, exhilaration, Distortion of senses	?	No	No?	No?
Psilocybin		3 (2-dimethylamino) ethylindol-4-oldihydrogen phosphate	Natural (from Psilocybe)	Hallucinogen	None	Swallowed	25 Milligrams	6–8 hrs.	Insightful experiences, exhilaration, Distortion of senses	?	No	No?	No?
Alcohol	Booze, Juice, etc.	Ethanol ethyl alcohol	Natural (from grapes, grains, etc. via fermentation)	Sedative hypnotic	Solvent, Antiseptic	Swallowed	Varies	1–4 hrs.	Sense alteration Anxiety reduction, Sociability	Cirrhosis Toxic psychosis Neurologic damage, Addiction	Yes	Yes	Yes
Tobacco	Fag, Coffin nail, etc.	Nicotinia tabacum	Natural	Stimulant-sedative	Sedative, Emetic (nicotine)	Smoked, Sniffed, Chewed	Varies	Varies	Calmness Sociability	Emphysema, Lung cancer, mouth & throat cancer, cardio-vascular damage, loss of appetite	Yes?	Yes	Yes

Figure 6–7

2. The extremely punitive criminal sanctions against the use of "pot" are being fought by a number of physicians, educators, and psychologists, and by the American Civil Liberties Union. The ACLU contends that to include marijuana with heroin and other dangerous drugs is unconstitutional because it denies marijuana smokers equal protection under the law. Severe laws complicate rather than help the task of persuading users to give up the drug. Findings from surveys indicate that more than 80 per cent of those who have used marijuana favor reducing penalties, compared to only 30 per cent who have never tried it. As expected, older people were far more likely to favor tougher penalties than younger adults and teenagers. The same thing occurred in an Oregon survey. It was Oregon, in 1973, that abolished criminal penalties for possession of one ounce or less and made it a civil offense, similar to a traffic violation.[20] The periodical *Consumer Reports* points out that the notion that arrest and imprisonment are the proper social responses to possession of a hazardous product or substance appears inconsistent with society's usual approach to products, even to hazardous products.[21] Moreover, alcohol and nicotine are both demonstrably harmful drugs, but society does not arrest and imprison those found to possess them. A year after the Oregon decriminalization of marijuana the Drug Abuse Council found that there was no "marihuana explosion" as predicted by opponents of decriminalization. In fact, the nonusers said that they did not smoke it chiefly for health reasons, and not fear of criminal penalties.

3. The long term effects of taking marijuana are not fully known. However, the more obvious reactions are rapidity of heartbeat, lowered body temperature, appetite stimulation, and body dehydration. Users may become talkative, loud, unsteady in coordinated movements, and drowsy. The effects last from two to four hours and vary from feelings of excitement to depression. The user finds it harder to make decisions that require clear thinking, and he finds himself more responsive to other people's suggestions. Reflex actions are reduced, making it questionable to drive while under the influence of the drug.

4. National Institute of Mental Health studies show that psychotic reactions sometimes occur, for unknown reasons, in some individuals who take smaller amounts. Marijuana should be considered primarily a sedative-hypnotic anesthetic, and its desired effects (anxiety relief and euphoria intoxication) and adverse effects (nausea and high dose perceptual alteration) are closely related.[22] It may be erroneous to classify marijuana as a narcotic. Goodman and Gilman's prime reference in the field of pharmacology, *The Pharmacological Basis of Therapeutics,* is unwilling to classify marijuana as either a narcotic or a hallucinogen, placing cannibis in a miscellaneous drug classification. It appears that the physiologic, pharmacologic and toxicologic effects of marijuana are not those of the drugs classified as narcotics.

5. There is some evidence of conjunctivitis, chronic bronchitis, various digestive ailments, and sleep difficulties among long-time marijuana users. Regular hashish users in two Eastern surveys report some impairment in physical health, as well as psychosis. More research is necessary. With the recent availability of synthetic THC (tetrahydrocannabinol) and the ability to determine the amount of THC in marijuana, it is now feasible to know the exact quality of the substance being studied.

6. Temporary intoxication with "pot," as with alcohol, poses no immediate threat to a normal individual. One or two "experiments" should cause little harm. Large doses,

---

[20]Pat Horn, editor of *Behavior Today,* reporting on information from the Drug Abuse Council, Washington, D.C.

[21]Consumer Reports, April, 1975, pp. 265–266.

[22]Frederick C. Meyers, "Pharmacologic Effects of Marihuana," *Journal of Psychedelic Drugs 2,* 1:31–36, Fall, 1968.

eaten or drunk, have extreme effects, including hallucinations and feelings of depersonalization, all the way up to a full LSD-trip-like experience. Moderate use over a long
period of time is open to question. Drawing an analogy to alcohol, it may be that many
people can smoke pot, as they are able to drink socially, all their lives without visible
harm. Too much pot, as with too much alcohol, may lead to self-destruction. Some
studies have indicated that "pot" smokers demonstrate an early diminution in self-
awareness and judgment along with slowed thinking and shorter spans in concentration
and attention.[23]

7. An individual who abuses one drug tends to abuse another. However, any association between marijuana and other drugs is due to the influence of personality and peer
group factors. There is nothing in grass that leads one to heroin. Moreover, there is no
evidence that pot creates a craving for heroin or anything else. One who is inclined to
lean heavily on marijuana, however, most likely has the potential for drug dependence,
and therefore may be in danger of developing dependence on more destructive substances.

8. Social control of marijuana is most difficult to handle via legal means when the
drug in question permits both use and abuse. The problem of penalizing the majority
because of the abuse of the minority has been ruled on by the Supreme Court (Volstead
Act). Prohibition is generally unsatisfactory. Thus, there is a continuing debate over how
to regulate marijuana so that the statutes are consistent with the abuse potential of the
drug, and so that constitutional rights of individuals are not violated. As it is, marijuana
laws seem designed to protect the individual against doing potential harm to himself.
They create, like adultery laws, a victimless crime.

9. Whether another intoxicant should be accepted into the culture is the question.
With millions of alcoholics all around, should another mind-altering chemical be added to
the existing problem? Should "grass" be legalized and controlled through licensing and
taxation? It may be that society will approach marijuana licensure in a two-step
process: first reducing the stiff penalties, and then weighing the public health risks
carefully, examining whether a licensure system might be the most rational way to control its use. Or society may turn its back on marijuana and concentrate on controlling
LSD, heroin, and amphetamines, and let the pot smoking fad die out.

THE COMMUNITY CHALLENGE

Meeting the local problem of alcohol and drug abuse requires a community effort.
The school simply cannot go it alone. Where special programs are functioning, the
school or some *ad hoc* committee of the school board has generally taken the lead in involving parents, clergy, medical personnel, and law enforcement officers in the development of this area of the health education curriculum. Working together, community "hot
lines" and emergency referral practices have been put in working order.

Government programs fail when local communities do not organize to meet the
problem. Moreover, in the past there has been a tendency to approach the problem by
increasing funds to hunt down the pusher, to discover and treat the drug addict, and to
set up drug identification and drug information centers. Obviously this is important, but
the vast majority of youth needs to become intellectually involved themselves in order to
understand the hazards. In Hartford, Connecticut, this took place in the form of high
school youths teaching seventh and eighth graders about the dangers of drug abuse. It

---

[23]Harold Kolansky and W. T. Moore, "Marihuana, Can it Hurt You?" *Journal of the American Medical
Association,* 232:923–924, June 1975.

was discovered that older students were held in high esteem by younger students; their thinking and acting regarding early drug experimentation was modified. Moreover, civic groups worked with the schools and the WHCT-TV station.

The Holland Patent Community Health Project in Holland Patent, New York, is an example of a school-community education endeavor to prevent alcohol consumption at an early age. The project involves individuals in leisure time pursuits, personal involvement in activities which enhance self-image and benefit the community, learning new skills for the home and work, understanding communication between age groups, and developing positive attitudes about oneself and others. Another model program is the Substance Education Program (Project PRIDE) of Dade County, Florida. Here, there is an instructional component leading to decision-making, an affective component leading to self-awareness, and an alternative activities component to counter the need for drug experimentation and use. Significantly, the program recognizes that the abuse of drugs is symptomatic of other problems facing growth. It is a "feeling program" with peer and teen counseling. There are places to drop in, socialize, and "rap" about problems—and the names of drop-in places sound like television shows—The Lighthouse, The Yak Shack, Ziggy's Place, The Open Door, The Way Up, The Place, Aquarius, and One Step Beyond. There are things to do in the community, and, best of all, there is solid community support.

From what has been said it is obvious that the community must be a part of the school's planning efforts, especially where *alternative programs* are being established. The National Clearinghouse for Drug Information has been asking:

What are alternatives for preventing drinking problems?

What are strategies for implementing alternatives?

A real case can be made for alternatives as an important route to drug prevention. If drug abuse is "a response to an experience deficiency," then realistic alternatives to drugs where young people find fulfillment and self-understanding is called for.[24] The task in every school-community situation is to develop alternative paths to the same student objectives—excitement, risks, heightened sensitivities, camaraderie, and stimulating discoveries. To make programs work local teams explore school-community opportunities, secure resources, mobilize peer groups that transcend drug-using boundaries, i.e., users and non-users who will help invalidate the oft-heard remark that "there is nothing around here to do." Finding alternative routes for young people is affective education. In fact, affective education is in danger of becoming an ephemeral fad if it does not find a solid base in which feelings and humanizing are a part of the alternative program.

Perhaps the greatest stumbling block to successful programs is the teacher who talks about "relating" to pupils, but has not discovered how to do it effectively. There has to be an in-depth communication quite unlike what occurs in other subject matter areas. For one thing, teachers must learn to overcome their fear of intimacy with their students and begin to personalize the discourse. Edgar Friendenberg, in his study of a Midwestern high school, *The Vanishing Adolescent,* found that most of the teachers were afraid of intimate relationships with their students. Most of them, he felt, were motivated by a fear that their aura of authority would be undermined. The students, therefore, were unhappy and called the program "irrelevant" to their lives.

To get through the maze of obstacles to learning in this difficult area, one must relate to boys' and girls' "search for identity." It has to be personal. It has to tie in with youth's *feelings* as they ask "Who am I?" and "What am I doing here?" Let them talk; let them question; let them search for answers with an instructor who sits in their group

---

[24]See especially the well-developed manual by the National Institute on Drug Abuse, *Alternative Pursuits for America's 3rd Century* (DHEW Pub. No. (HSM) 73–9158).

listening and doing very little talking. Allan Cohen has found this approach extemely effective. He has demonstrated that the sympathetic teacher with empathy immediately puts the class at ease. Students reveal their inner feelings and become willing to work personally toward changes in the society—political and social policy planning.[25] Cohen also subscribes to the belief that the most understressed objective in narcotic education today is the *provision of alternatives*. Instructors should abandon their defensive posture pertaining to drugs and put special priority on nonchemical means in reaching optimum interpersonal relationships, enduring values, and inner experience. Students will move away from drugs when something more satisfying comes along. Cohen finds that social involvement at the local level is an excellent substitute for chemicals. The user can stop cannabis if he wants to. The critical issue is to get him to want to stop. And if he has not started, perhaps he'll begin to turn in another direction.

ALCOHOL EDUCATION

In this era disease may be viewed ecologically as a maladjustment of the human organism to the physical and social environment. The chronic and degenerative diseases such as poor mental health, heart disease, and alcoholism are the "way of life" diseases. Studying them, therefore, must involve more than the usual laboratory approach; it must consider the importance of social epidemiology. Disease may be a medical entity, but illness is a social phenomenon.

Human beings are often agents of their own disease. They can hurt themselves more than the outside germ or infectious agent. This is the concept that must be put across in alcohol education. The medical cause of alcoholism may be ethyl alcohol, but the psychosocial cause is drinking. The popular booklet, "Thinking About Drinking" (U.S. Government Printing Office), is a valuable teaching aid simply because it encourages thinking about alcohol on a social basis—individual, family, and community. Heretofore, much of the alcohol education has met high resistance to factual evidence, with little appeal to reason. More progress is made when information is dispensed and discussed in the context of the social group.

Social drinking in moderation is acknowledged, and even accepted, as a part of the culture, and is weighed against the variety of alcohol-related ills—brain damage, shortened longevity, heart disease, chronic alcoholism and poor mental health, cirrhosis of the liver, lowered resistance to infection, fatal aircraft accidents, drunken drivers, drownings, industrial problems, and crime.

With the spectacular rise in alcoholism, accidents, and problem drinkers, it is important to start early in the junior high school to discuss the current pattern of living and to find out why people drink. Attention should be directed to why teenagers drink and when they first tasted alcoholic beverages. Most tasting is done by the age of 10. The first drink comes at about age 13. As many as 50 to 85 per cent of high school pupils, depending on the area, say that they drink at least occasionally. This does not necessarily mean that such early exposure to alcohol leads to a greater consumption in later years. Nor does it lead to delinquency in general. Most teenage drinking follows the adult pattern in the same community. Drinking parents have more drinking teenagers. The first exposure is likely to be in the home with parents. In New York, Wisconsin, and Kansas studies, one in four teenagers claimed to be "high" at least once during the month prior to the research. Beer is the most common beverage of drinking youth. Laws

---

[25]Allan Y. Cohen, "Inside What's Happening: Sociological, Psychological, and Spiritual Perspectives on the Contemporary Drug Scene," *American Journal of Public Health*, 59:2092–2095, November, 1969.

relating to teenage drinking appear to have little effect on the drinking practices. Many students seem to take delight in breaking such laws. However, problems associated with teenage drinking are related to family attitudes toward drinking. Jewish and Italian-American families, for example, frequently expose their children to alcohol at an early age, but when they grow up they have the lowest rates of alcoholism of any cultural groups in the United States. This is what Norman Zinberg and the National Institute on Drug Abuse favorably refer to as "social control."

In Vermont in 1882 students were educated against alcohol. The concern was alcoholism and the other negative effects on the human body. Today the emphasis is on safe drinking and responsible drinking. Essential understanding include:

It is not essential to drink. Respect the attitude of non-drinkers.

Excessive drinking does not indicate adult status, virility, or masculinity.

Uncontrolled drinking is an illness.

Safe drinking depends on specific physiological as well as psychosocial factors.

"Alcohol education" should not be restricted to "alcoholism education."

A particularly good way to initiate discussion, to which factual evidence can be introduced later on, is to set forth questions such as the following for upper junior high and senior high school students:[26]

What Does a Family Do IF
—a teenager who is allowed to drink at home assumes that he or she can drink anywhere?
—the parents are non-drinkers and their teenagers are wondering whether to drink?
—the teenager planning a party wants to serve beer?
—one of the parents drinks so much that alcohol interferes with his other daily living?

What Does a Girl Do IF
—she sees that her date is getting high at a party?
—she doesn't like drinking, but does like her date, who wants her to accept a drink?
—she doesn't like drinking, and her date smells of whiskey when he calls for her?

What Does a Boy Do IF
—he feels high when it's time to leave a party and drive his date home?
—his parents ask where he's going when he's headed for a beer party?
—his date is drinking more at a party than she can handle? (Does he hope she'll sober up before the party ends? Does he tell her she must stop drinking? Does he suggest leaving the party and taking her home immediately?)

Most education about alcohol—and certainly most of the films and literature available on the topic—still warn of dire results and tragic consequences and make them appear to be inevitable. The kids know better. They know that the majority of young people do not end up dead, or in the hospital, in jail, or pregnant from too much drinking. Such one-sided, negative kind of teaching substantially reduces the believability of all teaching.

Bedrock honesty must prevail, striking a balance between the conservatively alarmist and the defiantly radical viewpoints. Rose believes that the social aspects of alcohol can be set up to provide a variety of viewpoints. The social dilemma for the student is depicted here:[27]

Society promotes the use of alcohol through advertising, by showing parental and adult approval, and by consuming alcohol at acceptable functions such as cocktail parties and wedding receptions.

---

[26]These questions have been used in schools and are adapted from the booklet, *Thinking About Drinking*, available from the U.S. Government Printing Office, Washington, D.C.

[27]Janet L. Rose, "Providing A Variety of Viewpoints," *Health Education*, 6:18–19, March/April, 1975.

The school curriculum highlights alcohol use in relation to family breakdown, crime, destruction of health or of life, both for the individual and others, and costs to society for treatment and rehabilitation.

What, then, does the student conclude after viewing these facts? What should one think about society's attitude toward alcohol? What goes into making the right decision for oneself?

DRUG EDUCATION

More and more secondary school instructors are permitting young people to survey themselves about drug taking. Those who take antihistamines, tranquilizers, and pills for various allergies are recorded. So are those who are trying other drugs. In the Hartford Public Schools survey, drug experimentation began in the eighth or ninth grades. Many normal youngsters (in and about the home and school) readily reported their experiences. In one class of 56 boys and girls the following information was collected:

DRUG USAGE	NUMBER OF STUDENTS WHO HAVE USED THE DRUG
Marijuana	11
Heroin	0
LSD	4
Airplane glue	5
Pills (barbs & amphs)	6

Further study indicated that these pupils greatly lacked information about the psycho-physical effects of drug abuse. This comes as no surprise, because other participants in the "psychedelic revolution" are equally uninformed.

Consistent with the philosophy of teaching in anticipation of needs and concerns, the Glen Cove (New York) schools worked with the elementary grades on the proper use of drugs. Then a consultant met with all seventh through twelfth grade students to: (1) motivate those who had chosen not to become involved with drugs to continue that way, (2) motivate those who were experimenting with drugs to face up to the reality of what they were bargaining for and do something about it, and (3) motivate the regular users to reconsider, and if they could not make it on their own, to seek professional help. The program of group discussions was successful, partly because the instructor showed responsible concern for the pupils as human beings. Many students made appointments for further discussion during their free time. Reality Conversation groups were set up from among these students. In one six month period, approximately 1000 junior and senior high school students *voluntarily* made appointments for further discussion.[28]

It has been said that *people* can be divided into three groups: those who make things happen, those who watch things happen, and those who wonder what happened. In an effort to appeal to the first group, the Baltimore (Maryland) schools designed a program of study to go beyond the commonly used and misused drugs discussed in grade five. Starting in grade seven the emphasis is placed on pharmacology, psycho-social items, and interpersonal relationships. The viewpoint is that the more students *understand themselves,*

---

[28]Rose M. Daniels, "Drug Education Begins Before Kindergarten," *Journal of School Health,* 40:242–248, May, 1970.

the easier it will be to teach about narcotics and other dangerous drugs. The curriculum is as follows:

Drug Abuse Education Program
  Curriculum Content: Grade 7

I. Pharmacology
  A. Characteristics of drugs
    1. Drugs come in many forms, sizes, shapes and color.
    2. Substances may be introduced into the body by various methods (ingestion, implantation, injection, application).
  B. Effects of drugs
    1. Drugs may be used for beneficial reasons.
      a. Medical uses
      b. Research
      c. Veterinary science
      d. Agriculture
    2. Drugs may be misused causing
      a. Dependency
      b. Overdosage
      c. Unpredictable side effects
      d. Undesirable behavior
      e. Accidental death
    3. Drugs may be abused causing
      a. Depression
      b. Stimulation
      c. Distortion
      d. Intoxication
      e. Delirium
  C. History of drugs
    1. Chemicals have been abused and misused as far back as 4000 B.C.
    2. Some chemicals are abused more than others
      a. Volatile chemicals (glue, paint thinner, gasoline)
      b. Controlled drugs (depressants, stimulants, hallucinogens)
      c. Narcotic drugs (opiates)
II. Psycho-Social Aspects
  A. Recognition of different life styles
    1. Humans differ in racial, ethnic, and religious backgrounds.
    2. Life styles have merit for the individuals involved.

    3. Individuals are more alike than different.
  B. Role of the environment in the use of drugs
    1. Environment is a factor in determining which drugs are abused.
    2. Environment is a factor in determining the extent of drug abuse.
  C. Role of the individual in the use of drugs.
    1. Individuals differ in their involvement with drugs.
    2. Individuals differ in their reactions to drugs.
  D. Society's involvement with the drug problem.
    1. Society failed in the past to control the manufacture and use of drugs.
    2. Advertisement of drugs has filled the communication media.
    3. Drug education programs have been established in schools.
    4. Agencies for treatment of drug abusers are available.
    5. Laws to control the manufacture, possession, use and transportation of drugs have been passed.   *Guest Speaker*
III. Interpersonal relationships
  A. Personal adjustment
    1. Development of a worthwhile self-concept is necessary.
    2. Development of a sense of values is essential.
    3. Individuals need to feel successful.
  B. Peer interaction
    1. An individual must have a feeling of belonging.
    2. An individual must get along with his peers.
    3. An individual must be able to

withstand pressures of his peer group.
  C. Family relationships
    1. It is necessary for one to understand family problems.
    2. An individual must assume responsibilities as a family member.
    3. An individual must be able to accept his family.
  D. School and community relationships
    1. An individual must learn self-control.
    2. He must learn to understand other points of view.

    3. He must learn from failure and defeat.
  E. Role of the individual in society
    1. He must learn effective methods of problem solving.
    2. He must learn to release frustrations in a harmless fashion.
    3. He should learn to guide his natural curiosity into constructive channels.
    4. He must develop a life philosophy compatible with the society in which he lives.

One of the finest resource books containing summaries of factual information on the major drugs of abuse, and techniques and suggestions that experienced drug educators have found helpful in communicating with young people, is the *Resource Book for Drug Abuse Education.* It was developed by the AAHPER and the National Science Teachers Association and is available from the National Education Association in Washington. The Smith, Kline and French Company manual (Philadelphia, Pennsylvania) also contains numerous teaching ideas. Schools may subscribe free to *Alcohol and Health Notes* and *Grassroots,* updated drug education publications available from the National Coordinating Council on Drug Abuse Education and Information, Inc., 1211 Connecticut Ave., N.W., Washington, D.C. 20036. In addition, the following references are particularly valuable to the health and science teachers:[29]

Addiction and Drug Abuse Report, monthly newsletter on drug abuse, prevention, and treatment; write for further information (Addiction and Drug Abuse Report, 331 Madison Ave., New York, N.Y. 10017).

Alternative Pursuits for America's 3rd Century, resource book on alternatives to drugs. National Institute on Drug Abuse. Superintendent of Documents, U.S. Government Printing Office, Washington, D.C. 20402. $2.60 per copy DHEW Pub. No. (HSM) 79–9158.

Answers to the Most Frequently Asked Questions about Drug Abuse, pamphlet; other materials also available, including model curriculum guide; write for information (National Clearinghouse for Drug Abuse Information, 5454 Wisconsin Ave., Chevy Chase, Maryland 20015).

Drug Abuse and Your Child, Public Affairs Pamphlet No. 448, by Alice Shiller; suggests how parents can help youngsters stay clear of drugs (Public Affairs Committee, Inc., 381 Park Ave. South, New York, N.Y. 10016; $.25).

Drug Abuse: Everybody's Hang-up, 14 min., sound, color film; of special interest to parents, teachers, community groups (NEA Sound Studios, 1201 Sixteenth St., N.W., Washington, D.C. 20036; $90).

---

[29]Also see Chapter 12 for many additional sources to be used by the instructor and students.

Drugs of Abuse, pamphlet showing pictures of various drugs; catalog No. FS 13.128/a: D842 (Superintendent of Documents, U.S. Gov't Printing Office, Washington, D.C. 20402; $.20).

Teaching About Drugs: A Curriculum Guide, K–12, Comprehensive 200-page guide. American School Health Association; Kent, Ohio 44240.

What You Must Know about Drugs, by Harvey R. Greenberg; for junior- and senior-high pupils (Scholastic Book Services, 50 W. 44th St., New York, N.Y. 10036; paperback $.95; hardcover edition $4.75).

Youth and the Drug Problem, by Henry T. Van Dyke; written for high-school level but usable in junior highs (Ginn; paperback $1.59 net).

A Handbook on Drug and Alcohol Abuse, by Frederick G. Hofmann, Toronto: Oxford University Press, 1975.

Behavioral Objectives

(Junior High Level)

Illustrates that if properly used, drugs are of immense value to mankind.

Explains how the development of better drugs has decreased disease, extended the life span, and improved mental health.

Identifies prescription drugs as those that can only be legally purchased with a prescription from a medical doctor or a doctor of dentistry who is licensed to prescribe medication.

Tells why only a registered pharmacist is licensed to fill a prescription, left over medicine should be discarded, and time can change the strength and nature of a drug.

Names the numerous commercials on television, radio, newspapers and magazines that are designed to "sell" the public on the habitual use of unnecessary drugs: tonics, alkalines, pills, capsules, laxatives, pain relievers, and many others.

Examines the Federal Food, Drug and Cosmetic Act, which is designed to insure the safety and efficacy of drugs reaching the consumer.

Researches the literature to find that experimentation with drugs can lead to uncontrolled use of drugs; it may also lead to other individual health problems.

Chooses not to use drugs such as the stimulants (amphetamines) for "kicks" since the "side effects" may not be able to be dealt with—excessive nervousness, poor judgment, spasms, tremors, and hallucinations.

Explains how a number of narcotic drugs are used by physicians when treating patients to deaden pain and induce sleep; care is exercised against overuse.

Identifies a number of illegal drugs, all of which are capable of affecting a person's mood and ultimate well-being.

Explains how the craving for certain drugs is so intense in the addict that maintaining his drug supply becomes his main concern, leading to crime to support the habit.

Illustrates how various kinds of alcoholic beverages affect the body in different ways.

Writes that there is a relationship between all chemicals which have an effect on the mind—they either stimulate or depress at some level of the brain.

Describes how alcoholic beverages may result in personal and community health and safety problems.

Discusses alcoholism as a disease that has many causes; it affects people in different ways; it can be treated.

Acts out a common adolescent view of drinking as "adult" behavior; teenagers tend to imitate adults.

Explains how some young people resort to drinking as a way of meeting the unhappiness of failure.

Demonstrates how alcohol inhibits muscular coordination and judgment.

Tells how the excessive use of alcohol may affect one's ability to keep a job; accident rates increase when workers have been drinking, and the ability to concentrate, hear, see, and touch are impaired by alcohol.

Outlines how crime may be an outcome of the misuse of alcohol.

Essential topics (Drugs)	*Essential topics (Alcohol)*
Anesthetics	Manufacturing alcohol
Antibiotics	Physiological effects
Aspirin	Illness and death
Tranquilizers	Social problems
Amphetamines	Beverage consumption
Barbiturates	Legal controls
Antiseptics	Gang behavior
Morphine	Blood alcohol percentages
Codine	Youth-adult relationships
Heroin	Juvenile delinquency
Cocaine	Automobile and industrial accidents
Addiction	Alcohol and mental health
Commerical advertising	Peer pressure
Antihistamines	Attitudes about drinking
Hallucinogens	Alternatives to heavy drinking
Marijuana	Building self-image
Prescription drugs	
Non-prescription drugs	
Safeguarding drugs and their use	
Peer group practices	
LSD	
DMT	
Mescaline	
Psilocybin	
Dependence	
Government regulations	

Behavioral Objectives

(Senior High Level)

Uses drugs as medically directed; to do otherwise is to ignore years of research, testing, and quality control.

Details how it is possible to become addicted to drugs because of mental or social problems, feelings of inadequacy, or a low self-image.

Solves problems by seeking help from friends, counselors, clergymen, and physicians, which is more constructive than drug addiction.

Interprets research to show that withdrawal illness is the reaction of the body to the absence of the drug upon which the person has become dependent.

Explains how the U.S. Department of Justice has agents around the world attempting to reduce heroin traffic into this country.

Comments on the fact that the Supreme Court has ruled that drug addiction is an illness, and that the development of programs of compulsory treatment of addicts would serve the health and welfare interests of the state.

Illustrates, with examples from the literature, why most addicts are described as immature, easily frustrated, and incapable of assuming responsibility; in their rehabilitation they learn to face up to life's responsibilities without the use of drugs; the helping process is difficult and complex.

Depicts how the economy of the nation is affected by illegal drug production, drug traffic, and drug use.

Shows how alcohol may be used in a number of ways to benefit as well as adversely affect people.

Illustrates how the economy of the country is affected by alcohol consumption—industry, taxes, accidents, broken homes, welfare costs.

Outlines how the rehabilitation of alcoholics calls for community involvement.

Makes the decision to drink or not to drink; a mentally healthy person does not attempt to escape reality by the excessive use of alcohol.

Explains that there is a relationship between cirrhosis of the liver, pneumonia, tuberculosis, acute pancreatitis, longevity, and mental well-being.

Talks with former alcoholics to find that psychological-emotional treatment and rehabilitation are available through Alcoholics Anonymous.

Discovers that alcohol research is being carried on by many individuals and organizations; some are voluntary and some are public.

Refrains from drinking prior to school activities (dances, games, etc.) because it is in poor taste and frequently leads to trouble.

Essential topics (Drugs)	*Essential topics (Alcohol)*
Review major stimulants, depressants, hallucinogens, and other mood modifiers	Psychological effects
	Rehabilitation
Pharmacological controls	Legal limits
Drug traffic	Beverage content
Legal controls	Community problems
Physical dependence	Liquor advertising
Tolerances	Alcoholics Anonymous
Intelligent decisions	Research agencies
Economic influences	Alcohol taxes
Legislation	High school functions
Rehabilitation	Self-image and esteem
Socio-psychological determinants	Teenage consumption
Marijuana controversy	Traffic Safety
Withdrawal	Giving help with problems
Central nervous system	Alternative activities
Mood modifications	Marriage and family implications
Youth rebellion	
Meaningful education	

Suggested Activities

(Junior High Level)

1. Study the lives of health scientists who discovered life saving drugs. Diagram how these various drugs enter the body, travel the bloodstream, and reach their intended destination to help the individual. This can be done with penicillin.

2. Diagram the central nervous system in order to show how drugs and volatile chemicals affect the body. Invite a local druggist to extend the discussion.

3. Have students prepare a bulletin board display of newspaper and magazine patent medicine advertising.

4. Appoint a committee of three to call on several physicians in order to obtain a variety of drug company advertisements pertaining to drug products. These advertising items may also be found in medical and public health journals.

5. Study the meaning of such words as the following:

personality disorders, establishment, society, culture, self-discipline, social control, self-reliance, self-identification, individuality, conformance, euphoria, hallucinogen, sedative, pharmacology, nausea, lethargy, analgesic, depressant, tranquilizer, toxicity, neurotic, delirium, stimulant, narcotic.

6. Examine patent medicine and prescription drug labels. Indicate what kinds of side effects people should be alerted to with certain drugs. Show the wide range of human reactions, from mild rash to death, because of individual body chemistry.

7. Obtain Food and Drug Administration materials relative to drugs. Couple this with a talk by an FDA representative from the nearest regional office.

8. Set up a *value grid* to show how beliefs or actions fit the seven valuing process requirements. Have each student construct a value grid as shown below:

ISSUES	1	2	3	4	5	6	7

Then, with the student's help, name some health issues such as marijuana smoking, "speed" usage, drinking and driving, over-the-counter drugs, or any others. The students then list the issues on the lines under *issue*. Next to each issue they write down a few key words that summarize their position on that issue.

The seven numbers in the columns to the right represent the following questions:

(1) Are you *proud* of and do you prize or cherish your position?

(2) Have you *publically affirmed* your position?

(3) Have you chosen your position from *alternatives*?

(4) Have you chosen your position after *thoughtful consideration* of the pros and cons and consequences?

(5) Have you chosen your position *freely?*

(6) Have you *acted* on or done anything about your beliefs?

(7) Have you acted with *repetition,* or *consistency* on this issue?

Each student checks the appropriate box for each issue. They may also decide to leave the question blank. There is a personal evaluation to help students acknowledge the strength of their convictions and how they arrived at them.

9. To illustrate *peer pressure* as a factor in drinking, divide the class into groups of six.[30] Place a water-filled liquor bottle in the center of each group. Provide each group

---

[30]Adapted from the work of Ruth C. Engs and reported in Ruth C. Engs, S. Eugene Barnes, and Molly Wantz, *Health Games Students Play: Creative Strategies for Health Education,* Dubuque, Iowa: Kendall-Hunt Publishing Co., 1975.

member except for one in each group with a slip of paper which reads: "Under no circumstances take a drink from the bottle. Resist all efforts of anyone attempting to make you." Give the single member of each group a slip of paper which reads: "Take a drink and attempt to coerce anyone not drinking to do so." Request that no one share their directions with anyone else. Having asked all to read their directions, allow 10 minutes for everyone in the several groups to interact. When the game is stopped by the teacher, ask the "it" person:

    a. How does it feel to have this kind of pressure on you?

    b. How do you feel now?

Then ask the class questions such as

    a. What was happening in this activity?

    b. What is peer pressure? Why is it important to learn about it?

    10. Study the danger of drugs in sports—particularly the "pep" pills (amphetamines) which act to overstimulate the individual, lessening the sense of fatigue and constricting blood vessels. This is a particularly dangerous drug for athletes because it artificially heightens the strain on various physiologic systems already under special stress due to exertion.

18-year old French soccer player dies after game.   British cyclist rides himself to death.

---

    11. Sedatives, hypnotics, and certain tranquilizers can cause drowsiness while driving an automobile. "Speed" drugs can produce muscular tremor, dizziness, and hallucinations in which roadways appear that do not exist. Discuss *drugs and driving,* with a legal officer in class to act as moderator.

    12. Appraise for class lesson planning how much *knowledge* and *interest* students have in drug related areas. Two sample items are given from a 38-item checklist used by Oakley Ray[31] on p. 184.

    13. Organize a student survey of home medicine cabinets. Combine information obtained in class, and then discuss differences between prescription and non-prescription drugs.

    14. Post question:

WHY ISN'T "SPEED" USED BY ATHLETES?

Allow the answer to develop—that amphetamines are dangerous because of the hazardous effect of masking the signs of fatigue or exhaustion. Side effects include psychological dependence.

---

[31]Oakley S. Ray, *Checklist for Knowledge and Interest on Drugs and Drug Use,* in *Drugs, Society and Human Behavior,* St. Louis: The C. V. Mosby Co., 1972.

	KNOWLEDGE			INTEREST		
	none	some	adequate	none	some	great
Use of drugs						
a. To reduce appetite						
b. To reduce anxiety						
c. To increase wakefulness						
d. To aid in falling asleep						
e. To reduce symptoms of mental illness						
f. To reduce cold and allergy symptoms						
g. To reduce aches and pain						
h. To reduce mania						
i. To modify learning ability						
j. To increase pleasure						
Alcohol						
a. Physiological effects						
b. Use for medical purposes						
c. Use for nonmedical (recreational-social) purposes						
d. Possible adverse effects with moderate use						
e. Possible adverse effects with excessive or long-term use						

15. Collect pictures from advertisements for various drugs, e.g., aspirin, cough syrup, capsules for sleep, rubbing alcohol, nose drugs, inhalers, pain relievers, etc. Have students arrange pictures on a bulletin board under following headings:

FOR INTERNAL USE		
Ingestion	Inhalation	Injection
FOR EXTERNAL USE		

16. Illustrate the Texas billboard sign used in a social drinking campaign:

If you need a drink to be social, that's not social drinking.

17. Take sides in a debate affirming:

a. Stronger laws are the answer to the drug abuse problem.

b. It is better to join the gang than be a loner.

c. Marijuana should not be classified as a narcotic.

d. A 24-hour telephone service for young people to call to get help with a problem will not work because it will be labeled the "establishment."

18. Perform some experiments to answer basic questions:

BASIC QUESTIONS	EXPERIMENTATION
a. How do drugs affect the rate of an animal's heartbeat?	a. Test the effects of various stimulants and depressants, including beverages, on the pulse rate of *Daphnia* (water flea). Compare results and give conclusions.
b. What other effects may a drug have on an animal?	b. Observe the effects of amphetamines and barbiturates on the behavior and appetite of mice. Extrapolate these findings to human behavior.
c. How does the physician choose an effective drug for his patient?	c. Determine which antibiotic inhibits the growth of *Bacillus cereus*. Discuss the use of antibiotic discs to show growth-inhibition of pathogenic bacteria.
d. How fast do drugs act on the body?	d. Measure the time required for tablet disintegration in gastric and intestinal fluids. Relate the need for specific tablet coatings to the controlled ingestion of a drug.

A detailed example of experimentation on basic question (a) is as follows:

How do drugs affect the rate of an animal's heartbeat?

The small fresh-water crustacean called the Daphnia is a good laboratory animal in which to observe the effects of a drug on the rate of an animal's heartbeat. Daphnia are commonly found in ponds or streams, or may be purchased from any biological supply house.

The Daphnia is transparent, and you may observe the rapidly beating heart with a wide-field microscope. Place a Daphnia in a drop of water on a microscopic slide and focus under low power. Make three 1-minute counts and average the counts to determine the normal rate of heartbeat of the animals. This is the control.

a. Demonstration using a stimulant (amphetamine):

Crush one 5 mg. tablet of d-amphetamine sulfate, or one 10 mg. tablet of dl-amphetamine sulfate, or a similar stimulant, and dissolve it in 1 quart of water. Place a Daphnia in one drop of this weak solution on a microscopic slide. Take the average of three 1-minute readings of the pulse. Compare the reading with the reading obtained from the control Daphnia.

Discard the animal used with the drop of amphetamine solution, or flush it thoroughly with fresh water.

b. Demonstration using a depressant:

Make another weak solution of a drug, this time using a tranquilizer, such as chlorpromazine hydrochloride, or a more potent depressant, such as phenobarbital. A 10 mg. tablet in a quart of water will be suitable. Determine the average heart rate of the Daphnia under the influence of the depressant. Compare the reading with those obtained from the control Daphnia and from the use of amphetamine.

c. Demonstrations using beverages and o-t-c drugs:

Test other substances which may have a depressant or stimulant effect on the rate of heartbeat. Suggested substances are: tea, coffee, cola drinks, alcohol, cough syrup containing codeine, and over-the-counter (o-t-c) preparations for "inducing sleep." Classify the test substances under these headings: pulse unchanged, pulse increased, and pulse decreased.

   d. Evaluate the accumulated data. Answer the following questions:
   (1) If many different Daphnia are used, what is the control?
   (2) Could some factor other than the added drugs (or beverages) have caused the differences in heartbeat?
   (3) Which of the substances tested are stimulants; which are depressants?
   (4) If the concentrations of the drug solutions were changed, how would this affect the pulse?

   19. Set up a discussion pertaining to these issues:
   Teenagers use alcohol only to rebel.
   Teenagers aren't old enough to make decisions for themselves.
   Daily drinking leads to alcoholism.
   Liquor dealers and advertising are responsible for drinking among young people.
   There are laws against teenage drinking.
   The best place to learn about drinking is in the home.

   20. Discuss the following personality types which are prone to alcoholism:
a. lonely
b. inferior
c. anxious
d. dependent
e. passive or withdrawn
f. immature

   21. Collect advertisements from newspapers and magazines and determine whether they are effective on youth. Discuss the "half-truth" approach of some ads, such as the Canadian Club ad where the man who conquers some difficult obstacle or achieves a great sporting feat always reaches for a glass of CC whiskey.

   22. Sample class opinion regarding drinking myths.[32]

   — I drive better after a few drinks.
   — Most skid row bums are alcoholics.
   — Very few women become alcoholics.
   — You are not an alcoholic unless you drink a pint a day.
   — Most alcoholic people are middle-aged or older.
   — Alcohol is a stimulant.
   — "Ya gotta hand it to Joe. He can really hold his liquor."
   — Getting drunk is funny.
   — "Give him black coffee. That'll sober him up."
   — Today's kids don't drink.
   — It is rude to refuse a drink.
   — Alcoholism is just a state of mind.

   23. Assign groups of three students to build crossword puzzles pertaining to the drug use and abuse practices (see Figure 6–8).

   24. Collect newspaper clippings on accidents involving alcohol. Use these to introduce the topic of blood alcohol concentration. Check on State definitions of intoxication levels. (The probability of an accident increases rapidly from 0.08 per cent to an extremely high rate *above* 0.15 per cent.)

---

[32]Obtain the especially useful booklet, "Drinking Myths: A Guided Tour through Folklore, Fantasy, Humbug and Hogwash," United States Jaycees, Box 7, Tulsa, Oklahoma 74102.

Can you build this snowman?

ACROSS

3. Bean-shaped organs which might be injured by drugs
5. Marijuana is usually ————— but can be eaten mixed with food.
7. Taking drugs can be compared to getting caught in a spider's ————.
8. Hard drug from the poppy plant
9. Marijuana cigarette
10. LSD can be mixed with ———— or drinks.
12. Each time you take barbs you need ———— than before to get the same results
13. LSD (slang)
14. Some people take drugs because it is the latest ———.
16. Misusing drugs (2 words)
19. A person who sells illegal drugs
20. Body part with which you think, which may be injured by drugs
21. Teenagers are usually introduced to drugs by their ————————
23. Once you start taking drugs it is hard to ————
26. Where you might have to go for 2 to 10 years for having marijuana in Texas
27. Source of marijuana (2 words)
30. Where much marijuana is grown
31. Energy-giving amphetamines (2 words)
34. Because barbs slow you down, they are often called ————————
35. Possession of marijuana is a ———————— in Texas
37. Heroin is usually injected into a ————
38. Because amphetamines speed you up they are often called ————————
39. A good reason to take legal drugs is to help you get well when you are ————
40. Hallucinogens (such as LSD) are ———— ———— ———————— drugs
45. LSD is often eaten on this; you might put it in your coffee
46. One excuse people give for taking drugs is that they want to escape from ————————

DOWN

1. Initials of a drug which is a man-made chemical
2. Marijuana (slang)
4. Amphetamines (slang); also to go fast
6. Drug which comes from the hemp plant
8. Heroin (slang); Spanish is "caballo"
11. An overdose of barbs may cause ———————
15. Blood-pumping body part, which may be injured by drugs
17. Marijuana (slang)
18. Barbiturates (slang)
19. What people sniff besides glue to get high
22. Heroin is usually ———————— into a vein with a needle.
24. Marijuana (slang)
25. One dose of heroin
28. Source of heroin (2 words)
29. Marijuana cigarettes (slang)
32. A body part near the stomach which might be injured by drugs
33. What you do with glue to get high
34. Amphetamines used in weight control (2 words)
36. Heroin is a member of the ———————— drug family.
41. Opposite of smart
42. Some people take drugs to be "————"
43. The main thing people sniff to get high
44. Taking LSD now may someday cause your ———— to be born with deformities

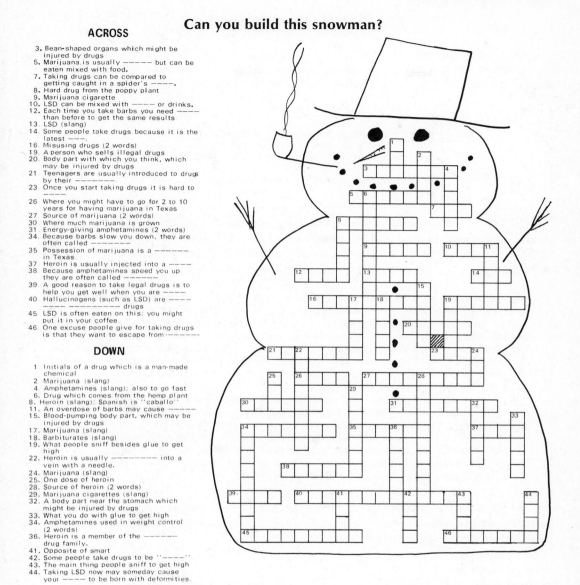

Figure 6–8   Drug education crossword puzzle. (Courtesy of Jana Whealdon, Lubbock, Texas)

25. Appoint three students, each to cover one of these topics of social drinking:

a. Social drinking is distinct and separate from alcoholism.

b. Social drinking is not harmful.

c. Social drinking is helpful.

26. Invite members of the armed forces, police department, clergy, and welfare department to discuss drinking problems as they relate to their areas of work in dealing with individuals, the family, and the public. Preface the visit with a discussion of the leading public health problems in America resulting from the alcohol problem.

Suggested Activities

(Senior High Level)

1. Raise the questions: "What does it take to *awaken* the American public to the alcohol problem? What is *social drinking?*" Post the following information on the bulletin board.

> Where does social drinking end and problem drinking begin? There's no simple answer. But here's a pretty good definition:
>
> *If you need a drink to be social, that's not social drinking.*

2. Try a "data and opinion" approach by reading the following. However, prior to reading paragraph two raise three questions: (1) How do you feel about the statement? (2) Is it too strong? (3) Is it what you would expect from someone teaching about drugs? A Mississippi state senator once addressed his legislature thus:

> You have asked me how I feel about whiskey. All right, here is just how I stand on this question: If, when you say whiskey, you mean the devil's brew, the poison scourge, the bloody monster that defiles innocence, yea, literally takes the bread from the mouths of little children; if you mean the evil drink that topples the Christian man and woman from the pinnacles of righteous, gracious living into the bottomless pit of degradation and despair, shame and helplessness and hopelessness, then certainly I am against it with all my power.

> But, if when you say whiskey, you mean the oil of conversation . . . the drink that enables a man to magnify his joy and his happiness and to forget, if only for a little while, life's great tragedies and heartbreaks and sorrows; if you mean that drink, the sale of which pours into our treasuries untold millions of dollars which are used to provide tender care for our little crippled children, our blind, our deaf, our dumb, our pitiful aged and infirm, to build highways, hospitals, and schools, then certainly I am in favor of it. This is my stand. I will not retreat from it; I will not compromise.

3. Reactions to alcohol vary considerably. Different people react differently to the same amount of alcohol. Ask the class to look into the following variables:
speed of drinking (see Figure 6–9)
type of beverage
food consumption
body weight
body chemistry
mood
attitude toward drinking
drinking experience
the situation

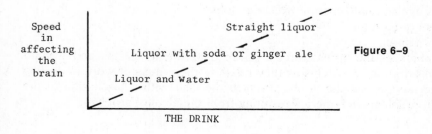

Figure 6–9

Speed in affecting the brain

Straight liquor

Liquor with soda or ginger ale

Liquor and water

THE DRINK

4. Initiate a teaching unit with the following quiz. This will ascertain feelings and facts—as well as myths and half-truths.

Circle TRUE or FALSE beside each statement.*

1. True or False: Alcohol is a drug.
2. True or False: Alcohol is a food.
3. True or False: In the body, alcohol is digested just as food is.
4. True or False: In the body, alcohol is burned up just as food is.
5. True or False: Because it is a stimulant, alcohol tends to pep a person up.
6. True or False: Everyone's body reacts the same way to the same amount of alcohol.
7. True or False: Alcoholic beverages can be fattening.
8. True or False: Alcohol in any quantity will damage organs in the human body.
9. True or False: A person can die of alcohol poisoning.
10. True or False: All alcoholic beverages are equally strong.
11. True or False: Liquor taken straight will affect you faster than liquor mixed with water or soda in a highball.
12. True or False: You'll get drunker on vodka or gin or rum than on the same amount of whiskey.
13. True or False: Switching drinks will make you drunker than staying with one kind of alcoholic beverage.
14. True or False: You can sober up quickly by drinking black coffee and dousing your head with cold water.
15. True or False: It's risky to drive a car right after having a drink.
16. True or False: Drunkenness and alcoholism are the same thing.
17. True or False: Anyone who drinks at all is likely to become an alcoholic.
18. True or False: Alcoholics can be helped.
19. True or False: There are certain symptoms to warn people that their drinking may be leading to alcoholism.

5. Post and study the following chart, which is based on 0.10 per cent as the legal

---

*The only **TRUE** answers are numbers 1, 2, 4, 7, 9, 11, 15, 18 and 19.

Figure 6-10

The operator of a motor vehicle is presumed by law to be impaired when the percent of alcohol in his blood is above a certain level. To drive legally the table below indicates how long a normal adult of given body weight must wait after drinking a given amount of whisky, to be safely within those limits. If the weight is between two of those shown use the lower one.

Drinks (1 ½ ounces) Consumed

Lbs. body weight	1	2	3	4	5	6	7	8
100	0	½	3½	6½	9½	12½	16	19
120	0	0	2	4½	7	9½	12½	15
140	0	0	1	3	5½	7½	10	12
160	0	0	0	2	4	6	8	9½
180	0	0	0	1	2½	4½	6½	8
200	0	0	0	½	2	3½	5	6½

Hours to wait after start of drinking

Prepared by Dr. Leon A. Greenberg
Rutgers University Center of Alcohol Studies

blood alcohol level. Some states have legal limits of 0.15 per cent. However, studies have shown that the level for safe driving by many people is well below the legal limit (see Figure 6-10).

6. Present a problem to be solved involving the separate processes of fermentation and distillation. Find out why fermentation will not produce alcoholic beverages over 20 per cent, while distillation may reach 50 per cent or more.

FERMENTATION		DISTILLATION	
Beer	4%	Rum	
Burgundy	10 to 14%	Gin	
Sauterne	10 to 14%	Vodka	} 40 to 50% (100 proof equals 50% alcohol)
Port	18 to 20%	Brandy	
Sherry	18 to 20%	Whiskey	
		(Rye, Bourbon, Scotch)	

7. Investigate alcohol comsumption and calories. Build on the following statements by applying them to real life situations in the home and community.

Alcohol is higher in calories than sugars and starches, although lower than fats. An ounce of liquor contains about 70 calories, the equal of a fried chicken drumstick. A 12-ounce can of beer contains about 150 calories, the equal of one frankfurter. The calories in alcohol can contribute to overweight. However, if alcohol is substituted for a balanced diet, the person may suffer from malnutrition.

8. Create a survey instrument to question senior high pupils about their drinking experience to date. Discuss findings with the class. Question both the validity and reliability of this technique, particularly as it pertains to the school survey.
Example:

WHAT KIND OF DRINKER ARE YOU?

Take This Test And Find Out For Yourself.

☐ 1. Do you think and talk about drinking often?

☐ 2. Do you drink more now than you used to?

☐ 3. Do you sometimes gulp drinks?

☐ 4. Do you often take a drink to help you relax?

☐ 5. Do you drink when you are alone?

☐ 6. Do you sometimes forget what happened when you were drinking?

☐ 7. Do you keep a bottle hidden somewhere . . . at home or at work . . . for quick pick-me-ups?

☐ 8. Do you need a drink to have fun?

☐ 9. Do you ever just start drinking without really thinking about it?

☐ 10. Do you drink in the morning to relieve a hangover?

HOW TO SCORE:

According to the National Institute on Alcohol Abuse and Alcoholism, a social drinker should have 3 or fewer "yes" answers. If you have four or more "yes" answers, you may be one of the nine million Americans with a drinking problem.

This test is not a foolproof diagnosis, but it is a rather good indicator. Four or more "yes" answers does not necessarily mean you are alcoholic, or even that you have a serious drinking problem, but it should be regarded as a real danger signal.

The drunk driver will kill 673 of us this week. Is your number up?

Figure 6–11

9. Investigate Alcoholics Anonymous, the worldwide fellowship of men and women who help each other to maintain sobriety and who offer to share their recovery experience freely with others who may have a drinking problem. (Materials are available from 305 East 45th St., New York, New York 10017.) Read several impressive case histories from *Young People and AA*. Discover the agencies that the AA is geared to work with in a typical community.

10. Young people and adults get hung up on words. Discuss such words as *dependence* and *addiction*. The word "addiction" has been pretty much discarded for "dependence." This is because a person can be addicted to something (gambling or alcohol drinking) involving some *psychological* dependence but *with or without* physical dependence.

Psychological dependence is a compulsive need for a drug to relieve emotional discomfort.

Physical dependence occurs only after prolonged usage, when the body tissues become literally dependent on the drug and cannot function properly without it.

11. Educate for moderate drinking by weighing the old expression "if you drink, don't drive – if you drive, don't drink" against the more realistic rule of current society: "No one should drive unless he has waited at least one hour for each cocktail, 'shot,' or bottle of beer beyond the first drink." Discuss the chart in Figure 6–12. Individual susceptibility to alcohol varies; this is indicated by wavy lines in the chart.

12. Initiate a discussion aimed at searching for the "why" behind the numerous newspaper headlines. Post several typical headlines on a bulletin board (see Figure 6–13).

Percent of blood alcohol	.01%		.05%		.10%		15% & Over
Number of drinks in an hour	1	2	3	4	5	6	7
Intoxicated?	Normally not		You may well be		Most persons are		You definitely are
If you drive a car	Take it easy		Use Caution		Don't		Absolutely not!

Figure 6–12

64 arraigned on So. Shore drug charges

Sixty-four youths, in-
cluding six juveniles, ar-
rested in drug raids in
Hull, Scituate and Cohasset
yesterday.

present
were
l
cc

re   continue

Figure 6–13

13. Role play real people. Obtain copies of "A Community at the Crossroads," complete with player's guide and film discussion guide. This may be obtained from the National Institute of Mental Health, National Audio-Visual Center, GSA, Washington, D.C. 20409. The film, *Understanding,* will be used. After the activity, solicit response to the following:

Many communities in America today are seeking ways of dealing with and solving "the drug prob-lem." A variety of "solutions" have been proposed. Please rank your agreement or disagreement with the following proposals.

	AGREE			DISAGREE	
a. Include drug education program in school curriculum	1	2	3	4	5
b. Increase penalties for drug use	1	2	3	4	5
c. Decrease penalties for drug use	1	2	3	4	5
d. Increase community mental health facilities	1	2	3	4	5
e. Establish self-help facility	1	2	3	4	5
f. Establish "hot line"	1	2	3	4	5
g. Create community-wide drug education program	1	2	3	4	5
h. Increase student participation in community and school planning	1	2	3	4	5

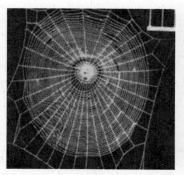 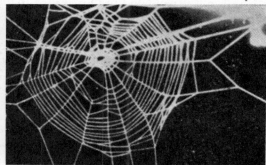

Figure 6–14   A common species of orb spider (*Araneus diadematus*) weaves an intricately symmetrical web which glistens with morning dew in the fields. When the spiders sip a weak drug solution from a syringe they freak out. Amphetamines, for instance, affect spiders like humans; they become hallucinatory, hyperactive, and so disoriented that they fail to make the correct actions, and weave the web in the wrong place. Spiders stoned on barbiturates weave smaller and more erratic webs. Both muscular coordination and brain control seem to be affected. (Psilocybin seems to cause the animals to lose interest in the process and quit early.)

14. Illustrate one effect from "tripping" on drugs by referring to animal research. Make an enlarged drawing of Figure 6–14.

> FREAKED OUT SPIDERS — from straight to stoned.

15. Prepare a student questionnaire similar to the Medford one on this page, in order to find out about drug use, rehabilitation, and prevention attitudes among high school pupils.

In order for the Medford Drug Action Council Inc. to do its job properly, we are asking you to help us by completing this questionnaire. The answers that you give us will help determine the direction which the council will take. Thank you for your cooperation. All answers will be treated confidentially.

1. Do you know what "Project People" is? ___YES ___NO (IF NO, OMIT 2 & 3)
2. Where have you heard about "Project People?"
   ___Newspaper, ___Posters, ___Friends
3. What would you like this program to offer? (check as many as you want)
   ___Hot-line, ___Rap counseling, ___Prof. counseling
   ___Drop-in center (counseling)
4. Would you like personal or drug related counseling available to you during the school hours? ___Yes ___No
   If yes, would you prefer:
   ___Trained student counselors   ___Trained teacher counselors
   ___Professional counseling   ___Trained adult counselors
5. Have you ever used drugs?
   ___Yes ___No   If yes, please check one:
   ___Experimented   ___Regular user
   ___Occasional User   ___Addicted

6. What drugs do you use:
   ___Marihuana   ___Barbiturates   ___Heroin
   ___Amphetamines   ___Acid
7. If you have a serious drug problem, are you willing to come to Project People for help? ___Yes ___No
8. Would you like to become a trained "rap" counselors for the Project?
   ___Yes ___No
9. Would you prefer to work the hot-line, lead group rap discussions, or lead individual counseling? (please circle one)
10. Would you like a drug education course incorporated with your curriculum? Ex. One semester course on drug education
    ___Yes ___No
11. Would trained adult counselors on the hot-line deter you from calling?
    ___Yes ___No
    If yes, explain:

12. Do you think the hot-line should operate seven (7) nights per week?
    ___Yes ___No
13. What hours do you think the hot-line should operate?

14. If you have used the hot-line, are you satisfied with the results of your conversation? ___Yes ___No
    If No, please explain:

15. Would you be in favor of a recreational drop-in center? ___Yes ___No
16. Would you be opposed to a drop-in center in a church? ___Yes ___No
17. Would you be opposed to uniformed Police officers patrolling the drop-in center? ___Yes ___No
    If yes, please explain:

MARIJUANA SURVEY QUESTIONNAIRE

1. How would you rank marijuana as a problem?
   - ————equal to narcotics (e.g., heroin)
   - ————equal to prescription drugs (e.g., tranquilizers)
   - ————equal to tobacco or alcohol
   - ————not a serious problem
2. Where did you get *most* of your information about marijuana?
   - ————personal experience
   - ————experience of others (e.g., clinical experience, experience of friends)
   - ————communications media (e.g., radio, TV, magazines, newspapers)
   - ————professional sources (e.g., conferences, clinicians, journals)
3. In your opinion, which of the following effects are produced by marijuana?

	Yes	No	Don't Know
a. Has habit-forming qualities (addictive)	————	————	————
b. Potentially poisonous (due to its high toxicity)	————	————	————
c. Decreases inhibitions	————	————	————
d. Develops increasing tolerance to the drug	————	————	————
e. Causes permanent mental disorders (e.g., insanity)	————	————	————
f. Lowers achievement	————	————	————
g. Provides unusual perceptual experiences (lightheadedness, time distortions)	————	————	————
h. Increases aggressions	————	————	————
i. Improves social interaction and sociability	————	————	————
j. Increases sensitivity (e.g., to food, music, sex)	————	————	————
k. Increases passivity	————	————	————
l. Worsens social relations	————	————	————
m. Increases sexual desire	————	————	————
n. Leads to other drugs (especially heroin)	————	————	————
o. Increases self-knowledge	————	————	————
p. Leads to mental deterioration	————	————	————
q. Any other effects (specify)			

4. How do you feel about present marijuana laws?
   - ————too strict   ————not strict enough   ————satisfactory
5. What position would you advocate concerning future marijuana laws?
   - ————a.   Not available legally under any circumstances
   - ————b.   Available by prescription only (and for medical research)
   - ————c.   Same availability and legal status as tobacco and liquor
   - ————d.   No restrictions on its use
6. What is your general attitude toward marijuana now?
   - ————favorable   ————unfavorable   ————mixed feelings
7. How often have you used marijuana?
   - ————never
   - ————tried it a few times
   - ————up to 3 times per week
   - ————more than 3 times per week
8. (a) If you DO NOT use marijuana, and it were legalized, would you then use it?
      - ————yes   ————no   ————undecided
   (b) If you DO use marijuana, and it were legalized, how would your pattern of usage change?
      - ————increased use   ————decreased use   ————remain unchanged
9. Have your attitudes toward marijuana changed?
   - ————yes, more favorable toward marijuana
   - ————yes, less favorable toward marijuana
   - ————no, unchanged
10. If you *have* used marijuana, at what age did you first use it?————————
11. Which of the following drugs have you *ever* used "recreationally" (i.e., not medically prescribed)?
   - ————Opiates   ————Amphetamines ("pep" pills)   ————Cigarettes (nicotine)
   - ————Mescaline   ————Tranquilizers   ————Alcohol
   - ————LSD   ————Sleeping pills   ————Coffee (caffeine)
   - ————Cocaine   ————Other (Specify) _____
12. What percentage of students do you think have tried marijuana?————%
13. Do you think that marijuana has potential for medicinal purposes?
   - ————yes (if yes, please specify below)   ————no   ————don't know
   _____
14. Do you think marijuana will be legalized within the next 5 years?
   - ————yes   ————no

16. Organize a group of high school students to visit some seventh and eighth grade classes to discuss drug abuse. Participation by speakers and listeners may be voluntary. This worked very well in the Hartford (Connecticut) public schools, where the average junior high school student held in high esteem the older boys and girls. Moreover, both junior and senior high pupils acknowledged that drug abuse is a teenage problem that teens can do something about.

17. Debate the legalization of marijuana. There is always danger in restricting freedom of choice in America. There is also danger in increasing the dosage of the active ingredient of cannabis (THC); it increases both the intensity and incidence of the psychomimetic effect.

18. Marijuana use has become a major health issue. There are legal and mental health considerations about which high schoolers have feelings. Reproduce and sample class opinion with the survey questionnaire.[33]

19. Appoint a small group to visit local druggists and read about barbiturates in general. Formulate lists of substances inducing sedation and sleep. Examples:

Barbiturates	*Barbiturate-like action*
Barbital (Veronal)	Chlormezanone (Trancopal)
Mephobarbital (Mebaral)	Meprobamate (Equanil, Miltown)
Phenobarbital (Luminal)	Mebutamate (Capla)
Amobarbital (Amytal)	Carisoprodol (Soma)
Butabarbital (Butisol)	Ectylurea (Levanil)
Hexethal (Ortal)	Chlordiazepoxide (Librium)
Pentobarbital (Nembutal)	Mephenoxalone (Trepidone)
Secobarbital (Seconal)	Bromisovalum (Bromural)
Hexobarbital (Sombulex, Cyclonal)	Diazepam (Valium)
Thiopental (Pentothal)	Buclizine (Softran)

20. Set up a question-answer period about drugs and drug abuse. Have certain pupils act as "authorities" in the area of a particular drug and be ready to give an answer to a question. Especially helpful to all concerned will be readily obtainable copies of the *Federal Source Book: Answers to the Most Frequently Asked Questions About Drug Abuse* (U.S. Government Printing Office). Most questions are set forth just about the way a pupil would ask them.

21. Arrange the class in a comfortable manner and play a tape. Throw out several questions after it is played. A good tape will bring forth discussion. Try the John Burt tape, *Tripping Out* (also available on LP record), Box 285, Sylvania, Ohio 43560. Try also *Marijuana, Hallucinogens, and Narcotics,* available from Educational Progress Corporation, 8538 E. 41st Street, Tulsa, Oklahoma 74145.

22. Demonstrate how drugs are used to treat brain tumors. Some 30 drugs have been helpful in various forms of cancer. A silicone rubber tube may be inserted into one of the brain ventricles or into the bed of the excised tumor. This tube is connected to a reservoir placed beneath the scalp. An anticancer drug is placed into the reservoir via a needle, and flows from the tube into the cerebrospinal fluid, where it diffuses into the brain. By pressing on the scalp skin covering the reservoir, the physician may pump the drug into the central nervous system at a predetermined rate (See Figure 6–15). (Drawing: U.S. Department HEW, Washington, D.C.)

23. Post marijuana "fables" for all to see. Following class discussion, post the "facts" (U.S. Government Printing Office, *Marihuana Fables and Facts*).

24. Ask students to recommend what additional community facilities are needed to help young people with their problems. Are there *alternatives* to drugs in the community that students can suggest?

---

[33]Adapted from a longer questionnaire employed by Richard H. Seiden, et al., "Patterns of Marijuana Use Among Public Health Students," *American Journal of Public Health,* 65:613–622, June, 1975.

ALTERNATIVE PURSUITS?

FABLES	FACTS
1. Marihuana is a narcotic.	Marihuana is not a narcotic except by statute. Narcotics are opium or its derivatives (like heroin and morphine) and some synthetic chemicals with opium-like activity.
2. Marihuana is addictive.	Marihuana does not cause physical addiction, since tolerance to its effects, and symptoms on sudden withdrawal do not occur. It can produce habituation (psychological dependence).
3. Marihuana causes violence and crime.	Persons under the influence of marihuana tend to be passive. Sometimes a crime is committed by a person while under the influence of marihuana. The personality of the user is as important as the type of drug in determining whether chemical substances lead to criminal or violent behavior.
4. Marihuana leads to increase in sexual activity.	Marihuana has no aphrodisiac property.
5. Marihuana is harmless.	Instances of acute panic, depression, and psychotic states are known, although they are infrequent. Certain kinds of individuals can also become over-involved in marihuana use and center their lives around it. We do not know the effects of long-term use.
6. Occasional use of marihuana is less harmful than occasional use of alcohol.	We do not know. Research on the effects of various amounts of each drug for various periods is underway.
7. Marihuana use leads to heroin.	We know of nothing in the nature of marihuana that predisposes to heroin abuse. It is estimated that less than 5 per cent of chronic users of marihuana will progress to experiment with heroin.
8. Marihuana enhances creativity.	Marihuana might bring fantasies of enhanced creativity but they are illusory, as are "instant insights" reported by marihuana users.
9. More severe penalties will solve the marihuana problem.	Marihuana use has increased enormously in spite of severely punitive laws.
10. It is safe to drive while under the influence of marihuana.	Driving under the influence of any intoxicant is hazardous.

3. SMOKING EDUCATION

Tobacco is a dirty weed, I like it. It satisfies no normal need, I like it. It makes you thin, it makes you lean. It takes the hair right off your bean. It's the worst dam stuff I've ever seen. I like it.

—G. L. Hemminger
Published in Penn State
Froth, November, 1915

Not long ago, James Reston underlined a condition of the collective psyche more potent than all the warning cries of apocalyptic earthquakes or urban chaos or nuclear Armageddons that pound human ears. Mr. Reston cautioned that

> ... something important is happening to the human mind. *It is being drugged by facts and diverted from reality*. Every hour and every day it hears and reads the most astonishing things but is not astonished. It is given the facts of the human condition, but it does not feel them or doesn't think it can do anything about them.

This is a disturbing thought. Does it mean that society ignores the staggering, even astounding fruits of competent nicotine and tar research? Does it miss the message because it doesn't care? Is it simply willing to join Hemminger's smoker and say "I like it"? Have people arrived at that unhappy state in present civilization where their judgment and potentially superb sensitivities are tarnished and dulled?

It has been known for years that tobacco smoking is a health hazard. Yet eliminating the practice has been next to impossible. In fact, it has increased over the decades, not because of powerfully permeating advertising campaigns and the narcotic effects alone, but because human response to a noxious agent depends more upon past mental and emotional experience than upon the particular and immediate stimulus. Moreover, cultural and interpersonal human pressures may be more threatening than physical or biological forces, and they may override intellect.

Smoking is a socially acceptable addiction which is encouraged more than it is discouraged. It is part of the way of life. The smoker smokes with his friends. He smokes to reduce anxieties and gain relaxation from tension. Huge industries profit from its use, and the government derives large revenues from tax on its consumption. Attempting, therefore, to separate the individual from "big business" and something which is so much a part of his life style is most difficult. Thus, the tobacco smoking mortality and morbidity statistics continue, frequently startling the reader—much too often only in an academic way.

The research findings are irrefutable. The statistics by themselves will not change behavior, but properly employed, they may help. With this in mind, the Surgeon General

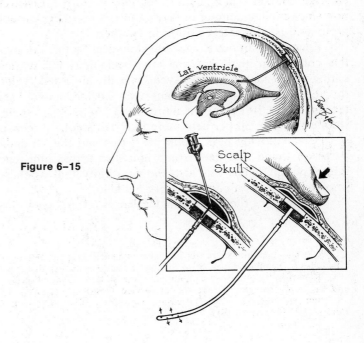

Figure 6–15

of the Public Health Service issued the now famous 1964 report, *Smoking and Health,* which associated cigarette smoking with higher death rates and death at earlier ages. In 1967, a follow-up report was issued, *The Health Consequences of Smoking,* and after this, some supplementary reports strengthening the conclusions reached in the earlier study. In addition to these concentrated findings, a great amount of information has come from the National Health Survey—a continuing study conducted by the National Center for Health Statistics of the Public Health Service. In carrying out the survey, interviewers each year visit 42,000 families and question them about illness, disability, and days absent from work because of illness. It has been well documented that there are considerably more chronic illnesses among the heavy smokers than among those who smoked fewer cigarettes or none at all. Smokers also reported more chronic conditions per person.[34] In fact, there are about 11 million more cases of chronic illness yearly in this country than there would be if all people had the same rate of sickness as those who have never smoked cigarettes. Research findings continue to link tobacco smoking with heart disease, hypertension, emphysema, oral and lung cancer, pregnancy difficulties, sinusitis, peptic ulcers, cirrhosis of the liver, accidental death from fires, and the more obvious economic losses related to days lost from work. On the average, the life expectancy of a non-smoking male of 25 is 6½ years longer than that of a male who smokes one or more packs a day. The age at which one starts to smoke is important. Men who started smoking prior to age 15 show a death rate from lung cancer nearly five times higher than those who begin after age 25.

It is difficult to read and appreciate paragraph after paragraph of facts relating to death and illness from cigarette smoking. Numerous excellent reports from both official and non-official health agencies have tables, charts, and graphs which depict the real extent of the problem.

TEENAGE SMOKING PRACTICES

Somewhat like adults, teenagers are a real mixture of humanity. Thus, there is no clearcut smoker's personality emerging from the research. While smokers differ from non-smokers in a number of ways, there is no single variable which is found solely in one group and is completely absent in another.[35]

Except for an occasional physiological factor, the overwhelming evidence points to the conclusion that smoking—its beginning, habituation, and occasional discontinuation—is to a large extent psychologically and socially determined. Status orientation of the teenager is more important than socioeconomic status of the parents. In fact, teenagers are 100 per cent more likely to smoke if their friends, brothers, and sisters smoke and only 50 per cent more likely to smoke if their parents or other adults smoke.

After studying peer group pressures and the "friendship patterns" of adolescents, Newman found that peer group influence grows and reaches its peak during the high school period.[36] There is also the possibility that when peer group needs are not met, smoking becomes a compensatory behavior.

The extent of teenage smoking varies from place to place, and although adult smok-

---

[34]Chronic conditions are those illnesses which last for a long time—months, even years. Asthma, tuberculosis, rheumatic fever, heart disease, chronic bronchitis, diabetes, and arthritis are all chronic diseases.

[35]Report of the Advisory Committee to the Surgeon General of the U.S. Public Health Service, *Smoking and Health,* Washington: Public Health Service, U.S. Dept. HEW, 1970, p. 40.

[36]Ian M. Newman, "Peer Pressure Hypothesis for Adolescent Cigarette Smoking," *School Health Review,* 1:15–19, April, 1970.

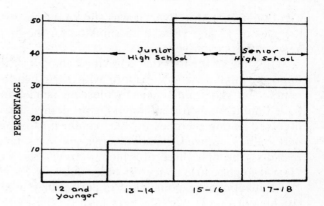

Figure 6–16   Age at which students begin to smoke. (Courtesy of John H. Arnett and Drexel University Study)

ing has dropped off owing to massive educational efforts, the youth statistics continue to rise—with the greatest number of individuals beginning to smoke at age 15 (see Figure 6–16).[37] It is the girls who have increased the most in every age group over a 6-year period. Kelson demonstrated this in a northwestern Ohio study.[38] The U.S. Department of Health, Education and Welfare, in a more extensive study found the same thing (see

---

[37]John H. Arnett, et al., "An 11-Year Study of Cigarette Smoking Habits of Students Entering Drexel University, Philadelphia," *American Journal of Public Health,* 64:120–128, February, 1974.

[38]Saul R. Kelson, "The Growing Epidemic," *American Journal of Public Health,* 65:923–938, September, 1975.

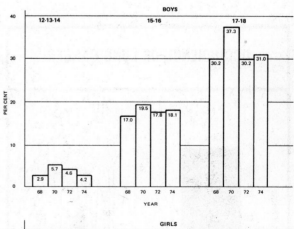

Figure 6–17   Percentage of regular teenage smokers, 1968–1974. (Courtesy of U.S. Department of Health, Education and Welfare)

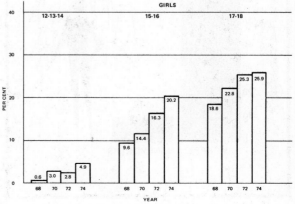

Figure 6–17).[39] Moreover, it was shown that every day over 3200 young people between the ages of 12 and 18 take up smoking for the first time—adding up to over one million new smokers each year.

In view of the fact that smoking behavior reflects personality and social forces, it is important that teachers explore with their health classes the various cultural components, peer group influences, adolescent needs, and other psychosocial variables which have ramifications for anti-smoking programs. This kind of instruction can become quite involved as one searches for reasons for not becoming a smoker, or for giving it up. Arnett's study showed that both boys and girls failed to start, or gave it up for several reasons—the first three of which were (1) "lack of enjoyment smoking cigarettes," (2) "fear it might cause cancer or other diseases," and (3) "athletic considerations."

Educational responsibility is particularly great in the smoking area. Too often, as Hochbaum points out, teachers harp on the evils of smoking, drinking, marijuana, and sex, and deny the satisfactions some adolescents derive from them—so much so that adolescents openly say that we do not know what we are talking about. Hochbaum illustrated this some years ago by referring to a well written but one-sided booklet he had a teenage class read. It was fairly well received until the readers came to a passage which told them that they were young and smoking should present no particular problem. It went on, " . . . All you have to do is to make up your mind not to take any more cigarettes." At this point, two of the teenagers immediately put down the booklet and

---

[39]National Clearinghouse for Smoking and Health, *Patterns and Prevalence of Teen-Age Cigarette Smoking: 1968–1974*, DHEW Pub. No. (HSM) 74–8701.

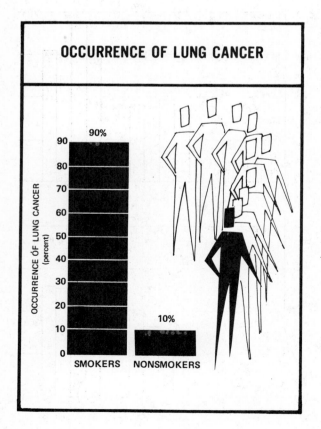

Figure 6–18 Incidence of lung cancer among smokers and nonsmokers. (Courtesy of U.S. Public Health Service)

remarked that the author "does not know anything about teenage smoking or he would not make such a stupid remark."[40] It happened that both of these students were already smoking two packs a day and had tried unsuccessfully to give up smoking. They didn't bother to finish reading the booklet. Because the booklet didn't fit reality, it lost the very readers to whom it was primarily addressed.

There is a fair amount of evidence that the vast majority of youngsters know that cigarette smoking is harmful to health. Many of the older youths are not impressed, because they see a world of "credibility gap" examples. Younger children accept facts with somewhat more certainty. What hurts the most, according to student statements, is having a teacher set a poor example by smoking, and thereby undoing most of his or her effectiveness. Significantly related to this is a study of smoking behavior and attitudes toward smoking education of teachers who smoke. Here it was discovered that smoking teachers were the least active in initiating student smoking behavior change, while ex-smokers were the most active.[41] Needed are in-service programs for teachers who want to stop smoking.

So often it is heard that a new approach is needed for smoking education. Since smoking is still sociably acceptable and heavy advertising tries to create an atmosphere of acceptance, it is not likely that the task of changing practices will become any easier over the next several years. Teacher training models can help. The Berkeley Unified School District model was created by the National Clearinghouse for Smoking and Health to reach fifth, sixth, and seventh grade pupils with an organization built around body systems: living and respiratory system for the fifth grade, heart and circulatory system for the sixth grade, and brain and nervous system for grade seven. The program is comprehensive, fosters critical thinking regarding the consequences of smoking, and culminates in an understanding of how abuses affect the intricate human machine. All units of study are correlated with other subjects and a variety of resource persons from the community. Parents and other family members are worked into the program. Much of the success is due to the preparation of the teachers in the model.

From the Nathaniel Greene Middle School in Providence, Rhode Island, to the Stephen F. Austin Junior High School in Amarillo, Texas, dramatic alternative ideas to smoking are being experienced. In both instances students quit smoking in great numbers, having been convinced of the wisdom of their decision. In a similar circumstance in Niagara County, New York, there was a tendency for smokers to reduce their levels of smoking even if they didn't stop altogether.[42] In this instance, it was made clear that one way of presenting the smoking topic does not fit everyone. Several quite distinct approaches must be made. A good example is the Creative Advertising Workshop at the University of Michigan where teenagers are being reached by recognizing their ability to see through phony approaches and appreciate well-directed satire and sarcasm. The program stresses the generation gap and builds smoking up as an old-fashioned practice belonging to the older generation.

Pupil involvement is always good teaching. One of the ways to do this is to have the class help prepare a survey instrument and then put it to use. This has been done in a number of schools and in a number of ways. To make the students aware of their own

[40]Godfrey M. Hochbaum, "How Can We Teach Adolescents About Smoking, Drinking and Drug Abuse?" *Journal of Health, Physical Education and Recreation,* October, 1968.

[41]T. L. Chen and William R. Rakip, "The Effect of the Teachers' Smoking Behavior on Their Involvement in Smoking Education in the Schools," *Journal of School Health,* 45:455–461, October, 1975.

[42]Herbert S. Rabinowitz and William H. Zimmerli, "Effects of a Health Education Program on Junior High School Students' Knowledge, Attitudes and Behavior Concerning Tobacco Use." *Journal of School Health,* 44:324–330, June, 1974.

QUESTIONNAIRE I

1. How does smoking affect the heart rate?
   Increase_____ Decrease_____ No effect_____
2. How does smoking affect body temperature?
   Raise_____ Lower_____ No effect_____
3. How does smoking affect blood pressure?
   Increase_____ Decrease_____ No effect_____
4. Is the risk of lung cancer less for non-smokers than for smokers?
   Yes_____ No_____
5. Name two respiratory diseases (diseases of the breathing system) other than lung cancer that are related to smoking.
6. Name three substances found in tobacco smoke, which are known to be harmful in large quantities.
7. Why do athletes endorse smoking in advertisements although they are not supposed to smoke?
8. Does smoking contribute to nervousness_____or to relaxation_____?
9. Explain the effect of smoking on the growth process.
10. Explain the effect of smoking on stomach ulcers.

smoking problems and feelings, the Cleveland Public Schools developed a first-class curriculum guide, *The Health Hazards of Smoking,* and set up two appropriate questionnaires. Questionnaire I is factual. Questionnaire II is designed to show pupil background and attitudes toward smoking. Both questionnaires have been used for several years to stimulate interest in the topic prior to a full discussion.

In order to take advantage of the survey findings, the Cleveland guide proceeds with its *Secondary Unit on Smoking* as follows:

I. What are the prolonged effects of smoking on the body?
   A. Lung Cancer
   B. Heart Disease
   C. Gastric and Duodenal Ulcer
   D. Respiratory Diseases (R.D.)
   E. Physical complaints more frequent with smokers than non-smokers.
      1. Smoker's Cough
      2. Shortness of Breath
      3. Hoarseness
   F. Allergic reactions in others

II. What are the immediate effects of smoking on the various parts of the body?
   A. Circulatory System
      1. Heart
      2. Arteries and Blood Vessels
   B. Respiratory System
      1. Lungs
      2. Bronchi
   C. Digestive System
      1. Salivary Glands
      2. Stomach

ANSWERS FOR QUESTIONNAIRE I

1. Increase
2. Lower
3. Increase
4. Yes
5. Pulmonary emphysema and chronic bronchitis
6. Ammonia, carbon monoxide, hydrogen cyanide, nicotine, pyridine, formaldehyde, arsenic
7. They get paid for it and perhaps were unaware of the health risk involved.
8. Nervousness
9. It affects the appetite which in turn affects body growth.
10. Smoking does not cause ulcers but it irritates them and interferes with the healing process.

QUESTIONNAIRE II

TO THE STUDENT: This is a survey on smoking among the students in the junior and senior high schools. We ask that you complete this form with honesty, neither holding back nor exaggerating the facts that pertain to you—only through your truthfulness will we be able to secure a report that will be of value to all of us.

THIS SURVEY IS PREPARED so that you *cannot* be identified as an individual. Please do not write your name on these sheets. Simply place a check in the appropriate space that refers to you.

1. I am a Boy_____; Girl_____.
2. I am in Grade 7_____; 8_____; 9_____; 10_____; 11_____; 12_____.
3. My age is 11_____; 12_____; 13_____; 14_____; 15_____; 16_____; 17_____; 18_____; 19_____.
4. Have you ever played on an athletic team either in school or outside of school? Yes_____; No_____.
    (a) If your answer is Yes, did any of your coaches advise you not to smoke during the season?
        Yes_____; No_____.
5. When you see advertisements in magazines of famous athletes smoking cigarettes, do you feel that if he smokes it must be all right?
        Yes_____; No_____.
6. Did you know that cigarette smoking may contribute toward:
    (a) Lung cancer and other chronic lung diseases?
        Yes_____; No_____.
    (b) Stomach ulcers and other digestive ailments?
        Yes_____; No_____.
    (c) Heart disease and hardening of the arteries?
        Yes_____; No_____.
7. Does information in question number six influence you not to smoke?
        Yes_____; No_____.
8. Does your father smoke? Yes_____; No_____.
9. Does your mother smoke? Yes_____; No_____.
10. Does an older brother smoke? Yes_____; No_____.
    Have no older brother_____.
11. Does an older sister smoke? Yes_____; No_____.
    Have no older sister_____.
12. Have you ever smoked, even once? Yes_____; No_____.
    (a) If your answer is Yes, please check about how many times you have smoked:
        Only once_____; Less than ten times_____; More than ten times_____.
13. Do you smoke now as a matter of regular course? Yes_____; No_____.
    If your answer is Yes, answer the following questions:
14. Do your parents know you smoke? Yes_____; No_____; I don't know_____.
15. Do your parents approve of your smoking? Yes_____; No_____; I don't know_____.
16. At what age did you start to smoke regularly? (Please print figure)_____
17. How many cigarettes do you smoke per day? One to five cigarettes_____; Half pack_____; One pack_____; More than a pack a day_____.
    Reason:
18. Why do you smoke? (It is possible that more than one reason be checked.)
    because my friends smoke_____
    because it seems to be "the thing to do" at my age_____
    because my friends will think I am "chicken" if I don't smoke_____
    because there's nothing wrong about smoking_____
    because smoking makes me feel "grown up"_____
    because my parents smoke, so why shouldn't I_____
    because my older brother and/or sister smoke_____
    because smoking seems to calm me down_____
    because smoking leaves a good taste in my mouth_____
    I smoke for other reasons than those listed above_____

Now turn this paper upside down on your desk and wait for it to be collected. Be certain that your name is not placed anywhere on this form. Thank you for your cooperation.

III. What chemical substances can be found in tobacco smoke?
  A. What is their effect on living tissue?
    1. Alcohol
    2. Acids
    3. Carbon Monoxide
    4. Tars
    5. Nicotine
IV. Why do people use tobacco?
  A. What constitutes the smoking habit?
  B. How extensive is the use of tobacco in the United States?
V. What forces exist that encourage the use of tobacco and cigarettes?
  A. Psychological Motives
  B. Social Pressures
  C. Advertising Media

VI. What are the social disadvantages and/or advantages (if any) of smoking?
  A. Additional Cost
  B. Discolored Teeth
  C. Bad Breath
  D. Discolored Fingers
  E. Fires (cause of)
  F. Automobile Accidents (cause of)
  G. Setting of Bad Example (by adults)
  H. Imposition on Others
VII. How can the smoking habit be stopped?
  A. Individual Level—Positive "Help" Program
  B. On the National Level—Federal Government Control
  C. Testimony of individuals who have stopped smoking; how they were able to succeed

Irwin, Crestwell, and Stauffer studied the effect of three different kinds of classroom activity on knowledge, attitudes, and beliefs about smoking.[43] They developed instructional objectives and content for seventh graders based on the concept that *"The cigarette smoking habit is a health hazard of sufficient importance for youth to resist the pressure to smoke."* From this, five central ideas or sub-concepts were arranged into a five-lesson sequence. The same curricular materials were used in three different teaching approaches:

Individual Study Approach—the students' own study and interpretation of the materials.

Peer-Led Approach—class discussion with peers.

Teacher-Led Approach—combination of individual and peer approaches and discussion with teacher in charge.

It was found that the Teacher-Led Approach was the most effective in situations where good discussion was possible. The Peer-Led Approach was the most effective in smaller classes. Individual Study was effective depending upon the particular class mode of learning. The five experimental lessons appear to change attitudes and beliefs, with a 130 per cent mean increase on the attitude belief scale. Moreover, the authors confirmed the need to avoid the school's traditional authoritarian and disciplinary roles in relation to cigarette smoking by pointing to the success of the Individual Study Approach.

Second-hand smoke is a new consideration today. The issue is the non-smoker who suffers in the presence of the smoker. There is a real effort underway in defense of clean air; it is an assertive effort built around:

1. *The right to breathe clean air*—a right that supersedes the right to smoke when the two conflict.
2. *The right to speak out*—to voice objections about discomfort and adverse reactions to smoke.
3. *The right to act*—through legislative channels and other legitimate means.

---

[43]Robert P. Irwin, William H. Crestwell, Jr., and Delmar J. Stauffer, "The Effect of the Teacher and Three Different Classroom Approaches on Seventh Grade Students' Knowledges, Attitudes and Beliefs About Smoking." *Journal of School Health, 40*:355–359, September, 1970.

An American Medical Association survey shows that approximately one out of six individuals is "sensitive" to second-hand tobacco smoke.[44] A variety of physical reactions results from inhaling second-hand smoke, including increased heart rate and blood pressure, and higher blood levels of cadmium and carbon monoxide. There is also a solid psychogenic dimension as smoke fumes annoy some people and cause mental distress, but do not particularly bother others. Rummel, Crawford, and Bruce found that when experimental subjects were divided into two distinct "attitude toward smoking" groups, there was a significant difference in the heart rate increase of those who objected ("disliked") to being in the presence of cigarette smoke, when compared with those who did not mind ("indifferent").[45] However, the psychogenic factor may have little to do with altering the biological effects of sidestream smoke. This smoke which emanates directly from the burning end of the cigarette, may have up to twice as much tar and nicotine and five times as much carbon monoxide as that which is inhaled by the smoker through the ciagarette. With this kind of ammunition the school has a real responsibility to educate non-smokers to speak up and look over the non-smoker's Bill of Rights (HEW-National Interagency Council on Smoking and Health). Attention can then be drawn toward how people everywhere *feel about smoking*. How popular will it be when "no smoking" signs appear in *all* public places, travelers request seating in non-smoking sections, and hotels and restaurants establish no smoking areas? It is only a matter of time before large masses of non-smokers will cease to be shy about defending themselves against inconsiderate smokers. The movement is well underway. Moreover, most people are basically considerate of others; so are the young idealists in secondary schools. Thus, the second-hand smoke detail should prove to be a powerful teaching item in which the humanistic approach to teaching is nicely combined with the study of peer-social status-popularity.

Behavioral Objectives

(Junior High Level)
Gives up smoking, or cuts down on the number of cigarettes smoked per day.

Explains how many countries have recognized the relationship between lung cancer and smoking, and some have taken measures to control the use of cigarettes.

Illustrates how no cigarette filter has been developed that can protect the smoker from the cancer-producing agents of tobacco.

Shows that since television advertising has been discontinued, it is more difficult to encourage teenage smoking.

Names individuals, including young people, who start to smoke because they and their friends do not understand scientific findings, and frequently are unconcerned with future illnesses resulting from smoking.

Lists the number of reasons why many people have made the decision not to smoke.

Demonstrates how smoking is more injurious to one's health if the individual smokes rapidly, inhales the smoke, and leaves a short butt end.

Discovers that in addition to lung cancer and other respiratory diseases, smokers have more other diseases than non-smokers.

---

[44]Useful classroom information may be obtained from the report of the Surgeon General, *The Health Consequences of Smoking,* Washington, D.C.: U.S. Government Printing Office (current copy), and *Second-Hand Smoke,* available from the American Lung Association and the Chicago Lung Association.

[45]Rose Mary Rummel, Marilyn Crawford, and Patricia Bruce, "The Physiological Effects of Inhaling Exhaled Cigarette Smoke In Relation to Attitude of the Nonsmoker," *Journal of School Health*, 45:524–529, November, 1975.

Portrays in graph form how smoking curtails length of life, can affect the performance of an athlete, causes chronic bronchitis, pulmonary emphysema, and cardiovascular disease, all of which are found more commonly in cigarette smokers than in non-smokers.

Essential Topics

Lung cancer	Smoking experimentation
Emphysema	Peer group influences
Cardiovascular disease	Tobacco advertising
Respiratory efficiency	Habituation
Carbon monoxide	Athletic performance
Tar and nicotine	Fire hazards
Second-hand smoke	Government regulations
Sociability—popularity	Lung tissue examination

Behavioral Objectives

(Senior High Level)

Eliminates smoking, or cuts down on the number of cigarettes smoked per day.

Draws bar graphs to show how the mortality ratio of cigarette smokers over non-smokers is particularly high for the diseases of chronic bronchitis, emphysema, cancer of the larynx, peptic ulcers, and heart and coronary artery diseases.

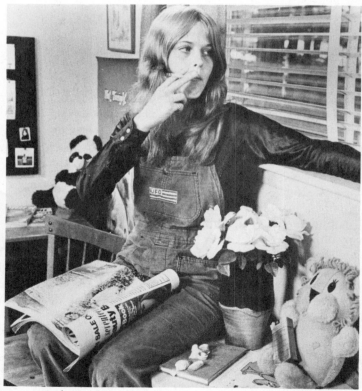

Figure 6–19 In "Trying Times," a program from the new school television series for 11 to 13 year olds entitled "Self Incorporated," Julie smokes without her parents' knowledge. "Self Incorporated" is produced by the Agency for Instructional Television. (Courtesy of Herb Jones, Ball State University)

Develops useful guidelines to help people who wish to give up the smoking practice.

Examines the role of a personal commitment, and notes that the reasons for smoking are largely psychological and sociological.

Takes part in local agencies concerned with the health status of Americans vigorously involved in anti-smoking programs.

Tells how leading scientific and medical groups in the country acknowledge the health hazards of smoking.

Analyzes why the sale of tobacco is presently essential to the economic well-being of certain areas of the United States.

Looks into the use of statistical evidence as a universally accepted scientific procedure in research.

Explains that although no true "smoker's personality" has been identified, there are distinct personality characteristics associated with smokers.

Draws a line graph to show that smokers who discontinue the practice have a total death rate considerably lower than those who continue to smoke.

Illustrates how the most comprehensive and widely accepted smoking reasearch has been conducted by the U.S. Government.

Encourages older students to set examples for younger boys and girls. There is an association here just as there is between students' smoking and parental patterns.

Essential Topics
Public establishment surveys
Mortality statistics
Research studies in detail
Tobacco industry position
Economic consequences
Autopsy studies
School smoking rooms
Breaking the habit activities
Personal commitment
"Smoker's personality"
Power of example
Animal experiments
Socioeconomic factors
Psychological issues
Second-hand smoke campaigns

Suggested Activities

(Junior High Level)

1. Conduct a survey to determine how many fathers, mothers, brothers, and sisters smoke and relate this to individual cigarette consumption. When this was done in the Bedford, Massachusetts, Schools, it was discovered that boys especially began to smoke if their siblings smoked.[46]

2. Set up a debate:

RESOLVED: Smoking rooms should be provided for students who smoke.

---

[46]Esther B. Kahn and Carl N. Edwards, "Smoking and Youth: Contributions to the Study of Smoking Behavior in High School Students," *Journal of School Health*, 40:561–562, December, 1970.

The National Education Association leaflets will prove helpful ("Smoking: The School's Responsibility" and "Cigarettes and the Schools").

3. Hang posters on strings suspended above the classroom. Six 9″ × 12″ posters are available from the American Cancer Society:

Is Cancer Any Reason To Give Up Cigarettes?

We'll Miss Ya, Baby.

Smoking Is Very Debonair.

Congress Has Acted: The Next Step Is Yours.

If You Figure It's Too Late To Quit.

Best Tip Yet, Don't Start.

4. Investigate through small group action the area of *second-hand smoke*. Approach it from the right to breathe clean air, the right to speak out, and the right to act. Materials are available from the U.S. Public Health Service, the American Lung Association of Boston, and the Chicago Lung Association.

5. Obtain several copies of the Surgeon General's reports of 1964, 1967, 1969, 1975, and a current copy, and examine the research findings. Several class committees may be appointed.

6. Obtain and show photomicrographs of cancerous and non-cancerous lung tissue. Excellent slides of real lung tissue may be obtained from Oscar Auerback, M.D., Veterans Hospital, E. Orange, New Jersey 07019.

7. Post newspaper and magazine tobacco advertisements. Consider truths and half-truths in advertising.

8. Help a small group of students set up a smoking machine. Figure 6–20 is from the New York State Health Curriculum Materials for grades 7, 8, and 9, Strand II, Smoking, p. 59. This can be a highly effective experimental device with which students can think of several experiments to conduct.

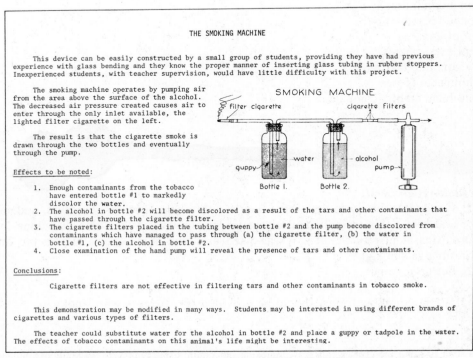

THE SMOKING MACHINE

This device can be easily constructed by a small group of students, providing they have had previous experience with glass bending and they know the proper manner of inserting glass tubing in rubber stoppers. Inexperienced students, with teacher supervision, would have little difficulty with this project.

The smoking machine operates by pumping air from the area above the surface of the alcohol. The decreased air pressure created causes air to enter through the only inlet available, the lighted filter cigarette on the left.

The result is that the cigarette smoke is drawn through the two bottles and eventually through the pump.

Effects to be noted:

1. Enough contaminants from the tobacco have entered bottle #1 to markedly discolor the water.
2. The alcohol in bottle #2 will become discolored as a result of the tars and other contaminants that have passed through the cigarette filter.
3. The cigarette filters placed in the tubing between bottle #2 and the pump become discolored from contaminants which have managed to pass through (a) the cigarette filter, (b) the water in bottle #1, (c) the alcohol in bottle #2.
4. Close examination of the hand pump will reveal the presence of tars and other contaminants.

Conclusions:

Cigarette filters are not effective in filtering tars and other contaminants in tobacco smoke.

This demonstration may be modified in many ways. Students may be interested in using different brands of cigarettes and various types of filters.

The teacher could substitute water for the alcohol in bottle #2 and place a guppy or tadpole in the water. The effects of tobacco contaminants on this animal's life might be interesting.

Figure 6–20 The smoking machine. (Courtesy of New York State Education Dept.)

Tar and Nicotine Content of Cigarettes

Federal Trade Commission, March 1975

(Ranked from low (1) to high (136))

NF—Non-Filter (All other brands possess filters)
M—Menthol
HP—Hard pack

RANK (tar)	BRAND	TYPE	TAR (mg)	NICOTINE (mg)
27	Alpine	King, M	13	0.8
45	Alpine	100mm, M (HP)	16	0.9
35	Belair	King, M	15	1.0
9	Belair	100mm	17	1.2
42	Benson & Hedges	Reg. (HP)	9	0.5
	Benson & Hedges	King (HP)	16	1.1
57	Benson & Hedges 100's	100mm	17	1.1
54	Benson & Hedges 100's	100mm, M	17	1.1
131	Bull Durham	King	28	1.8
123	Camel	Reg, NF	19	1.3
100	Camel Filters	King	19	1.3
1	Carton 70's	Reg.	2	0.2
3	Carton	King	4	0.3
2	Carton	King, M	4	0.3
119	Chesterfield	Reg, NF	24	1.4
132	Chesterfield	King, NF	29	1.7
82	Chesterfield	King	18	1.2
85	Chesterfield	King, M	19	1.2
104	Chesterfield	101mm	20	1.3
127	Domino	King, NF	26	1.3
116	Domino	King	23	1.2
33	Doral	King	15	1.0
23	Doral	King, M	13	0.9
37	DuMaurier	King (HP)	15	1.0
114	English Ovals	Reg, NF (HP)	22	1.5
133	English Ovals	King, NF (HP)	29	2.2
92	Eve	100mm	19	1.3
90	Eve	100mm, M	19	1.2
130	Fatima	King, NF	28	1.6
36	Galaxy	King, NF	15	1.0
124	Half & Half	King	25	1.8
134	Herbert Tareyton	King, NF	29	1.8
112	Home Run	Reg, NF	21	1.6
8	Iceberg 100's	100mm, M	9	0.6
44	Kent	King	16	0.9
38	Kent	King (HP)	15	0.9
87	Kent	100mm	19	1.2
81	Kent	100mm, M	18	1.2
7	King Sano	King	8	0.3
6	King Sano	King, M	7	0.3
97	Kool	Reg, NF, M	19	1.2
46	Kool	King, M	16	1.2
43	Kool	King, M (HP)	16	1.2
66	Kool Milds	100mm, M	17	1.4
25	L & M	King	13	0.8
83	L & M	King	18	1.2
110	L & M	100mm	20	1.4
94	L & M	100mm, M	19	1.3
77	Lark	King, M	18	1.2
96	Lark	100mm	19	1.3
129	Lucky Strike	Reg, NF	27	1.6
11	Lucky Ten	King	9	0.6
14	Lucky 100's	100mm	10	0.7
135	Mapleton	Reg, NF	30	1.2
118	Mapleton	King	24	1.2
72	Marboro	King (HP)	17	1.1
67	Marlboro	King, M	17	1.1
31	Marlboro	King, M (HP)	14	0.8
26	Marlboro	King	13	0.8
73	Marlboro	100mm	18	1.1
60	Marlboro	100mm (HP)	17	1.1
21	Marlboro Lights	King	12	0.8
5	Marvels	King	6	0.2
125	Marvels	King, NF	25	0.9
4	Marvels	King, M	4	0.2
39	Miyako	King	15	0.9
70	Montclair	King, M	19	1.4
79	More	120mm	17	1.4
88	More	120mm, M	18	1.5
20	Multifilter	King	12	0.8
12	Multifilter	King, M	10	0.7
64	Newport	King, M	17	1.2

Tar and Nicotine Content of Cigarettes

Federal Trade Commission, March 1975

(Ranked from low (1) to high (136))

NF—Non-Filter (All other brands possess filters)
M—Menthol
HP—Hard pack

RANK (tar)	BRAND	TYPE	TAR (mg)	NICOTINE (mg)
71	Newport	King, M (HP)	17	1.2
113	Newport	100mm, M	21	1.5
78	Oasis	100mm, M	18	1.2
80	Old Gold Filters	King	18	1.1
52	Old Gold Filters	King (HP)	17	1.2
103	Old Gold Straights	Reg, NF	20	1.2
121	Old Gold Straights	King, NF	24	1.5
117	Old Gold 100's	100mm	23	1.4
128	Pall Mall	King, NF	27	1.7
108	Pall Mall	100mm	20	1.4
68	Pall Mall	100mm, M	17	1.3
13	Pall Mall Extra Mild	King	10	0.7
10	Pall Mall Extra Mild	King (HP)	9	0.6
34	Parliament	King	15	0.8
32	Parliament 100's	King (HP)	14	0.8
49	Parliament 100's	100mm	17	1.0
107	Philip Morris	Reg, NF	20	1.1
126	Commander	King, NF	25	1.5
56	International	100mm (HP)	17	1.1
65	International	100mm, M (HP)	17	1.0
106	Picayune	Reg, NF	20	1.5
122	Piedmont	Reg, NF	17	1.2
136	Players	Reg, NF (HP)	31	2.1
40	Raleigh	King	16	1.0
120	Raleigh	King, NF	24	1.4
69	Raleigh	100mm	19	1.3
30	Raleigh Extra Mild	King	14	0.9
99	Safari	100mm	22	1.4
62	St. Moritz	100mm	19	1.1
84	St. Moritz	100mm, M	16	1.3
89	Salem	King, M	17	1.3
86	Salem	King, M (HP)	17	1.3
91	Salem Extra	King, M	18	1.3
74	Sano	Reg, NF	22	0.8
115	Silva Thins	King (HP)	22	1.1
51	Silva Thins	100mm, M	17	1.2
48	Spring 100's	100mm, M	16	1.2
111	Super M	100mm, M	21	1.2
59	Tareyton	King	17	1.2
109	Tareyton	100mm	20	1.3
102	Tempo	King	19	1.3
15	Tramps	King	11	0.8
75	Tramps	King, M	18	1.1
47	True	Reg, NF	16	0.9
16	True		11	0.6
19	True	King, M	12	0.7
22	True	100mm	13	0.7
24	True	100mm, M	14	1.0
53	Twist	100mm (HP)	17	1.2
18	Vantage	King	11	0.8
41	Vantage	King, M	11	0.8
63	Viceroy	King	16	1.0
29	Viceroy	100mm	17	1.1
50	Viceroy Extra Mild	King	17	0.9
101	Virginia Slims	100mm	19	1.3
61	Virginia Slims	100mm, M	17	1.1
58	Winchester	King, M	19	1.2
105	Winston	Reg, NF	20	1.4
98	Winston	King	19	1.3
93	Winston	100mm	19	1.3
95	Winston	100mm, M	19	1.4
28	Winston Lights	King	14	1.0

U.S. DEPARTMENT OF HEALTH, EDUCATION, AND WELFARE / PUBLIC HEALTH SERVICE
Center for Disease Control / Bureau of Health Education / National Clearinghouse for Smoking and Health

DHEW Publication No. (CDC) 75-8703

Figure 6-21 Tar and nicotine content of cigarettes.

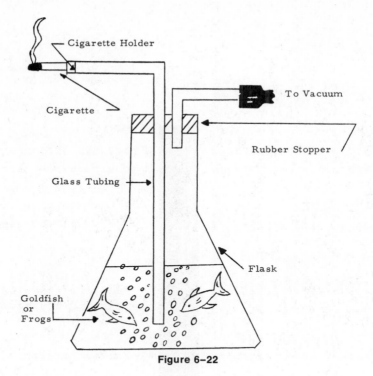

Figure 6–22

9. Locate issues of magazines published in the late 1950's showing athletic testimonials. Discuss the changes that have occurred since that time in attitudes of athletes, medical men, and others toward smoking.

10. Obtain from the U.S. Public Health Service the latest government ratings of tar and nicotine content of brands of cigarettes. (see Figure 6–21).

11. Experiment with the effect of smoking upon the heart rate. This is best done by students on their parents at home. The arterial pulse at the wrist is checked before smoking and after the third or fourth puff. When the cigarette is finished, the pulse is taken every 15 minutes until it returns to normal.

12. Demonstrate how the 300 toxic compounds in cigarette smoke (mostly lead, arsenic, nicotine, formaldehyde, and carbon monoxide) can affect fish when they are compelled to absorb the fumes (see Figure 6–22).

Equipment:
500 cc flask
glass tubing
water
2 or 3 goldfish
rubber stopper with glass tubing holes
a vacuum source (siphon or aspirator)
Procedure:
Hook a vacuum line (from an aspirator or siphon) to a burning cigarette in the manner described in the drawing. As the vacuum is applied, the smoke from the cigarette will bubble through the water. By the time three to ten cigarettes have been consumed, the toxic agents in the smoke, primarily nicotine, should begin to affect the fish, causing them to lose their equilibrium. As soon as the fish lose their equilibrium, and begin to roll to one side, they should be removed from the water and placed immediately in fresh water. If this is not done promptly, this experiment will be fatal to the fish. We urge that extreme caution be used so that the experiment is not lethal to the fish.

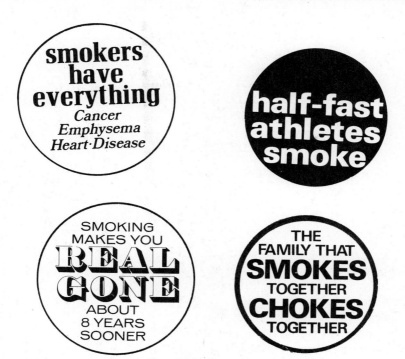

Figure 6–23

13. Distribute sample *Ban The Butt* buttons and other anti-smoking buttons, available from Spenco Medical Corporation, P.O. Box 6322, Salt Lake City, Utah 84106. Ask the class if they think these items have any value. Should a person make fun of the smokers? Will it cause anybody to cut back or not start smoking? This company also sells teaching specimens and teaching guides regarding smoking. Their highly successful mechanical smoker is a dramatic teaching device which channels smoke from a lighted cigarette into a plastic mini-lung. Every health instructor should have one of these aids to teaching (see Figure 6–23).

14. Breathing smokers' smoke may have detrimental effects. Non-smokers are now asserting their right to breathe clean air. The first Romanoff Czar in the seventeenth century never felt guilty when he said "no smoking," either. He usually sentenced smokers to having their nostrils slit. Talk about assertiveness! Have the class present pro and con statements related to the following:

> A smoker has the option whether or not to smoke;
> a non-smoker doesn't have the option whether or
> not to breathe.

Suggested Activities

(Senior High Level)

1. Set up a number of questions on one side of a bulletin board. The covered answers appear on the other side. (See diagram following.)

```
┌─────────────────────┬─────────────────┐
│     QUESTIONS       │    ANSWERS      │
│  ─────────────────  │     UNDER       │
│  ─────────────────  │     THIS        │
│  ─────────────────  │     DOOR        │
│  ─────────────────  │                 │
│  ─────────────────  │                 │
│  ─────────────────  │                 │
│  ─────────────────  │                 │
│  ─────────────────  │                 │
│  ─────────────────  │                 │
│  ─────────────────  │                 │
└─────────────────────┴─────────────────┘
```

Example questions:

Why do many adults continue to smoke?

Are pipes and cigars safe?

Is "cutting down" on smoking effective?

Is carbon monoxide in cigarettes very harmful?

Why do some people gain weight when they stop smoking?

2. Talk about early death. What are the viewpoints of class members about dying thirty to fifty years from now? How significant to students is the fact that the risk of death is about 70 per cent higher for men who smoke cigarettes than for men who do not? This should open up a discussion of research and human values. One could eventually ask, is a smokeless generation possible? Why or why not?

3. Investigate on an individual pupil basis, a number of studies comparing smoking habits and health status. The U.S. Public Health Service literature is a rich source for pertinent research. Problem-solving techniques can be worked out if there is a satisfactory school or community library.

4. In the Portland, Oregon, study of 22,000 high school pupils, each successive grade had a higher percentage of smokers than the preceding class. Post the Oregon information and invite the class to suggest a variety of reasons for the increase.

5. Start a noon-hour *kick-the-habit* clinic. Learn how to develop personal motivations for quitting, together with a variety of plans for doing so by obtaining materials (free) from American Lung Association of Boston. In this program peers work with peers, and teachers stay in the background as much as possible.

6. A task force was set up by the U.S. Public Health Service to attack the smoking problem. Have the class give their candid opinions of how well the following four areas of concern have been realized.

(a) Education of Youth to Prevent Smoking

(b) Influence of Professional Health Personnel

PERCENTAGE OF SMOKERS

CLASS	MALE	FEMALE
Freshman	14.5	4.6
Sophomore	25.2	10.6
Junior	31.1	16.2
Senior	35.4	26.2

TEST 3
WHY DO YOU SMOKE?

Here are some statements made by people to describe what they get out of smoking cigarettes. How *often* do you feel this way when smoking them? Circle one number for each statement.

Important: Answer every question.

	always	fre-quently	occa-sionally	seldom	never
A. I smoke cigarettes in order to keep myself from slowing down.	5	4	3	2	1
B. Handling a cigarette is part of the enjoyment of smoking it.	5	4	3	2	1
C. Smoking cigarettes is pleasant and relaxing.	5	4	3	2	1
D. I light up a cigarette when I feel angry about something.	5	4	3	2	1
E. When I have run out of cigarettes I find it almost unbearable until I can get them.	5	4	3	2	1
F. I smoke cigarettes automatically without even being aware of it.	5	4	3	2	1
G. I smoke cigarettes to stimulate me, to perk myself up.	5	4	3	2	1
H. Part of the enjoyment of smoking a cigarette comes from the steps I take to light up.	5	4	3	2	1
I. I find cigarettes pleasurable.	5	4	3	2	1
J. When I feel uncomfortable or upset about something, I light up a cigarette.	5	4	3	2	1
K. I am very much aware of the fact when I am not smoking a cigarette.	5	4	3	2	1
L. I light up a cigarette without realizing I still have one burning in the ashtray.	5	4	3	2	1
M. I smoke cigarettes to give me a "lift."	5	4	3	2	1
N. When I smoke a cigarette, part of the enjoyment is watching the smoke as I exhale it.	5	4	3	2	1
O. I want a cigarette most when I am comfortable and relaxed.	5	4	3	2	1
P. When I feel "blue" or want to take my mind off cares and worries, I smoke cigarettes.	5	4	3	2	1
Q. I get a real gnawing hunger for a cigarette when I haven't smoked for a while.	5	4	3	2	1
R. I've found a cigarette in my mouth and didn't remember putting it there.	5	4	3	2	1

HOW TO SCORE:

1. Enter the numbers you have circled to the Test 3 questions in the spaces below, putting the number you have circled to Question A over line A, to Question B over line B, etc.
2. Total the 3 scores on each line to get your totals. For example, the sum of your scores over lines A, G, and M gives you your score on *Stimulation*—lines B, H, and N give the score on *Handling*, etc.

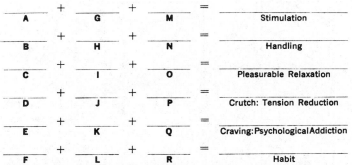

Totals

A + G + M =			Stimulation
B + H + N =			Handling
C + I + O =			Pleasurable Relaxation
D + J + P =			Crutch: Tension Reduction
E + K + Q =			Craving: Psychological Addiction
F + L + R =			Habit

Scores can vary from 3 to 15. Any score 11 and above is *high;* any score 7 and below is *low*. Learn from Part 2 what your scores mean.

Figure 6–24 Questionnaire "Why Do You Smoke?" (Courtesy of National Clearinghouse for Smoking and Health)

(c) Group Approaches to Control Cigarette Smoking

(d) Advertising and Promotion

   (Question: "Should *all* cigarette advertising be banned?")

   7. Administer the *Smoker's Self-Test.* This test may be obtained from the U.S. Public Health Service (Publication No. CDC 74–8716). It is an excellent teaching device. All student answers are clearly analyzed in a booklet. The test deals with a number of statements related to four essential questions:

(a) Do you want to change your smoking habits?

(b) What do you think the effects of smoking are?

(c) Why do you smoke? (Test No. 3, Figure 6–24.)

(d) Does the world around you make it easier or harder to change your smoking habits?

   8. Demonstrate, through class experimentation, the physiology of ciliary action in the tracheobronchial tree, and the effect of cigarette smoke on cilary action. Two fresh chicken tracheas are slit upward from below and pinned to a block of wood, so that the inside, with cilia, can be viewed. Put a small drop of India ink on the mucous membrane at the lower end, and place it in a moist chamber with the upper end elevated, so that the ink will have to travel against gravity (Figure 6–25A). Note the rate of travel with millimeter rule and stop watch. The ordinary rate is about 10 mm per minute. Do the same with the second trachea and blow smoke against the mucosa. The ciliary action will stop (Figure 6–25B). When the cilia are inactivated, the cancer-producing agents in the mucus stay longer in contact with the lining of the respiratory tract. For a full description of this and other experiments, see the American Cancer Society manual, *Biology Experiments for High School Students.*

   9. As group projects, build one or more smoking machines and follow directions in experimenting with living things.

(a) Test the effects of carbon monoxide in tobacco smoke on animal blood.

(b) Observe the biological effects of cigarette tars on white mice (See Figure 6–26).

   Procedures:

   Hook a vacuum line (aspirator or water pump) to a burning cigarette in such a manner that the cigarette is consumed in about 4 to 6 minutes. In the line, a trap containing glass wool moistened with acetone should be attached. This will collect most of the tobacco tars. The distillation of the tar can be facilitated by placing the bottle in an ice water bath during the course of the experiment.

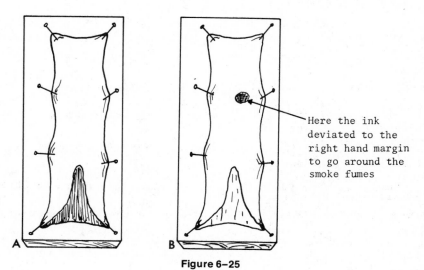

Here the ink
deviated to the
right hand margin
to go around the
smoke fumes

Figure 6–25

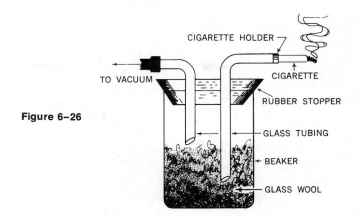

CIGARETTE HOLDER

TO VACUUM

CIGARETTE

RUBBER STOPPER

Figure 6–26

GLASS TUBING

BEAKER

GLASS WOOL

After the cigarettes (about 40 per day) have been smoked, the tar can be removed with additional acetone, using as little as possible to dissolve the tar. This solution should be allowed to stand for several hours in a fume hood to concentrate the tar.

The backs of mice should be trimmed with electric clippers to remove heavy hair growth. The tars from about three cigarettes can be applied by eye dropper twice daily to the clipped area, five days a week.

Tumors can be expected to appear in about 40 per cent of the mice in 6 to 9 months. These will be both benign and malignant tumors.

(c) Show the effect of smoke on the respiratory tract.

Put a salamander to sleep by soaking him in a solution of saturated Chloretone (chlorobutanol), diluted by adding nine parts of water, or in a 1 per cent aqueous solution of Tricaine (ethyl *m*-aminobenzoate methanesulphonate). As soon as it is asleep, cut off the head, open the chest and abdominal cavity, slit the lung longitudinally and snip it off. Keep the specimen wet with Ringer's solution. Examine the lung surface under the microscope to study the cilia beating. Blow a little smoke from a collection flask over the tissue and observe the effect it has on the cilia.

(d) Show the effect of smoke on the circulatory system.

Pith a frog and place it on its back on a frog board. Spread and pin the web of a foot over an opening in the board and examine the blood vessels under a microscope at low power. Keep the specimen moist with Ringer's solution. Place a tube from the smoke bottle in the frog's mouth and blow smoke in while someone is watching the rate of blood flow. If it is possible to count the blood cells going past a given point, you may notice several rate changes; faster, then back to normal, and maybe faster again and back to normal a second time.

(e) Perform some simple experiments:

1. Using a cotton pellet which has been saturated with tars from the smoking machine, wipe the stems of several growing plants. Keep some plants as controls to observe the differences.

2. Wipe a cotton pellet which has been saturated with tobacco tars on the tongue of a live frog and note temporary collapse.

3. Place a small fish in the water flask of a smoking machine and note how the nicotine poisoning causes the fish to roll to one side. As soon as this happens, place the fish in freshly aerated water to revive it. Substitute tadpoles for fish and observe the results.

4. Place a drop of solution containing paramecia on a microscope slide. With the low power of a microscope, observe the movement of these one-celled organisms. Blow smoke from collection flask on the preparation and note the effects on the paramecia.

5. Make a nicotine insecticide by soaking cotton pellets from the smoking machine or cigarette tobacco in water. Test and use as a spray on insects.

10. Show the film *Who Me?* (American Cancer Society) to the class. It relates to smoker's cough, x-rays and lung cancer, the Portland Study, inhaling, chemicals in cigarette smoke, the Surgeon General's Report, bronchitis, heart disease, and emphysema.

11. Form small groups of five students each to discuss the following statements from *health, individual rights,* and *legal* points of view:

a. There is undisputed knowledge that smoking is a causal factor in many debilitating, and often fatal diseases. Given this awareness, should smoking be condoned on school premises?

b. The National Association of Secondary School Principals (NASSP) suggests that student lounges may implicitly promote smoking in the public schools. Therefore, instead of establishing them, NASSP suggests that intensive educational programs be set up to reduce and finally terminate smoking in the schools—the programs should involve students, faculty, parents and the community at large.

12. Obtain a copy of the teaching curriculum "The Respiratory System and Smoking" from the Chicago Lung Association, 1440 W. Washington, Chicago, Illinois 60607. This is the most practical multi-media teaching kit available anywhere. There are transparencies, duplicating masters, and experiments covering a wide variety of respiratory and circulatory system difficulties associated with smoking.

4. SEX AND FAMILY LIVING EDUCATION

If a soul is left in darkness, sins will be committed. The guilty one is not he who commits the sin; but he who creates the darkness.

—*Victor Hugo*

In recent years, whenever the question of *relevance* in American education arises, the concern for human sexuality and the need to understand it comes to the forefront. Although it is both a powerful and popular topic, it is frequently dismissed as "explosive" or "controversial" when health curriculum materials are prepared. However, this is changing fast as hundreds of communities have not sidestepped this area, but have met Victor Hugo's challenge by providing facts where there were myths, peace of mind where there was insecurity, and light where there was darkness.

Because sex is an integral part of total personality, it becomes a multidimensional topic for educators. It is both biological and non-biological. It is concerned with human relationships and responsible boy-girl behavior, and as such, is fraught with problems as old as mankind. In fact, man's sexuality has always given him trouble. David Mace, Professor of Family Sociology at the Bowman-Gray School of Medicine, points out that sex, as a force within man, is bewilderingly ambivalent, " . . . now pulling him down, now raising him up; now stirring him to ecstasy, now driving him to despair; now endearing him to, now alienating him from, his fellows. . . . The elementary problem of our sexuality remains exactly what it has always been—how to reconcile our personal desires with our social obligations. And this, of course, is the fundamental problem of all human culture."

Human sexuality, says Hoyman, " . . . emerges from the complex ecologic interactions of hereditary and environmental factors and forces and the developing self."[47] It is partly inborn and partly learned, and as such, is influenced by almost every cultural detail in the society.

---

[47]Howard S. Hoyman, "Should We Teach Sexual Ethics in Our Schools?" *Journal of School Health,* 40:339–346, September, 1970.

Sex is popular. It is exciting. It is on display. It is the subject of art, books, plays, films, and jokes. It stimulates curiosity and sells everything from bras and perfumes to cigars and automobiles. While sex is being paraded in a highly genital-centered culture, young people are told not to let it bother them. Yet boys and girls frequently discover at an early age that they are a part of the "instant gratification" era; that one can have his pleasures now and pay later; hedonism, playboyism, and "Why wait till marriage?" make a certain kind of sense in a fast-moving, not always secure society. Certainly, if a society places *people* in the category of *things,* and values ability to *purchase* above the ability to *relate,* the young people will learn to behave accordingly.

The average student, in his early teens, probably spends as much time engaged with the mass media as he does in school. Various stages of love making are depicted on television, on movie posters, and in newspapers and magazine stories, comics and advertisements. Half-clothed people embracing are commonplace in his life. Sex is almost exclusively body oriented.

This is also a culture where young couples are thrown together at an early age — at drive-in theaters, in automobiles, at unchaperoned parties and overnight visitations. They are asked to be responsible without preparation. They are asked to act like adults while being treated as children — frequently being considered by their parents as too young to be told the "facts of life." Thus, thousands of youths grow up harboring false notions and myths pertaining to their sex and sexuality. Their education was less than adequate. And those who suffer from unwanted pregnancies, disease, unhappy friendships, and broken marriages have somehow been cheated.

Studies dealing with the pupil and his knowledge about sex and human relationships continually indicate a case of the "blind leading the blind," as uninformed companions in the peer group pass on sex information to be lived by. Thus, New York City boys, who are frequently sophisticated and old before their time, are unaware of how pregnancies occur, and Chicago teenage girls use a Coca Cola douche to prevent conception. Moreover, they will not seek answers from their parents. It is not uncommon to find only one-tenth of the students in a survey who get sex information from their parents. Yet, when encouraged, parents will attempt to talk more with their children — particularly if the children have had some sex education in the school or through a community agency. In the Unitarian Universalist Association study evaluating the growth of junior high schoolers who had taken a sexuality course, it was found that these pupils increased their level of communication with the members of their own immediate families to a large degree. Moreover, the "generation gap" frequently gets overplayed. To counter situations of child alienation there are many occurrences of parent and student agreement on sex education particulars.[48]

Illegitimate pregnancies and early forced marriages have long been on the increase among 14 to 19 year olds; they have doubled in 25 years. Over 500,000 teenagers give birth each year, and most are at risk educationally, socially, and psychologically. While one third opt for an abortion, a large number enter pregnancy-caused premature marriages.[49] Starting with 1000 pregnant schoolgirls a year, the school board in New Orleans developed an adolescent parent program that would continue the education of the girls and produce healthy babies. From this beginning, uniform statewide services are now available to adolescent parents.[50] But, the pregnancy problem is not going away. Since

[48]John A. Conley, "The Generation Gap In Sex Education: Is There One?" *Journal of School Health,* 44:428–437, October, 1974.

[49]Paul A. Reichelt and Harriet H. Werley, "A Sex Information Program for Sexually Active Teenagers," *Journal of School Health,* 45:100–106, February, 1975.

[50]Eileen Cowart et al., "The Louisiana Strategy: An Interdisciplinary Approach to the Programs of Adolescent Parenthood," *Journal of School Health,* 45:469–473, October, 1975.

1940, there has been a 500 per cent increase in teenage marriages. More than 4000 girls of ages 14 *and under* were married in the United States in a recent year. Depending on the particular piece of research pregnancies at the time of marriage vary from 50 to 80 per cent. For mothers under 20 there is a 30 per cent higher mortality rate for both infant and mother than for mothers aged 20 to 24. The divorce rate for teenage marriages is the highest for any age group; so is the suicide attempt rate. There is also a strong relationship between unplanned pregnancy and post-partum psychiatric symptoms.

The implications here are far reaching, especially as one views the unhappy marriages and broken homes. In one western state, the divorce rate is about one for every two marriages, whereas, for the country as a whole, there is now one divorce in every three marriages. Human relationships, and how to live together as a family, are more relevant than they have ever been. Unfortunately, uninformed and delinquent youths frequently grow up to become delinquent parents. If it is true that the trend today is to accept or be more tolerant of "permissiveness with affection" among youth at an early age, then education for sexuality and responsible living is a number one priority. The school, church, and home have a cooperative job to do. High school students who lack involvement in these three areas appear to be more permissive and irresponsible.[51] Significantly, in the country as a whole, a large number of individuals have intercourse in a fashion which suggests a weak personal relationship and an irresponsible attitude toward the partner. This is brought out in epidemiological studies of venereal disease contacts, where the "friend of the opposite sex" is the most frequent contact, but running a close second is a "stranger of the opposite sex." Suggestions of weak relationships may come as no surprise with premarital activity so common. A *Redbook* poll of 100,000 married women indicated that 80 per cent had had premarital intercourse, beginning at an average age of 17.[52]

Venereal disease is the number one communicable disease. Syphilis and gonorrhea are sweeping the country in an uncontrolled epidemic that is hitting hardest among those in the 15 to 24 year age bracket. It is a pandemic situation. It is estimated that there are one half million teenagers with venereal disease. Nationally, the incidence of gonorrhea has been rising 10 per cent every year since 1955, and probably fewer than one of every 12 cases is reported. For every boy or girl with the disease, there is at least one, and perhaps several, sex partners with venereal disease. Approximately 900,000 new cases of gonorrhea and 80,000 of syphilis occur a year. The disease is actually out of control, and there are more clinical complications appearing.

Some 14 million Americans have one disease or the other. They and the youths that follow them must be educated to report their problem, help identify contacts, and help bring venereal disease under control. Quite a variation exists among states and cities in the reported occurrences of the disease. The state of Texas and the District of Columbia have had the highest syphilis rates in their respective categories, and the state of Alaska and the city of Atlanta have had the highest rates for gonorrhea. The medical director of the American Social Health Association attributes much of this rise in VD to more sexual intercourse, especially among young people, and to the use of the pill instead of the condom, which has some prophylactic as well as contraceptive benefits.

There is another societal dimension which contributes to the sexuality attitudes and practices of youth. It relates to sex and authority. In middle class America, sex is seen

---

[51]Gerald Globetti, "Sexual Permissiveness Among High School Students," *School Health Review*, 1:29–31, April, 1970.
[52]*Newsweek*, September 1, 1975.

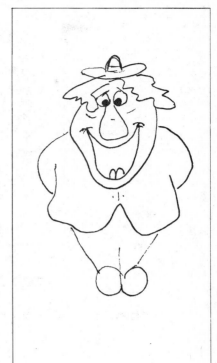

"As principal, I think you ought to know I read an article this month that says 42% of you young ladies will have had intercourse by the time you graduate. What you do on your own time is your own business. Just remember, we're educators here. Don't come running to us for any kind of information."

Figure 6–27   (Courtesy of Atlanta Adolescent Pregnancy Program)

by youth as something which officially belongs to authority, and authority belongs to legally defined adults. Like many other adult items, sex is withheld from youth until they accept the rules laid down by parents, clergy, and other oldsters. Marriage makes sexual intercourse legal and thus perpetuates the authority structure. Coupled with this is the strong tendency of adults to keep children and youth in the dark about sex information. Moreover, this is done over the long period between puberty and the socioeconomic readiness for marriage—a time when sexual drives are extremely intense, yet abstinence is generally held to be the ideal. With such a broad sex-authority situation, youths have tended to question the whole process, to shout hypocrisy, and, in many instances, to rebel and do their own thing when it comes to persons and sex. They want to be free to experiment, discover, and develop their own life styles and values. Such freedom of activity, without a corresponding understanding of human sexuality, has brought on many of the problems. Yet, youth studies show that young people want sex education, and they point out that it does not lead to promiscuous sexual behavior. In fact, in the Iver-

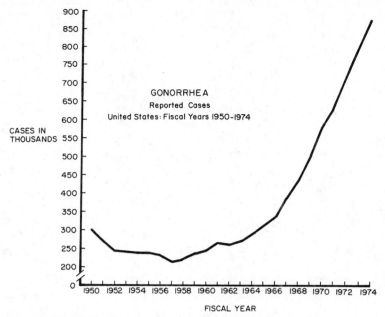

Figure 6–28   Gonorrhea: the most frequently reported communicable disease.

son study, an overwhelming majority of adolescents believed sex should be associated with love relationships.[53]

Related to this new freedom to be an adult at an early age is the confusion regarding male and female images. Today one can seriously ask: What is male? What is female? Where is the model or ideal to follow in a culture that supports a steady depolarization of the sexes? Should we teach now for similarities between sexes or for differences? Even love today is not based on "opposites," but on "closeness" and "sameness" in the unisexed and neutered society. Certainly, this area is ripe for discussion in secondary school classes, with implications for social studies and English as well as health education.

THE ROLE OF THE SCHOOL

Sex education in the school has been approved by a large number of national organizations.[54] In survey after survey—both locally and nationally—parents have made it clear to the schools that they should do the job and that they are better equipped.

At times, there has been some confusion as to just what sex education is. In earlier days, it was thought of rather coldly as biological and anatomical information. The new

---

[53]Sonya Rae Iverson, *Sex Education and Adolescent Attitudes,* Doctoral dissertation, University of Maryland, 1974.

[54]This includes the American Academy of Pediatrics, American College of Obstetricians and Gynecologists, American Medical Association, American School Health Association, American Public Health Association, National Education Association, National Congress of Parents and Teachers (PTA), National Council of Churches, National School Boards Association, American Association of School Administrators, National Student Assembly, Synagogue Council of America, U.S. Catholic Conferences, UNESCO, and U.S. Dept. of Health, Education and Welfare.

emphasis is on interpersonal relationships—a kind of education dealing, first-hand, with the realities of being human, with the most intimate feelings and deepest longings of the human heart. Moreover, sex education is to be distinguished from sex information. In the words of an American School Health Association committee, sex education "... consists of instruction to develop understanding of the physical, mental, emotional, social, economic, and psychological phases of human relations as they are affected by male and female relationships. It... emphasizes attitude development and guidance related to association between the sexes. It implies that man's sexuality is integrated into his total life development as a health entity and source of creative energy.[55]

It is somewhat obvious that sex education is a multidimensional topic, frequently calling for a multidisciplinary approach. It is, therefore, of equal concern to guidance personnel and to teachers of social studies, home economics, physical education, science, and health education. English teachers are especially interested in the area, for they discuss in class the assigned readings in contemporary literature. When the pupil asks, "What's a pimp?" or "What makes a woman become a prostitute?" the teacher needs a sex-related answer pertaining to moral and ethical values and she needs it right away.

For some school systems, what to call such an area of study, and where to put it, has created some concern. Across the country, the sex education course is identified by a number of names. At the State Department of Instruction level in Pennsylvania, it is called "Human Sexuality." In Oregon and numerous other places, it is simply called "Sex Education." It is called "Family Health" in Washington; "Life Education" in Rochester, New York, and Wellesley, Massachusetts; "Health and Family Life Education" in San Francisco; "Family Life and Sex Education" in Great Neck, New York; "Personal Ethics" in Winchester, Massachusetts; and "Sex and Family Living Education" in Bedford, Massachusetts. In the fall of 1970, the Dallas School District in Dallas, Texas, changed the course name from "Sex Education" to "Human Growth and Reproduction" because it seemed to offend fewer critics.

Regardless of what it is called, programs of sex education have the full support of numerous state boards of education. States such as Illinois, Pennsylvania, Connecticut, Iowa, and New Jersey were pioneers in working out strong policy statements for their school people to follow. The Illinois and Iowa statements are most complete in terms of definitions, needs, policies, guiding principles, objectives, and program suggestions. In the Illinois statement, there are sixteen excellent guiding principles and twenty-four general objectives worth studying by any person about to engage in curriculum planning in this area.[56]

The question of where to put the sex education program can usually be resolved in one of three ways, all of which are presently in existence:

1. A separate course
2. A part of health education
3. An integrated approach

For the already overcrowded curriculum, the separate course presents the usual difficulty of moving other subjects around so that adequate time can be given to sex education. This provides a certain in-depth concentration, but it tends to isolate a major health topic for concentrated study. One then asks, shouldn't alcohol and drugs or mental health receive the same treatment? Of course, it is possible to set up mini-courses where a topic is covered in concentrated form over a short period of time. Where there

---

[55]American School Health Association, Growth Patterns in Sex Education (Revised).
[56]The Illinois Sex Education Advisory Board, *Policy Statement on Family Life and Sex Education,* Springfield, Illinois: Office of Superintendent of Public Instruction, Revised.

```
                        R E S O L U T I O N


               SEX EDUCATION OF CHILDREN AND YOUTH*


                          Adopted by
                      House of Delegates
                   American Medical Association
                        July 15, 1969
```

Whereas, The traditional sources of sex information and guidance for young people are often inadequate; and

Whereas, The local public and parochial schools--as social institutions accessible to all young people, reflecting broad community support and with sufficient intellectual and material resources--can aid substantially in the development of sound individual codes of sexual behavior; therefore be it

Resolved, That the American Medical Association recognizes that the primary responsibility for family life education is in the home, but that the AMA support in principle the inauguration by State Boards of Education or school districts, whichever is applicable, of a voluntary family life and sex education program at appropriate grade levels:

   (1)   as part of an overall health education program;

   (2)   presented in a manner commensurate with the maturation level of the students;

   (3)   following a professionally developed curriculum foreviewed by representative parents;

   (4)   including ample and continuing involvement of parents and other concerned members of the community;

   (5)   developed around a system of values defined and delineated by community representatives comprising physicians, educators, the clergy, and other appropriate groups; and

   (6)   utilizing classroom teachers and other professionals who have an aptitude for working with young people and who have received special training; and be it further

Resolved, That local organizations be urged to utilize physicians as consultants, advisors, and resource persons in the development and guidance of such curriculum and that state and county medical associations be urged to take an active role in this participation.

*(By sex education is meant instruction to strengthen family life, to increase self-understanding and self-respect, to develop capacities for good human relationships, to build sexual and social responsibility, and to enhance competency for responsible parenthood. It is not concerned with sexual techniques nor sexual deviations.)

Figure 6-29 Resolution of American Medical Association.

are scheduled electives such courses as "Marriage and the Family" are quite popular. If one subscribes to the comprehensive or unified approach to health education, then the separate course plan is generally unacceptable. As it is, the numerous health misconceptions that have an immediate bearing on well-being and boy-girl relationships are being discussed in health education classes. Placing sex education in the health education course seems most practical, for it fits well into the health education sequence as one of the major health topics of the day. Strong support for this way of handling the subject comes from the American Medical Association. It is also highly recommended by the Joint Committee of the American Association of School Administrators and the National School Boards Association. Their point is that ". . . health is a unified concept. . . it cannot be achieved with a piece-meal approach," and ". . .including sex and family life

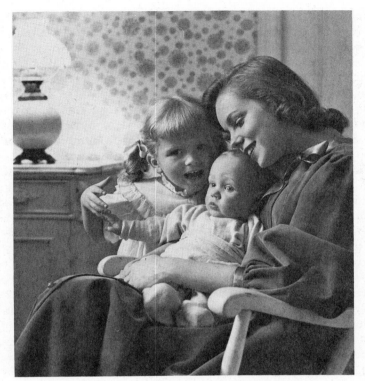

Figure 6–30   Family life education stresses the positive side of human sexuality. (Courtesy of Gerber Products Co.)

education with the other categorical health topics in one sound, interrelated, and sequential program. . . assures that all topics will be part of a long-range program."[57]

A third possibility is to correlate or integrate sex education with other subject-matter areas in the school. This makes it possible for students to think about sexuality and themselves from several viewpoints. There is a lesson to be learned about human emotions and enlightenment in an English class, as one considers why George Eliot had to publish under a man's name, or what D. H. Lawrence's concept of women and sex had to do with his writing. The contribution of history class to sex roles in the nineteenth century helps understand British politics, or the numerous reactions and implications of the women's suffrage movement. This requires very careful planning, so that all pertinent subject-matter personnel perform their functions adequately. This requires constant attention by a coordinator or supervisor in order for sex education not to be neglected. Although this has been done in a few instances, it is less satisfactory than assigning the responsibility to the health education teacher.

There is no crisis in sex education when the community of parents, clergy, physicians, and others understand what sex education is, what it is not, and what the school is planning to do.

A program that overlooks or ignores parental concerns is going to be shot down. Many parents have fears and an appalling amount of misinformation, as well as many

---

[57]Joint Committee of the National School Boards Association and American Association of School Administrators, *Health Education and Sex/Family Life Education*, NASB, Evanston, Illinois, 1969.

personal problems, which cause them to be most cautious before lending their support to a new school venture. This is especially noticeable if sex education is to be a new and separate course, and less of a problem where it is part of an ongoing health program.

There is no church pronouncement or position that can be legitimately quoted against sex education; there are priests, ministers, and others who are cooperative, even in a conservative locality, when they see that the school is also trying to advance acceptable moral and ethical values. Very helpful in this situation is the highly supportive *Interfaith Statement on Sex Education* developed jointly by the National Council of Churches, the Synagogue Council of America, and the United States Catholic Conference. It is available from all three groups and has had wide distribution.

The most acceptable and successful programs involving sex education topics are those in which help from the community has been obtained in all initial planning sessions. Official and voluntary health agency personnel should be included. Informed parents give support. Where there is concern, it is not over their children discovering the "facts of life." They'll support human reproduction, venereal disease, and other biologically oriented teachings. But they are frequently afraid of what a particular teacher may teach about boy-girl behavior. Very specifically, they wonder what may be taught pertaining to pre-marital intercourse. In our pluralistic society, this is never completely resolved. However, conflicting values can be explained and discussed. Any school that teaches sexual anarchy, position variations in sexual intercourse, techniques of sexual arousal, and detailed discussions of sexual perversion is headed for trouble. It is along these lines that well-meaning citizens are sometimes misled by a radical minority.

Another concern for parents, as well as for administrators, is the question of who shall teach about human sexuality. What is the attitude of the teacher? How interested in the topic is this person? Will he or she have special preparation? Is there an in-service opportunity to pursue the topic in detail?

A fully prepared health educator will ordinarily be capable of teaching a section of sex and family living education as a part of the health education curriculum. A state mandate for health education helps this situation. Some additional in-service work or study at a nearby university is frequently quite valuable. Ideally, the warm, sympathetic kind of person who relates well to adolescents is probably best suited to handle this area of the curriculum.

Reluctance on the part of some teachers to become involved in sex education can be expected. Hesitation may stem from lack of familiarity with content and uncertainty of ability to teach this subject. This is less apt to occur with teachers who are health education majors. However, when reluctance occurs, it should be acknowledged, with another teacher being scheduled for the sex education lessons—perhaps in a team-teaching sense. In at least one study, there is evidence to show that those teachers harboring the greatest number of misconceptions were least willing to teach controversial sex-related topics. Also, there were more misconceptions in the sociopsychological area than in the biological area.

There are professionals in the field of sex education who feel that there will have to be a new kind of teacher prepared—one who has been exposed to a variety of experiences in human awareness and can help others escape from their guarded inner selves. However, as desirable as this might be, it is not likely that specialists in sex education will be in great demand—particularly if the unified approach to health teaching continues to gain ground. What will continue is the need for special courses to boost the ability and confidence of health instructors. Fortunately, there is now an increasing number of teacher education programs offering both undergraduate and graduate courses pertaining to sexuality and sex education. These teacher understandings are called for quite specifically in the *Recommended Standards for Sex Education Teachers* issued by the Pennsylvania Department of Education. This same publication stresses that teachers should know their own feelings concerning sexuality, know the mores and customs of their community, demonstrate a wholesome attitude toward the dignity of man, and show a sincere trust and belief in the integrity of youth.

CONTROVERSY AND CONTROVERSIAL ISSUES—HOW SERIOUS?

What is controversial in one community is sometimes noncontroversial in another. This is especially true when a town or city has been properly prepared for the sex education program. Also, as indicated earlier, values differ widely in a pluralistic society. This is illustrated by observing two experts; one calls premarital relations particularly damaging to females, and the other refers to chastity as a form of ignorance and childishness. Likewise, there are bound to be parents at both ends of the scale on topics such as premarital relations, homosexuality, birth control, and abortion. Students do discuss these issues, if not in school, then outside. They are confronted with petting and coitus in learning to live with their peers. They seek answers. Just as there are parents who feel such a discussion will open curiosity doors and do more harm than good (for which there is no evidence), there are others more liberal, who feel that the open forum approach may safeguard boys and girls and help them avoid peer group and mass media pressures, and sexual exploitation.

Abortion and birth control are recognized as important public health issues. The various ethical views, as well as biological particulars, should be discussed in class. Pupils will learn that there are differences of opinion, and despite the population explosion and the rights of the female, there is no "absolutely right answer." Should a pupil press the teacher for his or her viewpoint or recommended practice in any of these controversial areas, the teacher need only explain that what is right for one person may not be right for another. The questioner should be reminded of the culture he is a part of, and the influences of his church and parents. In effect, the teacher is saying, "You know all the facts and viewpoints. Now, to find out what is the right practice for you, find out how your family and close friends feel. Then you can make your decision."

Since each new generation is responsible for helping to build the future, it will be necessary to teach youth in terms of moral and ethical values, and run the risk of being controversial somewhere along the way. How else can the three R's (*respect* for others, *reverence* for life, and *responsibility* for one's own actions) be conceptualized?

THE PROGRAM

There are many suggestions for secondary school programs in sex and family living education that have been worked out by committees and authors, and have been used successfully in school systems. Some of the more impressive contributions worth reviewing for program ideas are as follows:

Sex Education—A Working Design for Curriculum Development and Implementation, Grades K—12, The Education Council, 131 Mineola Blvd., Mineola, N.Y. 11501.

Steps Toward Implementing Family Life and Sex Education Programs in Illinois Schools, Springfield, Ill.: Superintendent of Public Instruction (Revised).

Education for Sexuality: Concepts and Programs for Teaching, 2nd edition, by John J. Burt and Linda A. Meeks, W. B. Saunders Co., Philadelphia, Pa., 1975.

Sex Education in the Schools, by H. Frederick Kilander, Macmillan Co., New York, 1970.

Family Life and Sex Education: Curriculum and Instruction, by Esther D. Schulz and Sally R. Williams, Harcourt, Brace, and World, Inc., New York, 1969.

Sex Education and Family Life: Growth Patterns and Reproduction, K—12, a complete curriculum guide (Revised).

Teaching About Family Relationships, by Richard Klemers and Rebecca Smith, Minneapolis: Burgess Publishing Co., 1975.

Understanding Human Sexuality, by Frederick Cohn, Englewood Cliffs, N.J.: Prentice-Hall, Inc., 1974.

Human Sexuality, 2nd Edition, by James Leslie McCary, New York: Van Nostrand, 1973.

Ideas and Learning Activities for Family Life and Sex Education, by Mark Perrin and Thomas E. Smith, Dubuque, Iowa: William C. Brown Co., 1972.

Family Planning Education, by Charles W. Hubbard, St. Louis: The C. V. Mosby Co., 1973.

Personal and Family Living for the Secondary School, Curriculum Resource Bulletin, Public Schools, District of Columbia, Administration Annex No. 7, North Street, N.W., Washington, D.C. 20007.

A Pioneer Program in Health Guidance in Sex Education, Glen Cove Public Schools, Glen Cove, N.Y. 11542.

Guide to Social Health Education, by grades, San Diego City Schools, San·Diego, Calif.

Sex Education: SIECUS Discussion Guide No. 1, Revised 1975. Publications Office, 122 East 42nd St., New York, N.Y. 10017.

A Curriculum Guide on Venereal Disease for Junior High School Teachers, Massachusetts Department of Public Health, Division of Communicable Diseases, Boston, Mass.

Teacher's Manual: A Curriculum Guide on Sex Education, Massachusetts Department of Public Health, Boston, Mass.

Guide to Health and Family Life Education, Grades K—12, San Francisco Unified School District, San Francisco, Calif. (A highly detailed and informative guide.)

Curriculum Guide for Family Life and Sex Education, Great Neck Public Schools, Great Neck, N.Y.

In programming secondary school content, it is frequently rewarding for the new teacher to probe student interests. In one major interest study of 5000 somewhat typical Connecticut school children, the questions and comments of youth provide extensive information for the development of appropriate programs.[58] Here are a few samples:

Junior High

"Why do some boys in this grade understand sex and giggle and laugh?" (Boy)

"What is so big about miniskirts and beautiful legs?" (Boy)

"There are dirty girls, sexy girls, girls with just looks, girls with a good personality, and girls who try to be something they aren't." (Boy)

"I'm not planning to marry. Should I date?" (Boy)

"When are most people sexually mature?"

"What about bathing and swimming during your period?" (Girl)

"Why do some men rape girls?" (Girl)

"You should know what happens if you have sex relations too young. You should know this before junior high school."

"When people are going to get married, why do they have a blood test?"

"Why are there so many unwed mothers?"

"How does early marriage affect children?"

"Why are some babies deformed?"

"Why is the government interested in abortions?"

"Does acting mature at 12 to 14 hurt your personality?"

"She is stuffing her bra. The boys know it, but they like girls for what they are. Should I tell her?" (Girl)

"Why is it that some boys shy away from being introduced?" (Girl)

"How can you get a boy to notice you and like you?" (Many girls)

"If you're a dud, like me, how can you become graceful?" (Girl)

"Is there such a thing as love at 13?" (Many)

"How do you know you're in love?" (Many)

"Why are boys in their early teens so dirty-minded?" (Girl)

"What should you do when a man tries to pick you up?" (Girl)

"How can you show a boy you like him without going too far?" (Girl)

"Parents have such different values from many children. How can you explain what's coming off and keep their trust?"

"Why does sex ring such an awful bell in parents' minds?"

Senior High

"Parents won't help us understand; schools should. Teach it before eighth grade, so kids will know more than I do."

"What is a Caesarian operation?"

"How can you help your child if he is defective?"

"What are lesbians?"

"Why can't I get anything done because of thinking of sex and girls?" (Boy)

"Why do newspapers put so much emphasis on sex and drugs?"

"Some boys and girls start messing around and give the girl a baby without ever knowing it happened." (Many)

"Boys and girls need mutual understanding of each other."

"There's no place a teenager can go to talk about sex relations openly."

"Why do people hide sex, if it's good and natural?"

"What is the role of the unwed father? What becomes of him . . . ?"

"Can you control your sexual emotions?"

"If a girl goes with a boy three years, knows that they are in love, that it's no kid stuff, is it all right to have intercourse?"

"Health is definitely concerned with sex."

"Are pre-marital sex relations bad? What happens to the mind and body?"

In the Arkansas study of secondary school level questions, many of the same concerns were voiced:[59]

"Can you die of VD if you've had it about a year?"

"Why is it always the boy's fault when a girl gets pregnant?"

"What do you do if you are a daddy at 14?"

"Can a girl get pregnant if she masturbates too much?"

"Can a girl have a baby from oral sex?"

"Why do girls become whores?"

"How can you convince a boy that just because you won't have sex with him doesn't mean that you don't love him?"

"How long should you date a girl before you try to get a little?"

Statements like these can be gathered from all corners of the country and spell out pretty much the same general concerns. They are both biological and socio-psychological. The psychological and sexual contents must be blended in a manner to advance psychological and psychosocial maturation (see Figure 6–31).

---

[59]*What Arkansas Teenagers Have Asked About Sex*, Little Rock, Ark.: Arkansas Family Planning Council, 1975 (P.O. Box 5149, Little Rock, Ark. 72205)

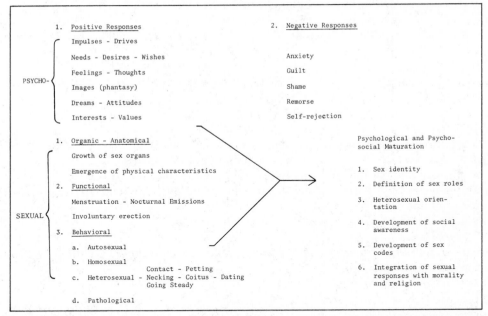

Figure 6–31   Structural analysis of psychosexual and psychosocial development in adolescence. (Courtesy of Massachusetts Department of Public Health)

Employing a conceptual approach to programming, the School Health Education Study set forth, as one of its ten major health generalizations, the concept that "the family serves to perpetuate man and to fulfill certain health needs."[60] From this were developed subconcepts, long range goals, behavioral objectives, and appropriate progressions and sequences for the teaching-learning experience. Transparencies and other teaching aids are a part of this program (Minnesota Mining and Manufacturing Co., St. Paul, Minn.).

The Cleveland, Ohio, schools worked from the above SHES concept to establish their own subconcepts. The following are for the ninth grade level and are a fine example of how to stress the family and the need for the personal responsibility at the junior high level.[61]

—The family is the basis for our society. It is a close group which usually experiences the five developmental stages of life: Infancy, Childhood, Adolescence, Adulthood, and Old Age.
—The interaction of the members of the family determines the family's living patterns.
—As the adolescent prepares for the world of the adult, he is developing a sense of identity.
—Dating is an accepted custom in our society. Parents are concerned for, and interested in, the behavior and welfare of their children.
—There are definite advantages and disadvantages in steady dating.
—Man develops his standards of beliefs and behavior according to the influences of his environment.
—Man needs companionship to reach his goals.
—The sex drive is a vital and complex force. It must be understood and controlled for a true and completely satisfying life.

[60]School Health Education Study, *Health Education: A Conceptual Approach,* Washington, D.C.: 3 M Educational Press, 1967, p. 66.
[61]Cleveland Board of Education, *Approaching Adulthood: Meeting Your Responsibilities,* Cleveland, Ohio, 1969.

—The adolescent years are the transition from childhood to adulthood.
—All growing bodies take time to attain physical maturity.
—Marriage provides for a deep exchange of love, thoughts, and feelings.
—Many factors can affect prenatal development and birth.
—A person's physical, social, and emotional successes are measured largely by his maturity.
—Young people today have more freedom than they had a generation ago.
—Society must understand one of history's oldest problems—venereal disease.

With the humanistic emphasis on reaching youth at the emotional level, considerable attention has been directed toward attitudes and values. Woody holds that there are seven basic attitudes that seem crucial to sex education and effective child rearing:[62]

1. Sexual organs and their functions are not inherently dirty, unsightly, or sinful.
2. There should be a consciousness about ensuring that the child's core gender identity be set to conform with his given sex at birth, as shown by anatomy and chromosomes.
3. Masturbation is a normal expression of sexual need in a variety of ages and circumstances for both males and females.
4. Sex education is an ongoing process between parents and child.
5. The advantages and disadvantages of pre-marital sexual behavior must be evaluated in the context of individual differences and one's unique mores, values, and environment.
6. Adolescents should have access to birth control information and methods.
7. Openness and clear communication about sexual matters are of great value in creating and maintaining meaningful relationships, and in learning how people can relate to each other as responsible and responsive human beings.

An especially important point that has been made by a number of school-community people is one that has to do with *parenting*—the education to be a parent. After all, there are a tremendous number of school-age parents. As of late 1975 there were just under 300 "Education for Parenthood" projects under HEW sponsorship. Jan Young, working in the Mankato (Minnesota) Public Schools finds that a young parent who understands his or her sexuality and growth and development is a better parent later on.[63] She exposes her students to attitude discussions, communicative skills, decision-making skills, how to cope with crises, and parental concerns. Fortunately senior high schoolers *do* think of themselves as potential parents and are receptive to sex education with this kind of concentration.

It is every bit as significant when dealing with sexuality as it is with other major health topics to have good teaching aids. There is a great amount of visual material available to put across biological fundamentals, boy-girl relationships, and parenting. Companies such as Guidance Associates and Sunburst Communications have superb films that promote real discussions (See sources in Chapter 10). Note the effect of a fine visual system in Figure 6–32. Here the slide projector focuses on two screens simultaneously so that the actual location of organs and processes can be shown along with the more typical slide. Here there are three interchangeable projection screen–forms: female pelvic reproductive anatomy, female breast anatomy, and male pelvic reproductive anatomy. Coupling these aids with good teaching can move a program a long way toward

[62]Jane Divita Woody, "Contemporary Sex Education: Attitudes and implications for Childbearing," *Journal of School Health*, 43:241–246, April, 1973.

[63]Jan Young, "Teaching Students About Their Future Role as Parents," *Health Education*, 6:13–17, September/October, 1975.

being effective. Sex and family living education calls for a warm, sincere teacher who relates well with youth. Eric Berne sums it up rather well when he says:[64]

"The main thing is that it should not be taught by frigid people, with some dried out members of the school board looking over their shoulders like kippered herring at a wake. In this situation, sex is like humor. Courses in humor, if they are given at all, should be given only by people who have laughed at least once in their lives and enjoyed it."

There are numerous examples of how the family, as a societal unit, is being stressed in recently developed curriculum guides. Also, individuals such as Kilander set forth junior and senior high school programs in an immediately useful manner (Chapter 5); Burt and Brower do not program the material, but they present excellent teaching units that can be adapted to local secondary school programs; Schulz and Williams treat both secondary periods separately and in detail. All three sources should be reviewed when programming is under way.[65] Also, the practice of carefully listing all behavioral objectives is very important. In the preceding chapter, the behavioral objectives for a major health topic were limited to the junior and senior high school levels. The assumption has been that there will be a progression from the elementary school years to the junior high level that will be smooth and sequential. This is far more apt to happen if *all* objectives, from kindergarten to twelfth grade, are set forth before program content details are de-

---

[64]Eric Berne, *Sex and Human Loving,* New York: Simon and Schuster, 1970, p. 19.

[65]H. Frederick Kilander, *Sex Education in the Schools;* John J. Burt and Linda Meeks, *Education for Sexuality,* 2nd edition (Section Four); and Esther D. Schultz and Sally R. Williams, *Family Life and Sex Education: Curriculum and Instruction* (Parts 3 and 4).

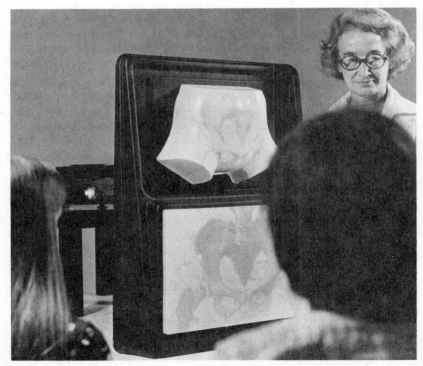

Figure 6–32 A relevant visual system to support instruction. (Courtesy of OMNI Educational System, Ortho Pharmaceutical Corp.)

veloped. In sex and family living education, this listing of all objectives is badly needed in order to limit the amount of material to be covered in the secondary school, as well as to give it more meaning. For this reason, the following full range of objectives are recorded; they have been used successfully by the author.

Behavioral Objectives

Kindergarten

Tells how one is a family member, and families do things together.

Explains that mothers and fathers are important too.

Illustrates how children and parents working and playing together help to make home a happy place to live.

Demonstrates how family members show love for each other.

Shows how to act as a member of a school family.

Tells how bodies are wonderful and there is nothing shameful about any part of the body.

Names the body parts concerned with elimination, respiration, movement, and thinking.

Demonstrates how to respect the privacy of others.

(Grades 1 to 3. Behavioral objectives applicable according to maturity and interests.)

Grades 1 and 2

Describes how a happy home life depends upon the contributions of each member of the family.

Cooperates in the home, sharing work as well as fun.

Cares for pets in the family or at school.

Accepts animals as part of family life.

Explains that all living things grow and reproduce.

Tells how both animal and human parents try to keep their young safe, fed, happy, and healthy.

Shows how several animals protect and feed their babies.

Recognizes that animals have babies like themselves.

Describes the many ways that happy families work and play together.

Names a variety of occasions when there are good times in a home and family.

Appreciates that boys and girls can play together, but that boys also play with boys, and girls with girls.

Explains how the family prepares for, cares for, and loves a new baby.

Grades 3 and 4

Observes how parents make a home a pleasant place.

Describes elementary reproduction: all living things come from other living things—illustrated by baby animals, plant life, and mothers and babies.

Shows how animals protect and feed babies in different ways.

Helps with family chores, and the caring of younger family members.

Diagrams how human beings grow in many ways—physically, mentally, and socially.

Describes the unique contributions of men and women to society.

Explains how children inherit the way they look from mother and father.

Describes the growth of the human being in the body of the mother—where life starts and develops.

Investigates the meaning of families as good neighbors.

Differentiates between the ovaries, testes, ovum, sperm, glands, hormones, and so on.

Distinguishes inherited characteristics from characteristics not inherited.

Grades 5 and 6

Details the start of life and how body cells begin from a single cell, which divides into two cells: terminology and structure.

Explains reproductive and growth process: egg cells, sperm cells, from egg to baby.

Describes elemental function of menstruation.

Investigates growth differences from 10 to 14 years of age: boy and girl differences; more rapid maturation of girls.

Recognizes the contributions of both sexes to family life and society in general.

Illustrates how at one time girls may be taller than boys, but later on the boys usually catch up to the girls in height.

Describes the continuing process of physical growth and maturation toward manhood and womanhood.

Explains how social, intellectual, and emotional growth are essential parts of the maturation process.

Tells the several meanings of adolescence.

Describes puberty and is aware of the physical and mental occurrences which have a bearing on peer group relationships.

Expresses the view that the uniqueness of boys and girls is seen in one's sexuality, not only through the reproductive process but within the framework of the family.

Junior High School Level

Grades 7 to 9

Human Behavior

The Family Unit

Reproductive Process

Dating

Human Behavior

Explains that although complicated by psychological and physiological functions, individual behavior can be controlled.

Self-directs intelligence to the solution of personal problems.

Experiences changes in energy levels and emotions.

Demonstrates that emotional health has a bearing on all behavior and happiness.

Discusses how personality develops as one works out a smooth relationship between self and others, including friends of both sexes, family, and society.

Acknowledges that there are different rates of development, and that there are normal patterns and differences in physical and emotional growth.

Expresses his emotions in a variety of situations, but with some control.

Explains how personal standards of behavior are influenced by how we see ourselves, what we wish to become, and how we interact with the many factors in the environment.

The Family Unit

States that because the society is always in a state of change, the role of the family members will change.

Justifies the fact that as parents and children make adjustments their family life becomes more healthful and a happier one.

Identifies the essential function of the family to provide identity, security, and love for all family members.

Explains how a variety of families from different cultures make up a particular community; the community, therefore, is only as strong as the quality of the individual family members.

Demonstrates the way families, working together, use a logical approach to find solutions to their problems.

Reproductive Process

Shows how physical development at adolescence is related to heredity and sexual maturity.

Diagrams how the male and female have a unique reproductive structure and function.

Describes how in the male the sex drive develops before or concurrently with the maturation of spermatozoa.

Explains that as the sex drive develops, it finds a natural expression through increased interest in associations with members of the opposite sex.

Acknowledges that girls and boys are biologically capable of mating and reproducing a number of years before they are mature enough to be responsible parents.

Outlines the way menstruation occurs normally in the absence of conception and fertilization.

Realizes seminal emissions are a normal occurrence during the growing up period.

Describes how expressing the sex drive through inappropriate means creates problems for the individual, the family, and the society.

Dating

Discovers that men and women, boys and girls learn to understand each other as sexual beings through the age-old custom of dating.

Helps formulate moral standards of conduct to relate to dating and the making of personal decisions.

Discusses the fact that the quality of boy-girl relationships while on a date is the responsibility of both the boy and the girl.

Practices control and illustrates how controlling the sex drive on a date is best understood and accomplished if the boy and girl both understand themselves biologically and emotionally, and also understand each other.

Accepts responsibility for the welfare of his dating partner as well as his own when dating.

Explains the many ways to be popular.

Applies the notion that there is a difference between being "sexy" and being feminine.

Discusses issues related to the statement that human sexuality has to do with what it means to be feminine or masculine.

Shows how premarital sexual experiences frequently result in unwanted pregnancies, venereal disease, and broken boy-girl relationships.

Senior High School Level

(Grades 10 to 12)

Human Relationships

Preparation for Marriage

Human Relationships

Demonstrates the manner in which emotional well-being encompasses a wide variety of emotional responses.

Explains in detail how human sexuality is concerned with the qualities of manhood and womanhood.

Illustrates how physiological sex drives differ between males and females and must be understood if an individual is to appreciate the feelings of companions.

Describes the wide variety of sources and samples of love. Terms such as "young love," "puppy love," "true love," "sexual love," and so forth have different meanings to people with different understandings.

Outlines how going steady has its advantages and its disadvantages.

Expresses an understanding of the fact that because parents are interested in the total welfare of their children, they usually express some attitude toward dating behavior.

Demonstrates self-respect by acknowledging the importance of setting limits for one's behavior while on a date.

Refrains from using too much alcohol which may create a personal situation where responsible sexual behavior is undermined.

Urges others to understand that venereal disease can be controlled in this country if individual cases are reported and treated.

Explains how prostitution is a social problem related to drug addiction, and to the hedonistic philosophy of Playboyism.

Discusses how the "new morality" need not ignore the virtues of respect for individuals and responsibility for one's own actions.

Acts in a given situation by a consideration of both the immediate and the long range consequences of his actions.

Explains that male and female homosexuality has to be understood for what it is; homosexual individuals are sometimes helped through proper psychiatry and counseling.

Preparation For Marriage

Shows how the choice of a marriage partner is influenced by many personal, economic, and societal factors. Understands that these should be thoroughly understood before two people decide to invest their lives and their resources in a joint enterprise.

Differentiates between a meaningful engagement and just going together.

Shows how a mature husband-wife relationship is based on mutual goals, giving of oneself without thought of return, and broad understandings of why the other person feels the way he does.

Analyzes how the premarital medical examination is designed to help a couple start married life in a state of optimal health.

Explains that the more a couple interested in marriage have in common, the better their chances of having a successful marriage.

Applies the idea that a society has to adjust to the problems brought about through overpopulation, divorce, abortion, and unwanted children.

Details family planning and how it means creating a family according to a purposeful design.

Tells how in order to provide for the total well-being of the family, children may be spaced at certain intervals; a large segment of the population employs contraceptive methods as a means of orderly family growth.

Passes along the information that physicians and other qualified advisers assist young people with specific information about family planning methods.

Describes how pregnancy requires the expectant mother to make a number of adjustments in nutrition, personal care, and emotional attitude.

Details how proper personal health practices, coupled with adequate medical care and vitamin and mineral supplements, enhance the prospective mother's chances of delivering a normal, healthy baby.

Recognizes that the birth of a couple's first child frequently requires a major adjustment for the husband and wife.

Expresses the view that the birth of the baby and the growth of the child during its first year help one appreciate and have a reverence for life.

Reacts positively to the proposition that one's personal standard of sexual behavior is complicated by a number of alternatives according to the culture, but it ultimately relates to a personal respect for the rights and feelings of others and the responsible actions of mature men and women.

Applies in actions the principle that a society is made whole and livable when the joys of family activity, planning, and fulfillment transcend the immediate gratifications of individuals.

Explains how parents have the major influence on the socialization and development of their children.

Practices the worthy use of leisure time and acknowledges its contribution to the full development of the individual and the family as a necessary attribute in modern society.

Space does not permit the detailed description of program content for each of the six junior-senior high school grades as it appears in several communities. Usually, a curriculum committee in a particular locality will divide a body of content suitable for the junior high school according to the number and extent of pupil exposures to sex education in the total health program. The same would be done at the senior high school level. This kind of flexibility is defendable, because there is no ideal or set program, and the needs of every town and city vary. In Great Neck, New York, where health education programs have been strong for a number of decades, the program content is spelled out as follows.[66]

Family Life and Sex Education

Suggested Content — Grades 7–9

A. Human Growth and Development
1. Principles of Growth and Development
2. Areas of Growth and Development
    a. mental
    b. physical
    c. emotional
    d. social
3. Factors Influencing Growth and Development
    a. parents
    b. culture
    c. sex
    d. intelligence
    e. race
    f. geographic area

B. Understanding of Self
1. Personality — Definition
2. Factors Influencing the Development of Personality
    a. heredity
       nervous system: normal — abnormal
       endocrine system: normal — abnormal
    b. environment
       childhood experiences
       family
       friends
       cultural sex expectations — sex roles

---

[66]*Tentative Curriculum Guide for Family Life and Sex Education,* Great Neck Public Schools, Great Neck, N.Y. Note that this program is tentative, leaving room for change as the local situation requires.

C. Maturation—Pubertal Stage—Male
   1. Differences in Physical Growth Patterns
      a. onset
      b. rate of growth
      c. role of endocrine glands
      d. expected and unusual changes of secondary sex characteristics
   2. Review—Male Reproductive Organs
      a. penis
      b. glans, penis, and prepuce
      c. testicles
      d. scrotum
      e. epididymis
      f. seminal vesicles
      g. vas deferens
      h. prostate gland
      i. urethra (dual function)
   3. Erection
      a. the mechanism involved
      b. causes
   4. The Sperm
      a. function
      b. characteristics
      c. seminal emissions
      d. nocturnal emissions
   5. Understanding Masturbation
      a. causes
      b. myths
      c. when harmful to an individual
   6. Emotional Reactions to Developing Male Sexuality
D. Maturation—Pubertal Stage—Female
   1. Differences in Physical Growth Patterns
      a. onset
      b. rate of growth
      c. role of endocrine glands
      d. expected and unusual changes of secondary sex characteristics
   2. Review—Female Reproductive Organs
      a. vulva
         clitoris
         labia (majora and minora)
         vaginal opening
      b. hymen
      c. vagina
      d. cervix
      e. uterus

      f. Fallopian tubes
      g. ovaries
   3. Menstruation
      a. attitudes towards menstruation
   4. Review—Conception and Pregnancy
      a. fertilization
      b. conception
      c. cell division and differentiation
      d. twinning
      e. embryonic development
      f. fetal development
   5. Review—Birth
      a. contractions (labor)
      b. amniotic fluid
      c. dilation of cervix
      d. delivery
      e. discussion of abnormal deliveries
   6. Emotional Reactions to Developing Female Sexuality
E. Human Behavior
   1. The Nervous System—Its Relationship to the Mind and to Behavior
      a. sensory nerves and perception
      b. motor nerves and response
      c. levels of behavior
         instinctive
         reflexive
         conditional responses
         emotional
         intelligent
      d. the brain in determining behavior
         unconscious behavior
         conscious behavior
   2. Basic Needs and Drives
   3. The Ability to Adjust
      a. problem solving
      b. getting along in school
      c. getting along at home
      d. getting along in the community
F. Emotions and Behavior
   1. Definition and Theories of Emotions
   2. Different Kinds of Emotions
   3. The Expression of Emotions
      a. vocal
      b. body activity
      c. spontaneous (autonomic) responses; e.g., blushing, perspiring, rapid breathing, increased heart beat
   4. Emotional Responses and the Endocrine System
   5. Emotional Maturity
      a. self-discipline

b. independence
c. acceptance of realities
d. acceptance of responsibility for self and others

G. Significance of the Peer Group
1. Fulfills Adolescents' Need to Belong
2. Bolsters Self-confidence
3. Provides Opportunity to Learn Social Graces in Heterosexual Settings
4. Influences Attitudes
5. Fulfills Girls' Precocious Interest in Dating
6. Helps to Establish Natural Heterosexual Relationships

H. Boy—Girl Relationships
1. Dating
   a. purpose of dating
   b. kinds of dating; e.g., double dating, single dating, "Dutch" dating.
   c. how to choose a date
   d. how to arrange a date
   e. what to do on a date
   f. dating etiquette
2. Going Steady
   a. purposes of going steady
   b. advantages and disadvantages
   c. parental reactions
3. Necking
   a. its purposes
   b. its effect on the boy
   c. its effect on the girl
4. Petting
   a. its purposes
   b. its effect on the boy
   c. its effect on the girl
5. Developing and Adhering to Valid Standards of Conduct
   a. resolving value conflicts

b. finding acceptable means of sexual behavior
6. Definitions and Discussions of the Following Terms:
   a. sexual relations
   b. sexual intercourse
   c. premarital relations
   d. premarital intercourse

I. Family Relationships
1. Roles Within the Family Structure
   a. the role of the mother
   b. the role of the father
   c. the role of siblings
   d. the role of other members of the family
2. Problems in Family Relationships
   a. those commonly experienced by adolescents
   b. the need for making appropriate adjustments to problems in family relationships
   c. finding acceptable solutions to such problems
3. Growing in Respect Towards Authority
4. The Development of Independence and Sound Judgment
5. Discipline
   a. parental controls
   b. developing one's own controls— self-discipline and responsibility
6. Developing Standards of Belief and Behavior
7. Developing Meaningful Friendships
   a. the extent to which friendships substitute for or complement family relationships
   b. resolving conflicts between one's family and one's friends

At this age, students want and need to know about premarital pregnancy, promiscuity, homosexuality, birth control, abortion, and venereal disease. When they are encouraged to discuss frankly their own questions and concerns, these and other topics will flow naturally from structured areas of content.

Suggested Content—Grades 10–12

A. Physiological Changes Through Adulthood
1. Review of Male and Female Reproductive Systems
2. Physiological Sex Differences
   a. sex hormones
   b. sex drive
3. Sexual Reactions
   a. erection
   b. orgasm

4. Menopause
B. Sexual Feelings and Sexual Maturity
1. Male-Female Psycho-sexual Differences
2. Characteristics of Healthy Sexual Maturity
3. Development of the Capacity for Mature Love
C. Factors Affecting Sexuality
1. Developmental Stages

2. Environmental Influences
   a. family
   b. social
   c. mass media
D. Cultural Mores
  1. Attitudes Toward Sex and Family Living in Other Societies (i.e., Scandinavian, tribal, Oriental)
  2. History of Sex and Family Life Practices in the United States
E. Sexual Variants and Aberrations
  1. Variations in Sex Practices
  2. Homosexuality
  3. Transsexuality
  4. Aberrations and Sex Laws
F. Determining Individual Sexual Values
  1. The Major Competing Value Systems
    a. traditional repressive asceticism
    b. enlightened asceticism
    c. humanistic liberalism
    d. humanistic radicalism
    e. fun morality
    f. sexual anarchy
  2. The Moral Implications of These Value Systems for the Individual and Society (i.e., the individual, the family, the democratic structure)
  3. Today's Sexual Behavior Patterns (i.e., dating practices, petting, premarital sex, promiscuity, double standard)
  4. Factors Influencing Changes in Attitudes Toward Sexual Behavior
  5. Possible Outcomes of Modern Sexual Patterns
    a. illegitimacy
    b. early marriage
    c. marriage vs. bachelorhood and the single woman
G. Preparation for Marriage
  1. Selecting a Marriage Partner
  2. Courtship
  3. Engagement Period
  4. Types of Marriage
    a. common law
    b. civil
    c. religious
  5. State Laws Governing Marriage
  6. Premarital Examination and Counseling
H. Marital Adjustments
  1. Psycho-sexual Adjustment
  2. Husband-Wife Roles
  3. Potential Sources of Conflict in Marriage
    a. career wives

    b. economics
    c. children
    d. in-laws
    e. religion
    f. racial differences
    g. infidelity
  4. Family Planning
    a. factors determining family size (i.e., health of mother, financial, educational, long range needs of each child)
    b. responsibility toward control of population explosion
    c. birth control
I. Human Reproduction and Parenthood
  1. Review of Conception, Pregnancy, and Birth Process
  2. Importance of Medical Care
    a. preconceptual
    b. pre-natal
  3. Husband and Wife Psychosexual Adjustments During Pregnancy
  4. Needs of the Newborn Infant
  5. Adjustments in Family Living Related to the Birth of a Child
  6. Parenthood
    a. mother and father roles
    b. causes and effects of single-parent households
    c. remarriage and step-parenthood
  7. Problems Occasionally Related to Planning for Parenthood
    a. sterility
    b. loss of child during pregnancy, or at birth
    c. birth of a handicapped child
  8. Possible Solutions for the Childless Couple
    a. adoption
    b. artificial insemination
    c. foster parenthood
J. Community Resources in the Area of Family Life and Sex Education
  1. Clergy
  2. Physician
  3. Psychological Services
  4. Marriage Counselors
  5. Health Agencies
    a. classes for prospective mothers and fathers
    b. prenatal and well baby clinics
    c. planned parenthood organizations
    d. homes for the unwed mother
    e. adoption agencies
    f. institutions for the handicapped
K. Critical Issues in Today's Society
  1. Abortion: Therapeutic and Criminal

2. Venereal Disease as a Social Problem
3. Illegitimacy — Its Impact on Society

4. Sexuality and the Law
   a. prostitution
   b. rape
   c. pornography

In Chapter 10, there is an extensive listing of sources that have been used by teachers. It should be carefully looked over. Particular attention should be paid to sources which involve students themselves. Stories and books for students to read are very important. Too many activites are classroom centered; the pupil often doesn't read enough on his own. The following brief list of references can supplement classroom studies very well (for other suggestions, see Chapter 10):

Junior High

Love and Sex in Plain Language
by Eric Johnson
Finding Yourself
by Marion Lerrigo
Moving Into Manhood
by W. W. Bauer
Teenage Sex Counselor
by B. Y. Glassberg
What Teenagers Want to Know
by Florence Levinsohn
How to Understand the Opposite Sex
by William Menninger
On Becoming a Woman
by Mary Williams and Irene Kane
Understanding the Other Sex
by Lester Kirkendall and Ruth Osborne

Are You There God? It's Me, Margaret
By Judith Blume
Somebody Will Miss Me
by Deborah Crawford
Sex and the Teenage Girl
by Carol Botwin

Senior High
How to Understand Sex
by Wayne J. Anderson
The Human Venture in Sex,
Love and Marriage
by Peter Bertocci
Sex, Love and the Person
by Peter Bertocci
When You Marry
by Evelyn Duvall and Reuben L. Hill

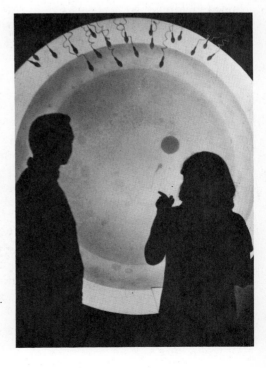

Figure 6–33 Greater Cleveland high school students view model of a giant, six-foot egg shown at the moment of conception. (Courtesy of the Cleveland Health Museum and Education Center)

Why Wait Till Marriage
by Evelyn Duvall
Young People and Sex
by Arthur Cain
The Art of Loving
by Eric Fromm
Life Can Be Sexual
by Elmer Witt
Love, Sex and Being Human
by Paul Bohannan
Telling It Straight
by Eric Johnson

How to Understand the Opposite Sex
by William Menninger
My Darling, My Hamburger
by Paul Zindel
Getting It All Together
by Michael Capizzi
Andy
by Phyllis A. Wood
Sex Facts for Teenagers
by Evelyn Fiore and Richard S. Ward
A Teenager's Guide to Life and Love
by Benjamin A. Spock

THE MENTALLY RETARDED

Health education for the mentally retarded is especially important. Sex and family living education sould be very much a part of these classes.

Although a boy or girl may be retarded in mental development, generally he or she will be quite like other children in physical development. During the adolescent period, many of the same problems arise that concern normal children. The difficulty is that the retarded youth cannot always handle them. When they are beyond his or her intellectual grasp, or they have not been discussed, it is possible for older people to take advantage of them—something that happens in almost every community, and sometimes contributes to the unwanted baby-welfare problem. The booklet, *How to Tell the Retarded Girl About Menstruation,* published by Kimberly-Clark Corporation in Neenah, Wisconsin, is very helpful. So is the publication, *A Resource Guide in Sex Education for the Mentally Handicapped,* second edition (American Association for Health, Physical Education and Recreation), which was specifically designed for teachers working with handicapped children.

Limited research indicates that physically and emotionally disabled children have a deficit in sex knowledge when compared to normal adolescents of the same age. Moreover, Bloom has shown that a course in sex education does not appear to be anxiety-producing to any harmful extent.[67]

✳ Suggested Activities

(*Junior High Level*)

1. Set up a student committee to poll fellow students about the three or four questions most often asked pertaining to human sexuality. An effective procedure is to collect these questions on small cards. This requires the pupil to think carefully and write out his question. This activity may be used in part to initiate a class discussion.

2. Show the filmstrips *Values For Dating* (Sunburst Communications) or *Tomorrow's Children* (Perennial Education, Inc.) in order to stimulate questions dealing with peer pressures, insights into different aspects of emotion, and to help students examine

---

[67]Jean L. Bloom, "Sex Education for Handicapped Adolescents," *Journal of School Health,* 39:263–267, June, 1969.

their own feelings. Assign out-of-class discussion time to investigate attitudes toward dating values, and different approaches to love.

3. Inquire about the advantages of family planning. How is it accomplished? Why? Is the world rapidly losing the power to feed itself? Does the population explosion affect the *quality* of life? Could a serious situation arise if the world population grows from 3.5 billion people in 1969 to 6.5 billion people by the year 2000? Collect estimates of population growth and food supplies available.

4. Post Paul Bohannan's definition of love before the class. Find out what the students think it means. It is for real — or just so many fine words?

> "Like 'life' in general, love embodies what appears to be contradiction: the satisfaction of the self through the satisfaction of the needs and desires of others."[68]

5. Obtain the *Materials Kit for Teaching Sex Education Classes* from the Cleveland Health Museum in order to make clear the basic principles of anatomy and physiology of reproduction from conception through the birth process (8911 Euclid Ave., Cleveland, Ohio 44106).

6. Put the poster shown in Figure 6–34 on the class bulletin board for all to see. Then raise the question of misconceptions related to menstruation. The teaching guide, *From Fiction to Fact,* is available free from Tampax, Incorporated, 161 East 42nd Street, New York, N.Y. 10017. Other teaching materials on menstruation may be obtained from Kimerly-Clark Corp., Neenah, Wisconsin 54957; Personal Products Corporation, Willows, N.J. 08850; and Scott Paper Company, Philadelphia, Pa. 19113.

7. Arrange, with student assistance, a simulated marriage. This is an activity that goes from the wedding ceremony, through having children to divorce. Select all players, i.e., partners, clergyman, family members, children, lawyers, and perhaps a neighbor or friend or two. Have non-performing class members prepare questions about the simulated marriage during the presentation.

---

[68]Paul Bohannan, *Love, Sex and Being Human,* New York: Doubleday and Company, 1969, p. 85.

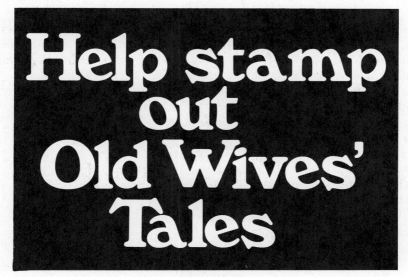

Figure 6–34

8. *Problem-Solving Project* for a group of three or four students: Examine a copy of Emily Post's *Etiquette* (revised by Elizabeth L. Post, New York: Funk & Wagnalls, 1965).

a. Ask students to choose from the book several rules of dating etiquette which they feel are old-fashioned. Discuss with the students their ideas about how dating mores have changed. Why were rules of dating etiquette developed in the first place? Why have they changed?

b. Ask each student to choose a rule for dating etiquette and write a parody of it. The parody should dramatize how values have changed.

c. Find an early edition of Emily Post's *Etiquette,* originally published as *Etiquette: The Blue Book of Social Usage,* by Emily Post in 1922. (Other early editions were published in 1927, 1931, 1934, 1937, 1940, 1942, and 1945.) Have students read the dating sections of one or more of these earlier editions, and ask them to compare the dating section in the newest edition with the earlier ones. Are there some early dating rules that still seem to make sense? Do they seem merely laughable? If, in activities (a) and (b), students have been harsh judges of Elizabeth Post's new dating rules, what do they think of her ideas after having read the earlier *Etiquette* editions? Did she write as good a dating section as she could have? How might she have improved it?[69]

9. Obtain audio cassettes from Spenco Medical Corporation (P.O. Box 8113, Waco, Texas 76710) on "Menstruation" and "Sex for Kids." Set up a small 8 to 12 person round table seminar. Play a cassette (16 to 20 minutes long) and be ready for student questions. Instead of answering questions assign library reading for answers.

10. Read parts of *Love and Sex in Plain Language* by Eric Johnson (Chapter 4). It explains rather simply that marriage provides for a deep exchange of love, thoughts, and feelings. What do eighth or ninth graders think of this concept? Is it too early or "on time" to think of what real love means?

11. *Role play* a family life situation where your parents have told you that they are getting divorced. Your younger brother or sister is distressed and wants to talk things over with you. How do you handle the situation? For your brother? Sister? Yourself? Appoint a "you," "brother," and "sister." Play the roles before the class. Then get into the topic of divorce and how it affects different families. How does the increasing number of divorces affect society? How is divorce treated in other cultures and times? (For assistance see Margaret Mead, *Male and Female,* New York: Dell Publishing Co., 1949.)

12. Prepare a short talk to be delivered to the League of Women Voters on the responsibility of each member of the community for education about and eradication of venereal disease. Assign class members to obtain local public health department literature on gonorrhea and syphilis.

13. Investigate "self-image" and feelings of security. Reproduce the following questions for individual consideration—*not for reporting to the class:*

a. Look at yourself in a mirror while undressed.
1. What do you see?
2. Do you like what you see?
3. How would you change your appearance?
b. Name what you like best about yourself.
c. Name what you like least about yourself.
d. Is it really important to change your image?
e. Who might influence you the most to change?

---

[69]Adapted from the teachers' guide to *Values for Dating,* Pound Ridge, N.Y.: Sunburst Communications, 1974.

f. Who would you most like to look like? Why?

g. Is it important for others to like you? Why?

14. Collect movie advertisements that appear in local newspapers. Note the ratings and the kinds of expressions used to "sell" the movie to the reader. Is there an emotional appeal here of some consequence? Is there a "sex pitch"?

15. Pre-test to evaluate class knowledge of human reproduction. After showing an appropriate film on reproduction, test again. Have each student note where he improved or failed to improve. Discuss these test changes with the class as a whole. What were the major changes shared by more than one or two students?

16. Have a group of girls develop a chart to rate their date. Have a group of boys do the same. Prior to doing this, it would be helpful to discuss factors thought important in choosing a good date.

Suggested Activities

(Senior High Level)

1. *Role play:*

Situation: You and your boyfriend/girlfriend are pretty serious. You are happy about that, but he/she does not want you to see anyone else—even just as friends. The security of your relationship is really nice, but you just are not ready to be that tied down. You discuss what to do with a friend.

Roles: you- Valerie/Vin (boyfriend/girlfriend- Wesley/Wendy) friend- Van/Vida.

Topics for Discussion:

How much control do local dating patterns have over your life? How much control do you have over them? Why do they exist in the first place? How do they differ from community to community?

How do dating and courting patterns differ with time and culture?

If you want to break a pattern what can you do? What are the long and short range consequences?

2. Create a double circle of students. The inner circle will discuss the following quotation; the outer circle may only observe. After 8 to 10 minutes call "Time," and without discussion change speakers and observers. After 8 to 10 minutes call "Time" and open the topic up to full discussion:

> "Love is the principal developer of one's capacity for being human, the chief stimulus for development of social competence, *and the only thing on earth* that can produce that sense of belongingness and relatedness to the world of humanity which is the best achievement of the healthy human being."[70]
>
> —*Ashley Montagu*

3. Post the three R's and inquire if they are truly achievable in this day and age.

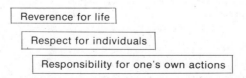

Reverence for life

Respect for individuals

Responsibility for one's own actions

Elaborate on how they relate to sexual behavior.

---

[70]Ashley Montagu in *Age of Aquarius*, by K. Jones, L. Shainberg, and C. Byer, New York: Goodyear, 1971.

RESPONDENT NUMBER

PLEASE — DO NOT WRITE YOUR NAME ON ANY PAGE

Directions

We all have beliefs and opinions about abortion and the following list of statements is an attempt to let you express your opinions.

Please remember that there are no right or wrong answers. This is NOT a test, but a list of items for collecting data. You are not asked to write your name. Your opinions will remain CONFIDENTIAL. Please answer all the statements as frankly and honestly as you can. Please respond to all items.

KEY: Circle the number next to an item which comes closest to your personal reaction to a statement as indicated in the following example.

EXAMPLE

1. If you strongly agree that abortion should be legalized, circle   5—Strongly Agree
2. If you agree that abortion should be legalized, circle   4—Agree
3. If you are undecided that abortion should be legalized, circle   3—Undecided
4. If you disagree that abortion should be legalized, circle   2—Disagree
5. If you strongly disagree that abortion should be legalized, circle   1—Strongly disagree

Circle the number next to the item which comes closest to your personal reaction to the statement.

		Strongly Agree	Agree	Unde-Cided	Disagree	Strongly Disagree
1.	Abortions are acceptable when the pregnancy is the result of incest (sexual intercourse between brother-sister, father-daughter, mother-son).	5	4	3	2	1
2.	Abortion should be treated legally as a form of murder unless it is performed to save the mother's life.	5	4	3	2	1
3.	Abortion is acceptable when it is reasonably certain that the fetus is malformed.	5	4	3	2	1
4.	An abortion is acceptable if the pregnancy seriously endangers the mother's life.	5	4	3	2	1
5.	I would not respect someone who had an abortion.	5	4	3	2	1
6.	Abortion would be acceptable if the couple expecting the child is in the process of divorce.	5	4	3	2	1
7.	An abortion should be available for a woman when she feels she already has as many children as she would like.	5	4	3	2	1
8.	It is the moral responsibility of any perfectly healthy woman to bear the child when she becomes pregnant.	5	4	3	2	1
9.	Abortion is acceptable if the mother is unmarried and does not wish to marry the baby's father.	5	4	3	2	1
10.	Abortion should be available to women who are threatening to commit suicide because of an unwanted pregnancy.	5	4	3	2	1

Figure 6–35 Discussion-provoking questionnaire developed by Sondra Wilcox, Middle Tennessee State University, Murfreesboro, Tennessee.

Illustration continued on opposite page.

4. Discuss predicting success in marriage. Highly associated items are (1) happiness of parents' marriage, (2) adequate length of courtship and engagement, (3) approval of marriage by parents and others, (4) ethnic and religious similarity, (5) maturity and similar chronological age.

5. Collect student opinions on courtship and marriage. These may be discussed openly in class. A more effective approach would be to use the 53-item questionnaire by

	Strongly Agree	Agree	Unde-Cided	Disagree	Strongly Disagree
11. The embryo is a human being at the time of conception.	5	4	3	2	1
12. Abortion is against my religious views.	5	4	3	2	1
13. Abortions are acceptable when the mother is mentally retarded.	5	4	3	2	1
14. Abortions are acceptable when the woman is married and pregnant and neither she nor her husband want the child.	5	4	3	2	1
15. I would strongly urge a close relative (sister or daughter) not to terminate any unwanted pregnancy.	5	4	3	2	1
16. Even if medical tests show that the developing fetus definitely is abnormal in some way I would not make abortion available to the mother.	5	4	3	2	1
17. An abortion is acceptable to me for any reason that a woman wished to terminate the pregnancy.	5	4	3	2	1
18. Abortion in any period of pregnancy is murder.	5	4	3	2	1
19. Abortion for unmarried women should not be made legal.	5	4	3	2	1
20. Abortion should be permitted because it is a lesser evil than giving birth to an unwanted child.	5	4	3	2	1
21. When there are serious financial burdens within the family, an abortion should be allowed.	5	4	3	2	1
22. Abortion of a human embryo is murder even if performed during the first trimester (first three months.)	5	4	3	2	1
23. My close friends would not approve of abortion.	5	4	3	2	1
24. Abortion is acceptable when the pregnancy is a result of rape.	5	4	3	2	1
25. The liberalization of abortion in the United States has sanctioned immorality.	5	4	3	2	1
26. Since abortions will take place whether legal or not they should be legalized so proper medical attention may be obtained.	5	4	3	2	1
27. An abortion should be available to a middle-age woman who has children of college-age and now is pregnant with an unplanned child.	5	4	3	2	1
28. Abortion denies the rights of the unborn child.	5	4	3	2	1
29. I would contribute time and/or money to an anti-abortion effort.	5	4	3	2	1
30. Since abortions have always been available to women with money, abortions should be legalized to avoid discriminating against those with less money.	5	4	3	2	1

Figure 6–35 *Continued.*

Landis and Landis, "Student Opinions on Courtship and Marriage" (J. T. Landis and M. G. Landis, *Youth and Marriage,* Englewood Cliffs, N.J.: Prentice-Hall, Inc., pp. 7–9).

6. Assign class members to investigate the extent of abortion reform. Since 1967, when Colorado liberalized its abortion laws, a great deal has happened. How does the class feel about this? How do their parents and other family members feel? How do the courts feel? How do students view this important social issue? Reproduce the Wilcox Abortion Attitude Questionnaire for class use (see Figure 6–35) or ask:

a. What are the pro-abortion and anti-abortion positions.

b. Does the absolute sanctity of any human life ensure the right of the fetus to independent consideration? Are there exceptions? Early Hebrew law indicated that one should not kill *unjustly.* Are there just situations regarding abortion—as with war killings, euthanasia, and capital punishment?

c. What are the needs of medical research concerning fetuses, administration of drugs, and the use of fetal tissue?

d. What are the implications for young people? Will difficult abortion opportunities create greater concern for contraception and sex education?

7. Establish student teams to survey local physicians about their willingness to report all venereal disease cases to the state department of public health. Gather pro and con opinions. Have some students contact the state department of public health officials for their statistics and viewpoints. Is reporting practice improving or staying about the same?

8. Discuss this concept of engagement: "Today engagement is viewed as a 'testing period' rather than a promise to marry." Carry this one step further by weighing the statement, "A broken engagement is better than a bad marriage."

9. Assign a student to elaborate on each of the five factors influencing twentieth century practices relative to sexual expression:

a. The great influx of *new knowledge,* the scientific era, Freud, the innovator, Havelock Ellis and Alfred Kinsey, motivation: love and affection.

b. The *emancipation of women in our culture*—this, coupled with the rise in *individualism*—with sexual behavior becoming more of a personal matter and less exclusively influenced by family and procreational considerations.

c. A *hedonistic philosophy*—"eat, drink, sleep, and be merry, for tomorrow we may die"—and "buy now, pay later"—and playboyism, which tends to reduce woman to a function or thing, thus dehumanizing and depersonalizing her.

d. Certain *medical advances,* chiefly, contraception and antibiotics for venereal disease.

e. The *free love campaign* which pervades the arts today and the so-called "new morality" allowing "permissiveness with affection."

10. Solicit student opinion on the extent of such practices as the "double standard" and "situation ethics." Is there a "new morality"? Is the Golden Rule still workable, or should we figure that individuals will always take advantage or exploit one another for their own satisfaction? Is there a place for "instant gratification"?

11. Research and discuss the achievements of medical science in the area of chemically controlling genetic characteristics. What are some of the moral and social implications of this line of research?

12. Look into the influence of one's religion on his point of view on sex. Is there a common ground of modern Protestantism, Roman Catholicism, and Judaism relating to children, love, marriage, family values, sex in marriage, sex outside of marriage, and other issues?

13. Administer a Dating Customs Survey. The one published by Schulz and Williams on p. 128 of *Family Life and Sex Education* is useful. A particularly effective dating survey instrument is the *Dating Problems Checklist* published by Family Life Publications, Durham, North Carolina.

14. Put on the one-act, 30 minute play entitled *Ring Around the Family.* It comes complete with a detailed discussion guide from the American Social Health Association and is a real commercial for family life education.

15. Debate woman's role in our culture today. Should women stay home and be housewives and mothers (Phyllis McGinley, *Sixpence in Her Shoe*) or get out of the kitchen and into the working world (Betty Friedan, *The Feminine Mystique*)? What answer does Katherine Millet have in her *Sexual Politics*? Does it mean anything that Bach and Beethoven were men? What did Freud have in mind when he said, "Anatomy is destiny"?

16. Survey pupils in the upper three secondary grades to see how many take their personal problems dealing with sexuality to their clergyman. A few years ago, a nationwide survey discovered that 42 per cent would turn to their clergyman for help. In 1969, a Temple University research team found that less than 2 per cent of Pennsylvania high school pupils would turn first to their clergyman. What would happen today?

17. Talk over with the class whether the following statements are true, half true, or false:

"Only men have the drive and clear thinking to make it to the top."

"Sensitivity and gentleness are female traits."

"A good demonstration of masculinity is skill in sports."

QUESTIONS FOR DISCUSSION

1. Teachers must be prepared to discuss the moral implications of such emotion-loaded sexual activities as masturbation, homosexuality, petting, pre-marital intercourse, and abortion. In the beginning, facts should be separated from moral implications. Then the clarification of value premises may follow. How do you feel about teaching this part of the sex and family living education unit?

2. From your readings and discussions, what would you prefer to call the course in sex and family living education? Where do you see it in the school curriculum—separate course, part of health education, or integrated with other subjects? Explain how you arrived at your conclusions.

3. Additional professional preparation is recommended in a number of states in order to teach sex and family living education. Do you think that this is really necessary for a person who has majored in health education? Elaborate.

4. Beginning teachers frequently think in terms of separating the sexes for the sex education unit, while experienced teachers keep boys and girls together for instruction. Why does this occur? How do you think it should be?

5. Most adolescents vacillate between telling the exact truth and "talking a good game" when asked about their behavior relative to mood modifiers. Although this is understandable, how does it affect classroom discussion and teaching goals?

6. Surveys conducted by the National Institute of Mental Health indicate more health problems among drinkers. There are also more money problems, job problems, family arguments and violence, marital break-ups, neighborhood troubles, and difficulties with the law among excessive drinkers. How do you think junior high school pupils will react to these alcohol-associated topics?

7. How does a teacher go about combating the many myths associated with alcohol drinking and drug taking? Is there a way to teach that may actually capitalize on such myths?

8. Very often among secondary school students there is a tendency to look somewhat askance at the professional viewpoint. It even may be considered an unwelcome tentacle of the "establishment." Why is it that a young person will accept the professional advice of the dentist, but hold in question the suggestions of a psychiatrist or psychologist about drug taking?

9. In his book, *Tobacco and Your Health,* Harold Diehl observes that there are a great many days of absences from work because of illness or injury—a figure considerably

greater among smokers. What appears to be the physiological basis for this research finding?

10. The list of tar and nicotine content in cigarettes is published and widely distributed periodically by the U.S. Public Health Service. What are the several ways this kind of information can be used with secondary school pupils?

11. The risk of death from coronary artery disease — which is the major killer of smokers and non-smokers alike — is 70 per cent greater for smokers than for non-smokers. What is the physiological relationship between smoking and the coronary artery? What experimental evidence is there to back up survey data and mass statistics?

12. How effective are posters? Are humorous ones more effective than the serious kind? Is there a certain way they can be displayed and referred to that enhances their value?

SUGGESTED ACTIVITIES

1. In the Mid-town Manhattan Study, Srole made an analysis of smoking and concluded that non-smoking, moderate smoking, and problem smoking are behaviors conditioned directly by both social and psychological factors, and that, in turn, the psychological factors are themselves importantly influenced by conditions in the family and other social realms during childhood and adolescence. (See Woody references at end of chapter.) Look up several pieces of research having to do with these factors. Can personality factors be separated from social factors? Must they be considered together?

2. Consider the personality and social variables related to the start of smoking in youth. Survey a number of junior high school pupils to find out how they *feel* about smoking. If they oppose it, is it because of the scientific facts, parental attitudes, or peer group practices? If they are for smoking, are they somewhat rebellious or independent in their thinking?

3. Investigate the intricate relationship of the medical aspects of marihuana smoking to the cultural and legal dimension. Examine sociological literature, the Volstead Act, and the current view of the U.S. Department of Health, Education, and Welfare. Weigh the findings of recent medical research against the constitutional right to do what one wishes in the privacy of one's own home.

4. In most communities there is a psychiatrist that the teacher may be able to involve in a class discussion about drug abuse, alcoholism, and mental health. Before doing this, seek an answer to the question, "What should be expected of psychiatry?" Should the psychiatrist appear early on the alcohol-drug scene, or be in the wings to be called when addiction and emotional confusion come about? Ask several medical people how they feel about this. How does the psychiatrist feel?

5. Review some curriculum materials designed for secondary school use. What kind of scope and sequence is there as one moves from grade seven to twelve? Look over the content, teaching suggestions, and references set forth for educators to use. See especially:
   Baltimore County Board of Education, *Drug Abuse Education,* Towson, Maryland
   Cleveland Board of Education, *Alcohol, Drugs, Narcotics and Tobacco,* Cleveland, Ohio
   Flagstaff Public Schools, *Narcotic and Drug Education,* Flagstaff, Arizona

Great Falls School District No. 1, *Tobacco, Drug and Alcohol Unit,* Great Falls, Montana

New York State Education Department, *Strand II: Sociological Health Problems,* Albany, New York

Rhode Island Department of Education, *An Educational Program Dealing With Drug Abuse,* Providence, Rhode Island

San Francisco Unified School District, *Drugs and Hazardous Substances,* San Francisco, California

South Bay Union School District, *Drug Abuse Education Unit,* Imperial Beach, California

Tacoma Public Schools, *Curriculum Guide for Drug Education,* Tacoma, Washington

6. Make a formal visit to some place where there is a real connection with youth and the drug culture: halfway houses, juvenile detention centers, courthouses, mental hospitals, drug treatment centers, folk churches, youth houses, rock music halls. Talk with youths, of course, but also talk with staff personnel. Get behind the formal structures to human feelings—feelings which result in attitudes toward society in general.

7. Participate in a workshop, in any capacity. It can be in education, law enforcement, psychology, pharmacology, sociology, or medicine. Moreover, it might be a workshop related to social service agencies or public health. Look for all aspects of the narcotic problem with a special searching for innovative ways to educate youth.

8. Examine several current official and non-official health agency leaflets, booklets, and literature designed to curtail tobacco smoking. See particularly U.S. Public Health Service and American Cancer Society materials. Do they appear useful to you? Effective? Superficial? Do they get down to the *feeling* or human *values* level?

9. Formulate a list of mental health area readings specifically oriented to (a) junior high youth and (b) senior high youth. Include magazine articles as well as books. The readings can be on any mental health or sex and family living education topic, as long as the reading level is appropriate for the secondary level suggested. This means that a number of references will have to be carefully read. Therefore, in order to efficiently screen articles and books, it will be helpful to establish a committee for this project.

10. Interview several teachers who are presently teaching such secondary school subjects as biology, home economics, social studies, English, and health education. Find out how they feel about teaching sex education, directly or indirectly. Do they feel prepared? Do they see the need? Would they take an in-service course to clear up misconceptions about the topic? Do they think they relate well to students?

11. Look over several junior high school books on sex education such as Duvall's *Love and the Facts of Life,* or Landis and Landis' *Building Your Life.* How do you see them being used beyond assignment for individual consumption? Will they help pupils at this age to solve problems, or do they need interpretation by teachers?

12. In the terms of the report of the Federal Commission on Obscenity and Pornography, it is difficult to prove that pornography or obscenity trigger individual antisocial acts. However, there are many parents who feel that such stimuli have not enhanced personal and psychological development, interpersonal relationships, or adaptive personality skills. How do you feel about this area? What are the implications for teaching? How do people feel about the influence of pornography on

youth? Is it less of a psychiatric concern and more an expression of the level of taste in the culture?

13. Conduct a poll of both students and faculty on sexuality possibilities for the future. How do they feel about the control of sex and intelligence of offspring? The predetermination of hereditary traits such as hair color and stature? Growing a fetus completely in the laboratory? What can be gained from your findings that will be of value in a senior high class?

14. Read George Orwell's *1984*, which was written in 1949. How does it compare with Aldous Huxley's *Brave New World* (1946) in terms of a pleasure-oriented projected world? Have any of these fictitious projections come true today? Elaborate. How might these books be used with a film, filmstrip, or discussion related to contemporary society?

15. Talk over the several means of presenting a controversial topic to the class. If possible, talk directly with health education teachers, to see just what they do and how effective they are. Consider, also, the orientation of parents and other community people. What you are seeking is a way of involving all pupils deeply and sincerely in the facts and ultimate value implications.

SELECTED REFERENCES

Altekruse Berger, Carol, and Patrick F. Altekruse Berger. "Death On Demand," *Commonweal*, 52:585–589, December 5, 1975.

Anspaugh, David J. "Learning Our Sexuality," *School Health Review*, 5:7–9, November/December, 1974.

Benell, Florence B. "Overcoming Teacher Reluctancy Toward VD Education," *Journal of School Health*, 40:483–486, November, 1970.

Broderick, Judith M. *Psychology of Women*, New York: Harper and Row, 1971.

Calderone, Mary, Sr. *Sexuality and Man*, New York: Scribners, 1970.

Chen, T. L., and William R. Rakip. "Are Teachers Prepared to Implement Smoking Education in the Schools?" *Journal of School Health*, 44:438–441, October, 1974.

Churan, Charles. "Redirecting Psychological and Social Patterns," Health Education, 6:14–16, March/April, 1975.

Conley, John A., and Thomas W. O'Rourke. "On Improving Instruction in Sex Education," *Journal of School Health*, 43:591–594, November, 1973.

Davis, Roy L. "Making Health Education Relevant In Elementary and Junior High Schools," *Health Service Reports*, 88(2):99–105, September, 1975.

Drole, L. "Social and Psychological Factors In Smoking Behavior: The Mid-Town Manhattan Study," *Bulletin of New York Academy of Medicine*, 44:1502–1513, 1968.

Einstein, Stanley. "Drug Abuse Training and Education," *American Journal of Public Health*, 64:99–105, February, 1974.

Forman, Ian. "Sex and Family Living," *American Education*, 5:11–13, October, 1969.

Fulton, Gere B. *Sexual Awareness*, Boston: Holbrook Press, 1974.

Fusco, Ronald A. "Mental Health Elective," *School Health Review*, 5:20–22, September/October, 1974.

Gadpile, Warren J. "Adolescent Sexuality and the Struggle Over Authority," *Journal of School Health*, 40:479–482, November, 1970.

Gagnon, John, and Bruce Henderson. *Human Sexuality*, Boston: Little, Brown & Co., 1975.

Gordon, Sol. "What Place Does Sex Education Have in the Schools?" *Journal of School Health*, 44:186–190, April, 1974.

Grams, Jean D., and Walter B. Waltjen. *Sex: Does It Make a Difference*, Belmont, Calif.: Wadsorth Publishing Co., 1975.

Greenberg, Jerrold S. "A Study of Personality Change Associated with the Conducting of a High School Unit on Homosexuality," *Journal of School Health*, 45:394–399, September, 1975.

Hafen, Brent Q. *Readings on Drug Use and Abuse*, Provo, Utah: Brigham Young University Press, 1970.

Hamrick, Michael. "A Role Playing Situation for Sex Education Issues," *Health Education*, 6:20–21, March/April, 1975.

Harmin, Merrill, Howard Kirschenbaum, and Sidney B. Simon. *Clarifying Values Through Subject Matter*, Minneapolis: Winston Press, 1973.

Hawkins, Barbara. "The Familylife Education Program in the Chicago Public Schools," *School Health Review*, 2:33–36, April, 1971.

Hoffmann, Frederick Y. *A Handbook on Drug and Alcohol Abuse,* Toronto: Oxford University Press, 1975.

Jones, Bert, and Nancy B. Stevens. "Overcoming Economic Barriers to Health Care," *Health Education,* 6:7–10, November, December 1975.

Klemer, Richard, and Rebecca Smith. *Teaching About Family Relationships.* Minneapolis: Burgers Publishing Co., 1975.

Kruger, W. Stanley. "Education for Parenthood and School-Age Parents," *Journal of School Health,* 45:293–297, May, 1975.

Lingeman, Richard. *Drugs From A to Z: A Dictionary,* 2d edition, New York: McGraw-Hill, Inc., 1974.

Louria, Donald B. "A Critique of Some Current Approaches to the Problem of Drug Abuse," *American Journal of Public Health,* June, 1975.

Maultsby, Maxie C., Jr., et al. "Teaching Self-Counseling," *Journal of School Health,* 44:445–449, October, 1974.

Morris, L. Mike. "Your Program—Not Mine," *School Health Review,* 5:27–30, November/December, 1974.

Omran, Abdel R. "Population Epidemiology," *American Journal of Public Health,* 64:674–679, July, 1974.

Perkinson, H. *The Imperfect Panacea: American Faith In Education 1865–1968,* New York: Random House, 1972.

Rosner, Aria C. "Drug and Alcohol Abuse Education: Opinions of School Principals," *Journal of School Health,* 45:468–469, October, 1975.

Samuels, Don. "Dade County's PRIDE Program," *Health Education,* 6:19–20, May/June, 1975.

Schlaadt, Richard G. "Implementing the Values Clarification Process," *School Health Review,* 6:10–14, January/February, 1974.

Seffrin, John R. "Teaching Teachers About Human Sexuality," *School Health Review,* 5:39–41, November/December, 1974.

Seltzer, Carl C., et al. "Smoking and Drug Consumption in White, Black, and Oriental Men and Women," *American Journal of Public Health,* 64:466–473, May, 1974.

Skolnick, Arlene, and Bruce Henderson. *The Family,* Boston: Little, Brown & Co., 1976.

Smith, Bert Kruger. *Aging in America,* Boston: Beacon Press, 1973.

Smith, Charles D., and Samuel Prather. "Group Problem Solving." *Journal of Physical Education and Recreation,* 46:20–21, September, 1975.

Solaro, Mary. "A Toast to Safer Driving," *Today's Health,* 48:61–63, December, 1970.

Sorenson, R. C. *Adolescent Sexuality in Contemporary America,* New York: World Book, 1973.

Sulzbacher, S. I., and Eugene Edgar. "Drug and Alcohol Abuse Education: Opinions of School Principals," *Journal of School Health,* 45:468–469, October, 1975.

Taintor, Zebulon. "The 'Why' of Youthful Drug Abuse," *Journal of School Health,* 44:26–29, January, 1974.

Tennant, Forest S., Jr., et al. "Effectiveness of Drug Education Classes," *American Journal of Public Health,* 64:422–428, May, 1974.

Weinstein, Gerald, and Marion Fantini. *Toward Humanistic Education: A Curriculum of Affect,* New York: Praeger, 1972.

Willgoose, Carl E. "Sequential K-11 Courses Replace Old Style 'Health,'" *Nation's Schools,* 85:80–81, March, 1970.

Woody, Robert H. "Smoking: Psychological, Personality and Behavioral Factors," *Journal of School Health,* 40:427–433, October, 1970.

Chapter 7

Area III—Environmental and Consumer Health

Components:
1. Environmental Health
2. Consumer Health
3. World Health
4. Health Careers

For several years there has been a resounding call to "ecologize"—a sense of urgency to do something about the environment by way of conservation and planning for the future. In considering the living space itself there is a deeper health concern for the consumer that is worldwide in scope. A part of this environmental effort relates to manpower and the need for specialized health careers that will help bolster the well-being of the world community. This chapter, therefore, brings together the health education implications of the four dimensions of environment, consumer, world health, and health careers.

1. ENVIRONMENTAL HEALTH

If one tugs at a single thing in nature, he finds it attached to everything else in the world.

John Muir

Something will have gone out of us as a people if we ever let the remaining wilderness be destroyed; if we permit the last virgin forests to be turned into comic books and plastic cigarette cases; if we drive the few remaining members of the wild species into zoos or to extinction; if we pollute the last clear air, dirty the last clean streams and push our paved roads through the last of the silence, so that never again will Americans be free in their own country from noise, the exhausts, the stinks of human and automotive waste.

Wallace Stegner

As one ponders the possibility that American society may not "make it" to the end of the century, there is a tendency to become ecologically oriented by persuasion. Automobile bumper stickers read *Ecologize Now;* and the key word of the 70's is *ecosystem.* There is a new word, *ecotactics,* but this movement concerning the science of survival dates back to such wilderness preservers as John Muir, who founded the Sierra Club in 1892. Today, the club's members are probably the most active ecotacticians in the country. They, along with others, see man not as the dominant creature he has always considered himself, but as a part of the environment, depending on all other forms of life. His long war with nature is finished. He must now combine with nature and fully recognize Charles Darwin's finding: species survive only by adapting to their habitats.

It has become clear that the basic theorem, that to every action there is an equal and opposite reaction, applies as much to biology as to physics. For those people who value life in an environment of quality and beauty, there is much to be done. It is late, but not too late. People with a common concern can get together. Even the Audubon Society, which was founded to protect wildlife, is saying, "We're not just worried about birds now. We're worried about people." In the last analysis, the solution to the health problems of a community will not be found in *Bacillus coli* counts or sulfur dioxide parts per million statistics, but rather it will come through the convictions and actions of concerned youth and adults. This will prevent what Alvin Toffler terms "future shock," the disease that comes from being in a world we are totally unprepared for, and from not having the physical and psychological resources to cope with it.[1]

Ecology is not a discipline. There is no body of thought and technique which frames an ecology of man. It must be, therefore, a scope or a way of seeing. Moreover, if environmental control fails, it will not be for lack of information. Books and articles are all about. One can literally read his way to a solution. This is particularly valid if it moves the community to (1) work toward making political leaders aware of the crisis, (2) undertake comapigns to delay excessive population growth, and (3) develop alternatives to the present way of life and view of the world.

There are many questions to be answered, however, that relate to the by-products of the civilization. Will the extinction of certain birds, blue whales and other animals, and vast numbers of insects have any significant bearing on world health? Can humans survive on a planet with a dead ocean? Will the continual release of ozone-damaging chemicals into the atmosphere actually reduce the barrier which shields the earth against harmful radiation from outer space?

Will life be pleasant 30 years from now? Will man have filters fitted into his tracheae? Will there be such things as required vasectomy, or euthanasia? Will ecological expedience require a kind of totalitarianism which will greatly limit freedom? These are serious questions to raise as one views the sordid present.

The wastes of society are everywhere. Solid waste means rubbish and garbage — newspaper, beer cans, broken glass, plastic bottles, ham bones, grass cuttings, old mattresses, junked cars. The daily throw-away average is now more than five pounds for each man, woman, and child. And when industrial and demolition wastes are included, the daily average becomes ten pounds per person. Disposal is the problem. Dumps account for about 90 per cent of the disposal; incinerators take care of the rest. The incinerators are in poor shape nationally; despite a general improvement, a great many lack adequate air pollution control devices. Moreover, these disposal systems are swamped with waste materials that will triple by 1980. The "throwaway" products glut the process. Tin cans rust eventually, but aluminum cans and plastic bottles are immortal.

---

[1]Alvin Toffler, *Future Shock,* New York: Random House, 1970.

Said a Chicago expert, "We're running in front of an avalanche—and it's already begun to bury us."

There is a *population problem* in a nation with no overall population policy. Although the birth rate was at a record low in 1974 there is no "zero population growth" in view. Women born during the 1950's "baby boom" are now of child-bearing age and the population will continue growing for a few decades. Unfortunately, the demographers, biologists, sociologists, economists, and resource analysts do not agree about the consequences of population growth, the urgency of controlling it, and the means that should be employed. In any case, growth in the natural world—and humankind is part of nature—when uncontrolled, unregulated, and when nature is not curtailed, becomes pathological and destroys its host. Already there are between three and four billion people on earth with a total of five billion predicted by 1990, and two-thirds of them are underfed, undersheltered, and without adequate water supplies. Moreover, there is a clear correlation between many forms of human disease and a crowded, dirty, noisy environment.

In the cities, loud, continuous levels of noise may damage unborn babies. Noise interferes with sleep, conversation, and school programs. The psychological effects are centered on fear and annoyance. If it cannot be eliminated, it should at least be contained. Although regulations regarding noise pollution are in effect a typical decibel count in a big city during rush hour averages 75. This is an exposure to noise over 10 million times as powerful as a whisper. People residing adjacent to a large airport have to bear jet noise that often reaches 100 decibels, or *10 billion times* the sound of a whisper.[2] Permanent hearing loss comes from repeated exposures to above-average sound levels. The 8-hour daily exposure to 80 or 85 decibels—not uncommon in factories—can lead to severe hearing damage.

As the population continues to expand, so does the number of big buildings designed to accommodate larger and larger numbers of people—in effect encouraging more people to move into the already overcrowded cities. In a children's game called Blockhead, one piles very light wooden blocks higher and higher and higher. The object is to see how far up one can go before the whole structure collapses. Von Eckardt pointed out several years ago that New York City has been playing this game for years, with the New York City Planning Commission calling for construction of additional downtown office buildings to house several hundred thousand more office workers—the last thing the city needs.[3]

Affluence and effluence tend to go together. In terms of polluting the environment and using up the Earth's resources, the United States is one of the most over-populated countries in the world. There simply is no place in the world where there is more pollution per person than in America. This country, with less than 2 per cent of the world's people, accounts for about 30 per cent of the poisons being dumped into the environment. It is an absurdity, therefore, to say that Americans are less of a drain on the earth than Chinese or Indians because they are so few in number by comparison. Classes in health education should collect figures and thoroughly discuss this point. Maybe Americans are indeed "ugly," particularly as they drop 16,000 pieces of *litter* on each mile of primary highway every month—costing 100 million dollars a year to pick up; it costs 500 million dollars a year to clean up public areas alone.

The requirement for *clean water* is everybody's business. It always has been. For decades, most school children, in discussing community health, have studied water sources, water purification, and sewage systems. They seldom discuss watershed areas,

---

[2]Decibels increase logarithmically, not arithmetically, so that a 10 decibel sound is 10 times as loud as a zero decibel sound, and a 20 decibel sound is 100 times zero, and so on.

[3]Wolf Von Eckardt, "The Perils of Concentration," *Saturday Review,* May 2, 1970.

water pollution, and water conservation. Few individuals realize that modern living demands vast quantities of clear water; 12 gallons every time someone takes a shower; 200 gallons to make one dollar's worth of paper; 65,000 gallons to manufacture one automobile; 320,000 gallons to irrigate just one acre of farmland, and 325 billion gallons of water every day to keep the cities, factories, and farms going. This figure will triple by the year 2000. Although more dams and soil and forest conservation can add to the supply, better use will have to be made of the water available.

It is interesting to learn that King Sennacherib of Assyria punished Babylon by dumping rubbish into its canals. Today our enemies need not poison us; we do it ourselves. Twenty or more *billion* gallons of dirty household water go down the drain every day. Industrial wastes, farm fertilizers, road salt, and storm sewer runoff add to water pollution. The water animals die out. The gamefish that require plentiful dissolved oxygen—trout, bass, bluegills, perch—leave the habitat to the carp and suckers that don't require much oxygen. A step further down, and only the bloodworms, leeches, and snails can survive. Moreover, the microscopic plants die off, leaving the pondweed and waterwort (Elatine). With more pollution, these plants die and leave the dying water to the blue-green algae—provided the poisonous wastes from paper mills, steelworks, and chemical factories do not extinguish every form of life.

The ocean can not be disassociated from water pollution. Undersea observation and photography indicate that the ocean is sick, very sick according to Jacques Cousteau.[4] From shrimp to whales to fish of all kinds, productivity has dropped off 40 per cent, while the ocean is treated by humans as "bottomless" and endless. Between the effects of

---

[4]See Jacques Cousteau, "The Perils and Potentials of A Watery Planet," Saturday Review/World, August 24, 1974. See also Thor Heyerdahl, "How To Kill an Ocean," *Saturday Review,* November 29, 1975.

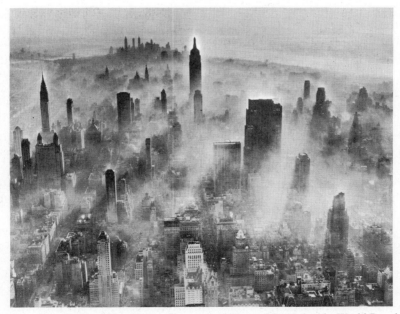

Figure 7–1   Population and pollution. (Courtesy of Planned Parenthood—World Population)

waste dumping and oil pollution, there are significant sublethal effects on marine life (see Figure 7–2).

Thermal pollution is a topic in itself. Approximately two-thirds of the total energy output from a nuclear power plant is in the form of waste heat. Because of this and the fact that nuclear plants must be large to be economically efficient, the heat output is enormous. In marine situations, commercially important shellfish and kelp beds may be severely damaged by additions of heated water. A rise in temperature markedly increases the metabolic rate, and hence the oxygen consumption, of fishes and other aquatic organisms, but also lowers the water oxygen-carrying capacity. Increased temperature accelerates bacterial decomposition, and this in turn, can greatly reduce oxygen reserves in an aquatic environment. The challenge in every classroom today is to make any student study of the water topic a fascinating one. Such items as water-borne diseases, water sanitation, water purification, water pollution, inland and coastal wetlands, water resources, and water recreation can become alive as they relate to individuals and families.

Another environmental peril began developing over a decade ago in Japan and Sweden. *Mercury pollution,* roughly 3 to 14 times the level ruled safe for human consumption, has commanded the attention of the U.S. Federal Water Quality Administration. Inorganic mercury, when it enters the human body, is converted by bacteria in water to methyl mercury. It collects in the red blood cells and may cause anemia. It is also linked with the nervous system and brain damage (numbness to limbs and tremors). Excessive fatigue, headache, loss of memory, difficulty in swallowing, and "punchdrunk" movements may occur. About a half million children undergo treatment for *lead poisoning* a year. Some 200 die and others become hyperactive. Unleaded gasoline and non-lead paint regulations have helped this situation. Another poison that is discharged into the environment, vinyl chloride, is yet to be measurably reduced. It is created chiefly through the manufacture of polyvinyl chloride resin used in industrial plastics. A relationship has been found with a rare and fatal form of cancer, angiosarcoma of the liver.

The *air pollution* facts have been staggering to observant citizens for some time. Dirty air rots and soils clothes. It cracks rubber, blisters and discolors paint, corrodes steel, rusts metals, and causes 500 million dollars worth of damage to crops and illness and death to livestock. It stunts growing vegetables, shrubs, and flowers. It makes eyes burn and may blur vision. In air inversion disasters, it causes "excess deaths over normal." It contributes to absenteeism due to colds; chronic bronchitis and bronchial asthma get worse on days of higher air pollution. It promotes a higher death rate among older people, especially those with heart ailments who must breathe a little harder. Lung cancer deaths double in a metropolitan area, even after full allowance is made for differences in smoking habits. The same is true for emphysema, the fastest-growing cause of death in this country. Chronic childhood allergic disease is made considerably worse in polluted air locations. Solutions to these problems are not simple. Students wrestle with smog (traditional and photochemical), inversion, fossil fuels, airshed, and urban climate and diseae. Yet, how can one eliminate the air pollution—8 per cent from homes, 11 per cent from power plants, 16 per cent from industry, and 65 per cent from automobiles, trucks, and buses?

The coastal waters today reflect the *pesticide pollution,* just as the rivers and streams froth with *phosphate detergent pollution.* The reproductive processes of a number of fish populations may be threatened by the high residue levels of chlorinated hydrocarbon pesticides in the eggs. High levels of DDT residues have been found again and again in fish, as well as in birds. Although DDT has been phased out in the United States, it continues to be used throughout the world because of its protection and aid to food crops. Pesticides are rough on eyes and lungs. Farm workers frequently suffer

Some sublethal effects of petroleum products on marine life

Type of Organism and Species	Type Petroleum Product	Concentration	Sublethal Response
Marine Flora Marsh plants	crudes and refinery effluents	Single or successive coatings	Inhibition of germination and growth. Repeated coatings cause disappearance of some plants (increasing order of tolerance: shallow rooted plants, shrubby perennials, filamentous green algae, perennials, perennials with large food reserves)
phytoplankton	crude Naphthalene	1 ppm 3 ppm	Suppress growth Reduction of bicarbonate uptake
phytoplankton	oil	10^{-1} 10^{-4} ppm	Inhibition or delay in cellular division
phytoplankton	kerosene	3 ppm; 38 ppm	Depression of growth rate
phytoplankton	Kuwait crude	1 ppm	Depression of growth rate
phytoplankton	Kuwait crude; dispersant emulsions	20-100 ppm	Inhibition of growth; reduction of bicarbonate uptake at 50 ppm
Kelp	Toluene	10 ppm	75 percent reduction in photosynthesis within 96 hours
Larvae and Eggs Pink salmon fry	Prudhoe Bay crude	1.6 ppm	Avoidance effects; could have effect on migration behavior
Black sea turbot	oil	0.01 ppm	Irregularity and delay in hatching—resulting larvae deformed and inactive
Plaice larvae	BP 1002	0-10 ppm	Disruption of phototactic and feeding behavior
Cod fish larvae	Iranian crude	Aqueous extracts from 10^3 ppm, 10^4 ppm	Adverse effect on behavior, leading to death
Lobster larvae	Venezuelan crude	6 ppm	Delay molt to fourth stage
Sea urchin larvae	extracts of Bunker C	0.1-1 ppm	Interference with fertilized egg development
Barnacle larvae	oil	10-100 $\mu l/1$ (ppm)	Abnormal development
Crab larvae	oil	10-100 $\mu l/1$ (ppm)	Initial increase in respiration
Fish Chinook salmon Striped bass	Benzene	5, 10 ppm	Initial increase in respiration
Crustaceans Lobster	crude, kerosene	10 ppm	Effects of chemoreception, feeding times, stress behavior, aggression, grooming
Lobster	La Rosa crude	Extracts	Delay in feeding
Mollusks Mussel	crude	1 ppm	Reduction in carbon budget (increase in respiration; decrease in feeding)
Snail	kerosene	0.001—0.004 ppm	Reduction in chemotactic perception of food
Clam	No. 2 fuel oil	Collected from field	Gonadal tumors
Oyster	Bleedwater		Reduced growth and glycogen content
Snail	BP 1002	30 ppm	Significant inhibition to growth
Oyster	oil	0.01 ppm	Marked tainting
Mussel	No. 2 fuel oil	Collected from field after spill	Inhibition in development of gonads

Courtesy of the U.S. Environmental Protection Agency, Environmental Research Laboratory at Narragansett, R.I.

Figure 7–2 Sublethal effects of petroleum products.

burns, rashes, blurred vision, dizziness, and nausea. Much of the ecological balance is threatened by the loss of bird, fish, and ground animal life destroyed by pesticides.

As progress is made toward smogless motoring, and urbanists realize their combined environmental problems and turn creative, the quality of life will improve. But as one problem is solved another may emerge. As smog is reduced by the advent of more nuclear power plants, there will evolve a greater concern for radiological health. Before long, 200 nuclear power stations will generate a third of the nation's electricity. Fortunately, the Atomic Energy Commission is charged with the responsibility to fix the standards of safety in the use of nuclear energy.

PLANNED AND PREVENTIVE CONSERVATION FOR HEALTH

Chiefly due to the extensive efforts of the U.S. Environmental Protection Agency (EPA) the average citizen is beginning to appreciate that there are basic interrelationships of the environment and the economy, energy, transportation, and land use. Emerging is the fundamental ecological concept that because everything is related to everything else, every choice involves a trade-off. Moreover, the ordinary person has learned to influence the process of decision-making.

The EPA administrator recently cited the major results of a national survey by Opinion Research Corporation:[5]

1. People at all levels of society have air and water pollution uppermost in their minds, even after the passage of stringent environmental protection legislation.
2. A high percentage of the public (60 per cent) believe that it is more important to pay the costs involved in protecting the environment than to keep prices and taxes down and run the risk of more pollution.
3. A large number (48 per cent) of people believe that the extra price for pollution devices on automobiles is worth it.
4. As high a proportion of the public (43 per cent) agree as disagree (44 per cent) with the proposition that cleaning the environment is important, even if it means closing down some polluting plants and causing some unemployment.

Of interest is the fact that the closing of some 69 plants caused a loss of 12,000 jobs, but against this negative figure, environmental protection has created more than a million new jobs. Millions of additional jobs can be provided—in water treatment plants, solid waste and resource recovery programs, mass transit, railroads, and much more.

In a recent address to the students and faculty of Boston University, Mrs. Martin Luther King, Jr., called attention, once more, to the kind of action that is needed in today's world. Quoting her late husband, she said: "We must learn to live together as brothers or we shall perish together as fools."

The appropriateness of these remarks for environmental health and conservation purposes should not strain the imagination of any teacher. Man has haphazardly and selfishly altered his environment. He must now accept the "challenge of the land" and work cooperatively with others to exercise controls.

Secondary school students are mature enough to investigate the community and government planning that is being done today. Perhaps this is more important than

---

[5]From remarks of Russell E. Train in *Environment News*, October, 1975, p. 2.

learning the chemistry behind sulfur dioxide poisoning or something else within the confines of the classroom. Wordsworth wrote, "Let nature be your teacher." Get out and see pollution first hand. Much is being accomplished that should be viewed, discussed, and acted upon.

Examples of planning and action include the following:

1. Ecology laws permitting any citizen to sue any polluter. First accomplished after heavy legislative lobbying in Michigan.

2. Procedures to require industries to report, immediately, any pollutants dumped into state waters (another Michigan first).

3. Temporary permits issued to polluters only when they demonstrate that they are working on the installation of an approved abatement facility or an alternative waste disposal system (Vermont).

4. Industrialists and agriculturalists, aware that much of the new technology is incompatible with the demands of the ecosystem, are sitting down to talk seriously about products, pollutants, and human well being.

5. The final word is not in on Lake Erie and the other Great Lakes. The road back to healthy lakes is underway, with the Federal Water Quality Administration working to demonstrate that sewage and factory effluent usually poured into the lakes can be diverted by pipe systems to fertilize barren lands. This could eventually build up an agro-industrial complex of respectable size.

6. Licensed smokewatchers employed by the Department of Environmental Conservation in New York make random smoke sightings and report violations to regular inspectors, who issue summonses on the basis of the information.

7. In planning to reduce automobile smog, a number of large cities are installing bicycle lanes. A non-polluting organization devoted to the cause is Bicycle Ecology, with headquarters in Chicago.

8. Townspeople, through citizens' groups, are seeking concrete action through the establishment of community natural resource development planning committees. Long range planning committees work with conservationists and public health officials to conduct land and water surveys, flood control and antipollution activities, and recreation surveys.

9. More Town Forests are being established, especially if the country is hilly—for "to rule the mountain is to rule the river," says a Chinese proverb. This action is being accompanied by more of nature's safety valves, such as flood plain zoning and green belt areas. Ground water is being mapped, and plans are being fashioned for its replenishment (recharge).

10. The Federal Water Pollution Control Administration is making grants for improving municipal waste treatment facilities; helping the states improve water quality standards; enforcing the laws against pollution of interstate or navigable waters; and providing expert assistance on difficult pollution problems.

11. Thousands of previously unconcerned youths and adults are joining conservation groups and the Audubon Society in an effort to unite against a common enemy.

12. Sludge, the black tarry stuff left at the bottom of the sewage-treatment settling tanks—and frequently destined to be sunk in a lake or the ocean—is now sold as excellent fertilizer (Milorganite). It is combustible, and can be turned into a gas and used to run machinery.

13. Through the use of natural gas in power generating stations and in other industrial applications, dangerous sulfur dioxide pollution is being reduced in a number of cities by several thousand tons per year.

14. Large chemical companies are searching for new ways to prevent pollution. There is an exchange of information with interested industries and communities. Helpful

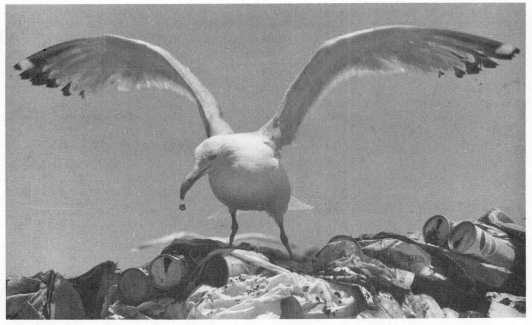

Figure 7-3   Is the open dump here to stay? (Courtesy of U.S. Environmental Protection Agency)

for teachers is the magazine *Environmental Science & Technology,* available by sub-scription (monthly) from the American Chemical Society.

15. A number of utilities have stopped burning soft coal or heavy fuel oil. More nuclear generators are being contemplated as civil law suits, based on real environ-mental damages, are brought to the courts.

16. Catastrophic oil spills, which kill birds and shellfish alike and spoil white beaches, command front page newspaper space. Planning exists to prevent these occur-rences.

17. Automobile built-in pollution control devices do some good. More planning is taking place. The speed-up of the flow of traffic through cities helps, for the faster an engine runs, the better its combustion. However, cutting down on the number of au-tomobiles in the city is the major objective today, with improved mass transportation fill-ing the travel need.

18. Since the acid atmosphere of air pollution decomposes library books, as well as art pieces, a great many well known libraries are spending considerable amounts of money to microfilm and microfiche decaying books and similar material.

19. Civic and cultural organizations are attempting to limit population expansion through birth control, abortion, and education for human sexuality.

20. Community leaders along the coastal areas are bringing oil drillers, fishermen, shippers, and others together to save the seacoast environment. Competition for coastal zones is intense. The surface is small—only 15 per cent of the United States land area. But 33 per cent of the population is concentrated on the coasts.

21. The relatively new government organization, *The Consumer Protection and En-vironmental Health Service,* is composed of the National Air Pollution Control Adminis-tration, the Food and Drug Administration, and the Environmental Control Administra-tion. Working together, they have made visible multipronged programs for improvements in environmental health.

The issues of environmental survival are not scientific, says Barry Commoner. They demand value judgments. The scientist cannot possibly determine that it is better to suffer respiratory disease in the city than to raise taxes in order to have a non-polluting transport system. This is a social and political judgment. The public conscience makes the choices imposed on us by the environmental crisis. Although the media have helped get the message of the scientific community to the public, there is much more communicating to do. Education and the social sciences are potential agents of reform. Most of the problems man encounters in dealing with his environment are problems of human behavior. Behavioral specialists, however, have provided very little information as to how people react to changes in their environment. New gauges are needed to measure environmental stress.

The *educational effort* and success of this major health teaching area will depend on how seriously the health curriculum developers view environmental problems. This chapter discussion, to this point, clearly indicates a substantial role for health educators, calling for a vastly greater scale of teaching than almost anything so far envisioned. New courses of study are needed in order to pull all the parts of the ecotactics topic together. Integrative and correlative teachings have to be planned. Both junior and senior high pupils will have to engage in a minimum amount of work-study with town or city planners, conservationists, and environmental quality professionals. Multidisciplinary classes will need exploration at the local level so that the school graduate will have explored the problems in terms of health, humanities, and natural and social sciences. This also means that much of what is now taught in public schools as conservation or community health is probably ineffective in itself and ill-adapted to present needs. All ramifications of environmental health have to be considered. A class discussion which overlooks the economic and perhaps uncomfortable political implications will miss the essential point. This concern is made realistic when one reads the story of the Vermont Public Service Board and its action to curb companies from promoting electrical consumption. The Board suggested that power is in short supply, costs are rising, and production of electricity adversely affects the environment. As is predictable, all power and energy sources came out against the regulation. Unexpected opponents, however, were newspapers and radio stations, who paused in their environmental crusades to send lawyers to the hearing to protect their advertising revenues generated by electrical promotion.

The root cause of environmental abuse — which must be considered by teachers and pupils — is the principle of fragmentation. In modern society, the fragmentation actions of people have outrun the principle of unity, and have produced the disorder of the moment. One has to learn that rational beings have to come together to solve the problems that their earlier disunity created. Teachers can be of help in fostering this view.

There is no ideal program. Somehow, all the ecological conditions referred to in this chapter have to be brought to the attention of junior and senior high school students. Upper grade level students will pursue details and solutions in greater depth. They will also study the environmental condition and practices in the light of personal and group needs and values in a culture frequently dominated by political expediency.

In the filmstrip, *Man's Natural Environment: Crisis Through Abuse* (Guidance Associates), the stirring song "America the Beautiful" is sung while photographs of a desecrated environment flash by. The mood is set for a comprehensive study of the problems and possible solutions for the several forms of pollution. The attempt is to create a climate for introducing program specifics. By being shown the death of Lake Erie, the Santa Barbara oil leak, the threats to the Everglades National Park, and the refuse problems of New York City, the pupil generates a viewpoint, and is at least partially prepared to examine proposals for meeting current ecological crises. From this point on, it is conceivable that a junior high school class could begin to put down on paper what *they* think they need to study. Working with the teacher, it is possible to create a skeleton outline for the total environmental health presentation. Such a programming approach has great value, for it affords students an "input" so that they become part of the process. Moreover, they are able to anticipate what is coming up in future class meetings.

Another way to program the topic is to introduce it as it was done in the Aspen Middle School—through an outdoor initiation into the nearby Rocky Mountains.[6] Here there was an openness honestly expressed as pupils observed the pure water tumbling down the stream. They looked more seriously at their natural environment. This paid off later when they returned to the classroom. The same down-to-earth approach to the environment can be accomplished through the Outward Bound program. In the New England area, Project Adventure is a highly successful school program that couples challenging outdoor activities with sometimes subtle environmental learning. The program began in the Hamilton-Wenham Regional School, Hamilton, Massachusetts; it is another concrete example of a superb *alternate pursuit* to learning. Experiences such as these may be introduced in the classroom prior to moving out into the community by viewing, listening, and discussing such materials as *Exploring Your Environmental Choices,* a kit with a listening tape, nine transparencies, and a decision-making model (Metropolitan Life Insurance Company). Another excellent multimedia kit, *The Human Environment,* concentrates on ecology, earth-space sciences, and health. (Nystrom, 3333 Elston Avenue, Chicago, Ill. 60618.) Particularly helpful in spelling out what is happening in the wider environment is the *Environment News,* available every month (free) from the U.S. Environmental Protection Agency, Rm. 2203, John F. Kennedy Federal Building, Boston, Mass. 02203.

Recently, the National Park Service set up, for educators and youth, the National Environmental Study Area Program. Available sites for day trips are located throughout the country, where teachers themselves conduct on-site classes, developing their own programs or using prepared curriculum guides. The enthusiastic and ingenious teacher usually finds such a rich study resource of great help in resolving biological and cultural relationships within the environment. Usually an advisory committee of educators and resource management personnel are available to help the teachers. In this program, especially designed for environmental education, the strand approach is used. There is some identification and classification work. Also required are open-ended investigations leading to problem solving.

Obviously the success in problem-solving depends upon motivations. Fortunately, in the environmental area student interest appears high. In several surveys, one of which was conducted in the Pittsburgh area, over 90 per cent of the students evaluated the environmental situation as serious.[7] Moreover, they were willing to make some personal sacrifices in order to help clean up their communities.

In expanding the older concept of community health into the ecologically oriented environmental health, it has been necessary for health curriculum personnel to structure course content in such a manner that all disciplines bordering on health education will be acknowledged. The result is a pretty big package. In many instances, it is not practical or even desirable to cover the total package in the health education course. Some integrative planning with other subject matter areas is required. (For assistance, see Chapter 10 on source materals for the instructor.)

---

[6]Gerald B. DeFries, "Will I Ever Catch Another Butterfly?" *Journal of Health, Physical Education and Recreation,* 41:41–44, December, 1970.

[7]John H. Kilwein, et al., "The Social Class of Young Adults and Their Views on the Environment," *Journal of School Health,* 44:196–198, April, 1974.

In terms of curriculum development, New York State, through the strand system, nicely combined environmental and community health into one area. An introduction to ecology comes at both secondary levels. It is supported by environmental and public health content as follows:[8]

ENVIRONMENTAL AND COMMUNITY HEALTH
GRADES 7, 8, 9

(Emphasis is on ecology and its development.)

I. History of Environmental and Public Health
II. Relationships Among Environment, Disease, and Health
III. Scope of Public Health
IV. Water and Water Pollution
V. Air and Air Pollution
VI. Radiation and Health
VII. Food
VIII. Space-Age Health
IX. Pesticides and Insecticides
X. Discovering Health Needs and Agencies in the Community
XI. Recent Progress in Medicine and Public Health
XII. Unsolved Problems in Medicine and Public Health

GRADES 10, 11, 12

(Emphasis is on relating epidemiology to ecology.)

I. History of Environment and Public Health
II. Definitions
III. Need for Healthful Environment
IV. Water and Water Pollution
V. Air and Air Pollution
VI. Radiation
VII. Food
VIII. Vector and Rodent Control
IX. Nuisances and Sanitation
X. Housing
XI. Pesticides and Insecticides
XII. Garbage and Refuse Disposal
XIII. Sewage Treatment and Disposal
XIV. Occupational Health
XV. Space-Age Travel and Health
XVI. Health Agencies in the Community
XVII. Cooperation Between Public and Private Health Agencies
XVIII. Sociological Aspects of Health
XIX. Solving Community Health Problems
XX. Recent Progress in Medicine and Public Health
XXI. Volunteer Services for Health Institutions
XXII. Unsolved Problems in Medicine and Public Health

ENVIRONMENTAL HEALTH

Behavioral Objectives

(Junior High Level)
Reveals how the existence of humankind will depend upon the ability to interact effectively with the total environment; human ecology is a study of this interaction.

Diagrams on paper how all parts of any environment, living or nonliving, are interdependent; their stability and existence are interconnected.

---

[8]The State Education Department, *Suggested Guidelines for the Development of Courses of Study in Health Education for Junior and Senior High Schools*, Albany, New York, revised.

Acknowledges through verbalization that the most constant characteristic of both the living and the nonliving parts of any environment is change.

Illustrates by example how all forms of life are characterized by the continuous interaction between heredity and environment.

Explains how individuals and groups relate to each other and their environment; this determines their characteristics.

Shows that the way a person perceives his environment influences the manner in which he uses it.

Arranges an exhibit to show that the process of living involves a continual interplay between the individual and water, air, soil, geography, climate, housing, and other physical items.

Analyzes the sociocultural environments to determine that certain persons have a higher incidence of disease than others; i.e., venereal disease, crime, and communicable diseases among the poor.

Applies the philosophy that the health of a country's population is considered to be the prime factor in its economic growth and development; poor standards of living and a low economy contribute to disease and illness.

Describes how the consequences of using insecticides, pesticides, and other such poisons in an overpopulated society present a number of complex problems.

Explains how federal, state, and local health agencies interact to create a favorable community environment.

Behavioral Objectives

(Senior High Level)

Describes how heredity and all the environments—biological, physical, social, and cultural—help mold the many characteristics and behaviors of an individual.

Sets forth the view that although stabilized by tradition and law, governments are changed by modification of the people's perception of the governmental function.

Tells how the concern for natural resources and technological advancement must be balanced so that all needs may be given proper attention.

Takes part in a project where medical science, industry, public health, and conservation personnel are actively engaged in research linking population, land areas, and various types of pollution to specific diseases.

Observes that as individuals have consumed the fruits of the environment at random, and increasingly triumphed over climate problems, pestilence, and famine, there has been created an environment which introduces new hazards to human health.

Analyzes how an epidemiological study of the characteristics and interactions of agent, host, and environmental factors helps determine the causes of disease, disability, health problems, defects, and death.

Realizes after field study that the impact of economic, demographic, social, cultural, scientific, and technological changes have not only improved man's health, but have also created additional health needs and a number of ecological problems—pollution, noise, neuroses, malnutrition, and so on.

Demonstrates how a number of social and cultural changes in the community have an ecological bearing on urban development, air and water pollution, mental illness, alcoholism, drug addiction, accidents, and other problems.

Suggested Activities

(*Junior High School*)

1. Through class action, develop a list of all the sciences which contribute to ecology. Then go back over the list and ask how each contributes.

2. After looking into water pollution, invite a sanitary engineer or sanitarian from the county health department to class as an outside resource person.

3. Post the U.S. Environmental Protection Agency poster (Figure 7–4) and raise the question about its truth. From this solicit EPA type art and photographic work pertaining to an ecological message.

4. Investigate the speed with which the local community is growing. Have students check the local hospital for number of births. What would be the population in ten years? Twenty years? Make a graph of net population increase of the town or city over the past fifty years. Try projecting the population for the future.

5. Set out with a tape recorder to record sounds in the community—natural and man-made, loud and soft, necessary and unnecessary, and so forth. How do the sounds affect animals? Humans? Do adults and youth agree on which sounds are noise? Play the tape for the students.

6. Make a map showing local and state parks, playgrounds, conservation lands, and other open space. Relate these spaces to such items as recreation, watershed, wildlife, wells, sewage, and waste disposal. In most communities a basic town or city map may be obtained from town or city offices.

7. Permit the environment to inspire certain kinds of writing by class members. Poems and stories of all kinds can be discussed and posted. The writings of Frost, van Doren, and Thoreau are all valuable.

8. Role Playing: Act out a water pollution situation by appointing a (1) builder, (2) farmer, (3) industrialist, and (4) boat owner. Ask the four persons to discuss the problem. Each is to speak of *his* concern not to pollute the water.

9. Study a local river that is polluted. Substitute this name for the Charles River in the box on page 267. Create a display by obtaining photographs and other artwork to support each statement.

10. Prepare a word bank that could be used in a letter-writing campaign about local water pollution. One class in Illinois investigated the water in streams and ponds around their town and came up with the following words :[9]

debris	radioactivity	refuse	unsanitary
aroma	detergent	stench	recreation
contamination	conservation	disease	disposal
natural resources	poisonous	slimy	oxidation
wildlife	mucky	thermal	perishable
communicable	unreplenishable	bacteria	sewage
pungent	consumption	pesticides	decay

[9]For more on this class activity, see Clifford E. Knapp, "Environmental Education Activities," *Instructor*, 81:52–62, January, 1971.

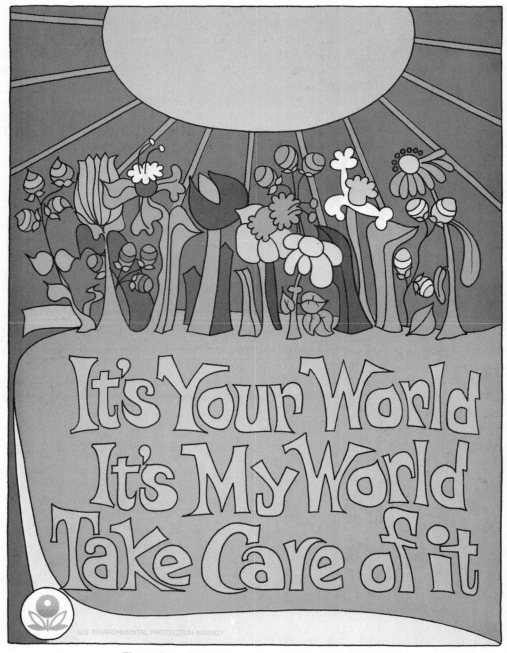

Figure 7–4   Environmental Protection Agency poster.

WE HAVE MADE the water of the Charles River so bacteria-ridden that we cannot drink it.
WE HAVE MADE the water of the Charles River so oily and irritant that we cannot swim in it.
WE HAVE MADE the water of the Charles River so unsupportive of life that we cannot fish in it.
WE HAVE MADE the water of the Charles River so malodorous and filled with refuse, and lined its banks with dumps and old junk, that we cannot contemplate its once natural beauty.

11. Prepare a questionnaire suitable for use in interviewing certain persons about water pollution in nearby streams or bodies of water. It should deal with sources of water, industrial wastes, fish and other aquatic life, water drainage from streets and hard top areas, governmental regulations and controls, and other subjects. Have some committees find out through personal interview how the following people feel about water pollution: town or city officials, a conservation leader, a local industry leader whose factory borders a stream, the public, the Audubon Society chapter, and others.

12. Send for a copy of the *Environmental Circle* (which depicts the various kinds of pollution and the effect on the total environment) from the New York State Department of Environmental Conservation, Albany, New York. It is an elaboration on the following and worth posting for all to see, as shown on the next page. In the circle chart the student will readily be able to connect the *three* pollutions. Number 1, for example, shows that open dumps bring about smoke and odors and cause drainage to surface waters. Likewise, in Number 8, agricultural manure causes odors in the air and nutrients in the runoff which slowly pollute streams and reservoirs.

13. Look at the following survey results, then survey segments of the public to see if they agree as strongly as the sample surveyed by the Opinion Research Corporation in late 1975.

"If we don't start cleaning up the environment now, it will cost us more money in the long run."
Agree   90 per cent
Disagree   7 per cent
Don't know   3 per cent

14. Examine, by small groups, some of the environmental health reading materials (see Chapter 10, and the references at the end of this chapter). The National Air Pollution Control Administration has many free booklets on air pollution (801 N. Randolph Street, Arlington, Va. 22203). See also free materials from the U.S. Department of the Interior; the report, "From Sea to Shining Sea," of the President's Council on Recreation and Natural Beauty; the United Nations report, "Problems of Human Environment," and the numerous inexpensive reading materials from Environmental Teach-In, 2000 P Street, N.W., Washington, D.C. 20036. See also *76 Ways You Can Help Save Your Environment,* Connecticut Department of Environmental Protection, Hartford, Conn. 06115.

15. Study how living things adapt to their environs by observing birds, animals, and humans. This could be diagrammed by a problem-solving group for classroom display. Consider both internal and external environments.

16. How does the press help? What do newspapers' editorials have to say about the environment and the health of the community? Show the film that was produced in cooperation with the Associated Press, *Man's Natural Environment: Crisis Through Abuse*—a real look at pollution.

17. Have the class find out how to test stream water for purity. How is the count taken? Appoint a group to check the quality of a nearby body of water or small stream every week for a period of time.

18. Look into where the air pollution comes from in a nearby city. Research results can be seen in the chart on page 269. Follow this with a study of the "greenhouse effect." Words such as airshed, fossil fuels, inversion, photochemical smog, and traditional smog will need defining.

NOISE AS A DESTROYER

---

19. Question: How does noise destroy anything? *Physical effects* demonstrated: British Comet, first jet airliner, grounded because sound vibrations caused fuselage cracks—acoustic fatigue of metal. *Psychological effects* shown: Noise annoys, spoils sleep, and, through fear, causes blood pressure changes.

LAND POLLUTION

1. Open dumps
2. Ashes and residue
3. Chemical wastes
4. Power plants
5. Septic tanks
6. Junk cars
7. Chemicals in soil and food
8. Agricultural manure
9. Erosion

AIR POLLUTION　　　　**ENVIRONMENTAL CIRCLE**　　　　**WATER POLLUTION**

1. Smoke and odors
2. Incineration—smoke and flyash
3. Industrial gases
4. Radiation and smoke
5. Sewage odors
6. Vehicle exhaust
7. Pesticide sprays
8. Odors
9. Dust

1. Drainage to surface waters
2. Processed water wastes
3. Chemical wastes and oil
4. Thermal pollution
5. Contaminated water supply
6. Contaminated rainfall
7. Chemicals in water
8. Nutrients in runoff
9. Silt in water

WHERE THE POLLUTION COMES FROM			
8% HOUSEHOLD	11% POWER PLANTS	16% INDUSTRIAL PLANTS	65% AUTOS, TRUCKS, BUSES

20. Construct a table model of a *sanitary* landfill—a smokeless, odorless, ratless engineering project to handle community solid waste. Canyons can be filled, as in Los Angeles. Hills can be built, as in Chicago, for recreational skiing.

21. Have the class, as a whole, design an environmental poster. It can be simple; it might look like Figure 7–5.

22. Arouse curiosity about the natural world by asking the class to *observe* an ecological situation, record what is seen, *interpret* what is seen, *communicate* it to others, and *define* the problem. This approach can be employed with a number of environmental health topics.

23. Declare the following statement and discuss it:

> "The population in the United States is simply living too high off the hog. Our affluence, our greed, our wastefulness, cannot be sustained."

24. Invite Audubon Society or Sierra Club people to visit class and lead a group in pursuing an environmental problem such as the relationship between the preservation of wilderness and mental well-being.

25. Establish a group to look over stamps that have been printed by various countries over the years. Those which refer to the environment should be brought to the attention of the class. See Figure 7–6.

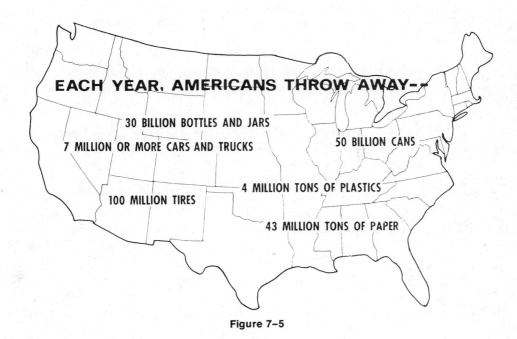

EACH YEAR, AMERICANS THROW AWAY--

30 BILLION BOTTLES AND JARS

7 MILLION OR MORE CARS AND TRUCKS

50 BILLION CANS

4 MILLION TONS OF PLASTICS

100 MILLION TIRES

43 MILLION TONS OF PAPER

Figure 7–5

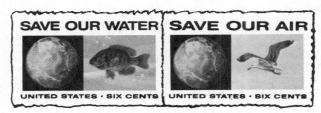

Figure 7-6

Suggested Activities

(Senior High Level)

1. According to the National Science Foundation and National Aeronautics and Space Administration (NASA) 14,700 windmills located 12 to 200 miles offshore would generate 159 billion kilowatt hours of electricity a year, four times as much as the six New England states used last year. Appoint several committees to look into harnessing the wind for electric power supply. Subdivide the topic.

2. Relate epidemiology to ecology. Obtain copies of *Vital Statistics of the U.S.* from the U.S. Government Printing Office. Invite an epidemiologist to class to tell about his work and how difficult it has become in overcrowded cities.

3. Arrange a class field trip to a municipal water treatment plant. Each pupil should prepare a report on types of treatment. In it, there should be some reference to water-borne diseases such as infectious hepatitis, typhoid fever, cholera, and other bacterial and parasitic diseases.

4. Examine the word *crisis*. How powerful is the word? Hawkins and Vinton examined the word and feel that the national ethic which places a high value on the biggest and best, causes individuals to ignore mere problems until they are termed *crisis*.[10] Prepare papers in this area for review by a class committee.

5. Investigate various methods of desalinization of sea water. Where are such methods now being used? Note lands with a severe water shortage or pollution which really need fresh water from salt water.

6. Check the local health department for figures pertaining to respiratory difficulties such as asthma, emphysema, lung cancer, and chronic bronchitis. Show how these diseases tie in with increased pollutants in the air. Mortality statistics are interesting, too. Diagram how these diseases relate to community, people, neighborhoods, industry, and so on.

7. Discuss the idea of using an Earthkeeping Seal of Approval for products which have no harmful side effects, and which create no disposal problems.

8. Check the quality of local drinking water. Where does it come from? What does the state think of it? In Vermont, one survey found 33,500 people in 66 separate communities to be drinking water that was "undesirable" for human consumption. see Figure 7-7.

9. Study the wetlands (coastal and inland), watershed areas, and flood plains. Seek help from the local conservation committee or State Department of Natural Resources.

---

[10]Donald E. Hawkins and Dennis A. Vinton, *The Environmental Classroom,* Englewood Cliffs, N.J.: Prentice-Hall, Inc. 1974.

Rate the observed areas in each of the 9 categories:

EARTHKEEPING
SEAL
OF
APPROVAL

	GOOD	FAIR	POOR
recreation			
wildlife			
water supply			
flood control			
agriculture			
nature study			
development			
aesthetic value			
historic value			

10. Post photographs and other pictures depicting environmental abuse: shore birds covered with oil, lead-poisoned ducks on a beach, rusting autos or appliances residing in a stream, a "no swimming—water polluted" sign. Under these pictures post the question:

WHAT CAN I DO?

11. Organize a planning committee to work with certain local groups interested in conservation and environmental problems. Boy and Girl Scout troops are always willing to respond to community "clean up" projects. Nationally, the Boy Scouts of America Launch Project (Save Our American Resources) can be given considerable support by older high school students.

12. Study town or city planning board activities in respect to land use. Find out about "cluster zoning." Is it really designed to conserve open space in new residential developments?

13. Have the class consider the effect of employing one of the following suggestions of legal experts relative to improving water quality. Also, ask the class, "Is there a local problem?" and "Can *we* act to do something?"

(1) Use the 1899 Refuse Act, which prohibits dumping into any navigable waterway in the country, except under permit from the Army Corps of Engineers. Half the fine (up to $2500) goes to those who give information leading to a conviction. In addition, the offender could receive a 30-day jail sentence.

(2) If you own land bordering on navigable water which is being polluted, sue for infringement of riparian rights. This means, in effect, that you may sue because the pollution is depriving you of access to or use of the shore, stream bed, and water bordering your land (your riparian rights).

(3) Use the laws most communities and states have regarding private and public nuisances. These can be especially effective against urban air polluters.

Figure 7–7

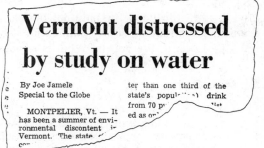

Vermont distressed by study on water

By Joe Jamele
Special to the Globe

MONTPELIER, Vt. — It has been a summer of environmental discontent in Vermont. The state c...

ter than one third of the state's popul... drink from 70 p...

(4) Federal officials and agencies can be sued for failing to carry out sworn responsibilities, or exceeding authority. One recent example is the citizens' suit against former Interior Secretary Walter Hickel, to prevent construction on the Trans-Alaskan Pipeline System.

(5) File a verified complaint with your state department of natural resources, or a similar agency. In Wisconsin, for example, six citizens filing a pollution complaint can force the state to hold a hearing within 90 days. Citizens there may also prod the state into administrative rule-making against alleged pollution, or file petitions for declaratory rulings. Conservationists banned DDT in Wisconsin through those methods.

(6) Last, most states have old laws against littering and dumping, not only on public highways but into waterways, as well. Although the fines are usually small, each offense can be pursued separately.

TEMPERATURE CHANGES AND HEALTH

---

14.   The Arctic ice pack controls the temperature of much of the Northern Hemisphere. Canada, especially, is concerned with oil pollution in this region. Some United States scientists fear a melting of the ice pack due to increased carbon dioxide in the atmosphere. Prime Minister Trudeau of Canada has some strong environmental protection viewpoints. Organize the class to look into this because it is an item suitable to debate.

15.   Employ students, canoes, boats, and trucks to clean up a nearby river. This will require class planning and cooperation with town or city officials. It has been done in many places. It is important to have local publicity, and help from fish and game clubs and other interested organizations. Class members can build a large chart of the river and mark accessible bridges, streams, mileages between points, location of pickup trucks, etc.

16. Develop an *Environmental Health Newsletter*.

ENVIRONMENTAL HEALTH NEWSLETTER "Have You Thanked a Green Plant Today?" (Ecograffiti)

Stress what *we* can do. (Recycle what we buy; make compost heaps from leaves, table scraps, lawn clippings, limestone, bones. A ton of newspapers recycled saves 17 trees.)

17.   Are "Save the Wilderness" groups overconcerned with conservation? Do they fail to balance industrial needs with open space needs? Investigate the literature of the Sierra Club and the Wilderness Society (Washington, D.C. 20005).

18.   Investigate the activities of the Conservation Law Foundation, Inc. (506 Statler Office Building, Boston, Mass. 02116). Their monthly *Notes* sheet is rich with legal illustrations pertaining to environmental health. Upper division students with a feeling for politics and law will enjoy this activity.

19.   Debate the pros and cons of such issues as "exploitation of Alaskan oil"; "the SST and trade balance"; "wilderness instead of minerals"; "public lands and mining laws," and "the need for national parks." Consider these topics from all angles—economics, government, social implications, industrial progress, conservation, and health.

20.   Look to the courts. What is happening these days?

In the Courts

Phoenix, Ariz.

Two university professors and their wives have brought a $2 billion suit for damages against six copper companies charging that smoke from their smelters is injurious to health, restricts visibility, and "damages the natural beauty of the environment."

Brooklyn

Six Brooklyn political leaders have filed suit against the Army Corps of Engineers to compel the corps to stop dumping sewage in the ocean within 100 miles of the New York and New Jersey shorelines. The plaintiffs charge that by permitting the dumping of sewage within five miles of Ambrose Light the corps has caused the contamination of 20 square miles at the entrance to New York Harbor.

Deepwater, N.J.

E. I. duPont de Nemours & Co. is suing the state of New Jersey, claiming that the state's prohibition against burning fuel containing more than 1 per cent sulfur is an "unconstitutional deprivation" of the company's property. DuPont maintains that, in setting the regulation, the state "wrongfully assumed that it was empowered to prevent, control, and prohibit air pollution without regard to balancing the substantiality of threatened injury against the cost to persons and the public at large of complying with regulatory measures." The cost to duPont of burning more expensive low-sulfur fuel is estimated at $900,000 a year.

21. Lay out a waterway in terms of water ratings. Sketch the streams on a map of the local countryside, and beyond—possibly to the sea. Place large visible letters along the way to indicate quality of water (see Figure 7–8).

Class A: Any use including drinking.

Class B: Fit for drinking after chemical treatment. All right for swimming and vegetable irrigation.

Class C: Fit for boating (most common water).

Class D: Suitable for transportation only.

Class E: Open sewer.

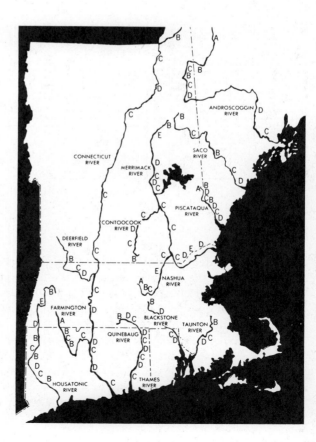

Figure 7–8

DECIBEL SCALE

EARDRUM RUPTURES 140	jet taking off
PAINFUL TO EAR 120	siren jet revving its motors for takeoff—maximum allowable for hearing roar of a two-engine prop plane
DEAFENING 100	thunder car horn at 3 feet—loud motorcycle loud power lawn mower
VERY LOUD 80	portable sander have to shout to be heard food blender continued daily exposure brings about loss of hearing noisy cocktail party impossible to use telephone
LOUD 60	city playground vacuum cleaner noisy office average traffic point at which use of the telephone becomes difficult
MODERATE 40	suburban playground all right for a restaurant average living-room
FAINT 20	quiet enough for courtroom or classroom private office a whisper at 5 feet
THRESHOLD OF AUDIBILITY 0	rustling leaves breathing

Figure 7–9

22. Post a decibel scale (Figure 7–9). Does it seem reasonable to the class?

23. Debate the socioeconomics of the following:
— The present course in the environment is suicidal.
— There is no way out except to reorganize industry and agriculture and make them compatible with the ecosystem.
— Surviving requires an alliance: scientists to produce the needed information; the media to spread it; the public to make the necessary decisions.

24. Collect poetry with an environmental health concern. Print some of the verses and post them for class members to see. Is the philosophy sound and the message clear? (See DeFries' article, "Will I Ever Catch Another Butterfly?" December, 1970, *Journal of Health, Physical Education and Recreation*.) The verse was written by John Denver.

2. CONSUMER HEALTH

In the words of Tom Hurt,[11] the typical American consumer is a "health illiterate." He or she is a prisoner of the immediate culture, a victim of both the old wives' tales of the past and current life styles, and of what the media would like the consumer to believe. How else can one excuse the purchase of a popular pain reliever that contains a little over one gram more aspirin than plain aspirin plus some caffeine but sells for four times the price of aspirin? Or the purchase of a worthless "cancer cure" electronic device, or sampling a hallucinogenic drug to "expand the mind," or simply eating something called "organic food" in the belief that it will be more nutritious than regular food? Or taking vitamin E for everything from gangrene to sexual dysfunction?

The Food and Drug Administration (FDA) has shown that 42 per cent of the population would not accept the word of scientists that a cancer "cure" is worthless. Moreover, they would not ban it by law. So they go on buying machines with multi-colored blinking lights and buzzing sounds as a cure-alls, but close their minds to the value of a varied diet of ordinary foods such as meats, fruits and vegetables, and dairy products. Superstitions continue, astrology gains additional followers yearly; there is a proliferation of gurus and spiritualistic groups; occult beliefs involving demons, sorcery, and witches flourish alongside the more scientific realm of parapsychology. Magical charms and mystical games have great appeal. And to make matters worse, the "victim" frequently comes away from these influences muttering, "I feel better; I must tell my friends."

Consumer health is that part of consumer education that pertains primarily to the health of the individual and the community. Not only does it have to do with all major health areas, but it relates as well to all physical and biological forces in society — forces that are manipulated or influenced by political, industrial, commercial, and economic considerations. Changing the health practices of the average adult consumer, therefore, is no easy undertaking, for the practices are generally rooted in a value system that tends to be more inflexible than flexible. Hope for change rests with the enlightenment of youth, where the forces of education have greater potential for altering health practices than those of consumer laws and legislation. Actually, changes in health practices are a combination of the two, as understanding citizens seek appropriate legislation to protect their well-being.

In educating for consumer health, it is important to think of health product safety and effectiveness in terms of human personalities and everyday living. What are the questionable products? Who uses them? Is it only the poor, the hopelessly sick, and the uneducated who permit the occult fad to capture their imagination? Do people risk their health and mental integrity for a cheap thrill? Was P. T. Barnum right when he said that people like to be fooled? Will mankind always flock to the quack, the guru, the swami or the fortune teller in search of a supernatural influence on their lives? What do the students think about all of this? Do they know how much quackery is thriving in this Age of Aquarius? Do they have a means of understanding that the more one seeks the oblivion of the spiritualist the more he loses touch with reality? Yet, young people in particular tend to be fascinated with what they can hear from the lips of a fortune teller. This does not mean that they are borderline psychotics. It simply means that Barnum was partly right and educators have a big task to tickle the appetite for rational thinking.

Consumer health education in secondary school has to take an in-depth look at the science of medicine. The essentials of "cause and effect" and the scientific method need

---

[11]Tom Hurt, "Positive Consumerism: Health Economics," *Health Education*, 6:2, November/December, 1975.

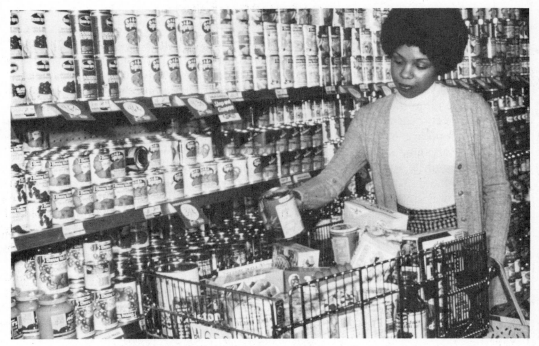

Figure 7–10 Nutrition labeling aids the consumer in making comparisons of the nutritional values and relative costs of different foods. (Courtesy of Cereal Institute Inc.)

to be reviewed using examples from the health domain to make a point. When there is an understanding of the relationship of medical research and expertise to the cure and control of disease and human misery, it will be possible to fully appreciate why an unscientific cult such as chiropractic is a significant health hazard. The book by Ralph Lee Smith, *At Your Own Risk: The Case Against Chiropractic*, should be required reading of senior students.

When the National Commission on Product Safety made its report, it made a strong plea for more well-informed consumers in America. Since the federal government cannot possibly fully check every consumer product from toothpaste to hot-water vaporizers, it is necessary for informed people of all ages to police themselves. This, of course, is very difficult to do in an age of heavy product advertising. A small fortune is spent on most products in terms of aesthetic appeal, testimonials, slogans, symbolism, novelty ideas, and comedy. Less overt in approach are the various hidden techniques appealing through family identification, the use of children, association with other products, nostalgia, "common sense," altruism, class distinction, humility, youthfulness, "naturalness" in preserving ecological balances, and sexual connotation.[12] Another hidden item underlying some advertising is an appeal to one's level of acceptability. Fear of not being accepted—not using a product others use—is capitalized on by the advertiser. In this respect, a study of social status and "keeping up with the Joneses" is as much a part of health education as it is of social studies.

Another phase of consumer health that may be readily correlated with economics and social studies in the senior high school is *health care*. In this era of big problems, the

---

[12]See the especially fine points made by R. Morgan Pigg, Jr., "Analysis of Health Advertising," in *Health Education*, 6:22–26, November/December, 1975. See also Chapter 2 in Warren E. Schaller and Charles R. Carroll, *Health Quackery and The Consumer*, Philadelphia: W. B. Saunders Co., 1976.

American physician and hospital services have received more than their share of abuse. Much of this is because large portions of the population have very little idea about medical training, services, and costs. They demand—and rightly so—personal, continuous, and comprehensive care of high quality, and at a reasonable cost. This, of course, is exactly what health professionals want, too. However, there has been a failure to meet public demands for cost control, comprehensive health insurance, uniform quality of services, and equality of access to these services. One asks, how much do young people know about all of this? They will soon be earning their own medical dollar. How is it being spent?

If the public is to effectively utilize the health care delivery system it must at some time investigate a variety of fundamental items. Out of a much larger list of such items, Vacalis determined the "essential" seven are:[13]

> Knowledge of sources of emergency help
> Knowledge to differentiate between legitimate and illegitimate medical practitioners
> Knowledge of the ways of selecting a physician
> Knowledge of the vaccination schedule for children
> Knowledge of the actions taken if medical aid is thought to be harmful
> Knowledge of the sources of psychiatric assistance
> Knowledge of the advantages and disadvantages of the different types of health insurance policies

Since there has been no slackening in the rise of health care costs, steps must be taken by health care providers and consumers to reduce direct and indirect costs of inpatient and outpatient treatment. Jones and Stevens point out that this is an educational undertaking in which the student studies the delivery of health care in the country by examining governmental roles, the providers and consumers of care, and the third party payers (Blue Cross, Medicaid, Medicare, etc.)[14]

A particularly helpful resource with suggestions for classroom teaching is *Consumer Health Education For Junior High Grades,* available from AAHPER (NEA), 1201 16th St., N.W., Washington, D.C. 20036. Note also that in Chapter 4, the area of consumer health was used to illustrate sub-topics and essential content in program planning. Pages 89 to 91, therefore, will be most helpful for the teacher preparing in this area.

Behavioral Objectives

(Junior High Level)
Discriminates between reliable and unreliable health information and advertising.

Determines that quackery and faddism are dangerous to health because they prevent people from following sound health practices and receiving adequate health protection.

Demonstrates the ways in which reputable physicians share their ideas, findings, and other pertinent information with the rest of the scientific community. Explains how the quack promises sure and quick cures.

Relates how self-diagnosis and self-treatment can endanger health; it sometimes occurs because of fear, false economy, and poorly understood illnesses.

Analyzes how agencies serve, protect, and inform the health consumer—some agen-

---

[13]T. Demetri Vascalis, "Determination of Vital Areas of Knowledge Needed for Wise Consumer Use of Health Care Services," *Journal of School Health*, 44:390–394, September, 1974.

[14]Bert Jones and Nancy B. Stevens, "Overcoming Economic Barriers to Health Care," *Health Education*, 6:7–11, November/December, 1975.

cies are UNESCO, the Food and Drug Administration, the Post Office Department, local health departments, voluntary health agencies, State health departments, and the Better Business Bureau.

Explains how standards for the processing of foods, drugs, and cosmetics are defined by the Food and Drug Administration; the advertising of these products is of concern to the Federal Trade Commission.

Utilizes magazines that sometimes rate health products; *Parent's Magazine, Good Housekeeping* and *Consumer Reports* are important to understand.

Discovers that emotional motives for purchasing health products and services may lead to unwise consumer behavior.

Analyzes teen fads, fashions, and other consumer trends having to do with such items as body weight and complexion aids.

Explains how teenage buying influence is considerable, both within and outside the family; some of this represents a striving for adulthood.

Essential Topics
Quackery and quacks
Health consumer
Ethical advertising
Consumer motivation
Teenage buying power
Food and Drug Administration
Federal Trade Commission
Teenage faddism
Harmful products
Medical ethics
Self-medication

Behavioral Objectives

(Senior High Level)
Discovers that there are a number of important differences between health specialists; the preparation, licensing, and certification of medical and paramedical personnel is very carefully supervised.

Explains how health services, as well as health products such as food, food additives, cosmetics, drugs, and medications are often selected on the basis of hearsay, emotional feelings, past experiences, and social forces and pressures.

Employs sound criteria to help make intelligent choices in providing for professional health care.

Tells how diagnosing and treating illness and injury are the responsibilities of qualified personnel.

Explains how expanding knowledge in every area of medicine has made medical specialties a necessity.

Analyzes the ways in which promoters of health products and services capitalize on consumer ambivalence—our expression of both positive and negative feelings about the same object or activity.

Demonstrates how behavior based on superstitions, ignorance or prejudice, rather than scientific evidence, can be expensive and harmful to the health consumer.

Studies various types of hospital systems, each serving its own particular function.

Illustrates how medical care is an important part of the national and family budget; because this care is costly, medical care insurance is increasingly necessary.

Essential Topics

Contemporary quackery and pseudoscientific practice
Medical care
Psychological considerations in buying habits
Myths and superstitions
Law enforcement
Hospital economics
Medical careers
Health insurance plans
Drug testing
Health and safety legislation
Health manpower
Patient-physician relationship
Cost factors in health care delivery system

Suggested Activities

(Junior High Level)

1. Role-play the health quack and the consumer. In order to bring out the various characteristics of quacks, act out some of the following quasi-medical propositions.[15]
   a. Claim to cure or alleviate a disease that puzzles physicians.
   b. Guarantee "satisfaction or your money back."
   c. Respond to an appliance, medicine, diagnosis, or other medical service offered by mail.
   d. Offer testimonials by "cured" or "satisfied" users.
   e. Claim the possession of secret formulas, secret ingredients, and secret methods.
   f. Demand medical service payment in advance.
   g. Claim endorsement by "high government officials."
   h. Offer a trial package free in a plain wrapper.
   i. Limit the supply for special customers.
   j. Indicate "doctor recommended," or "leading hospitals insist on it."
   k. State "proved by leading research laboratories."
   l. Use high-sounding academic degrees.
   m. Attack legitimate physicians, hospitals, nurses, or other genuinely professional personnel.
   n. Employ such items as hypnotism, magnetism, wonder drugs, "natural foods," and electronics to make quackery appear scientific.
2. Visit several antique dealers to find bottles that once contained such nostrums as Dr. Hosteller's Bitters.
3. Show and discuss the filmstrip *Mechanical Quackery*. This may be obtained from the American Medical Association or your State medical society. *The Exploited Generation*, available from Guidance Associates, is also worth seeing.
4. Examine mail order ads or offers and have the class determine the clarity of the statements made by asking themselves the question, "How much do I know about this advertised product?" Ads similar to the following can be found in many magazines (see Figure 7–11).
5. Assign a small group to read *Potions, Remedies, and Old Wives' Tales* by W. W.

---

[15]For more details on each of these propositions see Warren E. Schaller and Charles R. Carroll, *Health Quackery and The Consumer*, Philadelphia: W. B. Saunders Co., 1976, pp. 181–182.

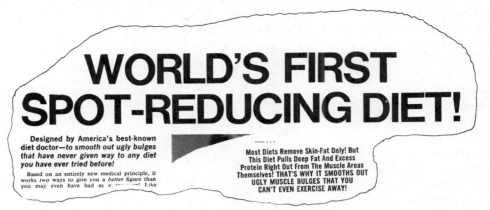

WORLD'S FIRST SPOT-REDUCING DIET!

Designed by America's best-known diet doctor—*to smooth out ugly bulges that have never given way to any diet you have ever tried before!*

Based on an entirely new medical principle, it works *two* ways to give you a *better* figure than you may even have had as a ~~~~~~! Like

Most Diets Remove Skin-Fat Only! But This Diet Pulls Deep Fat And Excess Protein Right Out From The Muscle Areas Themselves! THAT'S WHY IT SMOOTHS OUT UGLY MUSCLE BULGES THAT YOU CAN'T EVEN EXERCISE AWAY!

Figure 7–11

Bauer (New York, Doubleday and Co., 1969). Use the points made to help illustrate the weaknesses found in *Calories Don't Count* by Herman Taller (New York, Simon and Schuster, 1961). Put a copy of this pseudonutrition book on display.

6. Read and discuss nutrition labels. All fortified foods, and all foods *for which a nutrition claim is made,* must display nutrition information on the labels. Vitamins, minerals, additives, and weights will be the concern.

7. View the FDA film *The Health Fraud Racket.* It discusses how to spot quackery in the areas of food, drugs, cosmetics, and medical devices. (National Medical Audiovisual Center, Station K, Atlanta, Georgia 30334.) Also see the 27-slide series *What's New on Labels.*

8. Prepare point-of-view papers. Such topics as "What is Propoganda?" and "What is Quackery?" may be discussed by the class. Students may then read their papers to the class as a basis for discussion about the views.

9. Discuss health cultists. Mention that chiropractors may be the largest group of cultists in the United States. Point out that they, like other cultists, have an inflexible theory concerning a single cause of all human illness. Make it clear that ". . . in spite of available evidence, chiropractors believe that when people fall sick or become disabled, it is due to nerve roots being pressured because the backbone, or some section of it, has gotten out of line. And the single cure they espouse is to manipulate—twist, massage—the spine to bring it back into alignment."[16]

10. Visit the fresh fruit and vegetable section of a large supermarket or grocery store. Examine the produce. How appetizing does it appear? Is it fresh? Obtain copies of *A Narrative Guide for Consumer Tips on Fresh Fruit* from Sunkist Growers. The filmstrip by the same name is also valuable. It may be obtained without charge. The story of fresh fruits and vegetables may be obtained from United Fresh Fruit and Vegetable Association (see Figure 7–12).

11. Obtain from the FDA the *Consumer Protection* packets which consist of booklets, leaflets, and teaching suggestions suitable for health, science, and home economics classes.

12. List a wide variety of superstitions and myths that have something to do with

---

[16]Jacqueline Seaver, *Fads, Myths, Quacks—and Your Health,* New York: Public Affairs Pamphlet No. 415, 1968, p. 7 (381 Park Avenue South, New York, New York 10016).

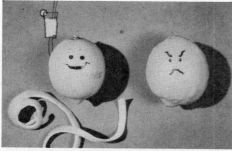

Avoid buying lemons with bruised, bumpy, wrinkled skins. This shows that they are either too old, badly stored or culls from the crop. Since you may want to use the peel as well as the juice, compare before you buy and select only the best.

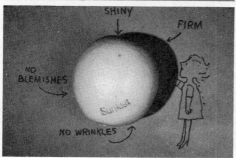

Can you tell when fresh citrus is fresh? It should be firm to the touch, without soft spots or breaks in the skin. Fruit that is fresh will not be spongy or wrinkled. Its peel will be shiny. Fruit that has been stored improperly will lose some of its flavor, juiciness and vitamin C. Even though a few pennies cheaper, it is not a good buy. Just as you have learned to identify consistent high quality in meats, boxed, canned and frozen foods by their labels, you can also identify high quality fresh citrus by its label.

Figure 7–12   Consumer tips on fresh fruit. (Courtesy of Sunkist Growers)

health and well-being. Here are a few that can be discussed to see if there is *any* truth involved:

People were healthier in the "good old days." (Were they — really?)

An apple a day keeps the doctor away. (How badly do we need the potassium found in apples?)

If a toad touches you you'll get warts. (Doesn't the skin protect you?)

"Natural" foods will do away with "that tired feeling."

You are what you eat. (An all-or-none rule?)

Aluminum cooking utensils are harmful to health.

Everyone should take vitamin pills just to be sure.

Natural "organic" fertilizers are safer than chemical fertilizers and produce healthier crops.

Sleeping with a dog prevents rheumatism.

A bad tooth should not be pulled during pregnancy.

Flowers will wilt if you touch them while menstruating.

13. Find out about Consumer Research, Inc. and Consumers Union, Inc. See the monthly magazine, *Consumer Reports*. Bring it to class for student use.

14. Send a committee to visit the Better Business Bureau. Bring literature back to class for committee report.

15. Ask the class to respond to the expression "teenage buying power." Are teenagers more easily motivated to buy than adults? How critical of the product are they? Are they selective in their choices? Create a questionnaire and survey both teenagers and storekeepers to find out what teenagers buy.

16. Look into non-ethical advertising. Visit the local postmaster to discover how the mails have been used locally to carry fraudulent schemes and the selling of nostrums. The postal inspector or divisional inspector may be willing to come to the classroom and tell of his personal efforts to safeguard the mails from medical frauds.

17. Solicit help on ways to engage in activities to combat health quackery and fraudulent advertising from the American Cancer Society and the Arthritis Foundation, Inc.

Suggested Activities

(Senior High Level)

1. Study the reasons why people are motivated to purchase goods. Classify these in one of three major areas: physical, emotional, and social. Construct a checklist; using this list, ask parents and peers why they bought a specific item. Cover several kinds of purchases such as cosmetics, clothes, cars, cameras, and food.

2. Arrange a bulletin board of advertisements displaying health products that provide outlets for various compensations. (Compensatory behavior involves those attempts by the individual to "make up" for real or imagined weaknesses or shortcomings in his psyche or physical being. Very often compensatory appeal may be found in hair restorers, acne cures, cosmetics, weight reduction preparations, and other such items.)

3. Distribute a variety of popular magazines, such as Newsweek, Time, and Sports Illustrated. Have the class count all of the health-related advertisements. Relate these ads to the recommendations (controls) of the Creative Code of the American Association of Advertising (available from the American Association of Advertising).

4. Pupil project: Discover the physician-patient ratio in the local town, city, or county. Is there an even distribution of physicians? Is there a shortage? Discuss what it means to people to have a physician near at hand. Consider private practice and group practice in terms of services. Also, consider health maintenance organizations such as Blue Cross–Blue Shield, Kaiser–Permanente, and Harvard Health Plan.

5. Require students to determine the cost of an ordinary appendectomy operation. Compare this cost for patients who have no insurance with that for those who have hospital insurance. Examine closely the particulars of a group hospitalization medical plan.

6. Appoint student groups of three each to survey the hospitals servicing their community. The survey should include:
   a. type of control/financing,
   b. nature of service provided,
   c. bed capacity, and
   d. number of physician members.

7. Debate the concept of national health insurance to cover everyone. Is it a "nebulous panacea" or a valid viewpoint?

8. Is there a consumer voice to be heard regarding:
   — the practice of medicine?
   — the problems of the hospital?
   — rehabilitation within the community?

> I have been asked whether I advocate community control of health services. I advocate a partnership of producer and consumer. I most certainly believe that there has not been enough consumer voice and influence upon the producers in medicine.
> —*John H. Knowles, M.D.*

---

9. Investigate the action of drugs in the body, and relate the ingestion of drugs to such items as self-medication, "the over-medicated society," the role of government regulations, and the process of "detoxification" by liver, kidneys, and lungs. Research the use of patent medicines. Is there proper value received here?

10. There are many ideas for consumer health activity. Let the class members suggest a few, and then agree to work as a group on one or two that seem interesting.[17] The best "idea response" comes when a previous consumer health reading assignment has been made to initiate this major area.

---

[17]See Carl E. Willgoose, "Instruction in Consumer Health," *Instructor*, 80:73–74, October, 1970.

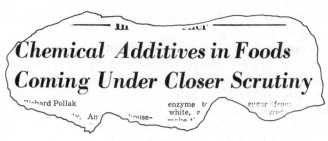

Figure 7-13

11. Investigate food additives. Look into FDA regulations pertaining to additives that (1) enhance flavor; (2) stabilize and thicken, such as starch, pectin, and gelatin; (3) neutralize or alter acidity or alkalinity; and (4) prevent oxidation and spoilage, such as sodium and calcium propionate which retard the growth of bread molds. How safe are the additives? What do we know about diethylstilbestrol for fattening beef cattle and sheep? Mercurial fungicide to treat wheat seed to prevent rot? Antioxidants to keep shortening from becoming rancid? See Figure 7-13.

12. Have the class look over the following list of ways the Federal Food, Drug and Cosmetic Act works to protect the consumer; then choose four or five of these to investigate:

1. Foods must be pure and wholesome, safe to eat, and produced under sanitary conditions.
2. Drugs and therapeutic devices must be safe and effective when used according to their directions. New drugs must be approved by FDA before they can go on the market.
3. Cosmetics must be safe.
4. Labeling must be truthful and informative.
5. Drug labeling must include warnings needed for safe use.
6. Drugs not safe for self-treatment are restricted to sale by prescription.
7. Drug plants must be inspected by FDA at least once every 2 years.
8. Antibiotic drugs, insulin drugs, and colors used in foods, drugs, and cosmetics must be tested in the FDA laboratories before they go on sale.
9. Chemicals added to foods must be proven safe before they are allowed to be used.
10. Pesticide residues which may remain on raw food crops must not exceed safe limits (tolerances) set by FDA.

13. Through some small class project, raise the necessary money to purchase eight or ten small cans of perishable hams (fully cooked, ready to eat and require refrigeration). Organize a ham tasting party for the whole class. Check all samples and compare for the following:

a. The taste—alone and on plain crackers after heating.
b. Remove all traces of loose fat and gelatin, and carefully weigh the resulting meat block (good hams are generally over 80 per cent edible).
c. Calculate the cost per pound of edible ham.

Possible samples are Armour Golden Star, Rath Hickory Smoked, Tala, Zwain Oak Smoked, Wilson's Certified Natural Hickory Smoked, Unox, Dubuque Royal Buffet, Wilson's Certified Honey Cured, Country Club Brand, Oscar Mayer, Krakus, A & P Super-right, Farmbest, Food Club, Swift's Premium, Morrell's Original Chef Brand Natural Hickory Smoked, Agar, Corn King, Morrell Pride, Armour Star, Hormel, and Cudahy Bar S. (From time to time canned hams are tested by Consumers Union, a nonprofit organization, and reported in *Consumer Reports.* See the October, 1970 issue, page 581. Also see the September, 1970 issue for a thorough run-down on how frozen fish sticks are tested.)

14. *Project:* Work up a questionnaire and survey the community for superstitions, myths, and misunderstandings pertaining to health. Have class members ask people from *all* walks of life. History is full of illustrations that scientific knowledge can co-exist with primitive reactions. Only recently we witnessed how the Nazis, in their quest for the so-called "pure" or Aryan race, took the discoveries of genetics and distorted, misinterpreted and transformed them into twentieth century "legalized" myth and superstition. Moreover, one should never forget that many of the intellectual elite are firm believers in such dubious notions as astrology, health foods, reincarnation, rejuvenation methods, chiropractic, and fatalism.

15. Twenty million Americans are injured each year by everyday things—exploded glass bottles, a short-circuited color television, top-heavy high chairs, unvented gas heaters, plastic bags. Ask the class to *research* these injuries. Is the prevailing maxim of the buyer-seller relationship "caveat emptor"—Latin for "let the buyer beware"? Can this be changed so that the *buyer is aware* and the seller had better *beware*?

"CAVEAT EMPTOR"

16. Obtain sample health care insurance policies and analyze them in terms of coverage. Build a chart showing the major categories of the insurance with advantages and disadvantages. Compare individual and family benefits.

17. Set up a "comparative shopping trip" for prescription drugs within the community. Note price differences from drug store to store. Consider the "discount" drug chains too.

18. Today in several sections of the United States the FDA has a "Consumer Phone" service, which will provide information about consumer protection at the moment. Assign a student to telephone for the consumer protection message of the week and report to class. See Figure 7–14.

19. Take a field trip to a nursing home, convalescent home, and retirement home for senior citizens. Evaluate them in terms of physical attractiveness, safety features, services, and attitudes and general atmosphere. (For a complete checklist of items see pp. 327–330 of Warren E. Schaller and Charles R. Carroll, *Health Quackery & The Consumer.* Philadelphia, W. B. Saunders Co., 1976.)

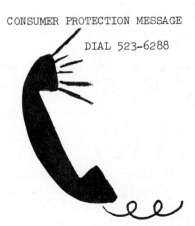

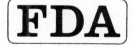

CALL EACH WEEK FOR
NEWS ABOUT:

Foods,
Drugs,
Cosmetics,
Medical Devices,
Hazardous Home Products,
and
Toy Safety

U. S. Food and Drug Administration, Boston District-------Region I

Figure 7–14

3. WORLD HEALTH

The concern for the larger community of man has become a major educational topic in an age when thousands of Americans are travelling half way across the world in a few hours. From South Africa to Ireland, from Ethiopia to Chile, there is a concern for human ecology, medical care, and social welfare. International health, therefore, is a topic for students to consider as they attempt to understand the many problems of people in a heavily populated and increasingly mobile world.

At both junior high and senior high levels, some part of the health education course should have to do with the health problems of the international community. The concept that world health is everybody's business needs wider acceptance. The "have" nations have a degree of moral responsibility for the "have not" nations. Moreover, the health and welfare of European, Latin American, African, and Middle Eastern peoples has in recent years come very close to the American scene—so much so that no pupil is isolated who dwells in northern Montana or southern Mississippi. Unrest in Canada affects Atlanta as well as Detroit. This is one reason why the United States Public Health Service, the State Department, the Department of Agriculture, and numerous other agencies of the Federal government are so active around the world. On the Mexican border alone there are 25 million people living in six Mexican cities and four of the United States; there are also 14 major twin-cities beginning in the west with Mexico's Tijuana and the United States' San Diego, and ending in the east with Matamoros-Brownsville. There is a cooperative health effort in this area, the responsibility of the United States–Mexico Border Public Health Association.

It is important to appreciate early that there is a price tag on the economic benefits that a nation derives from the control or eradication of a disease. For example, where malaria has been eradicated, new lands open to farming, forestry, and to a host of other industries. And because agricultural and forest products form the bulk of exports in developing countries, production increases, spurred on by further malaria eradication, lead to greater earnings of foreign exchange. So students in an eighth grade class in Iowa study the *Anopheles* mosquito and its resistance to insecticides—a major obstacle in eradication campaigns. They learn that OMS-33 is a better killer than DDT; however, because it costs about 15 times more than DDT, it is being used in limited operations. This is the way to make the very lives of people real. Child care centers in Latin America are real, too—an area of the globe where over 40 per cent of the population is less than 15 years old; an area where immunization against disease, nourishing food, water for drinking, and a decent place to live are on the way.

Americans have long been interested in world health. The mission of the famed Pan American Health Organization is to "combat disease, lengthen life, and promote the physical and mental health of the people." It is the oldest public health organization in the Western world, dating back to 1902. Its Pan American Sanitary Bureau functions as the regional office of the World Health Organization (WHO) in the Americas.

It could be argued that World Health as a topic should be included under the broad wings of Environmental or Community Health. This seems inappropriate, for when this was done in the past there was a strong tendency for health problems of the international community to be accorded a very light treatment. Given a variety of world-wide health topics to choose from, the average student's interest will quicken, especially when he begins to get answers to the question, "How does this affect me?" Moreover, the question will be answered in a more satisfying way if it is related to history, sociology, government, economics and political science, for the ultimate health of a citizenry is reflected in its culture, its industry, and the faces of its people.

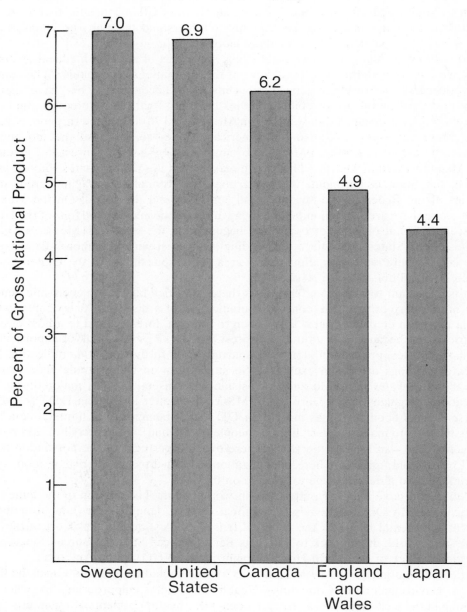

Figure 7–15 Total health expenditures as a percentage of gross national product. (From the Bureau of Research and Planning, California Medical Association, *Socioeconomic Report*, 12:5, 1972).

Behavioral Objectives

(Junior High Level)

Diagrams how communicable diseases may be spread throughout the world in a matter of hours because of the increased number of people travelling via rapid means of transportation.

Explains how the advanced nations of the world need to cooperate with the developing nations in disease prevention programs and eradication programs designed to control insects, polluted water, and general sanitation.

Demonstrates through documentation how the nutritional needs of the world have become overwhelming as the population has increased; malnutrition is a serious condition everywhere.

Shows the manner in which international health agencies bring modern scientific technology to bear on world health problems.

Illustrates the way the Pan American Health Organization, the United Nations, and the World Health Organization work cooperatively to improve world health.

Examines the way in which the culture of the people influences the nature and extent of international health problems.

Essential Topics

Disease control
Malnutrition
Family structure
Immunizations
Pen-pal projects
International cooperation
World Health Organization
Scientific technology
Economic stability
Occupations

Behavioral Objectives

(Senior High Level)

Describes the manner in which total health transcends local, state, national, international, and political boundaries.

Analyzes how regional health problems are influenced chiefly by cultural variations, economic differences, key occupations, geography, ecological balance, and technological development.

Demonstrates through research reports that only when the people of a country participate in a health program does it have a chance to be successful.

Depicts how older family members influence younger members; if patterns of behavior are based on superstitions and myths, the progress of world health will be delayed.

Discovers and expresses the view that programs for training health personnel are essential in the underdeveloped regions of the world.

Illustrates the fact that there are diseases which are potentially epidemic that need to be constantly controlled; when a disease is an epidemic there are many cases; when it is pandemic the cases are spread over a large geographic area.

Explains in detail how nutrition and mental health programs are greatly needed throughout the world; drug abuse and emotional disturbances are high on the list of mental health problems.

Essential Topics

Ecological balance
World climate
World health careers
Geographic population patterns
Native superstitions
Industrialization and employment
Regional health manpower
Primitive hospitals
Alcohol and drug use
Smallpox and malaria eradication
World power politics and health conditions

Suggested Activities

(Junior High Level)

1. On a world map, pinpoint the six regional offices of the World Health Organization. Raise the question of financial support for this operation. Should the United States continue to pay its share? In fact, is WHO doing the job it is supposed to do?

2. Obtain films showing the work of WHO in underdeveloped lands. WHO headquarters in Geneva, Switzerland, will supply a copy of its annual report and film listing if requested to do so. The film *Man Alive* is fine for describing WHO activities.

3. Through small group activity (three-person teams) gather information necessary to create a large wall chart depicting a variety of world health problems. One way to show the results of group work is to post problems by countries on a large map of the world.

4. Assign topics for individual research prior to class discussion:

Half the world goes to bed hungry.
Physician—rival to the witch doctor.
Smallpox: constant alert.
World fight against communicable disease.
Food for 1980.
Latin America, its health and development.

Suggested Activities

(Senior High Level)

1. Post a variety of short statements such as the following to arouse interest. At the head of the list state the question, "How Does This Affect Me?"

Healthy people create future beauty in Latin America.

Sweden is the safest of 36 countries in which to become a mother. The maternal death rate is only 11.3 deaths per 100,000 live births. It is several points higher in the United States. The death rate in Chile is 271 per 100,000.

> Gonorrhea, according to WHO, is sweeping the world and threatening to rage out of control. It is the No. 2 communicable disease in the United States (behind the common cold).

> The United Nations Commission on Narcotics has a world program against drug abuse and illicit narcotics traffic.

> The Africa of the bongo drums, the beads, the Voo-doo man and the topless mini-minis — the old travelogue version of Africa — is on the way out.

> Copernicus was born 500 years ago on the banks of the Vistula River. Today, the fish caught here stink of fuel-oil.

> Chemical and biological weapons pose a special threat to mankind because of their high degree of uncertainty and unpredictability.

2. Set up a class project to assist in an international health crusade to fight disease. The contagious disease of yaws can be cured with penicillin. This takes money.

> The students of Mount Royal High School in Quebec have set up an organization called SWAY (Students War Against Yaws); SWAY also means YAWS spelled backwards. Their aim is to gather funds for yaws control and so far WHO has received from this source more than $40,000 in eight years.

3. Employing the interview technique, have class members contact the "man-in-the-street" (teachers and fellow students as well as community people) and determine if most people are aware of world health problems. Prior to doing this, have class committees agree on the kinds of world health questions to be asked.

4. Look into disease transmission (a) generally, and (b) worldwide. Consider the effect of world public opinion. A flight of geese could carry diseases resulting from bacteriological warfare over frontiers far from the original site of combat. Now, are you interested in the state of health of people in Outer Mongolia or Dakar? See Figure 7–16.

5. Obtain copies of *World Health* (WHO official magazine) and *Gazette* (Pan American Health Organization). Focus on student-selected topics for discussion. Note the clarity of sketches and superb photographs in every issue.

6. Americans are so much alike that we tend to disregard the cultural gulfs separating people; this contributes to failures in intercultural health problems. Have the class find out how world health activities actually relate to the patterns of the culture. See L. Riddick Lynch, *The Cross-Cultural Approach to Health Behavior,* New York: Associated University Presses, 1970.

7. Invite an Action volunteer who has returned from a foreign land to class. Ask him to speak about heavily populated countries and the way large numbers of people affect the level of health.

8. Consider health manpower needs around the globe. Physicians, nurses, sanitarians, and trained health personnel of many kinds are in great demand, but are in short supply. Can anything be done to remedy the situation? Can people be trained in medicine

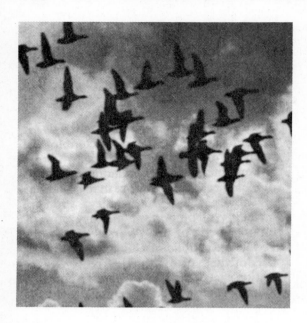

Figure 7–16

when over 40 per cent of the world's children do not even attend school? Check into the life of Albert Schweitzer. Was he successful in his medical efforts? Who was Dr. Thomas Dooley?

9. Start a learning resource center having to do with international health. Catalog materials received from UNESCO (United Nations) and WHO. They may be used for independent study.

10. Develop a model depicting the cycle of poverty. Materials may be obtained from Pan American Health Organization. Show how the poverty cycle affects productivity, population, economy, human motivation, and creativity. How does this affect disease control? How can this poverty cycle be stopped? An excellent reference for this topic is the April, 1969, issue of *World Health*. See also current editions of an encyclopedia.

11. Display on a large class bulletin board selected pictures and articles from newspapers and magazines that deal with hunger, poverty, and disease in one or several countries. News reports from Asia, Africa, and Latin America will be helpful.

12. Prepare a survey form designed to find out what high school students and teachers know about countries they or their friends have visited. Ask health related questions having to do with the extent of malnutrition; the frequency of people vaccinated against a disease; the cleanliness of city streets, buildings and people; food sanitation; medical and dental needs, and the extent of obvious myths, mysticism, and superstition.

13. Assign an independent study project to relate the health problems of Middle East countries to ideological and political power struggles. This same assignment can be given for countries such as Brazil, Chile, South Africa, and Northern Ireland.

4. HEALTH CAREERS

Health is big business. Employment in health industry and professions has multiplied by more than four times in the last 30 years. In the allied health fields alone (which excludes nurses, physicians, veterinarians, podiatrists, dentists, and optometrists) there has been a doubling of employment in a 10-year period. These people work in medical centers, hospitals, educational institutions, Federal, State and local government agencies, clinics, health care facilities, drug and equipment manufacturing firms, and numerous insurance agencies. It is a 100 billion dollar business involving 5.5 million people. All of this offers exciting opportunities in health careers.

New concepts, which are in part of health maintenance organizations, call for teams of professionals and auxiliary personnel to provide a variety of services on a pre-paid, insurance-type basis; these are proliferating and call for a health administrative staff. In addition, every hospital, large or small, has to have an administrator. Through 1980 it is expected that about 1000 new administrative positions will open. By the same date there are expected to be 185,000 jobs open in the drug industry, 114,000 in insurance, and 55,000 in insurance underwriting.

Health care in the years ahead will go beyond the hospitals and physicians' offices to the neighborhood health facilities, nursing homes, and the public, private, and voluntary ventures, all of which require manpower from the allied health professions. Environmental health opportunities are increasing year after year. Extended care facilities, preventive medicine, and out-patient treatment programs require nurses, physical therapists, occupational therapists, and many other health specialists who can work well with people in the community. As new laboratory and x-ray equipment continues to be developed for hospital use, the need for laboratory and radiologic technicians will double in only a few years.

The professional nurse supply has grown considerably in the last several years, but not in proportion to the population. In many high schools a real effort is being made to organize future nurse clubs. Physicians and nurses help raise scholarship money to boost this career field. Also, where the school nurse is active and known to the students she is able to "sell" her career. School nursing is a specialty, combining nursing skills with a background in both health and education—a multidisciplinary approach to health and health related problems. For an excellent description of her responsibility, see *This Is School Nursing,* distributed free by the National Council for School Nurses, 1201 16th Street, N.W., Washington, D.C. 20036.

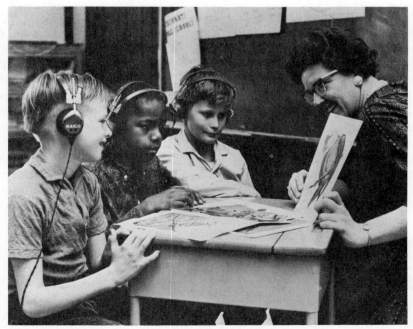

Figure 7-17 A health career—teacher of the deaf. (Courtesy of National Congress of Parents and Teachers)

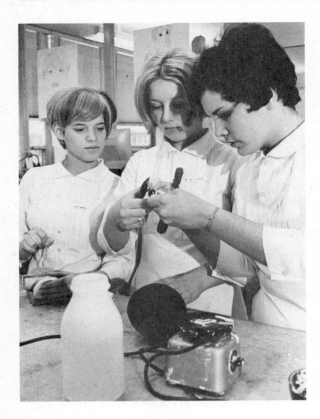

Figure 7–18 Dental assistants in training. (Courtesy of Ruth Byler, State Department of Education, Hartford, Connecticut)

It is now possible to begin training for a health career while still in high school, but the initial introduction to careers begins much earlier in the junior high school years. Information on training materials designed to prepare students for a wide range of health vocations is available from the U.S. Office of Education, Vocational and Technical Education, U.S. Department of Health, Education and Welfare, Washington, D.C. 20202. There is also information on health manpower training to be obtained from the Bureau of Health Professions Education and Manpower Training, U.S. Public Health Service. And new career entities are being developed right along to meet health needs. The nurse with advanced medical training is an example; she is prepared to take over a number of duties that were formerly the sole concern of the physician. Another example is physician assistants—a class of medical professionals who help physicians provide a wide variety of medical care services. Former military medical corpsmen, already trained in rendering care, now have a chance to continue their careers in the civilian world.

The junior colleges are preparing individuals in health careers to meet emergency medical manpower needs. Laboratory technicians, medical record librarians, and others may be prepared in a two-year college along with the medical emergency technician (MET). An MET serves in an emergency room or some other area of the hospital where there are life threatening emergencies.

A health career unit of instruction in the secondary school should function to get as many people as possible to work as volunteers or paid workers in the health field. Young people working in mental health institutions, hospital wards, rehabilitation units, and pediatric sections frequently do a better job than some of their professional counterparts, particularly if they are patient, pleasant, and like people. Throughout the nation there are more than 2000 hospitals making use of young volunteers. Their "lending a hand" makes it possible to free the staff for professional functions. It is a rewarding opportunity, and some hospitals accept volunteers as young as 14 years of age.

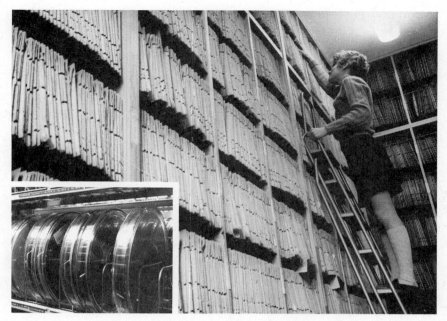

Figure 7–19 Medical librarian. Storage, old and new. The shelves hold records of a few thousand patients. Each reel and tape, in a plastic case, contains the records of 11,000 patients. (Courtesy of World Health Organization)

Treatment centers often welcome teenage volunteers to set up and participate in recreational projects. There are opportunities in camps to work with exceptional children. Mental health centers, civic clubs, churches, temples, and local volunteer health agencies that serve the mentally ill usually can recommend facilities that can use the help of young people. The Student American Medical Association encourages young people to participate in community health programs involving well-baby clinics, drug addiction centers, dental clinics, and many other projects that are needed in medically deprived areas.

It can be shown that health education as a teaching career can be most rewarding. There is a chance to bridge the gap between scientific health discoveries and man's application of them to daily living. There is an opportunity to develop individuals who are physically, mentally, socially, and spiritually sound, and to work toward these ends in school systems and public and voluntary health agencies. Sophomore students in a number of New York City high schools work directly with junior high school health education classes to gain first-hand experience with health concerns. This is frequently prefaced with a workshop about the health teaching career in which the following occurs:

— presentation by a group leader, usually with audiovisual aids
— completion of a worksheet by each participant individually
— discussion of the worksheet in small groups
— total group discussion which clarified and highlighted certain points

Behavioral Objectives

Explains clearly how there is a growing need for many more professional health workers, such as physicians, nurses, dentists, and pharmacists; there is also a need for more allied health personnel.

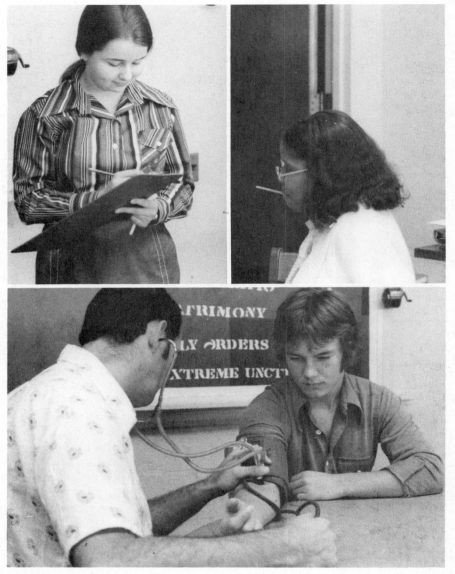

Figure 7-20   Health professions class in action. (Courtesy of Millicent C. Rhodes, Metropolitan Public Schools, Nashville, Tennessee)

Gives examples of how earning a livelihood by working in a health career field can be of great service to humanity, and can afford deep personal satisfaction.

Illustrates how academic preparation coupled with personality and interest sets the stage for the selection of an appropriate health career.

Differentiates between the many major fields of medical (M.D.) specialization, many more in dentistry, and several in nursing.

Describes how hospitals, nursing homes, rehabilitation facilities, and community health centers could not operate without the help of technicians, aides, helpers, and volunteers.

Essential Topics

Medicine and nursing

Dentistry and pharmacology

Medical technicians
Hospitals
Manpower shortages
Personal qualifications
Community health centers
Mental health organizations
Voluntary health associations
Health in industry
Education for safe living
Cooperative health services
Health education in schools and communities

Suggested Activities

1. Collect and pass around the class a wide variety of pamphlets and other materials on all fields which relate to health. Investigate grants, funds, and scholarships in health careers.

2. Examine the word "service." Show its relationship to emotional and social needs of mankind. Find example of how some of these needs can be met by helping others through careers in health.

3. Organize field trips to interview individuals in various health professions and allied health fields. Report back to class. Contrast the skills and needs of the physician with those of the licensed practical nurse or respiratory therapist. Compare educational qualifications necessary for various therapists and technicians.

4. Formulate two lists on the blackboard: (1) medical specialties requiring an M.D., and (2) allied health specialties not requiring an M.D. It is important to contrast the training and limits of responsibility of the psychiatrist with those of the clinical psychologist; compare the ophthalmologist with the optometrist, or the orthopedist with the podiatrist. Too often, apparently well educated people do not know the differences.

5. As a class project, assign each student one of the major *fields of medical specialization* recognized by the American Medical Association (see Figure 7–21). The specialties are described as follows:

Administrative Medicine. Serving in this field are those physicians who have administrative posts—in business, health programs and hospitals, for instance—which require the background of a physician.

Anesthesiology. This specialty field deals with the administration of various forms of anesthetic drugs necessary during surgical operations or diagnosis.

Colon and Rectal Surgery. This field is concerned with the diagnosis and treatment of disorders or diseases of the lower digestive tract.

Dermatology. The dermatologist specializes in the diagnosis and treatment of diseases of the skin.

Internal Medicine. The internist specializes in the diagnosis and nonsurgical treatment of diseases of the internal organs such as the heart, liver, and lungs.

Neurological Surgery. This branch of medicine is concerned with the diagnosis and surgical treatment of the brain, the spinal cord, and nerve disorders.

Obstetrics and Gynecology. This branch of medicine is concerned with the diagnosis and treatment of diseases of the female reproductive organs and also the care of women during and immediately following pregnancy.

Ophthalmology. An ophthalmologist or oculist is a physician—a Doctor of Medicine—who specializes in the care of the eye and all of its structures. He diagnoses and treats all visual problems. He prescribes whatever eye treatment is necessary, including

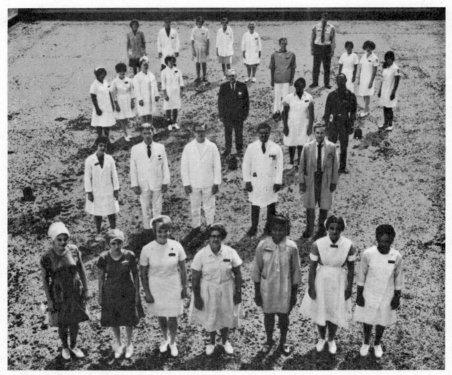

The Hospital Team

In many large hospitals, employees can be identified in two ways: (1) a badge giving name and job title, and (2) by the uniform. Diagram identifies the uniforms: (1) operating room technician, (2) infant nurse, (3) registered nurse, (4) nurse assistant, (5) station clerk, (6) student nurse, (7) licensed practical nurse, (8) social worker, (9) medical clerk, (10) intern, (11) resident, (12) staff doctor, (13) tray passer, (14) dietitian, (15) inhalation therapist, (16) x-ray technician, (17) chaplain, (18) maid, (19) housekeeper, (20) Service League volunteer, (21) male in-service volunteer, (22) candy striper, (23) in-service volunteer, (24) library volunteer, (25) transportation aide, (26) security officer, (27) medical technician, (28) physical therapist, (29) occupational therapist.

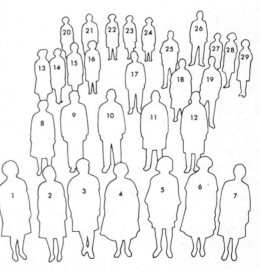

Figure 7–21 (Courtesy of Mr. Arnie Betts and the Northwestern Memorial Hospital)

the fitting of eyeglasses, contact lenses, optical aids for the partially sighted, and eye exercises (vision training, orthoptics).

Orthopedic Surgery. This branch of medicine is concerned with the diagnosis and medical or surgical treatment of diseases, fractures, and deformities of the bones and joints.

Otolaryngology. This branch of medicine is concerned with diagnosis and treatment of diseases of the ear, nose, and throat.

Pathology. The pathologist is engaged in the study and interpretation of changes in organs, tissues, and cells as well as alterations in body chemistry.

Pediatrics. This branch of medicine deals with the prevention, diagnosis, and treatment of children's diseases.

Physical Medicine and Rehabilitation. This branch of medicine is concerned with the diagnosis of disease or injury in the various systems and areas of the body and treatment by means of physical procedures as well as treatment and restoration of the convalescent and physically handicapped patient.

Plastic Surgery. This branch of medicine is concerned with corrective or reparative surgery to restore deformed or mutilated parts of the body or improve facial or body features.

Preventive Medicine. This specialty field deals with the prevention of disease and promotion of health through epidemiological studies and public health measures.

Psychiatry and Neurology. This field of medicine is concerned with the diagnosis and treatment of emotional disturbances, mental disorders, and organic diseases affecting the nervous system.

Radiology. This branch of medicine is concerned with diagnosis and treatment of disease through the use of radiant energy, including x-rays, radium, and cobalt 60.

Surgery. This branch of medicine deals with treatment of disease, injury, or deformity by manual or operative procedures.

Thoracic Surgery. This branch of medicine is concerned with operative treatment of diseases of the chest, those involving the heart, lungs, or large blood vessels within the chest.

Urology. The urologist specializes in diagnosis and treatment of diseases and disorders of the kidneys, bladder, ureters and urethra, and the male reproductive organs.

6. Probably the best paying profession today is dentistry. There are 100,000 dentists in this country and about 8000 of them are specialists in dental public health, oral pathology, oral surgery, oral roentgenology, orthodontics, pedodontics, periodontics, prosthodontics, and endodontics. See *Careers In Dentistry,* distributed free by the American Dental Association. Make clear distinctions between the following:

General Practice—Equivalent to the family doctor; trained in all phases of dentistry.

Oral Surgery—Practice limited to exodontia, complicated tooth removal such as impactions, and surgical procedures on the maxilla and mandible.

Peridodontics—Practice limited to surgical procedures upon the supporting structures of the teeth and occlusal equilibration.

Orthodontics—Practice limited to major and minor movement of teeth; work with maloccluded teeth.

Prosthetics—Practice limited to complicated or unusual appliances and tooth replacements; may include facial prosthetics for cancer patients.

7. Have someone find out about specialized work with exceptional children. Information on working with the blind may be obtained from the American Foundation For The Blind, 15 W. 16th Street, New York, N.Y. 10011. Speech therapy is another interesting area; therapists are at work in many clinics, hospitals, rehabilitation and treatment centers, public schools, and colleges.

8. Play the game Health Anagrams.[18] Distribute the list before the class meets so that the anagrams may be studied. Then divide the class into two teams. Work for 30 minutes and compare the scores of the two teams to determine the winner.

---

[18]Reported by Kathleen M. Siegwarth, "Health Anagrams," *Health Education,* 6:33–34, November/December, 1975.

1. Heston Satisgole	Anesthesiologist	25. T. S. Chime	Chemist
2. Les G. Trail	Allergist	26. Tod Roc	Doctor
3. Lenore Vut	Volunteer	27. Unis T. Tortini	Nutritionist
4. Sandie Sure	Nurse's Aide	28. Patricia Pylsthesh	Physical Therapist
5. Togol I. Scadir	Cardiologist	29. Nyle G. Gostico	Gynecologist
6. Hope Toast	Osteopath	30. Thom Toilgoes	Hemotologist
7. Lori N. Stouge	Neurologist	31. Scott Goily	Cytologist
8. Tobias T. Nicer	Obstetrician	32. Nat I. Eidic	Dietician
9. Phil O. Mostogoth	Ophthomologist	33. Stanlie Chet	Medical
10. Patti Goolsh	Pathologist	Comlodig	Technologist
11. Nate I. Picidar	Pediatrician	34. Caine Y. Xanchirt	X-ray Technician
12. Chris T. Stipay	Psychiatrist	35. Peter Lance	General
13. Sol Goitur	Urologist	Grantitoir	Practitioner
14. Gail T. Sodoir	Radiologist	36. Toni Priceset	Receptionist
15. Gib O. Loist	Biologist	37. Mort G. Sealdito	Dermatologist
16. Tania M. Torrids	Administrator	38. Mic A. Prade	Paramedic
17. Tad I. Porsit	Podiatrist	39. Sy A. Lant	Analyst
18. Seth Doorpit	Orthopedist	40. I. N. Rent	Intern
19. G. O. Nurse	Surgeon	41. I. C. Shypain	Physician
20. Rod Ryle	Orderly	42. R. E. Sun	Nurse
21. Ted Tins	Dentist	43. Pam C. H. Stair	Pharmacist
22. Thor Stondoit	Orthodontist	44. Morie T. Topst	Optometrist
23. Ricator Porch	Chiropractor	45. Cher E. Raser	Researcher
24. Gipsy T. School	Psychologist		

9. Investigate how large and influential health organizations plan to meet the need for more allied health personnel. Contact especially the American Hospital Association, American Medical Association, American Dental Association, American Physical Therapy Association, and American Nursing Association.

10. Interview health career people who are non-medical specialists, but have much to do with the recovery of the patient:

> dietitian   "candy striper"
> social worker   occupational therapist
> hospital chaplain   transportation aide

11. The career assistance program of the American Cancer Society is geared to career days, career clubs, and workshops. Moreover, students may visit local laboratories and talk with scientists and specialized technicians. Since the Society encourages phone calls, assign a committee to look into this field. The booklet "Teacher, Please Call Us!" is available to help teachers (American Cancer Society, 219 E. 42nd Street, New York, N.Y. 10017).

12. The recruitment film, *In a Medical Laboratory,* is distributed by the American Cancer Society for high school and college use. Invite a technologist or pathologist to school to answer questions after the film is shown.

13. Interest in physical therapy may be enhanced by having a few students examine the booklet "Around the Clock Aids for the Child with Muscular Dystrophy" (Muscular Dystrophy Association of America, Inc., 1790 Broadway, New York, N.Y. 10019).

14. Post the following prior to discussing the challenge of health research:

> "I implore you, take some interest ... in laboratories. They are the temples of the future ... there humanity grows better, stronger, greater."
>
> *— Louis Pasteur*

15. Appoint a student committee to compare the careers of the ophthalmologist and the optometrist. Since there is a shortage of vision care personnel, the pamphlet "What Is An Optometrist?" (American Optometric Association) will be helpful. For the teacher, the book by James R. Gregg, *Experiments in Visual Science* (Ronald Press), will add another career dimension.

QUESTIONS FOR DISCUSSION

1. The question was raised earlier in the chapter of whether a society can meet the pollution challenge without giving up anything. How do you feel about this? Will ecological expedience require a kind of totalitarianism that will greatly limit freedom?

2. Environmental health procedures require a great amount of unity between people of various backgrounds and interests. Each must look over the shoulder of the other and be of help. Charles C. Johnson of the U.S. Environmental Health Service writes, " . . . no engineer should be allowed into the world without an ecologist in attendance as a priest." Would you agree, or is this statement too strong to accept without reservation?

3. Politics is an area where ecological facts and human values sometimes collide: where interests compete and policy or stalemate results. Is there a way for this to be resolved? Can the quality of politics and the values of a society be tested and resolved by producers and consumers and by private and public sectors?

4. In such a multidimensional area, how can the teacher discuss a number of environmental health practices without offending some pupil whose family members are in some way contributing to one or another form of pollution? Also, what is your opinion of the teacher as a moralist?

SUGGESTED ACTIVITIES

1. Examine several health education curriculum guides for content in the area of community health. Appraise the content items for depth and breadth as they pertain to the more extensive topic of environmental health. In short, is community health a somewhat limited approach to the environment? Are public health and the role of voluntary health organizations stressed at the expense of such topics as conservation and urban blight?

2. Research indicates that polluted air has an effect on children and contributes to a higher rate of absenteeism (Irene B. Bury, "A Study of the Effects of Air Pollution on Children," *Journal of School Health,* 40:510–512, November, 1970). Inquire about the absenteeism rate in several schools located in areas that have heavily polluted air. Compare your count with a similar sample of children in a community relatively free from polluted air. What other findings can the school health service personnel provide?

3. Self-medication and the health of the consumer has always been an important topic for class discussion. Obtain copies of the following publications and prepare a teaching content outline covering the topic of self-medication:

    Food and Drug Administration: "FDA Fact Sheet on Self-Medication," Washington, D.C.: U.S. Department of Health, Education and Welfare.

    Food and Drug Administration: "We Want You To Know What We Know About Medicines Without Prescriptions," Washington, D.C., Superintendent of Documents, 1973.

    Editors of Consumer Reports: *The Medicine Show,* Revised Edition, Mount Vernon, New York: Consumer Union of the United States, 1974.

    Di Cyan, E., and L. Hessman, *Without Prescriptions — A Guide to the Selection and Use of Medicines You Can Get Over-The-Counter for Safe Medication,* New York: Simon and Schuster, Inc., 1972.

4. Prepare an up-to-date listing of allied health specialties that would be suitable for posting on a bulletin board for class viewing as one means of initiating a unit of work in the health careers field.

5. Investigate the proposals for stemming the flow of people into already crowded cities through the planning and development of rural areas. What are some of the health problems that would be eliminated by "new towns"? How would a senior high school class respond to such planning? Could they gather enough information to actually plan such a community and stay relatively clear of environmental health difficulties?

6. Work with a group of students to prepare a position paper on an impending legislative bill in the state which has to do with an environmental health concern. Acquaint them with the fact that government usually acts to solve only well-recognized and well-defined problems.

7. Examine a selected group of world health problems such as nutrition, parasitic diseases, water-borne diseases, ignorance, and superstition, and soon several people can become involved in selected areas of interest. After examining some problems apply the following question: How effective can the educational dimension be in helping to reduce the severity of these problems?

SELECTED REFERENCES

Abbott, Ellen, M. "Health Career Programs," *Journal of School Health,* 43:406–410, June, 1973.

Barrett, Morris, *Health Education Guide: A Design for Teaching, K-12,* 2nd edition, Philadelphia: Lea & Febiger, 1974.

Baugh, Robert J., and Carolyn B. Noe, "National Health Care: Consumer's Delight or Dilemma?" *Health Education,* 6:11–13, November/December, 1975.

Bundy, McGeorge. *Managing Knowledge to Save the Environment,* New York: The Ford Foundation, 1970.

Cromwell, C. "Organic Foods," *Journal of the American Dietetic Association,* 62:34–36, January, 1973.

Editors of *Consumer Reports,* "National Health Insurance: Which Way to Go?" *Consumer Reports,* 40:118–124, February, 1975.

Editors of *Consumer Reports,* "The Safe Approach to Laxatives," *Consumer Reports,* August, 1975, p. 508.

Editors of *Consumer Reports,* "Chiropractors: Healers or Quacks," *Consumer Reports,* September, 1975, p. 542.

Goleman, Daniel, "The Tranquility Box: A Consumer's Guide to Biofeedback Machines," *Psychology Today,* 9:132–135, November, 1975.

Hanlon, John J. *Public Health Administration and Practice,* 6th edition. St. Louis: C. V. Mosby Co., 1975.

Hawkins, Donald E., and Dennis A. Vinton. *The Environmental Classroom,* Englewood Cliffs, N.J.: Prentice-Hall, Inc., 1973.

Howell, Keith A. "Death and the Consumer," *Health Education,* 6:15–18, November/December, 1975.

Kennedy, E. M. *In Critical Condition,* New York: Pocket Books, Inc., 1973.

Marx, Leo. "American Institutions and Ecological Ideals," *Science,* November 27, 1970.

Masters, William H. "Phony Sex Clinics—Medicine's Newest Nightmare," *Today's Health,* 52:22–26, November, 1974.

Punke, Harold H. "Caffeine in America's Food and Drug Habits," *Journal of School Health,* 44:550–558, December, 1974.

Quinn, Nancy, and Anne R. Somers, "The Patient's Bill of Rights," *Nursing Outlook,* 22:240–245, April, 1974.

Rosen, S. "Beware of the 'Quackupuncturist' Who Operates for Profit," *Today's Health,* 52:6–7, 66–67, August, 1974.

Schaller, Warren E. and Charles R. Carroll. *Health, Quackery, and the Consumer.* Philadelphia: W. B. Saunders Co., 1976.

Smith, Ralph L. *At Your Own Risk: The Case Against Chiropractic,* New York: Pocket Books, 1969.

Stapp, William B. *Environmental Education: Strategies Toward A More Liveable Future,* New York: Halsted Press, 1975.

Turner, Alvis S. "The Environment of One World," *American Journal of Public Health,* 65:523–524, May, 1975.

Vivian, Eugene, and E. L. Henderson. "Environmental Education," *Instructor,* 50:52–61, Jaunary, 1971.

Weaver, Peter. "Are You Using Credit Wisely?" *Today's Health,* 53:42–44, November, 1975.

Willgoose Carl E. "Health Aspects of the Conservation-Recreation Effort," *Journal of School Health,* 38:359–365, June, 1968.

Chapter 8

Area IV—Safe Living

"Nothing of real value in the world is ever accomplished without enthusiasm and self-sacrifice."

—Albert Schweitzer

"The three great American vices seem to be efficiency, punctuality and the desire for achievement and success. . . . They steal from (Americans) their inalienable right of loafing and cheat them of many a good, idle and beautiful afternoon."

—Lin Yutang

In a culture where the "doctrine of progress" holds supreme, and a myriad of challenges to human endeavor spur individuals to strive toward greater goals, it is not surprising to find large numbers of men and women struggling to "move ahead" without thought of injury to self or society. Bold, brave people don't hesitate to act because of possible dangers, even accidents. On the contrary, Americans have thrived on challenges to life and limb as they sought Tocqueville's utopian myth—the "American Dream."

However, things are changing. There is evidence of relaxation and leisure, but perhaps not enough to satisfy Lin Yutang. Where man may have demonstrated a certain lack of sanity relative to personal safety in the past, there is emerging today another kind of progress—a variety of intellectual progress and sophistication that comes with the maturing of a civilization. Enthusiasm for an idea or effort is still welcomed. So is Albert Schweitzer's "self-sacrifice." The sacrifice, however, is a calculated one, for there are at least two ways to achieve a worthwhile goal: a reckless and hazardous way, and a safe way. Through action in government, industry, and schools, men and women are discovering that they can lead safe and happy existences, and be better off because of it. This does not limit freedom; it only enchances it. This is particularly true if one understands the significance of decisions. After all, as Lecomte du Noüy points out, ". . . if certain individuals make bad use of their freedom, so much the worse for them. . . . They were not evolved enough to understand."[1]

---

[1]Lecomte du Noüy, Pierre, *Human Destiny,* New York: David McKay Co., Inc., 1947, p. 17.

THE STATE OF AFFAIRS

The significance of a concern for safety is validated in dozens of ways as people of all ages work and play in an accident-ridden society that is frequently overcrowded and callous to the needs of others. Thus, safety education is relevant. It may be more relevant than sex and family life, or drug abuse, or venereal disease, or even five periods of high school English in one week. Anything which in one year killed 116,500 people and disabled 11.5 million others, and cost the country approximately 23 billion dollars, is certainly relevant.

There is no end to accident statistics. They are alarming because they bring about so much unhappiness; and they are enlightening because they point consumer safety engineers and educators in the direction of needed change.

Accidents are the leading cause of death among all persons aged 1 to 38 years. In fact, there is a person dying after an accident every 5 minutes in the United States. In the broad age category of 15 to 64 only heart disease and cancer take more lives. Note in Figure 8–1 how accidents are by far the leading cause of death among men 15 to 34 years of age. Note also that at ages 15 to 19 the loss of life from accidents is 12 times that from cancer and 40 times that from heart disease. It is this secondary school age period that needs attention. In the Hoover study the greatest number of accidents among junior high students were at the ninth grade level, with boys having twice as many accidents as girls.[2] Here the predisposing sources of injury were (1) being struck by a falling or moving object, (2) falling, and (3) tripping or slipping.

---

[2]Pearl Rollings Hoover, *The Epidemiology of Recordable Accidents Among Junior High School Pupils,* Master of Science, California State University, Northridge, California, 1972.

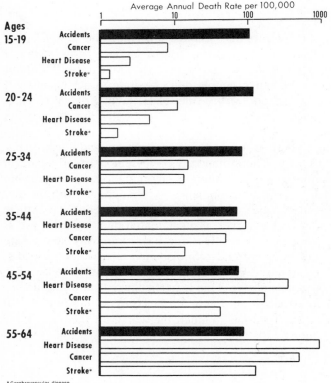

Figure 8–1 Accidents and other major causes of death among men of working ages. (Courtesy of *Statistical Bulletin,* Metropolitan Life Insurance Company, September, 1975)

* Cerebrovascular disease.
Source of basic data: Reports of Division of Vital Statistics, National Center for Health Statistics.

Type of Accident	Death Rate per 100,000						
	15-64*	15-19	20-24	25-34	35-44	45-54	55-64
Accidents—All Types	86.6	101.2	117.1	82.5	70.5	75.2	89.4
Motor vehicle	48.5	67.1	78.5	48.1	36.0	34.7	36.6
Traffic	47.6	66.0	77.4	47.3	35.3	34.0	35.7
Pedestrian	5.2	5.0	4.8	4.0	4.8	6.0	7.9
Drowning†	5.2	11.7	7.6	4.3	3.5	3.1	3.1
Falls	4.8	2.0	2.6	2.6	4.5	7.2	11.6
Fires and flames	3.3	1.3	2.3	2.5	3.3	4.5	6.6
Accidental poisoning by solids and liquids	3.2	2.5	5.8	3.9	2.5	2.0	2.5
Drugs and medicaments	2.1	2.0	5.0	2.9	1.5	0.7	0.9
Firearm	2.5	4.4	3.3	2.4	1.8	1.7	1.6
All other	19.1	12.2	17.0	18.7	18.9	22.0	27.4
Accidental deaths as a percent of all deaths	14%	63%	53%	39%	18%	8%	4%
Motor vehicle accident deaths as a percent of all accidental deaths	56%	66%	67%	58%	51%	46%	41%

*Adjusted on basis of age distribution of United States total population, 1940.
†Exclusive of deaths in water transportation accidents.
Source of basic data: Reports of Division of Vital Statistics, National Center for Health Statistics.

Figure 8-2 Mortality from leading types of accidents among men aged 15 through 64. (Courtesy of *Statistical Bulletin*, Metropolitan Life Insurance Company, September, 1975)

Yutang may laugh at American attitudes toward efficiency, yet both school work and the earning of a living are very much curtailed and made far less efficient at times owing to accidental injuries. In fact, nearly a third of all work days lost because of acute conditions are attributable to accidental injuries, according to estimates from the National Health Surveys. Motor vehicles, of course, cause the greatest number of injuries. Accidental falls are the second most frequent cause of disability. In terms of days lost from work, however, the accidental falls have a slight lead over motor vehicle accidents. A large number of the falls occur on one level, resulting from slipping on rugs, or tripping on sidewalks or floors. At the right time of year, ice is implicated as the cause of about a quarter of all falls on the same level. Frequently reported in every survey are accidents resulting from lifting, moving, or carrying objects, and injuries from machinery or cutting or piercing instruments.

It can be seen that many days are lost to disability caused by accidental injuries. Although the men do poorly in motor vehicle and industrial-type disabilities, the women have much more trouble with injuries due to falls and lifting-moving-carrying. (One might ask how many girls are in any way educated for such common tasks as the lifting, carrying, and moving of objects. Kinesiologically speaking, learning to move gracefully is a concrete move toward accident prevention.)

The most frequent injury caused by motor vehicle accidents is a sprain or strain. In accidental falls the most common cause of disability is a fracture, usually of the lower limb. There are obvious implications here for first aid programs.

Work injury rates vary considerably by industry. The most dangerous jobs are in manufacturing, with lumber and wood products industries leading the list and non-electrical machinery showing the safest on-the-job activity (U.S. Bureau of Labor Statistics). These figures are not as startling as they used to be, because manufacturing concerns have worked hard to establish safety records. By careful planning, a number of United States companies have set enviable records. The Du Pont chemical factory, for example, operated for 45 million man hours without a single disabling injury. A Houston construction firm spent several thousand dollars stringing a safety net around the base of a 50-story office building and found that the investment paid off in faster production.

HAPPINESS IS A SAFE ENVIRONMENT

How safe is it to walk the streets, or even cross the street? How can you kill 10 thousand Americans a year without public outrage? Simple. Run them down with 100 million cars.[3] The Injury Control Program of the Department of Health, Education and Welfare recently emphasized that each year more than 500,000 are injured on streets and highways as a result of a motor vehicle collision *without being either drivers or occupants of a motor vehicle.* They are over and beyond the 55,000 automobile deaths per year. They are pure pedestrian occurrences—most of which take place at night and could be avoided if people learned how to keep alert and walk on the proper side of the road. Each mile walked at night is *five times* as dangerous as the same mile walked in daylight. Sweden and Norway have an innovation which encourages pedestrians to use small reflective "tags" dangling from coat pockets. This appears to have reduced pedestrian deaths by over 20 per cent.

Death rates in automotive accidents have been substantially reduced by collapsible steering columns, break-resistant windshields, stronger door latches, more padding of interiors, and door guard rails. While seat belts have been required in vehicles for several years, "ejection" continues to be the number one cause of fatalities. The next major cause is the "second collision within the car," in which an occupant is thrown against some part of the automobile. In concluding a four year investigation of Michigan fatalities, Gikas showed that 53 per cent of the victims would have survived if they had been wearing seats belts.[4] Yet, even senior high school students discussing the seat belt issue will defend not wearing them in terms of "being caught in a burning car," despite the available evidence that this is not a factor when compared with all varieties of automobile accidents.

Where students live, around the home and neighborhood, can be pretty lethal. More than 150,000 disabling injuries and 850 deaths occur each year in bicycle accidents. This is partly due to the increased popularity of bicycling (there is one bicycle for every 2.4 registered motor vehicles). Almost as bad is the number of poisonings—mostly among children (500 deaths per year under age 5). Yet, older children seldom discuss this topic or learn to think in terms of younger brothers and sisters when they leave furniture polish, kerosene, bleaches, and other household items around. Every year, up to 2 million children ingest toxic substances. Children handle empty containers; teenagers work part-time in spraying operations. The three organic phosphorus esters (Malathion, DDVP, and parathion) account for thousands of accidents. Beyond the dispenser label, which many fail to read, where does understanding come from? Beyond an occasional warning, who explains the problems associated with aspirin, detergents, bleach, insecticides, analgesics, disinfectants, deodorizers, and polishes? Overdoses of aspirin still outweigh by six to one all other categories of ingestion accidents. Poison information centers and poison control centers help measurably, but they do not prevent the problem.

Senator Warren G. Magnuson of Washington has said on several occasions that "safety is hard to sell." This is one reason why reasonably knowledgeable people purchase fashionable fabrics that are flammable. Almost 200,000 persons are burned annually by flammable fabrics. When a little girl is seriously burned owing to a hazardous situation that should have been corrected, *or she should have known about,* everyone

---

[3]For an interesting study of deaths per *pedestrian mile,* see Susan P. Baker, "The Man in the Street: A Tale of Two Cities," *American Journal of Public Health,* 65:524–525, May, 1975.

[4]Paul W. Gikas and Donald F. Huelke, "Auto Safety Aids Are Saving Lives," *American Medical News,* October 26, 1970.

related rallies to her support. Blood is donated; newspapers write stories; money, clothing, and toys are sent from throughout the town or city. When she dies everyone in the community dies a little. Too often, little is done to capitalize on the situation and to upgrade safety education units in the local schools.

TO INSURE DOMESTIC TRANQUILITY

Engineers and others from the scientific disciplines unite to work on radiation safety problems and guard radiological health personnel from injury. Success is practically assured because most of the variables can be manipulated with some degree of certainty. However, when it comes to the poverty areas, the problem is complicated by intangibles such as ignorance, indifference, regulations, and despair. Education for safe living, in the end, must relate to the total condition of people.

People who live in overcrowded, dehumanized surroundings tend to be more violent; and violence—which has risen alarmingly in the United States—is dangerous. It is, in effect, another safety hazard. It disfigures society, making fortresses of portions of the city and dividing people into armed camps. Moreover, it poisons the spirit of trust and cooperation between people and substitutes force and fear for argument and accommodation.

In the final report of the National Commission on the Causes and Prevention of Violence, entitled *To Establish Justice: To Insure Domestic Tranquility,* it was set forth that there are internal dangers to a free society. These dangers need wide discussion, for they are health concerns. What is behind violence and violent crime? Should there be a means of "identification of specific violence-prone individuals..."? Should the recommendation that "concealable handguns, a common weapon used in violent crimes,... be brought under a system of restrictive licensing" be accepted?

Health education teachers at every grade level can profit from the findings of the

TABLE 8–1   National Commission on Product Safety Report

UNNECESSARILY HAZARDOUS	IN NEED OF POSSIBLE SAFETY IMPROVEMENTS
architectural glass	electric blankets
color television sets	electric dryers
fireworks	hot plates
floor furnaces which are gas fired	bath tubs
glass bottles	extension cords
high-rise handlebar bicycles	igniters (for cooking ranges and oil burners)
hot water vaporizers	lead paint
household chemicals	propane gas
infant furniture	footwear
stepladders	welders' eyeglasses
power tools	eyeglass frames
football headgear	swimming pools
rotary lawn mowers	recreational equipment
toys	boats
unvented gas heaters	automatic washers
wringer washing machines	aerosol containers
	cosmetics

National Commission on Product Safety. It is probably the most comprehensive account ever compiled of the perils one incurs by living in this technological age and highly mechanized culture.

Product categories reported included those shown in Table 8–1.[5]

Wide discussion is needed on injuries from toys and household products in general. Students, if given the opportunity, can predict the misuse of nearly every kind of item. Somehow the injury factor has to be resolved.

ACCIDENT PSYCHOLOGY

"Drugged by emotions, a man bent on avenging a supposed highway slight and a woman driver feeling sorry for herself take greater risks than Grand Prix racing champs."[6]

There is no question that some people have more accidents because they are accident-prone. Their mental state is such that they lack appropriate control of themselves. The emotionally disabled automobile driver, for example, is just as dangerous as the drunk. When emotions rise they frequently inhibit the brain's better judgment. They can also impair perception and block reactions. Frequently not appreciated by secondary school youth is that among youthful drivers, feelings of hostility and thrill-seeking can combine into a turbulent combination. Moreover, suicidal persons may drive a car to harm themselves as well as others.

Accident-prone individuals frequently fail to give proper attention to objects and practices in their environment. Their mind is elsewhere—a consequence of anxiety, depression, or emotional upset that could be caused by changes in job, school, residence, or personal relationships. There are also individuals suffering from long-standing paranoia. They are suspicious and figure that the world is against them, so they sometimes fight back with bloody revenge. In doing so, they sometimes mishandle familiar objects and trip over their own feet.

Accident psychology is an excellent topic for senior high school students to investigate. Among other things, it helps to make the mental health topic one that is practical and of consequence. It also helps to define outdated attitudes, values, and myths about preventing and controlling the problem. One can ask in dead seriousness: "Do accidents *really* just happen?" Is there so much apathy toward accident statistics that we don't have the inclination or time to separate accidents caused by hazardous products from those caused by maladjusted people?

Studying the reasons for accidents is difficult at best; and measuring accident-proneness is no exception. It is felt, however, that an understanding of human emotions under a variety of common circumstances is warranted. This may help to limit accidents due to guilt feelings and other inadequacies. It may also help the normal, adventurous young person who enjoys a challenge, but finds his controls less than adequate in a highly emotional state. Students who use hang gliders, ride motorbikes and snowmobiles, and take part in sports, have an opportunity to relate their own experiences to psychological factors. Skill is worth discussion time, too. Much of the fascination of such exhilarating avocations as parachuting, mountain climbing, motorcycling, and skiing lies in the skill and daring which the participant must display. The number of injuries each year

---

[5]The report did not concern itself with food, drugs, motor vehicles, insecticides, firearms, cigarettes, products with radiological hazards, and certain flammable fabrics.

[6]Stephen A. Framzmeier, "Driving Under the Influence of Emotion," *Today's Health,* 47:41, October, 1969.

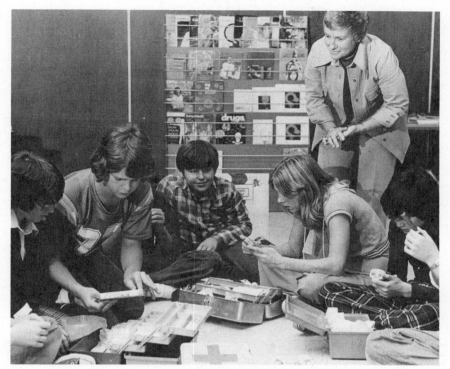

Figure 8-3 Assembling a first aid kit. Junior high school students are comparing items they have collected. (Courtesy of Loren Bensley, Jr., and Brad Fleming, Central Michigan University)

suggests that there is an inadequate appreciation of the hazards which these sports entail. Only one-fifth of the total deaths and injuries from mountain climbing involve experienced climbers.

EDUCATION FOR SAFE LIVING

It is hardly a new idea to prevent accidents by teaching people how to live safely. Fire drills and regulations supporting them appeared in the Boston Public Schools in 1900. San Antonio began safety instruction in its schools in 1913. Philadelphia and Detroit followed in 1916. By the following year, the American National Red Cross was introducing first aid programs into school systems. In 1918, St. Louis began curriculum studies to include safety in the curriculum. From 1920 on, a sizable amount of safety instruction was under way in many places, especially the states of Ohio, Pennsylvania, Missouri, Minnesota, Illinois, and Maryland.

Unfortunately, however, a close examination of health education outlines will show either no mention of safety and accident prevention or its placement is at the back of the outline. Rarely do teachers stress accident prevention. O'Rourke believes that much of this indifference is due to a lack of awareness of the scope of the problem.[7] Another reason may be an inability to present the safety topic in an interesting and challenging manner. Certainly the rules of safety can be taught in terms of conceptualized statements and observable behaviors. See the accompanying chart for an example.

---

[7]Thomas W. O'Rourke, "The Case for Positive Safety Education," *School Health Review*, 4:35–36, July/August, 1973.

Safety Rule	Behavior
Safety Rule Wear a life jacket while water skiing.	*Behavior* Demonstrate how to use a life jacket.

Conceptualized Statement

Life jackets support an individual who may be a poor swimmer or who may tire easily.

STUDENT ACCIDENT REPORT FORM

I.

School _____

☐ City   ☐ Exempted Village   ☐ Local (County)   ☐ Parochial

Mailing address _____

ENROLLMENT

Male _____
Female _____
Total _____

STUDENT INFORMATION

A. Name _____ *Last* *First* *Middle Initial*   B. Grade _____   C. Age _____

D. Sex - Male ☐   Female ☐   E. Teacher _____

II.   ACCIDENT INFORMATION

A. Time of Accident _____ A.M. _____ P.M.   Date _____

B. Supervised Activity?   Yes ☐ No ☐   C. If yes, teacher in charge _____

D. Nature of Injury

(May be completed after medical examination)

1. ☐ Abrasion	4. ☐ Concussion	7. ☐ Fracture	10. ☐ Sprain
2. ☐ Bruise	5. ☐ Cut	8. ☐ Laceration	11. ☐ Strain
3. ☐ Burn	6. ☐ Dislocation	9. ☐ Puncture	12. ☐ Other

E. Part of Body Injured

I. Head	II. Trunk	III. Arms	IV. Legs
1. ☐ Scalp	1. ☐ Chest	1. ☐ Shoulder	1. ☐ Hip
2. ☐ Back	2. ☐ Abdomen	2. ☐ Upper Arm	2. ☐ Upper Leg
3. ☐ Front	3. ☐ Back	3. ☐ Elbow	3. ☐ Knee
4. ☐ Eyes		4. ☐ Lower Arm	4. ☐ Lower Leg
5. ☐ Ear		5. ☐ Hand	5. ☐ Foot
6. ☐ Nose		6. ☐ Fingers	6. ☐ Toes
7. ☐ Mouth			
8. ☐ Tooth			
9. ☐ Neck			

F. Kind of Accident (check one only)

1. ☐ Animal bite or insect bite
2. ☐ Collision with student (Bump, etc.)
3. ☐ Contact with hot or toxic substance
4. ☐ Fall or slip
5. ☐ Fighting
6. ☐ Struck by auto, bike, etc.
7. ☐ Struck by object (swing, etc.)
8. ☐ Student collided with object (Door, etc.)
9. ☐ Other _____

G. Where Accident Happened (check one only)

1. ☐ Athletic Field	5. ☐ Hallway	9. ☐ Stairway
2. ☐ Cafeteria	6. ☐ Playground	10. ☐ To or from school
3. ☐ Classroom	7. ☐ Restroom	11. ☐ Vocational Shops and Labs.
4. ☐ Gym	8. ☐ School bus	12. ☐ Other _____

III.   CONTRIBUTING CAUSES

A. Environmental Factors (check one only)	B. Human Factors (check one only)	C. Agents (check one only)
1. ☐ Crowding	1. ☐ Active game	1. ☐ Animal or insect
2. ☐ Doors	2. ☐ Fatigue	2. ☐ Electricity
3. ☐ Drinking fountain	3. ☐ Fighting	3. ☐ Fire
4. ☐ Equipment	4. ☐ Horseplay	4. ☐ Gases
5. ☐ Floors	5. ☐ Lack of training or experience	5. ☐ Liquids
6. ☐ Hard surface	6. ☐ Preoccupation	6. ☐ Recreation equipment
7. ☐ Lighting	7. ☐ Running	7. ☐ Pencil
8. ☐ No handrail	8. ☐ Violation of rules	8. ☐ School equipment
9. ☐ Weather	9. ☐ Other _____	9. ☐ Solids
10. ☐ Other _____		10. ☐ Student
		11. ☐ Vehicle
		12. ☐ Other _____

Figure 8–4

Illustration continued on opposite page.

There are two major roles to be considered in the Education for Safe Living programs. One is the role of the community, and the other the role of the school. The community has its role to play in establishing and enforcing safety regulations and giving adequate publicity to hazardous situations. Operations are maintained for police and fire protection, building inspections, highway safety, gas and power lines, and emergency care units in local hospitals. The concerned community will also follow up certain accidents, so that they may be prevented from recurring. A city health department, for example, may survey the problem of lead poisoning in children, with emphasis on the defects in institutions which make this problem possible, and what can be done about them. Also, agencies work together; they work *with* community residents to control ac-

---

IV.   ACCIDENT DESCRIPTION

Describe the accident in your own words. Please give all details so that this accident report may be used to prevent other similar accidents.

V.   POST ACCIDENT INFORMATION

A. Was first aid given? Yes ☐ No ☐ By whom _____

Describe _____

B. Was parent or other responsible person notified? Yes ☐ No ☐ By whom _____ Time _____

If no, explain _____

C. Does health record indicate tetanus immunization currently effective? Yes ☐ No ☐

D. Was student sent home? Yes ☐ No ☐ If yes, was he accompanied? Yes ☐ No ☐

E. Was student sent to physician? Yes ☐ No ☐ Name of physician _____

F. Was student sent to hospital emergency room? Yes ☐ No ☐ Name of hospital _____

G. Days absent _____

VI.   ACTION TAKEN TO PREVENT SIMILAR ACCIDENT

                 I. Instructional   II. Policy, or Corrective Action

1. ☐ Discussed at staff meeting   1. ☐ Environmental changes effected
2. ☐ Discussed in each class as part of regular 2. ☐ Notified school safety committee
        instruction   3. ☐ Safety rules amended to prevent recurrence
3. ☐ Discussed with parent   4. ☐ Safety specialist invited to school to assist
4. ☐ Personal instruction given to student   in safety program
5. ☐ Personal instruction given to teacher in charge 5. ☐ Suggest closer supervision
6. ☐ Presented as a subject of assembly program

                              III. Other

                        1. ☐ No action taken

VII.

Signed _____ Title _____

Teacher _____

Other Witnesses _____

_____

Ohio Department of Health, Accident Prevention Unit
4966.10 Rev. 9-68

Figure 8-4 *Continued*

cidental deaths and injuries as well as violence and other unhealthful conditions. These activities are planned so as to involve the cooperative efforts of industry, local government, citizens, and school teachers.

The role of the school is to work within the community safety education framework. School building inspections are made by specialists. The health and safety of youth in the school environment, however, is everyone's interest. There is a way for this interest to relate to instruction.

Most schools today require the filing of accident report forms. After a year or two, these forms may be reviewed in order to find out what kinds of accidents are occurring in the schools. Most of these accident report forms provide a good amount of information useful in the classroom (Figure 8–4). Unfortunately, they are often stored away and forgotten.

A particularly fine feature of the Ohio report form is as follows:

ACTION TAKEN TO PREVENT SIMILAR ACCIDENTS

I. Instructional

1. ☐ Discussed at staff meeting.
2. ☐ Discussed in each class as part of regular instruction.
3. ☐ Discussed with parent.
4. ☐ Personal instruction given to student.
5. ☐ Personal instruction given to teacher in charge.
6. ☐ Presented as a subject of assembly program.

II. Policy or Corrective Action

1. ☐ Environmental changes effected.
2. ☐ Notified school safety committee.
3. ☐ Safety rules amended to prevent recurrence.
4. ☐ Safety specialist invited to school to assist in safety program.
5. ☐ Suggest closer supervision.

III. Other

1. ☐ No action taken.

THE PROGRAM

As in all other major health areas, the total scope of the safety program should be spread out from kindergarten to twelfth grade, in order to plan progressions and not to omit important considerations at various grade levels.

In most schools, safety education is not a separate subject. It is usually a part of the health education course. From time to time, and depending on local circumstances, safety has been treated separately. This has occurred in highly industrialized communities and farming areas where accident rates have been high. However, what is needed in Detroit, Michigan, may not need a great amount of attention in the hills of Tennessee. Likewise, New Hampshire has capitalized on firearm safety at the early junior high school level because hunting is so popular among youths in the state.

Driver education is a topic all by itself, taught by a specialist who is familiar with mechanical and electrical teaching devices and other program aids. It is not usually a part of the safety units in the health education course. This does not preclude reference to driving accidents and problems in the health class. In fact, where a school does not have any driver education program, an effort will have to be made to include some of the special content under safety in the health classes.

In a number of schools the *first aid* emphasis is so complete at each secondary level

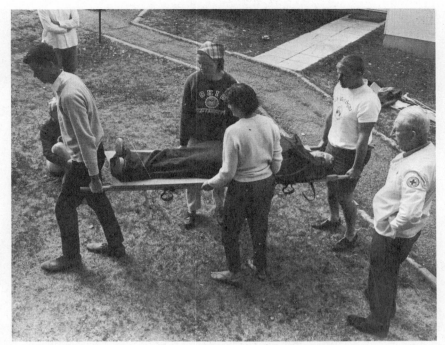

Figure 8–5 Students in a first aid course practice carrying a victim with a litter. (Courtesy of American National Red Cross)

that the major area is referred to as first aid and safety. Some schools find it very practical to plan programs in cooperation with the local chapter of the American Red Cross.

Of especially sound value is a high school course in *emergency medical services*—those that take place between the time of the incident and the time the victim is brought into a hospital for emergency medical *care*. This is more than a standard first aid course. It can be as much as an 80-hour course in Emergency Care and Transportation of the Sick and Injured, worked out by the American Academy of Orthopaedic Surgeons. Certainly, it should include cardiopulmonary resuscitation (CPR), the emergency technique demanded when heart and lungs fail. It includes mouth to mouth breathing and rhythmic pressure on the heart—a technique which must be practiced to be effective (see Figures 8–6 and 8–7). Superb practice equipment can be obtained from several sources. Resuscitation Annie and Resuscitation Andy are training mannequins available from Dyna-Med, P.O. Box 2157, Leucadia, Calif. 92024. The Resusa-Kate mannequin (24-inch baby) and the Med-E-Train mannequin are available from Simulaids, Tinker Road, Woodstock, N.Y. 12498. The latter mannequin is so life-like it can bleed, has a carotid pulse, a CPR indicator to teach the exact amount of pressure needed to supply oxygenated blood to the brain, and a broken bone simulation arrangement.

The high school *safety council* is an excellent teaching organization, wherein the gathering of knowledge and behavior ideas is indirect. By being concerned with the day-to-day hazardous conditions and accidents, the members of the council learn much about their immediate world and how to live in it without becoming a statistic of some kind. The task of the safety council is to reach the entire student body and thereby effect certain helpful changes in the life of the school.

At the secondary level the proposed program should center on the following assumptions:

1. A great number of accidents can be prevented.

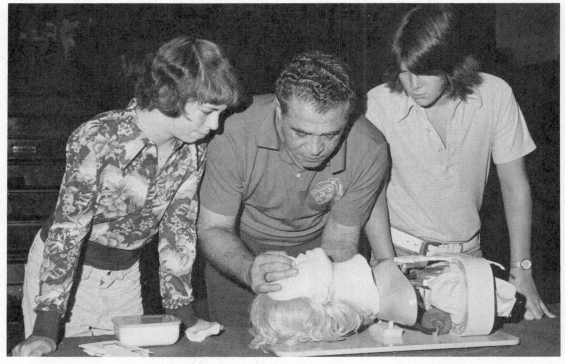

Figure 8–6 Mouth to mouth resuscitation instruction in Sunland Junior High School, Jacksonville, Florida. (Courtesy of American Alliance for Health, Physical Education, and Recreation)

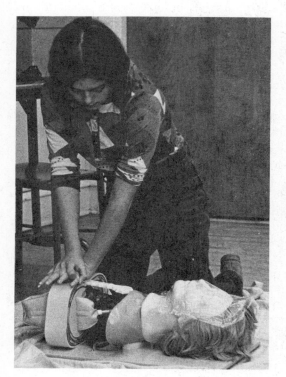

Figure 8–7 Eighth grader practicing cardiopulmonary resuscitation on Atomic Anne, the "dummy," in a medical emergency lesson. (Courtesy of Tacoma, Washington, Public Schools)

2. Accidents can be averted if people are aware of hazards and desire to follow safe practices.

3. One should assume the responsibility for his safety and for the safety of others.

4. It is desirable to appreciate the aesthetic characteristics of a healthful environment.

5. Frequent re-evaluation and readjustment of safety practices are essential to safe living.

The program guides in a number of towns and cities are well constructed. This is particularly true in such places as Philadelphia; Trenton, New Jersey; and Rochester, New York. The State Education Department materials of Pennsylvania, New York, Florida, and Indiana are also well presented. The recommended programs are somewhat alike in safety and accident prevention. They vary from very little exposure to first aid to a graduated first aid experience, junior high through senior high. In the Rochester program there is a combination of both safety practices and first aid early in the junior high school.[8]

ROCHESTER, NEW YORK, JUNIOR HIGH SCHOOL SAFETY AND FIRST AID MEASURES

A. Accidents and their prevention
1. In the home:
   falls, poisons, fire
2. In the school:
   a. gymnasium, play areas, pool, home economics rooms, shops, laboratories, classrooms, and in and around the building.
   b. fire drills and air raid alerts.
3. In the community:
   agencies dealing with safety— Chamber of Commerce, Police Bureau, Settlement Houses, Youth Board and Recreation.
4. Year round recreational areas: commercial, amusement centers, swimming areas, playgrounds, parks, boating and sailing areas, skiing and water skiing areas, and hunting and fishing areas.
5. At work:
   safety in various types of occupations.
6. On the highway:
   driver, passenger, and pedestrian safety; bicycle and vehicle safety.
B. First Aid
1. Wounds:
   types, first aid, follow-up care.
2. Mouth to mouth artificial respiration.
3. Other injuries:
   severe bleeding, poisonings, bone and joint injuries, shock, burns, bites, and stings.
4. Conditions:
   heat and cold—sunstroke, fainting, heat exhaustion, frostbite, exposure.
5. Basic bandaging.
6. Basic transportation.
7. At the scene of an accident.
8. First aid supplies in and away from home.

---

[8]Junior High School Curriculum Materials, *Health Education Grades 8–9,* City School District, Rochester, New York.

In the Philadelphia schools the safety area is outlined at both secondary levels, and is followed by a survey test to determine where pupils are weak on first aid information. Safety content for a combination of grades 10, 11, and 12 is as follows:

PHILADELPHIA, PENNSYLVANIA
GRADES 10, 11, 12
SAFETY

I. Introduction
   A. Nature of safety problem.
II. Vehicular Safety
   A. Characteristics of drivers
      1. Undesirable qualities:
         a. egotism
         b. show-off
         c. over-emotional
         d. rationalization
         e. thwarted
      2. Desirable qualities:
         a. driving skill
         b. ability to adjust
         c. maturity
         d. good social attitudes
   B. Safety education for the driver
      1. In school
      2. By insurance companies and agencies
      3. Through state and federal programs
         a. vehicle code
         b. road signs and signals
   C. Conclusions
      1. Driving is a privilege conferred by society.
      2. Obligation to others using highway.
III. Occupational and School Safety
   A. Incidence of hazards in industry
      1. Least in well organized and highly mechanized plants and occupations.
      2. Highest in farming

   B. School safety
      1. General safety regulations for school activities in the following areas:
         a. gymnasiums, locker and shower rooms
         b. lunch rooms, recreational areas, and lounges
         c. outdoor sports and recreational areas
         d. laboratories, shops, and classrooms
         e. corridor, stairways, and exits
IV. Accidents in the home
   A. Frequency
   B. Types
      1. Falls
      2. Electrical accidents
      3. Burns, scalds
      4. Explosions, asphyxiation
      5. Poisonings
      6. Minor accidents (cuts, bruises, scratches)
   C. Emergency precautions
V. Other Accidents
   A. Transportation (except private car and travel)
   B. Recreational accidents
   C. Falls, exclusive of home (ice, poor sidewalk maintenance, etc.)
First Aid
   Survey Test (followed by outline of content)

NEW YORK STATE

GRADES 7, 8, 9 SAFETY EDUCATION	GRADES 10, 11, 12 FIRST AID AND SURVIVAL EDUCATION
I. The Accident Problem	I. Transportation of the Injured
II. Safe Behavior	II. Automobile Accidents
III. Safety in the Home	III. Conditions Resulting from a Nuclear Explosion
IV. Safety in the School	IV. Chemical Warfare
V. Safety in Physical and Recreational Activities	V. Natural Catastrophes
VI. Safety at Work	VI. Psychological First Aid
VII. Safety in Driving and Walking	
VIII. Safety in Civil Emergencies	

If space permitted, it would be advantageous to set forth the detailed content outline from the New York State guides. This would show a gradual progression of topics from grades 7, 8, and 9 to grades 10, 11, and 12. Only the major headings are shown in the accompanying list.[9]

Behavioral Objectives

(Junior High Level)

Illustrates how new inventions and discoveries create hazards in the environment.

Explains that potential dangers are inherent in many activities; activities such as walking, bicycling, and boating can be safe or unsafe; with proper precautions most injuries can be avoided.

Demonstrates the way prompt care given in emergencies can save lives and prevent further injury.

Demonstrates a knowledge and practice of safety rules in recreational activities to prevent accidents.

Articulates and shows how water safety instruction can prevent needless accidents and develop skills for leisure hours.

Shows why accurate knowledge is important in handling an emergency situation.

Charts evidence to show how accidents are caused by a combination of events, each of which may be subject to human control.

Explains that individuals cannot always live safely by themselves since the attitudes of others affect them.

Acknowledges that the major causes of injuries in the home are falls and fires.

Participates and explains that through the close cooperation of students and school personnel, safety hazards in the school environment can be significantly reduced.

Demonstrates how there should be two persons in a boat for water skiing, one as the operator and the other as the observer.

Explains that the main task of a babysitter is to prevent accidents and injury while providing adequate care for children.

Tells how the atomic and nuclear weapons are the most destructive weapons ever created by man.

Diagrams the manner in which various kinds of storms are capable of mass destruction of property and injury to people.

Shows a number of ways in which first aid includes only immediate and temporary care until professional assistance can be obtained.

Illustrates a number of rules used in physical education activities designed to develop good safety practices.

Explains how smoking in bed is a prime contributor to house fires.

Behavioral Objectives

(Senior High Level)

Tells how the application of safety practices in industrial, recreational, and school activities adds to their enjoyment and value by helping to prevent accidents.

Explains that as civilization expands and the environment is further explored, new hazards are added to man's health.

---

[9]Strand V Education for Survival, *Safety Education for Grades 7, 8, and 9,* and *First Aid and Survival Education for Grades 10, 11, and 12,* Albany, New York: The State Education Department, 1970.

Demonstrates how the application of emergency medical procedures enhances survival when major disasters occur.

Acknowledges that total community planning is needed to establish effective environmental controls which consider all factors affecting man.

Analyzes the great impact of forces involved in many automobile accidents; there is usually more than one type of injury, and these are frequently of a complex rather than simple nature.

Shows how penetrating radiation has damaging effects on the body tissues.

Illustrates how injuries occurring from tornadoes, hurricanes, earthquakes, and winter storms include almost every type.

Explains the way an emotionally upset person may present a danger to himself as well as to those around him.

Outlines how violence, which sets the stage for injuries, may be brought about by such items as overcrowded living conditions, dehumanized populations of people, and general fear and distrust of one's fellow man.

Speaks out, and makes clear that safe automobile driving includes the use of seat belts and shoulder straps, abstinence from alcoholic beverages, and a respect for the rights of others.

Practices correct sport and recreational skills, coupled with courtesy during the activity, in order to realize more fun and fewer mishaps.

Depicts clearly that the highest liability insurance premiums are paid by the 16 to 25 year age group because of their high accident rate.

Promotes the concept that industries make provisions to promote the physical welfare of their employees by researching items such as the effect of fatigue upon production, health, and safety.

Examines the number of safety standards and legal factors involved in the construction of buildings, roads, bridges, and other structures.

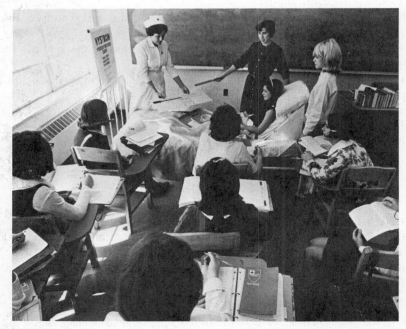

Figure 8–8   Home nursing course—a community service. (Courtesy of American National Red Cross)

Visits several official and non-official health agencies which are directly concerned with such areas as child safety, automobile safety, industrial safety, and school safety; they advance the concept of public responsibility for the prevention of accidents.

Suggested Activities

(Junior High Level)

1. Promote home safety by giving a slide presentation designed to test pupil knowledge of hazardous home situations and how to avoid or handle them. The National Safety Council (425 N. Michigan, Chicago, Ill. 60611) has a 16-page script to accompany the slides for *What's Your Home Safety I.Q.?*

2. Create a bulletin board display of news clippings depicting fires, falls, drownings, auto mishaps, bicycle accidents, airplane crashes, and freak accidents. Encourage all class members to contribute.

3. Engineer a fire drill. Have some pupils practice using a fire extinguisher.

4. Demonstrate and practice a variety of first aid skills. Solicit help from the personnel of the local chapter of the American Red Cross.

5. Request that each class member make a written inventory report of the contents of the medicine chest in his home. This may be extended to an inventory of first aid supplies.

6. Appoint a small group to prepare discussion content for the following statement:

"Most accidents are man-made and can be prevented."

7. Visit the office of the school nurse or person who collects school accident reports. If possible, scrutinize the reports over the past year or two and look for such items as kinds of accidents, locations, parts of body affected, and time of day. Return to the classroom and discuss the consequences of the accidents and what might be done to prevent them from recurring.

8. Consider the establishment of a school safety council. Prepare a list of projects that might be the responsibility of the safety council. Invite the class to comment on how effective such a council might be. Could it be just another committee?

9. Talk over safe driving and sportsmanlike practices. Make this real by street corner observations. Ask the class to analyze neighboring intersections and report some of the observed driving behaviors. Note evidences of anxiety, anger, and emotional outbursts.

10. Display a chart showing the number of accidental deaths and injuries to pedestrians. Discuss jaywalking as a contributing factor. Note also that at least a quarter of all pedestrian accidents involve alcohol consumption by the pedestrian. Is jaywalking a problem in the *local community?* Do "walk" lights help reduce the accident rate very much?

11. To clearly define accidents, present two situations:[10]

Situation A: When an airplane crashes, investigators search back in time from the scene of the crash to try to find the point at which the situation went out of control. That is where the accident happened, not where the plane crashed.

Situation B: A tornado. Since the weather cannot be controlled, it is not possible to prevent these kinds of natural events. But one can reduce the consequences of these events by taking shelter, building stronger buildings, fleeing from the storm, and so on.

---

[10]It is the contention of a number of people from the National Safety Council that safety suffers from a lack of clear definition. See article by Kenneth F. Licht, "Safety and Accidents – A Brief Conceptual Analysis, and a Point of View," *Journal of School Health,* 45:530–533, November, 1975.

Having discussed the situations, submit the following definition for consideration:

> AN ACCIDENT IS A SUDDEN UNPLANNED
> EVENT WHICH HAS THE POTENTIAL FOR PRODUCING
> INJURY OR DAMAGE

12. Stress the cooperative action in a school to eliminate safety hazards. Identify special provisions the school has made for:

safety of handicapped children
safety while changing classes or during school dismissal
safety in unorganized games
school bus and school traffic safety

13. Build a display of different types of protective sports equipment. When the display is complete, have different pupils explain to the class how each particular piece of equipment protects the wearer against injury. Such items as the following are readily obtainable:

hockey helmet
football shoulder pad
archery arm guard
soccer shoe
downhill ski binding
fencing mask
baseball batting hat
scuba diving suit
shin pads
hockey gloves
athletic cup supporter
eyeglass protector

14. Prepare a checklist in school that can be duplicated and given to each pupil to take home. Such a home safety checklist will supply information that can be tabulated and discussed in a later class. For example, see Table 8–2.

15. Practice mouth to mouth resuscitation on a mannequin. If the school does not own one (such as Resuscitation Annie), it may be possible to borrow one from the local chapter of the American Red Cross.

16. Study the places where bone fractures are apt to happen in a community. Where

TABLE 8–2   Home Safety Checklist

	YES	NO
Is the house kept neat and tidy?		
Are floors slippery?		
Are steps and railings safe?		
Is there adequate lighting?		
Are steps clear, not slippery?		
Are there safety rails on the sides of the steps?		
Does placement of furniture cause hazards?		
Is there an emergency phone number list?		
Are electric wires carelessly placed?		
Are combustible items away from the stove?		
Are cupboards cluttered?		
Is a rubber mat used in the bathtub?		
Is the medicine cabinet out of reach of children?		
Are home tools used and stored properly?		

Figure 8–9

THE SAFETY IDEA IS OLD

Long before man, prehistoric animals herded together to protect one another. The ancient cave man built a fire at the mouth of his cave to safeguard his family, and he probably had rules of fire prevention. Four thousand years ago King Hammurabi of Babylon made a safety law: "If a builder builds a house for a man, and does not make its construction firm, the builder shall be put to death."

do most breaks occur in an individual? Secure copies of x-ray film from a local hospital or physician's office to show what breaks and hairline fractures look like. Breaks due to skiing accidents are particularly interesting.

17. Obtain several copies of the Johnson and Johnson programmed text, *First Aid (Revised)* (200 Madison Ave., New York, N.Y. 10016). More than 25 topics are covered in an interesting fashion. Distribute individual copies to students to work on independently.

18. Appoint a group to design charts for bulletin board displays to show insects that bite or sting. Poison ivy, poison oak, and poison sumac may also be displayed, preferably in colored picture form rather than the real leaves.

19. Establish safety and first aid vocabulary lists. These lists can be used in a number of ways. In fact, a game situation can be created by having one person give a definition and having another person suggest the vocabulary word.

20. Discuss building regulations in a town or city. How regulatory should they be? Ask the local building inspector or one of his assistants to come to class to lead the discussion. See Figure 8–9.

21. Display the sign in Figure 8–10, and open up a discussion of home poisonings. Over 500,000 people—mostly children—are accidentally poisoned a year by household products. Have the class report stories *they* have heard about. Examples:

"A two and a half year old girl ingested cough medicine. The mother gave the medicine to her child during the night and left the bottle on the kitchen counter."

"A two year old boy swallowed furniture polish. The mother had given him cough syrup which was the same color as the furniture polish. He meant to take the cough syrup."

"A two year old boy swallowed bleach. His cousin had been using it in the bathroom and had placed it in a cup."

Figure 8–10

HAPPINESS

IS A

SAFE HOME

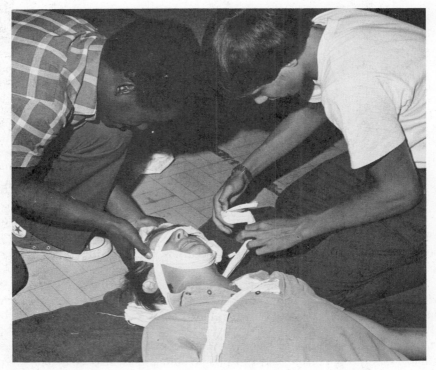

Figure 8–11 Safety education program on the spot in Jacksonville, Florida. (Courtesy of American Alliance for Health, Physical Education, and Recreation)

"A 15 month old child ingested nitroglycerine tablets that had been put on the top shelf of the medicine cabinet. Mother did not know the child could climb."
"A 16 month old boy swallowed mothballs. He had gotten into a dresser drawer. His mother was unaware that he could open drawers."

22. Look over the excellent films available from Aetna Life and Casualty Company, having to do with highway safety, seat belts, and recreation safety. They are appropriate for junior high school viewing.

Suggested Activities

(Senior High Level)
1. Plan an in-depth study of drinking and driving. With class committees outline suggested content using scientific input from a county or state law enforcement agency. This can be supplemented with an excellent film which shows *exactly* what alcohol does to the driver: *How Drinking Affects Driving,* available from Media Five, 1011 N. Cole, Hollywood, Calif. 90038.
2. Look into research pertaining to human engineering. What are the limitations of human sensitivity to environmental hazards? For helpful suggestions have a student review several volumes of the McGraw-Hill Company texts, *Product Engineering.* This reading activity could be done in connection with the reading of *Consumer Reports* magazine.
3. Carry out a Driver Education Survey in the school that will sample the opinions

TABLE 8-3   How Do You Feel Toward Driver Education?

a. I oppose high school driver education. □
b. The reasons I oppose it include:
    1. There is no evidence that it reduces accidents. □
    2. It is not the school's job. □
    3. It tends to have kids drive sooner than otherwise. □
    4. It's too expensive. □
    5. Other reasons. □
c. I favor high school driver education. □
d. The reasons I favor it include:
    1. It helps reduce traffic accidents. □
    2. It helps develop good attitudes and citizenship. □
    3. Every beginning driver needs instruction, and the schools are the logical
       institution for this task. □
    4. Schools have a legal and moral responsibility to teach general safety, and
       driver education is part of that over-all responsibility. □
    5. Other reasons. □
e. Driver education should be:
    1. Financed by the state or federal government. □
    2. Financed with school funds, the same as any other course. □
    3. Financed at least in part by the individual student. □
    4. Financed entirely by the student. □

of sophomores, juniors, seniors, teachers, and administrators. Find out how effective people feel driver education to be. Sample questions are shown in Table 8-3.

4. For many people this has become an outdoor world of parks, recreation, and conservation. Study some of the potential hazards in such an environment. For example, there are 132 species of snakes in the U.S.; only 19 are poisonous—rattlesnakes, copperheads, water moccasins, and coral snakes. Poisonous plants, of which there are more than 700, can also be discussed, such as poison hemlock, wild carrot, jimsonweed, and buttercups. See Table 8-4.

5. Administer a school safety quiz to find out how much high school pupils actually know about accidents and safety practices. An already prepared 160-item test, *How Much Do Your Pupils Know?*, is available for reproduction from the National Safety Council.

6. Have a committee examine the sample materials on fire protection available from the National Fire Protection Association (Boston, Mass. 02110). Their tests, leaflets, booklets, posters, and audio-visual items are quite extensive and for the most part are well designed for school use. Their safety checklists and suggested activities for children of all ages are appropriate for study by senior high school students.

7. Set up a home electrical survey for each class member. In a recent Ohio study, four out of five homes were inadequately wired, with electricity being second to smoking as a cause of fires (see Figure 8-12). Such a survey will acquaint students with their house circuit box and the wattage it takes to run appliances (a circulating fan requires 85 watts, while a deep fat fryer or roaster takes 1350 watts).

8. Experiment with fabrics and fire. Burn some fabrics in a controlled laboratory situation. Investigate each of the following factors by examining wearing apparel and textiles:
    a. Synthetic fibers and cotton, linen, silk, and rayon
    b. Weight and weave of material (tightly woven articles burn more slowly)
    c. Surface of the fabric (fine fibers ignite more readily)
    d. Design of the garment (close fitting garments are less hazardous)

9. As a group, review sample pedestrian safety materials from the American Automobile Association. Have a class committee evaluate the materials for use with younger children. In short, begin to saddle older children with a certain amount of re-

TABLE 8-4　Potentially Dangerous Plants

PLANT	TOXIC PART	SYMPTOMS AND TOXICITY
Yew	berries, foliage	fatal—foliage more toxic than berries
Golden Chain	seeds, pods	next to yew, the most poisonous of trees
Poison Ivy	leaves, berries, stem	serious skin rash from bodily contact
Poison Sumac	leaves, berries, stem	same as above
Deadly Nightshade	berries	poisonous to children
Jimsonweed	seeds or flower nectar	poisonous to children
Castor Bean	berries (seed)	one or two castor bean seeds near lethal dose for adults.
Larkspur (delphinium)	seeds, foliage, roots	digestive upset
February Daphne	berries	very poisonous
Foxglove	leaves	can be fatal
Rhubarb	leaves	raw or cooked leaves cause severe poisoning, convulsions, coma
Wisteria	seeds, pods	mild to severe digestive upset
Hyacinth Narcissus Daffodil	bulbs	nausea, vomiting, diarrhea
Dumb Cane	stalk	throat irritation and swelling of tongue
Poinsettia	leaves	poisonous if eaten
Lantana	berries	poisonous to children
Philodendron	leaves	contain an irritant
Mistletoe	berries	fatal
Jerusalem Cherry	berries	may be poisonous
English Ivy	leaves, berries	can be fatal

sponsibility for younger brothers, sisters, and friends. For senior high pupils, the films *The Final Factor* or *Emergencies in the Making* (AAA) should stimulate automobile safety.

10. Research sun tanning and the laws of heat and the human skin. Does sun worship make sense or can it be overdone? For a list of brand-names of tanning lotions and their effects as sun preparations, see spring-summer editions of *Today's Health* and *Consumer Reports.*

11. Consider a project to test the engineering of ski bindings. Considerable help can be secured from a local ski shop where machines are available to test the toe and heel stresses and relate them to release capabilities. Both forward fall release and torsional release can be related to leg fractures if appropriate x-ray film is available. For winter sports enthusiasts, this can be a very worthwhile project. (See also Outwater and Ettlinger, "The Engineering of Ski Bindings," *Medicine and Science in Sports,* 1:200–204, December, 1969, for currently useful diagrams of lines of force and mathematical equations.)

12. During or following a "cold snap," discuss the effect of wind on freezing conditions involving the skin. For example, according to the U.S. Army Wind Chill Index (Table 8–5), the effect of a 30 mph wind at 10° F is the same as being exposed to a temperature of −33° F on a calm day. This may be related to outside work and recreation, and to frostbite.

13. Chart, for display, the various circumstances associated with leisure time. Recreation is big business. Added to this is the fact that more people have a greater amount of leisure time than ever before. Investigate "Danger Days"—e.g., Christmas with 900 or more deaths over three days due to motor vehicle accidents. Trains and buses are the safest means of travel, followed by airplanes. Turnpikes are the safest roads, while two thirds of the people are killed not far from their own homes.

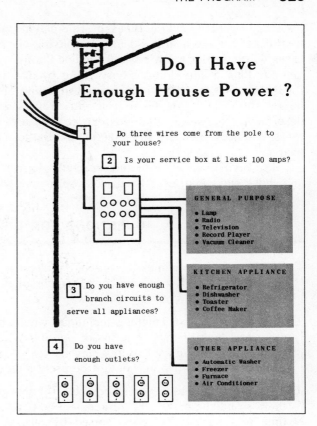

Figure 8–12 Education for running a home. (Courtesy of Ohio Dept. of Health)

14. Display the three E's:

ENGINEERING
ENFORCEMENT
EDUCATION

Have three different student groups prepare statements in each area related to accident prevention and safety.

15. Collect current accident statistics from government reports, from voluntary agencies such as insurance companies, AAA, and the National Safety Council, and from news clippings. Post the figures for all to see. Do the class members *believe* the figures? Is there some feeling that they may be a little higher than they really should be? Do people usually trust statistics? If there is a "credibility gap," is this the fault of the statistician or research worker, or the fault of the reader?

TABLE 8–5 U.S. Army Wind Chill Index

Equivalent temperature in cooling power on exposed flesh under calm conditions.

TEMP	30	20	10	0	−10	−20	−30
Wind (Miles Per Hour)							
10	16	2	−9	−22	−31	−45	−58
15	11	−6	−18	−33	−45	−60	−70
20	3	−9	−24	−40	−52	−68	−81
25	0	−15	−29	−45	−58	−75	−89
30	−2	−18	−33	−49	−63	−78	−94
35	−4	−20	−35	−52	−67	−83	−98
40	−4	−22	−36	−54	−69	−87	−101

Wind speeds above 40 mph have little additional chilling effect.

16. Organize several types of role-playing accident situations requiring first aid treatment. Initiate a first aid unit by having class members come in contact with the cases without prior knowledge of the conditions. What should be done?

17. Play a situation-response game by dividing the class into pairs. One student reads the description of an emergency situation; his partner has two minutes to tell what he or she would do. Then, roles are reversed as another emergency situation is described. Emergency situations can be built around drownings, fires, heat exhaustion, recreation accidents, and so on (see Engs, Barnes, and Wantz reference at the end of this chapter).

18. Invite a speaker on nuclear energy to lead a class discussion about intense light and shock wave injuries. Also discuss burns, and the social implications of a nuclear age.

QUESTIONS FOR DISCUSSION

1. Employing health games to stimulate interest in safety is practiced by some teachers. A question arises as to whether this technique can be overused, especially with high school students. What is your view?

2. How effective as a teaching technique would it be to have a class visit a large toy store and look at toys in terms of possible hazards? Glass, pins, sharp edges, electrical units, and other features may be visible and hazardous. Could the class profit from such a field trip or would it be useless unless the toys could be taken apart?

3. How much of a topic for senior high school investigation is accident-proneness? Is there so much apathy toward accident statistics that we don't have the inclination or time to separate accidents caused by hazardous products from those caused by maladjusted people?

4. Human ecology and environmental hazards go hand in hand. How do you see this relationship being discussed in the classroom? Would it be more effective in the junior high school or senior high?

5. In establishing goals for the late seventies, many writers, even when they are quite practical in their suggestions, fail to say anything substantial about the need for attention to safe living. Why is this? Is it, perhaps, that safety is a less than popular topic?

6. Would adult education for parents of school-age children be workable? Could child psychology, child safety, and such topics be taught in a meaningful way so that accidental injuries to children and youths could be reduced? What do you think of the idea?

7. How would you involve a senior high school group in planning for emergency medical services? How might they be motivated to get started?

8. Is there a way to use the school nurse or physician in the junior high safety program that will dramatize the seriousness of accident prevention? How might this be accomplished?

SUGGESTED ACTIVITIES

1. Safety is used in several contexts, which makes a difference in how it is received. Examine safety in the context of health, security, accident prevention, and accident mitigation. For help, review the Licht reference at the end of the chapter.

2. Human engineering as applied to accident prevention and safety education has become an in-depth kind of business. Examine some of the copies of *Consumer Reports* for examples of product information discovered through careful research. See also some of the back volumes of the McGraw-Hill Company publication *Product Engineering*.

3. Interview a representative from the American Automobile Association about the future of automobile driving practices and accidental deaths and injuries. What are the next steps to insure driver safety? Realistically, can accident statistics be reduced very much as the population grows and overcrowding continues?

4. Several years ago the safety people associated with the Health Education Division (now American Association for the Advancement of Health Education) of AAHPER broke away and started the Safety Division. It was felt that safety as a topic was big enough to stand on its own along with health education. Interview several health teachers and see if they think this was a worthwhile happening. Should safety have stayed within the division concerned with all health education? Is it any more important than mental health or drug education?

5. In every major health topic it is the express wish of the teacher to have pupils become personally involved. The more pupils one teaches, however, the more difficult it is to realize 100 per cent student involvement. Suggest some ways in which safety education can be made personally effective to pupils. Relate it to their status, to their peers, and to their day-to-day activities.

6. Plan a visit to a local school to see what is done in terms of environmental safety by school health services, custodians, administrators, and classroom teachers. Find out how often fire drills are held. Is there a school safety council? Are accident records kept? If so, what are they used for? Compare your findings with those of others doing the same investigation.

SELECTED REFERENCES

Clarke, Kenneth S. "Values and Risk-Taking Behavior: The Concept of Calculated Risk," *Health Education*, 6:26–29, November/December, 1975.

Engs, Ruth C., S. Eugene Barnes, and Molly Wantz. *Health Games Students Play: Creative Strategies for Health Education*, Dubuque, Iowa: Kendall-Hunt Publishing Co., 1975. Chapter 12.

Kraus, Jess F., et al. "The Effectiveness of a New Touch Football Helmet to Reduce Head Injuries," *Journal of School Health*, 40:496–500, November, 1970.

Licht, Kenneth F. "Safety and Accidents—A Brief Conceptual Analysis, and a Point of View," *Journal of School Health*, 45:530–534, November, 1975.

Mayshark, Cyrus, "Curriculum Development and Research for Safety Education." *Health Education*, 7:28–32, May–June, 1976.

Rinear, Charles E. "Emergency Care in the Inner City," *Health Education*, 6:6–10, May/June 1975.

Russell, Robert D. *Health Education*, Washington: American Alliance for Health, Physical Education and Recreation, 1975.

Thygerson, Alton L. "Safety In Health Education: Some Precautions," *Journal of School Health*, 44:508–511, November, 1974.

Willgoose, Carl E. "Educating for Safety," *Instructor*, 81:62–63, February, 1971.

Yamaguchi, Seiya, et al. "Factors Affecting the Amount of Mercury in Human Scalp Hair," *American Journal of Public Health*, 65:484–488, May, 1975.

Chapter 9

Effective Methodology and Teaching Aids

"I have found by experience that what my hearers seem least to relish is analytical technicality, and what they most care for is concrete practical application. So I have gradually weeded out the former, and left the latter unreduced; and, now that I have at last written out the lectures, they contain a minimum of what is deemed "scientific"... and are practical and popular in the extreme."

— *William James*

In his search for "what holds attention" William James set forth in grand style what he believed to be the substantial considerations in teaching. His classic work of 1899, *Talks to Teachers on Psychology,* demonstrates fairly well the differing orientations of teachers — some leaning toward a scholarly emphasis, and others toward an emphasis on life-adjustment.

Hofstadter and others have made the point that the teaching emphasis on life-adjustment has led to anti-intellectualism.[1] Others have followed suit and claimed that the "science" supporting the subject matter area has suffered. Yet, the voice crying for James' "concrete practical application" of knowledge with its relationship to the everyday lives of people is heard again and again through the years. The result is a persistent problem. This disparity undoubtedly has much to do with the troubles of education, and why there are over a million secondary school dropouts each year. When questioned as to why they left school, these students tell the researchers in so many words that they were not in any way "moved" or "turned on" in school; no one raised their level of interest.

TEACHING AS AN ART

There was once a teacher
Whose principal feature
Was hidden in quite an odd way.
   Students by millions
   Or possibly zillions
Surrounded him all of the day.

---

[1]Richard Hofstadter, *Anti-intellectualism In American Life,* New York: Alfred A. Knopf, 1966, p. 320

When finally seen
By his scholarly dean
And asked how he managed the deed,
   He lifted three fingers
   And said, "All you swingers
   Need only to follow my lead.
   "To rise from a zero
   To Big Campus Hero,
   To answer these questions you'll strive:
     Where am I going,
     How shall I get there, and
     How will I know I've arrived?"

—Robert F. Mager[2]

Seeking improved ways to teach is a never-ending search. It is the business of the teacher, every bit as much as setting goals and defining the curriculum, for teaching is both a science and an art. Science is analytical: it breaks things up, seeks detail, and looks for causes. Art, on the other hand, is engaged in giving *meaning to experience;* it puts things together—synthesis rather than analysis. An education that will reduce venereal disease or mental health statistics, or teach the sexes how to live together in co-operative harmony, is an education that has to be real. Unfortunately, much of education isn't real; it isn't taught in relation to life at the moment, and students are simply unimpressed. If it isn't exciting, rigorous, and demanding, then emotional abandonment will prevail. Teaching as an art, therefore, cannot be fully developed unless it gets close to the person. Joseph Conrad said it very well in *Lord Jim* when he pointed out that youth must experience events that "... reveal the inner worth of man; the edge of his temper; the fibre of his stuff; the quality of his resistance; the secret truth of his pretenses, not only to himself, but to others." Getting at this is what method is all about.

METHODOLOGY AND HUMANISM IN EDUCATION

The meaning of the word *method* is interesting. In a cold, organizational sense, Webster defines it as "orderly procedure or process ... orderly arrangement." This is hardly an adequate meaning of the word unless one relates it to expected outcomes. It is the manner in which something is done in order to get somewhere. Or, as the popular song went from several decades ago—"It ain't what you do; it's the *way* that you do it."

Charles Silberman, writing in *Crisis in the Classroom,* points out that an uncomfortably large number of teachers never ask *why* they are doing what they are doing. Obsessed by lesson plans, controls, and routines, it becomes very difficult to get away from conformity and docility and encourage individual curiosity, creativity, and spontaneity. The better schools, says Silberman after completing his Carnegie Corporation study, are those which draw heavily on the ideas of Swiss psychologist Jean Piaget, who demonstrated that the student is the principal agent in his own education, and that learning is likely to be more effective if it grows out of what interests the learner, rather than what interests the teacher.

The preoccupation with the information half of the learning equation has dehumanized schools, alienated youth, and produced a system which is frequently irrelevant for many students. Emerson was aware of this when he wrote his essay of 1837, "The

---

[2]Robert F. Mager, *Developing Attitude Toward Learning,* Palo Alto, California: Fearon Publishers, 1968, p. VII.

American Scholar," which asserted the need for an education "by nature, by books, and by action." The key word was "action" in concert with the virtues of humor, understanding, and acceptance of individual differences. In its day this was a rather humanistic approach. In later years Julian Huxley sounded the same concern when he condemned science for isolationism and for not being " . . . a part of the total human process, in common harness with emotion, value, and purpose."[3] Looking to the year 1997 Kahn and Weiner see education meeting needs when it is ". . . worldly, naturalistic, realistic, visual, illusionistic, every-day, amusing, interesting, erotic, satirical, novel, eclectic, syncretic, fashionable, technically superb, impressionistic, materialistic, commercial, and professional."[4]

It is clear that the affective and humanistic dimension must accompany the cognitive elements in methodology. Indeed, health knowledge can be advanced in a way that will enhance self-concept, increase achievement motivation, clarify values and promote better human relations. Very much needed is:

1. Conviction that the teacher should serve more as a *facilitator of learning* than an imparter of information.

2. Conviction of the *dignity and worth of students*.

3. Attitude of *respect* for "different" individuals and life styles.

4. Conviction that the teachers' *personal decisions* concerning health actions are legitimately held.

5. Skills in *problem solving and decision making*.

6. Skills in working with problem students individually.

7. *Experiential learning* in which the learner shares more of the responsibility than merely sitting passively.

8. *Intrapersonal skills* for knowing oneself and handling inner feelings.

9. *Interpersonal skills* for relating effectively to others, including a sensitivity to nonverbal communication.

Indeed, awareness makes a difference in teaching. Good and Brophy demonstrated that instructional failure frequently occurs, not because of pupil indifference, but because of a lack of awareness of what transpires in the classroom.[5] Teachers, more than ever, are like actors in their concern with communicating and providing experiences for others. Very often the effectiveness of the communication will depend on how good an actor the teacher is. To say he needs to be a good actor does not mean that he has to use gimmicks and personality to persuade his students to a particular point of view, but simply that he must be free enough to use his own capabilities to express what he feels about his own subject matter. Too often among the health topics of the day, inability to express enthusiasm, love, and anger is interpreted by students as a lack of interest. Constantly on show, being observed and imitated, the teacher should be conscious of what it is he desires to communicate. Being detached and without a show of emotion causes students to quickly sense and be suspicious of a dichotomy between what the teacher says and what he feels.

Methods courses exist to unite the young and the old in imaginative considerations of learning. The school imparts information, but it imparts it imaginatively. Whitehead makes it clear that " . . . this atmosphere of excitement, arising from imaginative consid-

---

[3]Julian Huxley, *Knowledge, Morality and Destiny*, New York: Harper and Row, 1960, p. 250.

[4]Herman Kahn and Anthony J. Weiner, "The Next Thirty Years," *Daedalus*, 96:707, Summer, 1967.

[5]Thomas L. Good, Bruce J. Biddle, and Jere E. Brophy, *Teachers Make a Difference*, New York: Holt, Rinehart and Winston, 1975. p. 231.

erations, transforms knowledge. A fact is no longer a bare fact: it is invested with all its possibilities. It is no longer a burden on the memory: it is energizing as the poet of our dreams, and as the architect of our purposes.[6]

THE CREATIVE FORCE

Two roads diverged in a wood, and I—
I took the one less travelled by,
And that has made all the difference.

— Robert Frost

Thinking in terms of setting forth over the "less travelled" road was an act quite in keeping with Robert Frost that could well be considered a pronounced departure from tradition—literally a creative undertaking by a poet sympathetic to change.

In Shirley Jackson's eerie short story, "The Lottery," a village holds a drawing each year to decide whom they will stone to death. One character in Jackson's story raises a question about why the villagers continue to carry out this inhuman ritual, but an elder quiets him with, "We have always had a lottery."

So it is with numerous school practices. We have, indeed, always had them and have not seriously questioned them or researched their worth. Under such rigid circumstances creativity can hardly exist.

The process of creative renewal always implies an appeal from a tradition as it *is* to a tradition as it *ought* to be. The life force of a tradition is a spiritual reality—a kind of Promethean energy to vastly improve the nature of things. The creative individual, therefore, seeks a better way of reaching his objectives without being tied to the sciences, practices, and popular views of the moment.

Creative thinking in the health education area can be developed to a point where decisions for change are made, both in the program and in the health practices of youth. Inventive approaches are a possibility almost anywhere. There is some degree of creative drive in each person if it can be aroused.[7]

Rollo May, psychotherapist and author, joins forces with others in calling for a much more in-depth level of approach, if the real feelings of youth and adults are to be reached. He sees no other way to change value systems pertaining to aggression, violence, and communication.

In his deliberations, May points out that there is a tendency, in most circles, to deny that we engage in aggression and violence. Such expressions of inner drive seem too extreme to accept readily. Yet, aggression and violence are basic to the human power of the individual. This is the power to affirm oneself, or to be so moved as to assert oneself. People who know where they are going, or are at least quite determined, assert themselves in a number of ways all the time. However, when the need to assert oneself is blocked, the stage is set for aggressive behavior. And when there is no outlet here, violence follows.

This human creative power, or underlying drive, comes from what Socrates talked about in 399 B.C. when he was being tried for teaching false *deimon*. The deimon, says May, is below the conscience level—halfway between man and God (a kind of spirit)—a

---

[6]Alfred North Whitehead, *The Aim of Education and Other Essays,* New York: The New American Library of World Literature, Inc., 1949, p. 97.

[7]For further elaboration on creativity, see *Creative Teaching in Health,* 2nd edition, by Donald A. Read and Walter H. Greene, New York: Macmillan Company, 1975, Chapter 5.

natural power within a person. The Greeks looked upon the deimonic as the creative power of a person. It can go awry and become a destructive entity (evil), or be harnessed for good. The word is related to the Latin word "genius." Thus, brightness, creative power, and drive tend to go together.

In the struggle for human morality, there is a tendency to leave the deimon behind. But humans still push for what they want. Man still fights. William James was probably correct when he said there *is* an attraction in war. To arrive at a state of law and order and away from war and war-like behavior, one has to substitute James' "moral equivalent" of war. In short, there must be an outlet for powers and drives that will be individually satisfying. Evil will still be evil, and mankind will not completely solve the problems of violence, but he can put it into perspective and use it constructively, by transforming it into creativity.

Most students have some avenue through which the health-related message can be introduced. Once this is accomplished, it is not uncommon for a spark of a talent to become known. Discovering and nuturing creative talent is one of the imperatives of education. Failure to develop any human talent today is a personal tragedy. However, unless the teaching method provides ample time for pupils to examine, explore, discover, and "find themselves," there will be little hope that any great number of students will have a creative experience.

CHANGING HEALTH BEHAVIOR

Favorably influencing health practices is difficult at best. The trouble is that many of the early established patterns of behavior and their underlying beliefs and views are (by the secondary school years) deeply ingrained and frequently quite resistant to change. The student, with all his attitudes and practices gained from multitudinous sources, is not necessarily well-informed. With a hodge-podge of correct information and misinformation on hand, he stands before the teacher. He requires an integrated view of health and health behavior—easier said than done.

Changing health behavior is dependent on a combination of variables. Seven significant behavioral influences are as follows:

1. A number of *social influences* are required for the integrated view of health. Forces having their roots in the home, community agencies, and the peer group are important considerations. It is worth recalling that the burden of bringing up the next generation does not fall wholly on the shoulders of the home and school. There are many influences to be engineered. Effecting a cooperative approach is sometimes hard to do as life in the modern community becomes more and more impersonal, and people only a few blocks from a pupil's home are total strangers.

2. Positive *teacher characteristics* have much to do with rapport and learning. It may require a more at-ease and responsive person to teach health. In the Menninger Foundation paper, it was pointed out that many educators have such a strong sense of commitment, self-sacrifice, and dedication that they are tense and border on a "superego" orientation rather than a reality orientation with youth. In her research into the characteristics of teachers best suited to work closely with the health problems of youth, Juhasz found that "the ability to communicate and carry on frank and open discussions with students" was mentioned most frequently.[8] This was followed by "warmth, sensi-

---

[8]Anne M. Juhasz, "Characteristics Essential to Teachers in Sex Education," *Journal of School Health,* 40:17–18, Jaunuary, 1970.

tivity and availability of teachers." Non-authoritarian teaching techniques followed these, and last (not first) was "knowledge" of facts and resources.

3. The instructor's knowledge of *motivational techniques* makes it possible to move the class from the initiation phase into the mainstream of the study with some degree of sophistication. Motivational research indicates that in most cases, once students get their "feet wet" and their curiosity is tickled, they can be expected to stay reasonably interested in the material. Initiating a unit of instruction, therefore, has much to do with understanding and ultimate practices. Organizing a favorable experience around the person, early in the health unit, takes a certain amount of expertise, especially in those schools where classes run large and facilities are crowded. Even in such situations, varying the teaching methods as different major health units are introduced can be helpful in stimulating pupil interest and motivation. In one seventh grade, the instructor was a bit unhappy with his teaching and felt that the class was half asleep much of the time. So, the next day, when he was to introduce the topic of body structure and function, he had three boys arrive at the classroom five minutes late, carrying the human skeleton. One supported the head and shoulders, another the hips, and the third, the legs and feet. As they ambled into the room with their "subject," the class came alive, and questions came from all directions—including students who hadn't been heard from for weeks.

4. It is time-consuming, but teacher-student *cooperative planning* of health lessons pays off in student involvement later on. Obviously, not all health topics will be set up via such an arrangement, but if several are treated this way throughout the year, it will command the attention of a number of pupils who would otherwise be likely to warm up slowly to the topic. In a cooperative planning session, a small group of students, working in a comfortable area around a table, adds subtopics and ideas for experience to a skeleton outline put together by the instructor. There is a sharing of comments. If the instructor remains patient and permits the students to do much of the searching and questioning, most of the basic points and issues will be brought up. Perhaps the most significant feature is that students respond very well when they feel that they have a voice in their own educational affairs. Moreover, by the time boys and girls reach high school, they pretty much know that youth can be divided into three groups: those who make things happen, those who watch things happen, and those who wonder what happened. Also, students who are successful anywhere, school included, know that they are responsible for their success. It is when they feel that others are responsible for their success that they don't feel adequate. And it is at this point that they begin to dislike processes and other people. Needed for everybody are actual "happenings" which are looked upon as favorable. Self-fulfillment does not come without experiencing success.

5. Pupils must be given *concise directions specifying the learning tasks* they are expected to perform, and the criteria to be employed for appraising task performance. This means that there must be access to credible information in all major health topics—both controversial and non-controversial.

6. The *multi-media approach* in health instruction should prevail. Not all students are equally impressed with a single approach such as a filmstrip or a field trip. Motivational research again makes it clear that by mixing the media throughout the length of the course, and by permitting student planning, interest may be generated and maintained.

7. There is an *art of listening* that some teachers know little about in their effort to tell the class all they know. Socrates listened intently; it was his most immediate form of living. Both he and Mahatma Gandhi engaged in the art of listening—a most trying thing to do when listening to the irrational. By waiting and listening, Socrates and Gandhi were able to trust their opponents, and in so doing, gain their respect. School teachers in the classroom discussing the drug scene have found the same thing to be true. When they listen well, the students rapidly begin to feel that the teacher is interested in *them*—and this is the point where real education begins.

METHODOLOGY OF HEALTH TEACHING

Because good programs have been discarded in the name of change, there is a fair amount of risk involved in innovation. But the risk must continue, for this kind of freedom to think and act is the finest criterion of humanness. In fact, says Paul Tillich, "... man becomes truly human only at the moment of decision."

In an effort to discover what determines favorable decision-making, numerous individuals have experimented with ways to present and teach health topics. For years, it was considered appropriate to set up a list of remote goals and specific objectives to work toward. Then it was discovered that these frequently ended up being "teacher oriented goals," so curriculum content and teaching techniques were geared to "pupil outcomes." Often these outcomes were structured only in terms of knowledges and attitudes to be achieved. They were usually so fact dominated that it seemed more realistic later on to write them down in terms of broad generalizations or concepts. Throughout much of this objectivication history, there has been little done with *behavioral objectives* — statements that describe what the student is expected *to be able to do.*

The advantage of defining teaching objectives in terms of competencies and observable student behavior is that it helps in the selection of an appropriate method of teaching. Also, when a choice of teaching strategy has been made without performance objectives, there are no empirical means for determining the degree of effectiveness of the strategy used. Individuals in industry, banking, space programming, and the military who embrace a systems approach lean heavily on concrete objectives to which their activities can be related. Spelling out instructional goals in terms of overt behavior also communicates to the student what is expected of him. Research by Dalis, carried on with high school students, showed that it was possible to enhance students' achievement significantly by providing them with precise instructional objectives in advance of instruction.[9]

In Los Angeles County, an effort has been made to improve health instruction in the form of a research plan, Project Quest — New Designs for Innovative Approaches to Health Instruction. Using the "systems approach" with behavioral objectives, there was found to be a significant improvement in all health goals in all grade levels. In the research, each goal was divided into related component parts and then gradually to the smallest concrete tasks that became the structure for lesson plans. An example of the breakdown is as follows:[10]

> *Mission and Goal 5:* The Health Educated individual copes with contemporary health problems.
> *General Objective or Major Function:* The student makes wise decisions about harmful substances.
> *Measurable Objectives for High School Students:*
>
> (1) Given instruction in causes and effects of smoking on the body, the student will develop at least four strategies to help him refrain from smoking cigarettes.
> (2) Given research background on smoking habits of people, the student will develop at least five psychological reasons why people smoke.

Although the affective and action domains are extremely important, the cognitive domain has much to offer if it is concerned with some student reasoning and problem

---

[9]Gus T. Dalis, "The Effect of Precise Objectives Upon Student Achievement in Health Education," unpublished doctoral dissertation, University of California, Los Angeles, 1969.

[10]For description in detail, see Charles Nagel, "A Behavioral Objective Approach to Health Instruction," *Journal of School Health,* 40:255–258, May, 1970.

TABLE 9–1   Cognitive Domain

LEVELS	CATEGORIES	DENTAL HEALTH EXAMPLE
First Level	*Knowledge* is recognized. It is *received* and passively attended to.	Toothbrushing is discussed. The students may be listening.
Second Level	*Comprehension* occurs and a *satisfying* response is given.	The student is aware of the topic and will enter the discussion.
Third Level	Skillful *application* of knowledge occurs, and the student *values* the activity, seeking ways to respond.	Toothbrushing is believed important and worth the time spent.
Fourth Level	*Analysis* and *synthesis* occur, and *conceptualization* of values takes place.	The student starts to make choices— whether to brush his teeth after eating or to go out immediately and join his peers.
Fifth Level	*Evaluation* of knowledge and skill occurs, and values are organized into *characterization* of the individual.	The decision is automatic; the teeth are brushed *before* joining peers.

solving. Knowledge can be acquired in a sequence that is comprehended, applied, analyzed, synthesized, and evaluated (see Table 9–1).

The *decision making* level is the down-to-earth place where it is demonstrated that the lessons have been learned. To aid in this process the College Entrance Examination Board developed *Deciding*—a decision-making program for junior and senior high school students.[11] Many thousands of students have used the exercises, group activities, simulations, role playing, and discussion guides to help make decisions that apply to their personal and vocational lives. The *Deciding* curriculum can be employed well in the health instruction area. It is divided into three units, Values, Information, and Strategy, with the following content areas:

— Identifying critical decision points
— Recognizing and clarifying personal values
— Identifying alternatives and creating new ones
— Seeking, evaluating, and utilizing information
— Risk taking
— Developing strategies for decision making

Particularly useful for teachers with health concerns is the way the program handles *alternatives* and *strategies*. Students are encouraged to take a hard look at the several alternatives at a decision point. Suppose, for example, the alternatives have to do with the nutritional topic of overweight. A plan of action might be set up using the four steps of the *Deciding* program.

The Situation: You have been told by your physician that you are considerably overweight and should do something about the condition. Do you know all the alternatives?

---

[11]College Entrance Examination Board, Box 592, Princeton, N.J. 08540.

Follow the steps to identify the alternatives:

Step 1: Define the decision including when it has to be made.
Step 2: Write down the existing alternatives you know about now.
Step 3: List the sources of help in discovering new alternatives.
Step 4: Add the new alternatives to those you have already identified.

The culminating act of the decision maker is to move from the alternative steps to a *choice*. Then follows the plan of action — strategy. Students need to have an opportunity (self-motivated by now) to examine several strategies in a health problem situation. At this point every problem can be subjected to the four strategies of the *Deciding* program:

1. "Choose what you desire most" (regardless of risk, cost, or probability)
2. "Choose to avoid the worst" (minimizes the maximum disaster)
3. "Choose the most likely to succeed" (the highest probability of being successful)
4. "Choose both the most likely and most desirable" (high probability and high desirability)

SUCCESSFUL HEALTH TEACHING METHODS

It has been said that the clever teacher can use almost any method of teaching and make it work. Perhaps so. However, for every clever teacher, there are dozens who are less than clever and have to choose carefully the manner in which they present a topic. Fortunately, there are a number of methods to choose from.

In reviewing the major teaching methods in terms of which one to select, it is important to keep in mind three fundamental questions:

1. What can secondary school students learn largely by themselves?
2. What can they learn from explanations and demonstrations largely by others?
3. What can they learn from personal interaction with other students and the teacher?

The opportunity to work by oneself can be a rich and rewarding learning experience for the right student. A one-man project coupling library study with a downtown visit may be hard to surpass as a means of understanding some health dimension. In another situation, it may be much more effective to have a group activity in order to register breadth of opinion. Comments on a number of methods and their appropriateness for health education follow.

Guided Discovery. There is some question whether this is a particular kind of method, or whether it is an on-going practice in all good teaching, and, therefore, a part of all methodology. In fact, conceptual learning is more apt to take place when learning experiences are rich in opportunities to discover interesting things heretofore unknown by the pupil. Woodruff touches on this point when he discusses concepts as generalizations, from very simple things to high-level abstractions. The discovery process helps the learner make meaning of things he has seen or otherwise perceived in his experience. The process insists that the student, not the teacher, inquire, compare, draw conclusions based on the comparisons, and thus discover enough to reflect or make decisions. Thus, it is the instructor's task, as each new health topic is introduced, to foster *the process of inquiry,* which reflects the need to find a solution, an answer. This is the kind of discovery that Bruner writes about. It need not be great; small discoveries are valuable.[12]

---

[12]Jerome S. Bruner, "The Art of Discovery," *Harvard Educational Review,* 31:20–32, 1961.

The focus of discovery can involve subject matter facts, relationships (similarities and differences), ideas, certain rules and systems, movements, and viewpoints. From an instructional concern, the emphasis is on the word *guided*. In short, the discovery is planned ahead of time and is insured by having the pupil follow certain steps—clues or questions—arranged in such a way that the student will gradually discover the concept or relationship. Arranging a sequence of experiences in step fashion requires that the major health area content be structured to permit inquiry and exploration. Then, to accomplish this end may require three or four teaching methods. Throughout the sequence of steps, the student responds to the clue or question and moves on. The teacher never tells the answer, always waits for the pupil to respond, and always reinforces the response. When students fail to respond, it indicates an inadequate design of the clue. The immediate and individual approval given after each step acts as a continuous motivating force to keep investigating.

EXAMPLE OF GUIDED DISCOVERY IN HEALTH EDUCATION

Topic: Human heart (Body Structure and Function area).

Purpose: To discover how a coronary heart attack occurs.

Question 1: What happens when a coronary heart attack takes place?

Anticipated answer: A white wax-like substance, cholesterol, enters the coronary artery in the heart and stops or reduces the normal flow of blood. (*Response:* "Right!")

Question 2: How can the build-up of cholesterol be reduced in the body?

Anticipated answer: By eating a low fat diet, taking regular exercise, and keeping relatively free from psychologically stressful situations. (*Response:* "Good!")

Question 3: Where does one go to have a thorough examination and find out more about how to prevent a coronary heart attack?

Anticipated answer: A cardiologist. (*Response:* "Excellent choice of specialists.")

Question 4: Is there one near here?

Anticipated answer: Yes. On Main Street near the hospital. (*Response:* "Right!")

Question 5: Would you like to talk with him?

Anticipated answer: Yes. Soon, if possible. (*Response:* "Good idea. Let's go.")

In the above process, the discovery that a cardiologist is a pretty important person is brought out, and it moves the student to want to do something about it. At this point, a trip to the hospital to talk with the specialist is in order (Field Trip Method). Earlier, following Question 2, the clues to diet, activity, and stress could have been brought out via a colored film strip (Audio-Visual Method) or a small group search through library materials (Library Method).

The essential point in the guided discovery method is that the student be guided—not told all the answers. He must taste, touch, smell, hear, and see for himself. By making incorrect responses and discovering correct answers himself, he finds out how to satisfy his own curiosity.

Brecht, the playwright, substantiates this method in *Galileo*. In the opening scene, he shows the great Italian scientist Galileo Galilei, in the early 1600's, teaching a young boy the particulars of the movement of the earth about the sun. As he initiates the lesson, there is no lecturing, no explanation; instead, Galileo asks the lad to examine his device for showing the way the planets move about the sun. "What do you see?" says the great man. "Count the bands. How many are there?" When doubting Thomases and scientists came to visit him, he taught the same way. When each would gaze into the crude telescope, Galileo would ask, "What do you see? Describe to me what you see." This not only awakened interest, but also tied the observer securely to the topic because his own *trusted senses* were involved. What he saw was real to him; it was not something someone described to him in mere words and phrases. It became a part of him and was not lightly considered and soon forgotten.[13]

Value Clarification.   The basic work of Raths, Harmin, and Simon considered several ways in which values can be transmitted, and concluded that student thoughts and later accomplishments can be linked together.[14]

In the clarifying approach to values it is acknowledged that the values held by an individual at any time are relative, personal, and situational. In addition, there is no attempt to transmit the "right" values. There is a distinguishing difference between value *teaching* and value clarification. This needs interpretation in many localities, otherwise certain individuals think that value clarification is teaching someone values and the question quickly arises—what values? The task is to assist the student in clarifying his or her own values relative to a health situation. Students examine their experiences and those of others and think critically about them; they share perceptions with their peers and learn ways to apply their value skills in their own lives.

Several broad value skills that can be advanced through classroom techniques are:

Choosing
1. Seeking alternatives when faced with a choice.
2. Looking ahead to probable consequences before choosing.
3. Making choices on one's own, without depending on others.

Prizing
4. Being aware of one's own preferences and valuations.
5. Being willing to affirm one's choices and preferences publicly.

Acting
6. Acting in ways that are consistent with choices and preference.
7. Acting in those ways repeatedly with a pattern to one's life.

Observe that these seven skills are progressive. Activity starts with an appraisal of a situation and noting alternatives. From this develops an affirmation of choice. The decision has been made, and from this evolves the behavior change—a change that one is committed to and makes room for in one's life style.

Questions are phrased in keeping with the Raths-Harmin-Simon seven essential and progressive value skills. See example chart for the topic of overweight and obesity.

A number of teachers like to prepare *value sheets,* which consist of a number of pertinent questions for each student to grapple with prior to becoming involved in future discussion. Osman finds that the value sheets are not always appropriate for discussions; he prefers his students to respond in writing, privately and deliberately.[15]

There are numerous techniques used to experience choosing, prizing, and acting. Perhaps the most common is the coat of arms approach to a health problem or situation.[16] Greenberg adapts the Simon-Howe-Kirschenbaum materials to the mental health area by asking the student to respond to each of the following questions by drawing, in the specific area of the coat of arms, a picture, design, or symbol.

---

[13]From *Health Education in the Elementary School,* 4th ed. by Carl E. Willgoose, Philadelphia: W. B. Saunders Co., 1974, p. 278.

[14]Louis E. Raths, Merrill Harmin, and Sidney B. Simon, *Values and Teaching: Working With Values in the Classroom,* Columbus, Ohio: Charles E. Merrill Publishing Co., 1966. See also Sidney B. Simon, Leland W. Howe, and Howard Kirschenbaum, *Values Clarification: A Handbook of Practical Strategies for Teachers and Students,* New York: Hart Publishing Co., Inc., 1972.

[15]Jack D. Osman, "Use of Selected Value-Clarifying Strategies in Health Education," *Journal of School Health,* 44:21–26, January, 1974.

[16]Jerrold S. Greenberg discusses this technique from a health research view in "Behavior Modification and Values Clarification and Their Research Implication," *Journal of School Health,* 45:91–94, February, 1975.

VALUE SKILLS SAMPLE QUESTIONS

1. *Choosing freely*
   a. Do your parents realize that you are considerably overweight?
   b. How do your friends feel about your weight?

2. *Choosing from alternatives*
   a. Was there more than one reason for gaining weight?
   b. Did anyone encourage you to ignore weight gain?

3. *Choosing thoughtfully and reflectively*
   a. Have you thought about the hazards of obesity?
   b. Does it bother you that obese people have more heart and movement difficulties?
   c. Can you explain how you might grow up heavier than you are now and not suffer any illness from obesity?
   d. Do you have some feelings about having chosen to ignore overweight?

4. *Prizing and cherishing*
   a. Would your life be different *without* extra weight to haul around?
      Would it be different *with* it?
   b. Do you really prize overweight?
   c. Would you want your younger brother or a good friend to become obese?

5. *Affirming*
   a. Would you be willing to give a short talk to a class about the hazards of obesity?

6. *Acting*
   a. What will you do first to help others reduce their overweight?
   b. What will some of your friends say when you try to persuade others to reduce?

7. *Repeating*
   a. Indicate what you have done so far to help others?
      How often?
   b. Have you plans for doing more?
   c. Are you glad you are doing something about overweight and obesity? Would you do it again?

1. What do you regard as your greatest personal achievement to date?
2. What do you regard as your family's greatest achievement?
3. What is the one thing that other people can do to make you happy?

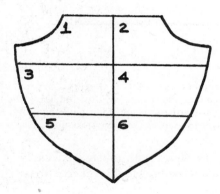

4. What do you regard as your own greatest personal failure to date?

5. What would you do if you had one year to live and were guaranteed success in whatever you attempted?

6. What three things would you most like to be said of you if you died today?

In the junior high school the *values grid* works well in providing a strategy for value clarification. Here personal beliefs and actions are measured to see how they fit the seven requirements of the process. The pupil fills in a grid with health issues such as drinking and driving, abortion on demand, use of seat belts, and so forth.

ISSUE	1	2	3	4	5	6	7

Adjacent to each health issue the pupil writes in a few key words that summarize for him or her a position on the issue. The seven questions (see p. 336) can be written on the board for all to see. Students are not called to defend their responses; only to consider the firmness of their convictions and how they arrived at them.

Values, of course, can be examined simply by voting—a raising of hands on an issue; or by groups of three pupils thinking about and sharing a difficult choice recently made; or acting out a feeling or belief:

EXAMPLE:

"All those who wear seat belts move to the rear of the room. All others move to the front of the room."

EXAMPLE:

"All those who would prefer to give up cigarettes rather than alcohol go to the rear of the room. The other way around to the front of the room."

This technique, as well as various individual movements in line formations, makes value indicators visible as individuals make choice freely. Such opportunities for expressing decisions make alternatives real and interesting. Another activity closely related to the above is the *reaction scale* (The Number Line) in which everybody lines up along the wall, physically placing themselves along a scale rating feelings on an issue:

Imaginary Scale for: _____

Number
Line   1   2   3   4   5   6   7   8   9   10

EXAMPLE:

React to a drug statement or sexuality statement—or any health issue or feeling. Simply request individuals to place themselves in position along the imaginary number line in terms of depth of feeling toward the issue. One could respond to a statement written in above, such as, *"Love isn't love until you give it away."*

Jack Osman uses superb slides with music, especially in the mental health, drugs, and smoking areas to draw out feelings (gut level reactions). After exposing the students to this multimedia presentation they are asked to write a *one word feeling* that they experienced in each of the four areas of the circle. Then they take one of the feelings and describe, elaborate, or explain it in two sentences.

Help is available for the teacher in the value clarification area. In addition to the works already noted, there are excellent value oriented curriculum guides. Four examples follow:

You and Your Decisions, San Diego County Schools Office, San Diego, Calif., 1974.

The Coronado Plan, Teachers Guide, Coronado (California) Unified School District, 1971.

Comprehensive Health Education Guide, Butte County Schools Office, Oroville, Calif., 1974.

Values-Oriented Approach to Drug Abuse Prevention Education, Orange County, (California) Schools Office, 1971.

Problem Solving. This is a natural extension of the guided discovery technique of teaching. However, instead of receiving questions and clues from the teacher, the student seeks answers completely on his own. This calls for greater self-discipline and self-involvement, and not all students are initially capable of such personal control. The instructor who knows the students will turn many of them loose to pursue a health topic beyond the "surface of the observed to the underlying structure of regularity"—a phrase coined by Jerome Bruner in his discourse on good problems and the related skills of relevance.[17]

To make something like nutrition or mental health meaningful, one has to *do* something with it. Bruner proposed this with physics in his early curriculum work and made a name for himself. He showed that what seemed to be at work in a good problem-solving "performance" is some underlying competence in using the operations of physics. Therefore, in doing a health problem such as nutrition planning or investigating a downtown mental health facility, the actual performance along the way is as important as the solving of the problem.

As an open-end process where there is always the possibility of another solution, problem solving can become constantly renewed as one goes on from one problem to another in a self-perpetuating process of discovery. This is highly desirable in a high school health education class. It has a chance of working if the problems that are presented are relevant:

Relevant

To the subject matter
To the readiness and experience of the class.
To the readiness and experience of the individual

---

[17]Jerome Bruner, "The Skill of Relevance or the Relevance of Skills," *Saturday Review,* April 18, 1970.

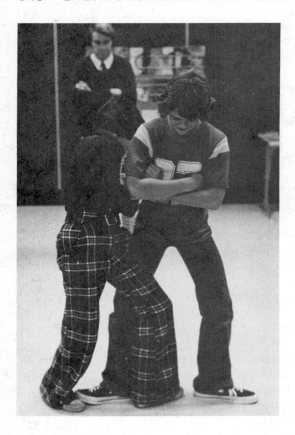

Figure 9–1 Non-verbal activity demonstrating reactions to conflicts of individual freedoms. (Courtesy of Loren Bensley, Jr., and Brad Fleming, Central Michigan University)

Secondary school students have found that solutions to problems such as the following are within their grasp:

A. Hospital costs in a few years will be $400 per day in rural areas and $600 in cities. The chancellor of the University of California Medical Center predicts a $1000 per day figure for major urban areas. Search for the reason behind these statements. What are the problems?

B. How can people be a social force for health in the marketplace? How effective are ordinary people? Consider the need to improve automobile safety. Should a non-profit group be organized to identify safe cars and safety-minded manufacturers?

C. Has a person a "right to die"? The United Nations is studying whether physicians should let people with incurable diseases die, instead of prolonging their lives with modern medicine. How serious is this issue? How do medical men, philosophers, and theologians feel? What appears to be the best practice for all concerned?

Incidentally, problem solving by teams is more effective than problem solving by individuals. Also, members of problem solving classes in health education have scored significantly better in gains of specific problem solving skills than did those in lecture classes in health education.

Jigsaw Puzzle Method.   The procedure here involves each student in a small group holding a piece of information. The information is useful only when it is combined with the information held by the other members of the group. Each student masters his or her information so that he or she can teach it to the others. Mastering the information usually involves some library study or general discussion with individuals outside the group. Problems that are examined this way bring home the idea that each member has a unique contribution to make through cooperative enterprise.

Lecture and Group Discussion.   A carefully prepared health talk can supply essential information on a topic and set the stage for an appropriate visual aid or series of problem questions. Employed every now and then, it can be quite effective—especially if the lecturer is a good speaker. Where the lecture method is overworked, it fails sto stimulate pupil learning. In fact, there is some evidence to suggest that it may even be instrumental in creating a kind of negative learning—a negative reaction to what is said because of the way it is said, which "spoils" a fresh positive approach to the subject at a later date.

When a lecture is followed by a preplanned class or small group discussion, the effect can be quite noticeable. Several pieces of research have demonstrated that group discussion as a method is more effective than the lecture method in influencing positive health practices, and in securing long-term motivation among the individuals. More personal decisions to amend health behavior occur through a weighing of facts in discourse than in listening to a lecture on what should be done.

Dialogue is a building process that can move readily through the following five points:

1. *Understanding.* The teacher asks enough questions to bring out information.

2. *Clarifying.* Ask thought-provoking questions to test a hypothesis or two.

3. *Exploring Alternatives.* Raise the possibility of alternative actions open to the students.

4. *Exploring Consequences.* Raise questions that will cause the students to consider the consequences of the alternatives that are open.

5. *Exploring Feelings and Making Choices.* Raise discussion points concerning choices and consequences open to individual class members.

A rewarding discussion meeting is one in which the student feels he took part and

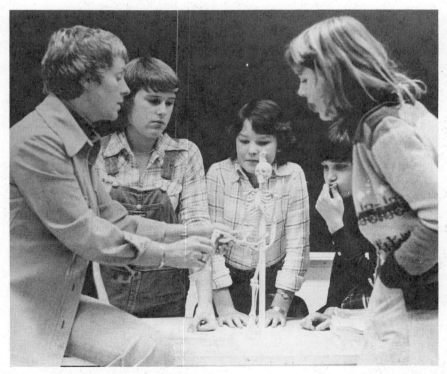

Figure 9–2   Small group instruction captures attention. (Courtesy of Brad Fleming, Central Michigan University)

made a contribution. When this occurs, he looks forward to going again. This can be engineered by a good leader—one who keeps questions moving so that they don't "die." Rephrasing a question frequently helps the group. At this point, the leader has to be careful not to take too active a part in the discourse. He can direct and still remain nicely in the background. It will be difficult to do, because most teachers have the facts on hand and the "message" to bring—quite often to individuals who would rather talk about it than hear about it.

Sometimes health questions, together with several possible answers, are distributed to the group to structure the discussion when it seems advantageous. This question-answer technique is a good practice to follow when some variety seems to be needed. It also provides a little more structure to the meeting and acquaints all students with exactly what is being studied.

Contract Approach. This is a method of teaching in which a binding agreement is made between two or more parties—usually pupil and instructor. It is designed to give a student choices in selecting learning activities as well as the grade level he wishes to achieve. The student may have a highly structured program or may have complete freedom. He may follow grade level requirements or substitute independent learning activities. Details are spelled out in the contract, and the contract is renegotiable. Failure to meet the contract specifications simply means that the student receives the grade he has achieved.

TABLE 9–2   Sample Contract

PREFACE STATEMENT

I, _____,
do hereby agree to be responsible for my own grade and work during the first six-week grading period in health education. I wish to contract for a grade of _____.

RENEGOTIATION CLAUSE

I also understand that I may, at any time during the six-week grading period, renegotiate the terms of said contract.

INDEPENDENT STUDY CLAUSE

I understand that I may substitute an individual study project during the six-week grading period for any or all of the above named requirements. I understand that the project proposal must be submitted in outline form giving the following details:
   a. What I am trying to find out;
   b. how I intend to approach the problem (resources and procedures); and
   c. how I plan to evaluate and report my findings.
Substitution value for individual projects will be agreed upon by the signers on the basis of time, effort, and worth of the project.

Student's signature

Teacher's signature

For the teacher, grading is a matter of pass-fail in accordance with the contracted grade level. If a student contracts for a "C" grade but does "B" work, he gets the higher grade. The real advantage is a teacher-student learning partnership. Flexibility is built in, as students are permitted to determine wholly or partially the degree of independent study (or any other self-designed learning activity) in which to engage. The contract form can be set in any style, but it must contain questions that ask: *What do you want to learn; how are you going to do it; and how do you plan to report your learning?* A sample contract is shown in Table 9–2.

Another form of contracting in health education, which works well where behavioral objectives are clearly spelled out, was tried quite successfully by Schley and Banister at the junior college level. However, there is no reason why it wouldn't work equally well in junior and senior high schools. In this plan, the student studies the objectives and directions for achieving an "A" grade, "B" grade, or "C" grade. As the studies are pursued the student knows the grade level toward which he or she is progressing and can adjust accordingly—depending on interest in the topic, time available, and general motivation.

The learning method is superb. The student (1) participates in an audio-tutorial instruction program presented by tape, filmstrip, or semi-programmed text; (2) performs a personal involvement activity, and (3) participates in a group discussion session. Since the discussion period comes last, the students are well prepared with questions and comments and are generally eager to take part. They will tell about their health performance activities and will listen to others. Also, grade requirements relate to the number of small group discussion sessions attended and class quizzes. Schley and Banister report excellent results from this method of teaching some sixteen major topics in health education. A sample of multimedia requirements for the unit on "stress" appears on the following page.[18]

Independent Study. As already indicated, independent study can play a major role in such teaching techniques as guided discovery, problem solving, and contracting. It is also a method of teaching in its own right.

With schools organized for mass education, it is difficult to individualize instruction. As an outgrowth of the Trump plan—in which large groups, small groups, and independent study were recommended—a number of junior and senior high schools teaching health education today have flexible schedules and a host of new time arrangements to serve the purposes of individual pupils. There is evidence that permitting youth to look at all the data available about a problem and draw their own conclusions will have a greater impact on behavior than almost anything else. It takes time to get at the basis of a health concern—more time than a class can spend. Through independent study, a number of pupils can work outside the class and even outside the school to chase down in-depth details. Youths who plead to be allowed to "do their own thing" are happy with this approach to health education. There is a lesson here to be learned by the instructor. When John Gardner was Secretary of HEW, he showed his support for this procedure when he remarked, "We have been giving children cut flowers when we should have been helping them plant and grow their own."

Field Trips. Moving out into the community is an old teaching practice that has had a good amount of success. Yet, there are thousands of secondary teachers who never leave the classroom from one year to another. Every pupil should depart from the classroom several times during the school year, and not just those students working on

---

[18]Robert A. Schley and Richard E. Banister, "Behavioral Change in an Academic Setting: How It Works," *School Health Review*, 1:13–16, November, 1970.

WEEK #5: REACTION TO STRESS

How does stress affect us? What can we do to reduce its undesirable effects upon us?

A. Objectives for a C grade

For a C grade you will be able to *identify* by recognition or recall:

1. Two classifications for stress reactions
2. The role played by the autonomic nervous system in physiological reactions to stress
3. The name of nine body organs or systems that are influenced by the autonomic nervous system
4. The effect of the autonomic nervous system on each of the nine body organs or systems studied
5. The influence of physiological and psychological stimuli in producing an emotional state
6. Six of the eight guidelines for making adjustments to stress situations

B. Directions for a C grade

1. Go to the library materials center, ask for the audio-tutorial unit *Reaction to Stress*, complete the worksheet, and bring it to your next scheduled group discussion session.
2. Identify three stresses you feel are most bothersome to you and write them down on the back of your worksheet.
3. Go to the library materials center, ask for the book *Health for Effective Living* and read on page 86 eight guidelines recommended for making adjustments to stress situations. Write them down on the back of your worksheet.

C. Objectives for a B grade

For a B grade you will be able to *recognize* and describe in writing:

1. One behavioral situation that reflects an abnormal physiological reaction to stress
2. A course of action that could improve the situation you described
3. A technique by which the proposed course of action could be put into practice

D. Directions for a B grade

1. Complete the assignment for a C grade.
2. Write a one page report on one real or imaginary health practice or condition related to emotional stress that you recognize to be in need of improvement. For credit your report must:
   a. Describe a specific health practice or condition needing improvement
   b. Recommend a course of action that will help improve the health practice or condition
   c. Explain how you would put your recommendations into practice

E. Objectives for an A grade

You will *perform* one personal health practice improvement or bring about one personal health practice improvement in another individual, that results in improvement of physiological reaction to stress.

F. Directions for an A grade

1. Complete the assignment for a B grade.
2. At some time during the course present to the members of your small group *evidence* that you have brought about an improvement in your health practices or have improved the health practices of another individual with respect to physiological reaction to stress.

G. Individual study session

1. Library materials center—audiotutorial unit *Reaction to Stress* (tape, filmstrip)
2. Campus or community—personal diary of daily stress situations

H. Small group session

1. You will come prepared to report, compare and discuss the information describing
   a. The stresses you identified during the previous week
   b. The type of adjustments made to these stresses
   c. The particular adjustment mechanisms used, and
   d. Your suggestions for lessening the effects of stress in the future
2. An open discussion will focus on possible cause and effect relationships between particular adjustment mechanisms that students use and the needs they feel, as indicated by audiotutorial unit *Appraising Mental Health*.

I. Supplemental reading

1. "Attaining Emotional Adulthood," Chapter 10, *Quality of Living*, Davis et al.
2. *Rope of the Mind*, Meerloo.

(Courtesy of Robert A. Schley and Richard E. Banister)

their own problems through independent study. A sign in a northern Minnesota classroom reads as follows:

The Community is the Classroom

In this school, field excursions were encouraged and taken to visit blind people, a health magazine headquarters, a birth defects institute, the accident ward of a hospital, a cancer program at a television station, a narcotics guidance council headquarters, and a county health department to check on the seriousness of the Asian flu.

Field trips are costly in terms of time, and they should therefore be carefully planned to achieve certain objectives. Upon returning to the classroom, there should be a follow-up discussion to recall the highlights of the trip and the purpose it served. Some teachers require pupils to make notes on what they saw and discovered on the trip. This is permissible, provided the notes will be used later in a class discussion session, and that note taking doesn't detract from what one sees and hears on the trip.

Parents as well as community leaders must accept field trips as worthwhile. They should be informed that they may be used to initiate or culminate a unit, to enhance accurate observations by employing all senses, and to afford pupils the opportunity to plan and implement the health program.

Experiments. Health teaching experiments performed by students themselves as part of a modified laboratory period have greater value than those demonstrated by the teacher. Too often the demonstration method of teaching is like an entertainment of some kind and without lasting value. In a proper experiment, there is a problem to solve. It is organized for study. It should be introduced in such a way that the pupil is curious and wants to solve the problem. Then, with the chance to test and try things out first hand, answers can be found. It is better if the pupil is not told what will happen. There should be some thinking and speculation before proceeding too far. When finished there should be an appraisal of findings in terms of everyday health practices. Care should be taken not to make sweeping generalizations and claim a great deal from the results. Most school experiments contribute an idea or two; they seldom are so thorough that they *prove* anything beyond a doubt.

The health education field is rich in opportunities to manipulate the environment and employ one's senses to see what will happen. Such activity quickly builds an appreciation for the health career fields. Experimentation with blood, smoke, drugs, foods, and so on sets the stage for questions relating to biochemistry, physiology, nutrition, and a number of medical and paramedical areas. They also help students understand, through the application and appraisal of knowledge, that the key to unlock health problems is more and better basic research.

In every major health area, there are suitable experiments in which to engage. Unfortunately, even the simple ones are often not tried or even demonstrated. A number of them can be performed very well by students. A few easily completed examples follow:

A. Relate dental plaque on the teeth to brushing practices by carefully brushing the teeth to remove all food particles. Then rinse the mouth with a coloring agent solution. A harmless coloring agent may be secured from Procter and Gamble Company. Where the brushing has missed a food particle, there will be bright red coloring, indicating how difficult it is to brush teeth thoroughly at any one time.

B. Study the mechanics of breathing and how the lungs respond to different pressures. Use the bell jar to demonstrate breathing action.

C. Study the absorption of liquid in the intestines. Try the following:
  1. Copy the circles in Figure 9–3. (Be sure the outside dimensions of both circles are the same.)
  2. Lay the paper on a piece of soft material or corrugated cardboard.
  3. Measure the inside of each circle with a piece of string. (Use pins to hold the string in place.)
  4. Which string is longer?
  5. If a liquid were flowing through both circles, in which one would more of the liquid touch the sides of the circles?
  6. If a liquid could be absorbed through the sides of the circles, in which circle would more liquid be absorbed?

D. Appraise personal level of physical fitness by taking a physical fitness test under the supervision of the physical education instructor; analyze the results.

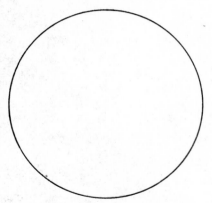 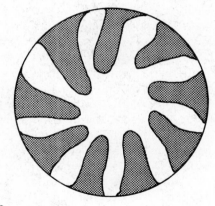

Figure 9–3

E. Examine disease-producing bacteria. Using the microscope examine the species listed in Table 9–3 or similar ones.

F. Look over bruised fruit for a consumer health lesson. Observe how decay begins.

1. Obtain two firm, sound oranges, and one that has already started to get moldy. Rub the point of a sharp knife over the spot of mold on the moldy orange. Pierce the skin of one of the good oranges with the knife point, and set the orange aside.

2. Thoroughly wash the blade of the knife with soap and water and dry it. To be certain it is free of germs, place the point of the knife in an open flame. Pierce the skin of the second orange with the knife tip and set the orange aside. Cover both oranges, and watch them for several days.

G. To comprehend the mechanics of cardiorespiratory efficiency, administer the Harvard Step Test or the Carlson Fatigue Test, and question the meaning of the findings. (For particulars, see *Evaluation in Health Education and Physical Education* by Carl E. Willgoose, New York: McGraw-Hill, 1961, pages 112 and 117.)

H. Administer reaction time tests to various classifications of pupils: fatigued vs. energetic, breakfast eaten vs. breakfast skipped, endomorphic build vs. ectomorphic build, and any other categories you can think of.

I. Examine throat cultures as a laboratory technician would do. Cultivate the bacteria in class.

J. Study human cilia and their contracting action, which moves fluids and foreign particles such as dust along a body tract. This can be done on a frog digestive tract or the trachea of a chicken.

K. Employing the high power microscope, observe the flow of blood through the tail of a goldfish in order to see living red corpuscles and the circulatory pattern.

L. Perform several nutrition related tests to detect such items as starch, protein, fat,

TABLE 9–3 Pathogenic Bacteria

GENUS	APPEARANCE	EXAMPLE
Bacillus	rod-shaped	Typhoid fever bacteria
Coccus	sphere-shaped	Staphylococcus bacteria
Spirillum	corkscrew-shaped	Rat-bite fever bacteria

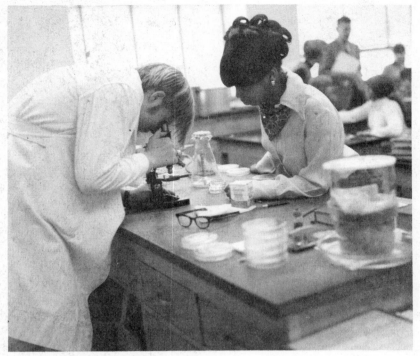

Figure 9–4   Laboratory experimentation. (Courtesy of Ruth Byler)

and acids. These may be combined experiments which are elemental enough to be reviewed at the junior high school level.

M. Evaluate postural controls in rats exposed to alcohol (reflexes relative to staggering and keeping the body in a right-side-up position). Food in the stomach vs. an empty stomach can also be checked. (For a complete description, see pages 182 and 183 in *Teaching About Alcohol* by Frances Todd, New York: McGraw-Hill, 1964.)

An experiment is best organized when it is concisely presented in four parts:

Purpose
Equipment and materials
Procedure
Discussion

After completing the experiment, there should be an opportunity to respond either in writing or verbally to some questions, appraising the results and applying them to living practices. Examples of more detailed experiments designed to stimulate question-answer discussions are as follows:

EXPERIMENT

Purpose: To collect tobacco tar in a smoking machine.
Equipment and materials:
Gallon jar with two-hole stopper
Small jar with two-hole stopper
Glass delivery tubes
Cigarette holder
Shallow pan
Cigarettes

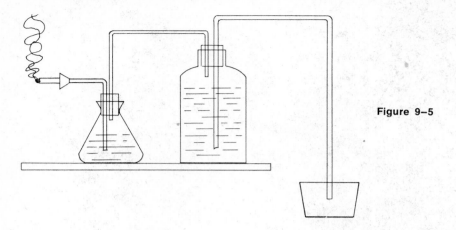

Figure 9–5

Procedure: Fill the large jar with water; the small jar should be half full. Then assemble the apparatus for separating the tar and place a lighted cigarette in position. Siphon some water from the large jar by sucking water from the outlet tube. As the water flows to the pan, the cigarette will burn and tar will be gathered in the small jar. (If a hand pump is available, the tar collecting apparatus need consist of only the small jar.)

Discussion: Points to be raised and questions asked by student and instructor.

EXPERIMENT

Purpose: To show the effect of smoking on the lungs.
Equipment and materials:
Flask
Large jar
Two-holed stoppers
Glass tubing
Rubber tubing
Y-tube
Pinch clamp
Cotton pellets or strands of glass wool
Cigarettes

(This smoking machine is similar to the one above except that a Y-tube is used to collect the tar deposits.)

Procedure: Insert small pellets of cotton or strands of glass wool in the straight section of glass tubing between the cigarette and the Y-tube. Also place loose pellets of cotton or glass wool at all points of the Y-tube. Observe whether more tar precipitates at the Y-shaped bifurcation than elsewhere. Compare the Y-shaped bifurcation with the

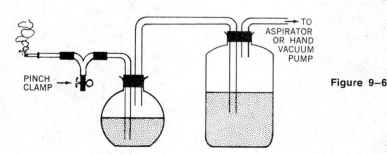

Figure 9–6

structure of the bronchial tree in the lungs of humans. (Note: There is a greater frequency of occurrence of lesions at the bifurcations than elsewhere in the bronchial epithelium of heavy cigarette smokers.)

Discussion: Comments and questions by student and instructor.

EXPERIMENT

Purpose: To examine the role of protein and carbohydrates in rat nutrition.
Equipment and materials:
Wire-bottom rat cages.

FOOD	CONTROL	PROTEIN-FREE	CARBOHYDRATE FREE
Casein	25%	0%	25%
Sucrose	58%	58%	0%
Vegetable fat (e.g., Crisco)	10%	10%	10%
Wesson salt mixture	4%	4%	4%
Cod-liver oil	1%	1%	1%
Non-nutritive fiber	2%	27%	60%

Six (6) young rats weighing about 50 g. each.

Three types of prepared diets using the nutrients shown in the accompanying chart. Include drinking water with each diet.

Sucrose (cane or beet sugar) and Crisco may be purchased at the grocery store; cod-liver oil, at the drug store. Biochemical suppliers will have the other items.

Procedure: Two rats are placed on each diet. They should be weighed daily and observed for any differences. Continue the experiment until the control rats weigh twice as much as any of the animals on the experimental diets. After this, the four experimental rats are placed on the control diet and observed as long as practicable. The animals must be handled gently so as not to frighten them. There should be clean, fresh water for drinking, and if wire-bottomed cages are not available, platforms of half-inch mesh hardware cloth should be made to raise the animals off the cage floor. Individual amino acids may also be studied in this type of experiment.

EXPERIMENT

Purpose: To show the effect of amphetamine derivatives on the central nervous system.

Equipment and materials:
Four (4) adult mice
Two wire-bottom cages
Drinking water
d-Amphetamine sulfate
Weighing scales

Procedure: Divide the mice into a control group and a test group. Daily record the weight of each animal and measure its intake of water and food. (Mark or weigh a bottle of drinking water each day for each animal. The amount of liquid needed to return the drinking water to the original mark on the bottle is the amount of water consumed by the mouse. To weigh the bottle before and after use may be easier, since 1 milliliter of water weighs 1 gram.) During the entire demonstration, offer the same daily diet (solid food) to each mouse. Continue record-keeping for a few days. Then, add *d*-amphetamine sulfate to the drinking water of each mouse in the test group at the dose rate of 5 milligrams per kilogram of body weight per day. Continue this treatment with the drug for 2 to 3 weeks, and daily measure the body weight and the amount of liquid consumed. Make careful observations of any change in the behavior of the mice in both groups. A maze or a slowly revolving wood dowel may be used in activity tests for the mice.

Discussion: Raise the following questions:

(1) What would probably happen if the amphetamine concentration in the drinking water were increased? Decreased?

(2) What effect, if any, did the drug have on the body weight of the mice? Did the eating habits of the mice in the test group change?

(3) Did the amphetamine treatment have any apparent effect on the behavior of the mice? Did the same mice show sharp changes of behavior as well as a loss of appetite?

(4) What other effects did the amphetamine apparently have on the mice? Do you think any of these effects should be considered harmful? If a human body responded to amphetamine in the same way, would the effect of the drug be considered "harmful"?[19]

Brainstorming.   As a teaching technique, brainstorming has not seen much action in secondary schools. It has a history going back to some of the early experimentation of Alex Osborn, who taught in terms of "applying the imagination." It is acknowledged that people have many ideas on a topic—good, bad or otherwise—that need to be brought out in a group meeting so that they will "spark" other ideas from those in attendance.

There is evidence that a "free-wheeling" brainstorming session can really get a class going on a health problem. Everyone has a chance to throw out his idea and no one can be wrong; criticism of ideas is withheld until later.

Steps to Successful Brainstorming in the Health Classroom

A. Select the Problem.   Problems should be chosen which are real and of particular concern to the age group with whom you are working. Students could well assist in the selection process.

B. Decide on the Number of Participants in Each Group.   Beginners' groups seem to function well with four to 10 members. With good leadership, larger sessions could well be organized. The deferred judgment principle can also be used individually.

C. Ask for Volunteers or Appoint at Least One Recorder for Each Group.   The function of the recorder will be to write, in brief form, all ideas as they are presented. Ideas may come too rapidly as the brainstormers gain experience. It may be necessary to have two recorders, each one jotting down every other idea.

D. Give Instructions Clearly.   Emphasize the deferred judgment principle and the need for quantity of ideas. You may want to point out some of the expected results. Encourage combination of ideas.

E. State the Problem and Prime the Students.   Present a few questions that will stimulate group thinking along a variety of approaches. A session might well begin with the teacher saying something like this: "New automobiles are required by law to have seat belts. We've read about how many lives could be saved each year if people would only use them. Some insurance companies agree to pay double medical cost to those per-

---

[19]The same experiment can be nicely used to demonstrate the effect of barbiturates on behavior. Phenobarbital in the drinking water works well. By performing both experiments, the effects of stimulants and depressants can be viewed.

sons injured in an auto accident while wearing the seat belt. We've all seen announcements on television and heard jingles on the radio reminding and encouraging people to use this safety device. In spite of all this, many seat belts are never used."

"Now, what can we do to help establish the good habit of using the seat belt?"

"Should we have windshield blinds that would be retracted only when the seat belt is fastened?"

"Maybe we could have the service station attendant hand a flyer to each customer with the slogan, 'We cherish our customers — use your seat belt — come again soon.' "

"Perhaps each traffic light should have a 'fasten your seat belt' sign that would flash and become visible when the traffic light is red and people are waiting for it to change."

"Or what would you suggest?"

F. Turn the Class Loose Brainstorming. Record all ideas. Beginning sessions should last from 8 to 10 minutes.

G. Stop and Evaluate All Ideas That Have Been Presented. The brainstorming group may evaluate their own ideas, or another group may be selected.

Textbooks and Workbooks. In recent years, there has been a partial return to the use of workbooks and similar study materials in which the pupil is directed to think, read, try things out, and write about the topic. This is usually more effective when the workbook relates to a more detailed section of a textbook. Thus, by combining textbook, workbook, and the suggestions in the teacher's manual, it is possible to involve students in a fair amount of purposeful activity.

As long as the workbook doesn't become a "crutch" for the teacher and a kind of "busy work" substitute for more meaningful activity, it can be accepted as one more means of putting a health topic across and getting a pupil response. A proper workbook for a secondary school class has to be more than a few pages of blank spaces to be completed. It should be attractive, have some pictures, charts, and diagrams, and call for some in-depth searching by the youthful user. Read, in his workbook, uses cartoons effectively to stimulate attention, and then proceeds with questions designed to call for an application of knowledge.

When it comes to an appraisal of textbooks for health education, they have always been under fire. They have been criticized for being in error, for having poor pictures, and for telling too much to the reader and thus preventing individual discoveries from taking place. Yet, if a textbook doesn't supply the needed information, where else does a pupil go to find the written word? The encyclopedia, magazine, and other library sources are helpful, of course, but the basic textbook for health education classes is still very much needed as a fundamental source of information.

Television and Videotaping. In a number of schools, educational television has been used to bring a message to a large number of pupils, to bring the community and its issues into the classroom, and to stimulate thinking and discussion of health topics. However, instructional television (ITV) has not achieved a central place in education. This may be due to the poor way it was used in some classrooms.

Closed circuit television has worked very well where there are large health classes, especially when the lesson involves small, near-at-hand items that cannot be seen very well from the front of the class, but can be shown clearly on the television screen. This kind of television is costly, so it is usually well-planned for selected audiences. It is not without criticism. Some students complain that there is no contact with the instructor. When properly handled, there is always an instructor on hand to answer questions during time allotted from the TV presentation. Perhaps the best way to use closed circuit TV is to follow the presentation with discussion or problem solving activity.

With the popularity of videotaping, it is possible to record the class on a field trip and play back the tape when the students return to the classroom. People like to see themselves in action. They also profit from viewing things on tape that couldn't be viewed individually in laboratories away from the school. These include electron micro-scope pictures, animal quarters where inoculations are demonstrated, laboratories where tissue cultures are prepared, automobile accident scenes where injuries occur, and many other health related occurrences. Class discussions and experiments can also be put on tape. Also, where there are large classes, the overhead television camera with a zoom lens is a very useful instrument; it allows the teacher complete control in showing pic-tures from textbooks or journals and in demonstrating microscope or first aid techniques.

In a study of middle and junior high school students, it was found that groups ex-posed to videotape teaching in health topics scored significantly higher on a health knowledge test than the control groups. Also, about two-thirds of the pupils responded that videotapes had taught them something new in an attractive fashion.[20]

Games and Simulation Techniques.   Unquestionably, games result in greater student involvement than conventional classroom methods. The simulation game is a strategy in which the participant usually plays a predesigned role in a makebelieve world that may or may not be similar to the real world. Three excellent sources of games and game ideas are:

> *Health Games Students Play: Creative Strategies for Health Education* by Ruth Engs, S. Eugene Barnes, and Molly Wantz (Kendall/Hunt, Dubuque, Iowa, 1975).
>
> *Simulation and Gaming,* Sage Publications, Beverly Hills, Calif. 90212.
>
> *Contemporary Games* by Jean Belch (Gale Research Co., Detroit, Mich., 1974).

Gilbert employs the simulation technique very effectively.[21] Students like it because they are kept busy following the information on the assignment they have selected. Moreover, the situations are real life situations and they will be tested later.

Conference-Portable Telephone.   Here the whole class can talk on the telephone with the help of Bell Company equipment at a modest rental fee. The set is a telephone with loudspeakers built in, and two microphones added. The students hear the phone through the loudspeaker, and they can ask questions through the microphones. A senator can explain pending health legislation, a meat inspector can describe some of his problems, and dozens of other issues can be aired for all to hear and respond.

Additional Techniques.   There are a number of other ways to make health instruc-tion interesting and productive. After a while, teachers prefer a certain technique; it works well for them. If someone doesn't like to work with white rats, he shouldn't have to. Each teacher has to try a number of methods and find the one that he can handle best.

The following are additional means of teaching: (1) The *class workshop* takes time to organize, with exhibits of materials, photographs, charts, and other materials, but it provides a concentrated experience worth attempting—particularly for a topic such as drugs and drug abuse for which there will be displays, speakers, and question-answer ses-sions. (2) *Dramatizations* offer a means of variety frequently welcomed by the pupils. A class play such as *Leave It To Laurie* (American Cancer Society) is hard to surpass as a method of initiating serious discussion of the problem of cigarette smoking and health. When the play or skit is being put on for others, care should be taken to choose mature, well-adjusted students for serious parts. (3) Closely related to dramatizations is the tried and true technique of *role playing.* There is some value here, as individual pupils think out how they would *feel* and *act* if they were less than well mentally, emotionally, or

---

[20]William Zimmerli et al., "A Pilot Program Using Video-tapes as a Health Education Medium with Students in Grades Six to Nine," *Journal of School Health,* 39:343–346, May, 1969.
[21]Glen G. Gilbert, "A Working Model for Simulation Techniques," *Health Education,* 6:10–12, May/June, 1975.

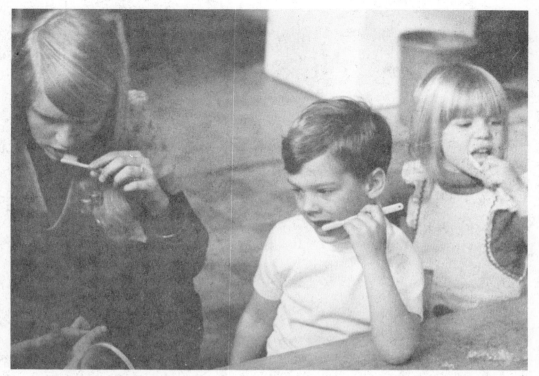

Figure 9–7   Youth to youth method. High school student teaches brushing technique for controling dental plaque to preschoolers.

physically. Role playing is somewhat akin to dance as an art form when the "actors" show joy and happiness in contrast to despair, worry, and over-anxiousness, or when they act the part of the distraught parent or pleased schoolchild. Role playing is an excellent technique for the exploration of health concepts. After the class is sensitized to the situation there is spontaneous dramatization, followed by a switching of roles; then follows a discussion and reaction leading to evaluation, where conclusions are reached. (4) When a story read in class, the *narrative,* is acted out, discussed, or written about, it too has value in promoting health concerns. (5) Youth to youth activities are particularly effective when secondary students involve themselves in teaching health concepts and behaviors to younger children. The THETA program in the Portland, Oregon, public schools has been very successful, primarily because the students doing the teaching were well prepared.[22] In their study of poor nutrition and eating patterns, Frankle and Heussenstamn discovered that teenagers are more effective teachers of their peers than adults.[23] In the San Diego area they have been very helpful in reducing drug abuse among youthful clients.[24] (6) The health fair has great potential for education in cooperative communities. Exhibits, displays, posters, literature, demonstrations, and so on are organized around a theme. There may be opportunities for eye and ear tests, hypertension checks, urine tests for diabetes, and a chance to view films and ask questions. The

[22]John K. Ellis and Michael S. Brock, "THETA: Teenage Health Education Teaching Assistants," *Health Education,* 6:21–22, May/June, 1975.

[23]Reva T. Frankle and F. K. Heussenstamm, "Food Zealotry and Youth," *American Journal of Public Health,* 64:11–18, January, 1974.

[24]A. Gartner et al., *Children Teach Children: Learning by Teaching,* New York: Harper and Row, 1971.

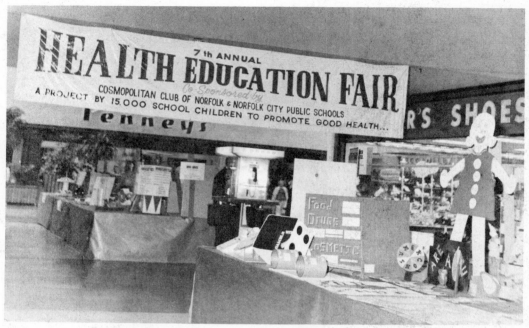

Figure 9–8   The health fair. (Courtesy of Norfolk, Virginia, Public Schools)

secret to success is in careful planning and publicity. A clearly detailed procedure has been written by Snell.[25] For many years, the Norfolk (Virginia) City Public Schools have had an annual health fair that involves the whole school system, with appropriate clinics, projects, student exhibits, and awards (see Figure 9–8).

TEAM TEACHING IN HEALTH EDUCATION

When two or more teachers work cooperatively to instruct and evaluate large groups, small groups, and individual students, the team effort is sometimes more productive than one teacher working alone. Sometimes two heads are better than one in planning and organizing a health lesson, even if only one teacher is to do the actual classwork. It also requires very careful planning and is sometimes bolstered by persons employed as teaching aids who perform some of the clerical duties.

A real advantage in the health area is that a particular teacher may feel strong in something like nutrition or the prevention and control of disease, but feel quite uncomfortable teaching about alcohol and drugs. Through team planning, one teacher may complement another by handling all of the alcohol and drug classes, while the other teacher covers the nutrition and disease units. In this fashion, each teacher uses personal strengths and has found a practical way to overcome weaknesses.

In a research project involving sophomore high school students, Schlaadt was able to show that the team teaching method is as effective as the traditional method in increasing health knowledge.[26] Moreover, pupils of superior mental ability who were

---

[25]Margaret Snell, "How to Plan and Present a Community Health Fair," *Journal of School Health,* 45: 580–590, December, 1975.

[26]Richard G. Schlaadt, "An Analysis of the Effectiveness of Team Teaching Compared to Traditional Teaching of Health to High School Sophomore Students," *Research Quarterly,* 40:364–366, May, 1969.

taught health education by the team teaching method showed a statistically significant gain over students of superior mental ability taught by the traditional method. This indicates, as some educators have suggested all along, that top pupils can profit measurably from extra attention — the kind that could be directed to them in a team teaching situation.

PROGRAMMED INSTRUCTION

This is a system of individual pupil instruction in which program elements or materials are carefully constructed in sequences of small steps to achieve near-at-hand instructional objectives.

Although much was claimed for this teaching technique when it first appeared, it has not received wide acceptance. Behavioral Research Laboratories programmed a *First Aid* manual which the Johnson and Johnson Company makes available for grades six to eight at a small cost. It comes with a filmstrip and a teacher's manual. Progress tests also are available from Behavioral Research Laboratories. These can be used with other health topics in the BRL series: *Body Structure and Function, Personal Health, Safety, Nutrition, and Prevention of Communicable Disease* (BRL, Box 577, Palo Alto, California 94302). An informative book, *Effective Teaching with Programmed Instruction,* is also published by BRL.

Considerable skill is required to prepare effective programs. Except for a few master's and doctoral theses, little experimentation has been done to develop and show the worth of programmed materials in health education. Hart showed that with first aid ma-

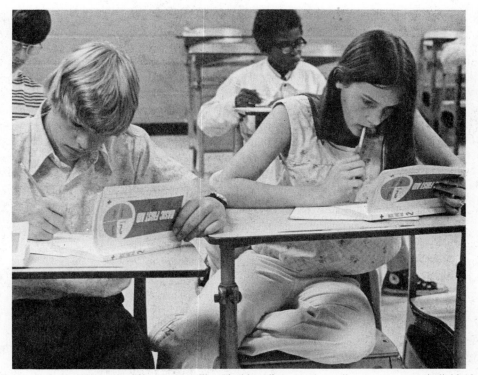

Figure 9-9 Self-instruction in Jacksonville, Florida, allows each pupil progress at an individual rate. (Courtesy of American Alliance for Health, Physical Education, and Recreation)

terial they were at least as effective as regular classroom teaching.[27] Earlier, Hurt and Martin discovered essentially the same thing, but they found that the fewer hours needed to study programmed materials were an added incentive for the students.[28] However, the finest treatment of the subject, with full explanations by competent people, is in the booklet, *"Programmed Instruction in Health Education and Physical Education."*[29] The first chapter, by Loren Benseley of Central Michigan University, is the most informative seen anywhere.

FLEXIBLE SCHEDULING

Effective teaching requires flexibility throughout the school. In the secondary school, the fully self-contained teaching unit hardly exists anymore. There is freedom today to move around, to vary the size of the class both within and between courses, in keeping with the nature of the topic. There is also provision for varying frequencies of exposure to health teaching and for varying lengths of time. In this respect the *module* plan is becoming a common operation. Here, a group of students (module) study for varying lengths of time. A module may go from 15 to 30 minutes. Classes may meet for one or several modules in a flexible scheduling system of organization. The advantage here is one of closer attention to detail, concentration, and small class size. There are times when it is better to have three 20-minute modules of 15 pupils each than to have a traditional 60-minute period with all 45 pupils. Obviously, modular scheduling takes more planning than almost any other teaching technique. In terms of health education, there is little research to affirm or deny that this flexible arrangement of students and time is any more productive of behavior change than the more traditional organizations.

CORRELATION AND INTEGRATION PRACTICES

Every student of educational methods writes about the virtues of correlating and integrating subject matter materials. In reality, however, very little of this activity occurs in strongly departmentalized junior and senior high school programs. For one thing, it takes time and effort to bring teachers of various subject matter fields together to see how they can be part of a total operation. It also requires some conviction that the effort will be worthwhile. Very little research has been done which shows the real value of these practices. Moreover, there are local experiences in many communities which indicate that when health topics (such as accident prevention, mental health, nutrition, alcohol and drugs) are integrated or correlated with other subjects, they are literally lost. In fact, experience shows that the quickest way to give lip service to the existence of a health education program is to say that it has been integrated with biology, general science, home economics, and physical education. This is probably one of the main reasons that *direct health teaching* with scheduled periods has been found to be significantly superior.

There is only one way for the correlation and integration relationships and activities

---

[27]Burton B. Hart, *The Effectiveness of the Programmed Instruction Components in the Standard First Aid Course Multimedia System Adopted by the American Red Cross,* Ph.D. thesis, The Ohio State University, 1972.

[28]Tom Hurt and Gary Martin, "A Comparison of Three Instructional Approaches in Health Education," *Journal of School Health,* 44:504–506, November, 1974.

[29]Authors: Loren Benseley, Mary Ost, Robert Clayton, John Redd, Mildren Barnes, A. Bruce Frederick, Einar A. Olsen, Thomas Eraul, Cyrus Mayshark. Washington, D.C.: American Association for Health, Physical Education and Recreation, 1970.

to really work, and that is to have a person assigned the task of helping to organize and supervise the procedure from start to finish.

There is a difference between correlation and integration. *Correlation involves the use of other areas within the school program by which health education is taught.* Health education, therefore, may be correlated with science, social studies, and language arts. For example, obesity as a health topic may be correlated with biology, where constitutional endowment and genetic predisposition to conditions such as obesity are covered. Also, when something like mental health is being studied, the English teacher may be advised to point to several illustrations of the conditions in the literature, and the physical education instructor could briefly refer to mental well-being through the medium of recreation and relaxation and even the nature of such terms as "fair play" and "sportsmanship."

The integration activity is a little different. *Integration involves an organization of learning experiences around a central object.* It differs from correlation by relating parts to the whole. The whole—even the "whole" person—is like a giant mosaic. Within the school, many forces are brought to bear on the health topic, carefully preplanned and executed.

STUDENT LEADERSHIP

For years, students have contributed to the teaching procedure by helping out in laboratories, shops, and physical education classes. In numerous situations, student leadership has been a significant contribution. Such activity can hardly be called a teaching method, but it does make it possible for the instructor to engage in more involved activities requiring complicated organizations of subject matter, audio-visual media, outside class projects, appraisal activities, and so forth.

Using pupils who enjoy the subject and have leadership characteristics makes good sense. They can assist with surveys, build exhibits, set up equipment, help with demonstrations and dramatizations, be group discussion monitors, and contribute their behind-the-scenes ideas about class procedures and the effectiveness of lessons. They can even do some teaching, especially in those communities where secondary school students visit the elementary grades and help with the younger children.

DEMONSTRATION PROJECTS

From a methodology viewpoint, the health education instructional program in any locality needs examining. In Florida, a multi-county health education project was launched to study some 15,000 students in an effort to improve the quality of health education in grades K to 12. Not only was the effectiveness of the programs in meeting objectives judged, but the methods used were also assessed.

Workshops and meetings were held with parents and teachers. Community resources were coordinated. A demonstration of a well-planned, sequential program of health education was presented by a fully qualified staff. The plan was to have this model program become a catalyst for the future evaluation of health education in the State of Florida.

During the evaluation period for the demonstration project, it was determined that the experimental groups experienced significant changes in knowledge, attitude, and behavior. This was attributed not only to fully qualified teachers, but to the conceptual approach in teaching and a great deal of interest by administrators and parents concerned. The implementation of the project findings by the end of the first year was so effective that two of the project counties expanded it to other schools within their counties. Moreover, requests for help in improving school health programs came from all over the state. The demonstration project proved, as is frequently the case, that programming and methods can be improved if adequate time and preparation are provided to try out new ideas. Running pilot programs from time to time is good teaching.

RELATING INSTRUCTIONAL MATERIALS

MORE ON THE MEDIA

The videotapes, filmstrips, charts, and other media are always a part of the methodology discourse. Whatever the method employed to teach a lesson, the media are a means to make it work more effectively. A lecture without a short film can be deadening; with it students may view descriptive material which makes the lecture more meaningful. Even when the experimental method is employed, a short filmstrip presentation before the laboratory work begins may set the stage for student experimentation by arousing curiosity and an ultimate concern for particulars.

Goodlad has pointed out that the most promising instructional materials "...are those which are designed to be responsive to the explorations of the student; enable the student to be self-propelling; extend the range of stimuli to several senses; provide alternative means to common ends; and free the teacher from burdens of routine correcting and testing.[30] The audio-tutorial format, in which the student might view a film, meet in a small discussion group, and finish up with individual study, would meet the Goodlad criteria.

Success with present-day audio-visuals requires teamwork. No longer can the individual teacher exist in isolation, planning and implementing his own teaching exercises. Sophisticated instruments and techniques of audio-visual education demand new allies—technicians, producers, and others—and thus the "center," "office," or "library of learning resources" was born. A number of schools have such a center, but without a staff—which sometimes makes it more of a storage location. This doesn't help the new teacher who needs someone to talk to about the use of media. Also, there is a certain amount of lethargy in this area. Teachers have been heard to say:

> "I'm against audio-visuals because they're 'canned,' and anything that is canned loses the living experience."
> "If a student really wants to learn, he can learn from a lecture."
> "The trouble with putting my presentation on videotape is that I have to plan it out in advance."
> "The trouble with being on videotape is that my colleagues pick my presentation apart."
> "I would enjoy teaching, if it weren't for the students."

Not only does the center or laboratory produce automated lectures and other materials for teachers and make a variety of equipment and materials available; it also conducts research related to learning and cross-media utilization. This is because the philosophy behind the multi-media approach is that there exists, at the moment, no single audio-visual tool with a monopoly on communication.

---

[30]John I. Goodlad, "The Educational Program to 1980 and Beyond," in *Designing Education for the Future: No. 2* by Edgar L. Morphet and Charles O. Ryan, New York: Citation Press, 1967, p. 54.

In the larger schools, teachers are putting in more and more time in the materials centers, designing teaching programs for future classroom use. Working with a multimedia specialist as program designer, specific ideas are translated into a number of specific drawings, recordings, charts, photographs, and so on. Visual designs for an overhead projector may be sketched in the rough. Pictures from magazines and other sources are collected to be copied; film and filmstrip descriptions are studied for appropriateness; short recordings may be made to augment the "live" remarks of the instructor. In a carefully organized presentation, the instructor can employ electronic cue pulses to start and stop the tape recorder and all of the projectors. Slides can be changed with random access, and any combination of visuals can be shown. Although such activity takes time to plan and to subject to some obvious experimentation, it is generally well received by the students.

APPRAISING THE MEDIA

The use of films, audiotapes, videotapes, or any other similar medium to educate young people in health education depends upon a number of factors, including classroom *climate*. The media will be most effective when the students are ready for them.

All instructional media should be considered as *aids* to learning. They are not expected to serve the total teaching task. Properly employed, however, they should contribute to conceptual thinking, have a high degree of interest for students, be close enough to reality to stimulate self-activity, provide some continuity of thought, and make possible some experiences not easily obtained through other materials. One way to appraise teaching aids is to ask several questions.[31]

Do the materials give a true picture of the ideas they present?
Do they contribute meaningful content to the topic under study?
Is the material appropriate for the age, intelligence, and experiences of the learners?
Is the physical condition of the materials satisfactory?
Is there a teacher's guide available to provide help in effective use of the materials?
Do they make students better thinkers, critical-minded?
Do they tend to improve human relations?
Is the material worth the time, expense, and effort involved?

The value of a teaching aid has less to do with the nature of the aid and more to do with *how* it is used with students. Many an excellent filmstrip has been abused by showing it too often, or at an inappropriate time. Likewise, good posters and pictures have been employed to put a point across, but were not clearly explained to the viewers. The general rule of thumb to use in choosing a teaching aid should be to ask the question, "How will I use the aid?"

There is an opportunity for the health education teacher to keep up to date in the use of instructional media by occasionally referring to the following printed materials:

Periodicals
Audiovisual Communication Review, Washington, D.C. 20036: Dept. Audiovisual Instruction, NEA, 1201 16th St., N.W.
Audio-Visual Instruction, Washington, D.C. 20036: Dept. of Audio-Visual Instruction, NEA, 1201 16th St., N.W.
Educational Screen and Audiovisual Guide, Chicago 60614: 200 Lincoln Park West.
EFLA Film Review Digest, New York, Educational Film Library Assn., 345 E. 46th Street, 10017.

---

[31]From Edgar Dale, *Audio-Visual Methods in Teaching,* revised, New York: Dryden Press, 1964.

Journal of School Health, Kent, Ohio 44240: The American School Health Assn., 515 E. Main St. Each issue has a section entitled: "New Teaching Aids."

Children's Record Reviews, Woodmere, N.Y. 11598: Five issues a year. Box 192.

Printed Materials

Educational Film Guide by J. S. Antonini, New York 10452: H. W. Wilson Co., 950 University Ave. Index of instructional subjects.

Educator's Grade Guide to Free Curriculum Materials by Patricia H. Suttlea, Randolph, Wisconsin 53956: Educators' Progress Service.

Educator's Guide to Free Films by Mary F. Horkheimer and John W. Diffor, Randolph, Wisconsin 53956: Educators' Progress Service.

Educator's Guide to Free Tapes, Scripts and Transparencies by Walter A. Wittuh and Gertie H. Halsted, Randolph, Wisconsin 53956: Educators' Progress Service.

Educational Media Index, New York 10000: McGraw-Hill Book Co. Wide range of instructional materials.

Educational Television Motion Pictures, Bloomington, Indiana 61701: NET Film Service, Audio-Visual Center, Indiana University. Educational TV programs available to schools.

Educator's Guide to Free Filmstrips by Mary F. Horkheimer and John W. Diffor, Randolph, Wisconsin 53956: Educators' Progress Service.

Library of Congress Catalog: Motion Pictures and Filmstrips, Washington, D.C. 20036: Issued quarterly on educational films and filmstrips by title and subject index.

U.S. Government Printing Office Films for Public Educational Use, Washington 20036: U.S. Dept. Health, Education and Welfare. From U.S. Government Printing Office, $2.75.

Filmstrip Guide by J. S. Antonini, New York 10452: H. W. Wilson Co., 950 University Ave.

For information dealing with instruction equipment, see the *Audio-Visual Equipment Manual* by James D. Finn (New York: Holt, Rinehart and Winston, Inc.), and *The Audio-Visual Equipment Directory* by James W. Hulfish, Jr. (Fairfax, Va.: National Audio-Visual Association).

For information pertaining strictly to health education, see *A Directory of Selected References and Resources for Health Instruction* by Mary K. Beyrer (Minneapolis, Minn.: Burgess Publishing Company, Revised).

Because of the multidimensional nature of health education, there is a wide variety of choices in each category of instructional materials. Very often, when certain materials are not listed under health education, they may be found under such headings as science, biology, social studies, and home economics. Also, much that has been prepared for people who teach the handicapped and disadvantaged is listed under special education materials, and is of value to health education instructors.

FILMS, FILMSTRIPS, SLIDES, OPAQUE PROJECTOR, OVERHEAD PROJECTOR

The visual materials are probably the most effective of all the teaching aids when used properly. This means that they must be shown with some degree of skill, previewed, and programmed into the instructional unit. It is a good practice to point out concepts to be gained from a film, filmstrip, or slide before it is presented. When using a more difficult visual aid, the assignment may require ten or fifteen minutes and the use of notes, as well as chalkboard diagrams. New vocabulary may be presented, where the pupil must master new words if he expects to profit fully from the aid.

Pictures, films, filmstrips, and slides frequently become outdated in a rather short time because of costumes, hair styles, automobiles, outmoded slang and other properties

AUDIOVISUAL AIDS EVALUATION FORM

Title_____Produced by_____

Running Time_____min. Filmstrip_____Slides_____

B & W_____Color_____Previewer_____Date_____

A. Technical Qualities

	Excellent	Good	Fair	Poor
1. Quality of camera work	____	____	____	____
2. Organization and development of content	____	____	____	____
3. Sound accompaniment	____	____	____	____
4. Condition of print or slides	____	____	____	____
5. Presents subject clearly	____	____	____	____

B. Instructional Qualities

	Excellent	Good	Fair	Poor
1. Accuracy of information	____	____	____	____
2. Correlation with course of study	____	____	____	____
3. Importance of subject matter	____	____	____	____
4. Develops desirable attitudes	____	____	____	____

   5. Objectionable or irrelevant elements   None_____ Few_____ Excessive_____

C. Other Considerations

   1. How will the film be used?   Introduce a unit_____
                                            Summarize   _____
                                            Cover a specific concept   _____
                                            Other   _____

   2. Will the film require a lengthy class preparation before it is shown?
                Yes_____ No_____

   3. What follow-up activities will be necessary after the class has viewed the film?
                Discussion_____Projects_____

   4. At which grade levels would the film be most appropriate?

    ____K-3   ____4, 5, 6   ____7, 8, 9   ____10, 11, 12

   5. General rating of film: Excellent_____Good_____Fair_____Poor_____

D. Comments: Use reverse side of form.

used. Pupils turn these kinds of media off quickly, even if the information is technically correct. Occasionally, a film or filmstrip will have incorrect scientific content due to new research, which is constantly being carried on in the health sciences. As an example, the film "Human Heredity" states that there are 48 chromosomes rather than 46. The instructor could acknowledge this error and point out that despite this discrepancy, there are other important scientific facts which the film presents well.

The *motion picture* is difficult to beat as a means of making teaching content real. This is particularly so when the presentation is pre-planned, followed through, and evaluated. A brief suggestion is to proceed somewhat as follows:

Know the film. To know the film, it is advisable for you to preview it. This will make your presentation much more effective.

Prepare yourself by asking yourself such questions as: What material will I review with the group before they see the film? What topics do I think this particular group will want to discuss? How much time will I devote to the discussion period? What refresher material do I need for my own information?

Prepare your group by telling them that: they are about to see a film showing . . . after the film showing there will be a discussion period at which time certain aspects of the film will be emphasized . . . they should save questions and comments for the discussion period.

In using films there is, in addition to the quality, another consideration. Some take the sociological approach, warning the viewer against such items as the loss of income, status, dignity, even freedom (if jailed) in a drug addiction film. Other films are purely descriptive—giving details, but leaving the student with his own thoughts about broad consequences. Some films are dramatizations, some documentaries, some lectures, some cinematic essays. Most are a combination. The teacher will have to decide on whether to project cool scientific detachment or a tone of moral outrage. Should a film be propaganda, supplying the moral element to the classroom's dispassionate discussions? Should a film, because it lists many physicians as consultants, be considered unimpeachable authority? Or should it be questioned, and, if necessary, demolished in the presence of its audience? As recorded here, of course, these are loaded questions. Unfortunately, many good films dealing with drugs, sexuality, drinking, and smoking are similarly loaded.

One teacher, who has used health films for years with secondary school youths, says, "Be wary of films on popular topics—drugs especially. Don't trust a film to be good just because someone says it is; no film is good for every school situation." Also, don't hesitate to use only portions instead of complete films, filmstrips, or tapes. Imaginative teachers have put together excellent shows by combining parts of several films. Many feel that all films should be shown twice, with a discussion period in the middle and perhaps another one following. It is worth considering. Lacey has an excellent chapter entitled "What to Do When the Lights Go On," in which he discusses film quality and inner meanings.[32] When a student responds to a film with "Fantastic movie!" Lacey quickly utters, "Define your terms."

An exceptional teaching aid is the silent cartridge *loop film*. This is a short (several minutes) presentation to drive home a point. Shown on the single-concept film projector, it can be used along with overhead transparencies, films, and filmstrips.

The evaluation form shown here can be used to appraise films, filmstrips, and slides.

Most of what has been said about motion pictures applies equally well to *filmstrips* and *slides*. Although fine colored slides are available, there is a distinct advantage in using filmstrips. They are inexpensive, easy to project, and are available in a wide variety of health topics. In fact, almost every media supply house has an extensive listing of filmstrips—from the more traditional ones dealing with nutrition and dental health, to the so called "hot topics" of the day. Most need careful previewing to establish the appropriate grade level. There has been a tendency for some filmstrip producers to create copy that will be useful in several grades. This seldom works well. Most of the time, the voice, script, and pictures cannot be extended to reach the levels of understanding for several age groups. Filmstrips, therefore, should be designated as junior high level or senior high level. Moreover, the teacher's guide accompanying the filmstrips should also be zeroed in on one secondary level or the other.

The *opaque projector* has many routine uses in the health laboratory or classroom. The light from any flat picture, photograph, newsclipping, chart, or graph may be reflected directly on the screen. It is possible to show student papers, drawings, diagrams, art work, and so forth where everyone can appraise them.

---

[32]Richard A. Lacey, *Seeing With Feeling: Film In the Classroom,* Philadelphia: W. B. Saunders Co., 1972. Chapter 2.

The *overhead projector* has been well received in most schools over the last decade because the teacher can face the class and project various kinds of transparencies onto a flat screen behind him for all to see without difficulty. By sketching, writing, or drawing on cellophane with a ceramic or wax pencil, it is possible for the class to see details more clearly than on the more traditional blackboard or other chalkboards.

A number of *transparencies* are available from voluntary health agencies, commercial organizations interested in health products, and distributors of teaching materials. The earlier chapters in the text have made reference to specific transparencies appropriate for the several major health topics. (See also Chapter 10 on source materials.) Single health topics are generally treated in sets of ten to twenty transparencies with a teacher's guide to follow. The teacher-created transparencies are also effective, especially if they have been prepared in a materials center with the help of a media specialist. A very effective transparency is the overlay type, in which two or three transparencies are hinged so that they can be laid over the original, thus adding a dimension of progression to the discussion.

TELEVISION, VIDEOTAPE, RECORDS AND TAPE RECORDINGS

The use of *television* as a means of communicating with youth has had a thorough testing during the last decade. The big questions remain to be answered: "Has it changed teaching?" and "Is it good enough to change teaching?" Perhaps it could be, for it is a powerful, informative, socializing, and mobilizing force both inside and outside the school.

Two decades of research have explored virtually every way that television could affect classroom teaching, and, in general, there is no significant difference between television and conventional instruction. This was probably due to the fact that the class did little more than sit in front of a television set. This may be why Megahey found that live instruction is more effective than televised instruction when the student is required to recall health information.[33] It has been demonstrated that television *can be* an effective teaching tool when new patterns of presentation, increased pupil participation, and improved techniques are worked out to hold attention.

Open circuit, educational television (ETV) and closed circuit, instructional television (ITV) have been dealing with such health topics as water pollution, drugs, mental health, and sex education, with good results reported out of such widely separated cities as Minneapolis, Minnesota; Spokane, Washington; Winnetka, Illinois; Portland, Oregon; and Port Washington, New York. Television can bring into the classroom short flashes showing clergymen, physicians, and other members of the community sharing their opinions on a current health topic. This may be the most efficient way to give coverage to such local problems as sewage in a river, heavy industrial smoke in the air, abortion, conservationists alarmed over the environmental scene, public health officials fighting venereal disease, interested citizens organizing to reduce accidents or combat health quackery, and many other topics.

In recent years, the *videotape* has become a popular teaching aid, not only in the heavily populated schools to bring a topic to a mass of pupils, but in a microteaching manner to three or four students who may be engaged in a health project and working largely by themselves.

There is obvious value in using professionally made videotapes in a program and, at

---

[33]Michael E. Megahey, *A Comparison of Televised and Direct Instruction In A Required Health Course,* Master's Thesis, Pennsylvania State University, 1972.

times, projecting a movie film through the school's closed circuit system. There appears to be an even greater value in creating videotapes which engage students directly in the preparation. There is much to put on tape as one visits local, private, and official health agencies, factories, hospitals, and similar locations. Portable equipment is easily moved about and detailed photography is possible. When the class returns from such a field trip into the community, the videotapes serve as discussion-provoking media, complete with pictures of the students themselves in action.

In a western New York study of 1087 students enrolled in grades 6, 7, 8, and 9, it was demonstrated that carefully prepared videotapes on alcohol, quackery, and smoking were more effective than the traditional class lessons.[34]

In terms of knowledge gained and ability to identify positive health information, the students exposed to the videotape teaching were significantly ahead of the control groups. It seems reasonable to assume that students using videotapes develop a heightened sensitivity to the health topic because of the closer relationship to community life situations. They see themselves as *part* of the scene, instead of viewers of the other fellow's scene from the cool, academic environment of the classroom.

With innovative projects involving instructional technology appearing in many schools today, it is not uncommon to work out multi-media approaches to health lessons by bringing the videotape recorder into play along with other equipment. Students in West Hartford, Connecticut, schools go to a carrel, put on headphones, dial a three digit code, and listen to audiotaped instruction. At Oak Park High School near Chicago, students dial in the same fashion for videotaped instruction. In numerous colleges and secondary schools, pupils have the freedom to visit a learning center and view a combination of tapes, films, living displays, and film cuts on a television monitor.

Using *tapes, cassettes,* and *disc records,* it is possible to bring to the classroom or learning center a wide variety of health topics — to be listened to *en masse* or in individual or small group listening areas. For some time, filmstrips and records have been used together. Tapes or cassettes and colored slides can also be programmed through the efforts of the teacher and media specialist. Student projects to develop the slides locally and filter in the audio comments can be an effective learning technique. Moreover, slide-tape programs can be stored and used at a later date by other students. There are also occasions when the instructor may wish to have a slide-tape combination function by itself.

There are numerous student uses of recording equipment that may contribute to health education learning. When it is not feasible to bring certain people into class, it is possible to send a two or three man committee into the community to tape record an interview. In one school, the students taped a whole legislative hearing on noise pollution and human efficiency at the state house some twenty miles away. When the tape was introduced in class, it was received more enthusiastically than almost any other kind of presentation during the school year. On another occasion, class members taped a series of radio and television commercials to be used in a discussion dealing with "truth in advertising" as a part of the larger unit on consumer health. In one county, students in four different schools viewed a particular tape, then took part in a discussion with each other and a teacher located at a fifth school via amplified telephone devices.

---

[34]William Zimmerli et al., "A Pilot Program Using Videotapes as a Health Education Medium With Students in Grades Six to Nine." *Journal of School Health,* 39:343–348, May, 1969.

TEXTBOOKS, PERIODICALS, PAMPHLETS,
AND CLIPPINGS

Junior and senior high school students need an opportunity to search through a variety of materials when they study a particular health topic. A library shelf of selected items is helpful, but most of the time it is not situated in a way to encourage any great amount of use. Ideally, a special health education workshop room or laboratory should be provided where projectors, screens, and certain films, filmstrips, slides, and tapes may be used along with a variety of health textbooks, newspaper clippings, periodicals, and pamphlets. Even with a minimum amount of space, an area off to one side of the classroom can be arranged for displays, posted charts and clippings, and several other pieces of material.

Textbooks are used by many teachers. In some cases, the whole program is built around them. More and more, however, they are being employed to supplement classroom activity. In this instance, they function as a source of scientific information. In this respect, the following textbooks have proven to be quite useful:

Junior High School

Bauer, William W., et al., *The New Health and Safety,* Glenview, Ill.: Scott, Foresman and Company, Revised.

Diehl, Harold S., et al., *Health and Safety for You,* 4th edition New York: McGraw-Hill Book Co., 1975.

Jones, Evelyn G., et al., *Living in Safety and Health.* Philadelphia: J. B. Lippincott Co., Revised.

Pounds, Eleanor T. et al., *Safety for Teenagers,* Glenview, Ill.: Scott, Foresman and Company, 1973.

Buxbaum, K. L., and S. Lindenmeyer, *What You Should Know About Venereal Disease,* New York: Harcourt, Brace, Jovanovich, 1975.

Fordor, J. T., *Health and Your Future,* River Forest, Ill.: Laidlaw Bros., 1975.

Rosenberg, E. B., H. J. Gurney, and V. K. Harlin, *Modern Health Investigations,* Boston: Houghton Mifflin, 1976.

Senior High School

Haag, Jesse H., *Focusing on Health,* Austin, Texas: Steck-Vaughn Co., 1974.

Lawrence, Thomas G., *Your Health and Safety In A Changing Environment,* 7th edition, New York: Harcourt, Brace & World, Inc., 1973.

Nicoll, James S., et al., *Health Today and Tomorrow,* River Forest, Ill.: Laidlow Bros., 1975.

Otto, James, et al., *Health and Safety for You,* Glenview, Ill.: Scott, Foresman and Company, 1970.

Miller, B. F., and B. L. Stackowski, *Investigating Your Health,* Boston: Houghton Mifflin, 1974.

The validity of textbooks as a moving force in changing health behavior is difficult to assess. Certainly, well written books that are able to command the attention of youth will do as much to bring about new health comprehensions and practices as some of the other aids to teaching. Unfortunately, many texts are not appropriate for a number of pupils in a designated grade. Sometimes, there is a range of six or seven years between the least and most competent readers at the seventh grade.

A *pamphlet* can supplement textbook information very well if it has an eye-catching cover and a simple message. Thousands of these are used yearly to accompany other written materials (see list of pamphlet sources in Chapter 10).

When a variety of pamphlets on related topics are spread out on a classroom table, they will be read. If the pamphlets are obtained from reliable organizations, the facts presented are usually accurate.

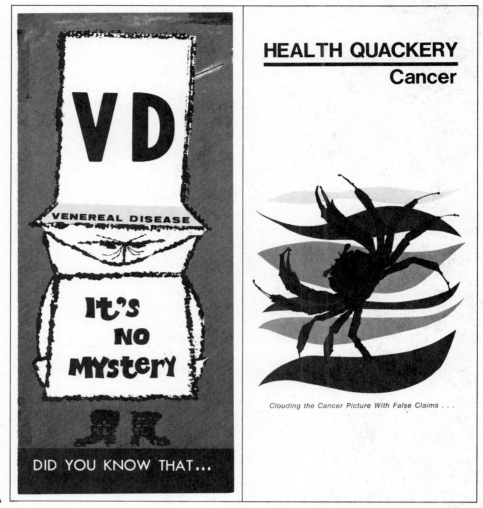

Figure 9–10　Pamphlets arouse curiosity. (*A*, Courtesy of Ohio Dept. of Health; *B*, courtesy of American Medical Association)

Another classroom or health workshop item is *periodicals*. With thousands of them on the library shelves, there is hardly an issue that doesn't make some kind of reference to one or more of the major health areas. Numerous classroom projects come alive with charts, pictures, and articles from magazines. *National Geographic, Newsweek, Time,* and *Reader's Digest* are among the most popular. Health articles appear also in *Family Health, Consumer Reports, Sports Illustrated,* and *Psychology Today.* Frequently, one of these magazines will simplify a difficult health phenomenon or process better than it could be done in a textbook or on film. *Current Health* is the monthly school magazine for secondary school pupils that explores different high interest topics each month. It is a useful class and library periodical which may be obtained from Curriculum Innovations, Inc., Highwood, Ill. 60040.

Newspaper clippings can be used just as well with older youths as they can with youngsters. Very informative material for background information and class display may be found in big city papers and Sunday supplements. Over the years, the New York Times has been a first class source for health education. Also, most articles written by medical writers are scientifically accurate; this is because they are written by people who follow the advances and experimentations of medical science rather closely and belong to their own highly reputable association of medical writers.

HOW WE IN THE UNITED STATES GET OUR CALORIES

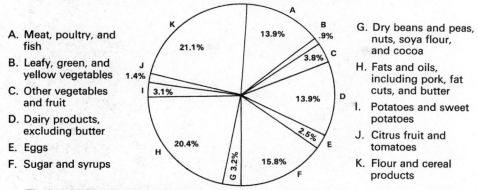

A. Meat, poultry, and fish

B. Leafy, green, and yellow vegetables

C. Other vegetables and fruit

D. Dairy products, excluding butter

E. Eggs

F. Sugar and syrups

G. Dry beans and peas, nuts, soya flour, and cocoa

H. Fats and oils, including pork, fat cuts, and butter

I. Potatoes and sweet potatoes

J. Citrus fruit and tomatoes

K. Flour and cereal products

A 13.9%
B .9%
C 3.8%
D 13.9%
E 2.5%
F 15.8%
G 3.2%
H 20.4%
I 3.1%
J 1.4%
K 21.1%

The CALORIE CONTRIBUTIONS of various classes of foods to the average American diet.

Figure 9–11   The pie-graph tells something at a glance. (Courtesy of General Mills, Inc.)

PICTURES, POSTERS, CHARTS, AND GRAPHS

An attractive *photograph* catches the eyes of the students passing the bulletin board. In fact, all good pictorial materials can be employed to put an idea or story across. Vivid, realistic pictures that stop the viewer in his tracks can be found if enough newspapers, pamphlets, and magazines are searched. Helpful are such pictures as au-

Figure 9–12   The bar-graph has long been a favorite. (Courtesy of U.S. Public Health Service)

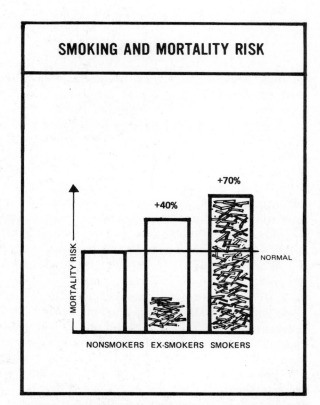

SMOKING AND MORTALITY RISK

+70%

+40%

NORMAL

MORTALITY RISK

NONSMOKERS   EX-SMOKERS   SMOKERS

The risk of death for ex-smokers is intermediate between that of smokers and nonsmokers, and it decreases with an increasing length of time following cessation of smoking.

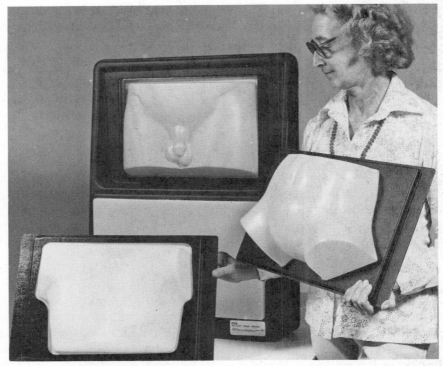

Figure 9–13 Relevant visual system cutaways for dual screen projection. (Courtesy of OMNI Educational System, Ortho Pharmaceutical Corp.)

tomobile wrecks, fire scenes, drug arrests, suicide attempts, starving children, oil covered waterfowl, and polluted air. Secondary school students frequently enjoy taking their own "health shots" for classroom display.

By far, the most effective bulletin board item is the *poster*. A considerable amount of money has been spent by numerous health industries and organizations over the years to develop, print, and distribute just the right kind of poster. Hundreds of these are available for little or no cost from most of the voluntary health organizations, state health departments, insurance companies, and the various special groups associated with such fields as nutrition, mental health, alcohol, cancer, heart disease, safety and accident prevention, and communicable disease control. See examples in Chapter 10.

Posters vary in size. Most of the time, it is better to have a size of about 22 by 28 inches—big enough to see and remember. Usually they depict one essential idea.

When several ideas are depicted and certain facts are organized in lines or blocks, the poster-like display becomes a *chart*. The American National Red Cross chart, *Blood as a Medicine,* is a good example. Here a 100 per cent figure of a test tube is broken down into descriptive blocks showing plasma (54%), white cells and platelets (1%), and red cells (45%). This teaching aid, big enough for posting, serves both as a poster and a chart. Another useful wall chart which can be mounted at the front of the room is distributed by the Johnson and Johnson Company and describes the six basic emergencies which occur most frequently: stopped breathing, bleeding, broken bones, burns, poisoning, and shock.

Especially useful and interest-provoking is the Relevant Visual System (RVS) of OMNI Education (190 W. Main St., Sommerville, N.J. 08876), in which a slide projection focuses on two screens simultaneously. Interchangeable projection forms permit detailed enlargements and cutaway sections for the study of such items as breast cancer and reproductive anatomy. See cutaway section examples in Figure 9–13.

MODELS, EXHIBITS, AND MUSEUMS

These three instructional entities frequently go together. A good *model* may be part of an exhibit in a health museum or elsewhere. The model is useful, because it is so accurate that it is almost real. It can be taken apart, handled, and thoroughly examined. Although the model is only a copy of the real human part or system, it can help create understandings that might be difficult to present otherwise. Several biological supply houses sell a wide variety of models suitable for junior and senior high school classes. An excellent life-size plastic heart model may be obtained from the pharmaceutical firm, Merck, Sharp and Dohme (West Point, Pennsylvania 19486). It is constructed of 22 pieces, sturdily molded in such a way that it can be separated into halves for internal study. A 20-page illustrated teacher's manual accompanies each heart model. Another source of life-size scientifically accurate models is the Cleveland Health Museum. Models of the uterus with fetus and birth process are available in light-weight polystyrene.

Models can be used to make an *exhibit* more interesting. They may accompany an automated film of some body function. A special side table or display case exhibit, shown at the time a certain major health topic is being studied, can be very effective. However, a good exhibit takes time to prepare and to dismantle. This is one reason why teachers tend to shy away from continually changing exhibitions of materials pertaining to a current health topic. Yet, with student help, the exhibit—like a bulletin board—can be changed frequently to foster student attention.

A proper exhibit should not try to tell everything; rather, it should focus on a central idea. It should be well lighted, colorful, and should employ several media such as slides, transparencies, models, and tape recordings—provided there is enough space so that everything isn't crowded together. Whenever possible, some kind of motion should be added to the exhibit to attract the eyes of the viewer. A simple battery and turntable arrangement can be used in a number of ways. In a dental health exhibit, for example, a phonograph turntable was covered with red paper and used to hold four different sets of plaster of Paris impressions of maloccluded teeth. This was very effective, because on the small screen just behind it was being shown a color transparency of maloccluded teeth anchored into the upper and lower jaws.

In an effort to research the effectiveness of health exhibits, Christie pretested ninth and tenth grade students just before the exhibits were placed in the schools.[35] Nothing was said in class about these, and the pupils were unaware that they were to be tested later. Yet, after post-testing, some 85 per cent of the students improved their performance as a result of observing the health exhibits—significant beyond the 0.01 level of confidence. Moreover, girls were slightly better than boys, and middle-class students showed greater gains than those from the lower socioeconomic group.

Most schools do not build their own museums. If they attempt to do so, there is a strong tendency for them to take up valuable space, gather dust, and become outdated. Using *permanent museums* is the answer, for these organizations keep current, are well-staffed, and exist to serve the public—chiefly by providing a place for school people to visit, study, and carry on some limited research. Several of the most famous health mu-

---

[35]Tasso G. Christie, "Educational Effectiveness of Health Exhibits," *Journal of School Health,* 40:206–209, April, 1970.

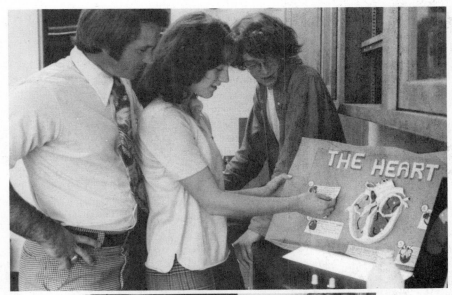

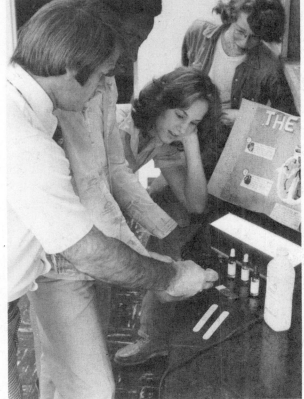

Figure 9–14 Instructor and students prepare an exhibit. (Courtesy of Millicent C. Rhodes, Metropolitan Public Schools, Nashville, Tennessee)

seums, used by thousands of youths every week, are the Cleveland Health Museum (Ohio), the Museum of Hygiene and Medicine (Rochester, Minnesota), the Dallas Health Museum (Texas), the Lankenau Hospital Health Museum (Philadelphia), the Hinsdale Health Museum (Chicago), and the Reading Hospital in Reading, Pennsylvania.

A characteristic of an effective museum is the existence of a combination of continuing exhibits in the fundamental health areas, and special exhibits designed to focus on the immediate health concerns of the month. Thus, in the Cleveland Health Museum, such items as the famous Dickinson models depicting human birth and the larger than life-size "talking lady" are always on display; new materials may take the form of exhibits pertaining to the drug scene and to air and water pollution about the city of Cleveland. For the teacher, the advantage of using a health museum centers on being able to use the museum staff as a superb source of accurate information, in a setting the school would have trouble trying to duplicate. Also, museums frequently make certain kits of health materials available on loan to schools.

QUESTIONS FOR DISCUSSION

1. Examining feelings that surround pupil interests can be approached by the use of film, says Richard Lacey in *Seeing With Feeling: Film in the Classroom.* Is there evidence that there are better ways to get at student feelings?
2. Robert Mager, in his book, *Developing Attitude Toward Learning,* describes how some teachers "overkill" the subject by spending a great deal of class time presenting material beyond the ability of the pupils to understand. He then speaks about the pupils experiencing "subject matter avoidance tendencies" which may do the student more harm than good. What do you think Mager means?
3. In the last quarter century, the word *creativity* has been used a great deal in educational literature. What exactly does it mean in terms of day-to-day student activities in the classroom? Give some examples of creative health activity and indicate how it differs from any other kind of activity.
4. Here and there are evidences of success with programmed instruction. Find out from your readings how "success" has been measured. Also, is "success" knowledge oriented or behavior oriented?
5. There are some teachers who use very little of the media, yet appear to be effective in holding class attention and making health education a vital subject. What might be several reasons for this apparent success?
6. Are not simulation games and role playing somewhat alike? How are they different? How might you use one teaching technique in a situation where the other technique would be inappropriate?

SUGGESTED ACTIVITIES

1. The Coleman study, conducted under the aegis of the U.S. Office of Education, involved a survey of about 650,000 pupils in some 4000 schools. It placed great emphasis on social environment in pupil achievement and found that schools have little influence on achievement that is independent of pupil background and general social context. It also found that the impact of the teacher was the most important element in the school. Interview several teachers from a depressed area to see how they view the Coleman report. Compare your findings with class members.

2. Alternative forms of education are needed everywhere in order to reach all kinds of students in secondary schools. Read about alternative efforts and suggest teaching examples that will also embrace the humanistic education concept.

3. Examine a number of junior and senior high school health education textbooks in a curriculum library. Are they attractive? Are they detailed enough so that the pupil will not have to fall back on the encyclopedia for accurate information? Do they provide so many of the answers early in the special chapters that there is little opportunity for the *discovery method* to work? Give your comments.

4. An effective teaching aid, when used sparingly, is the cartoon. It can provide a message in a humorous and subtle manner that is difficult to match through the use of other media and materials. Look through the popular magazines and newspaper pages and locate a number of health related cartoons. Categorize them into major health topic areas for future use as eye-catching bulletin board material.

5. From time to time, self-instructional devices, or so-called teaching machines, have appeared. It is likely that more will appear in the future to better present health programs in small steps for individual instruction. If these cheat-proof machines are really effective in improving learning, why are not more of them available? Search the literature and talk with teacher preparation faculty members about this situation. In short, try to establish some reason why teaching machines are not being used to any great degree.

6. Visit a school which uses portable videotape equipment for teaching health. Examine the organization and witness programs in action. How well are they received by pupils? Try to evaluate the process.

SELECTED REFERENCES

Allen, Dwight, W., and Jeffrey C. Hecht. *Controversies In Education*, Philadelphia: W. B. Saunders Co., 1974.

Brown, George I. *The Live Classroom*, New York: The Viking Press, 1975.

Clarke, Kenneth S. "Values and Risk-Taking Behavior: The Concept of Calculated Risk," *Health Education*, 6:26–28, November/December, 1975.

Ensor, Phyllis, and Richard K. Means. *Methods Handbook for Health Education*, Boston: Allyn and Bacon, Inc., 1974.

Fusco, Ronald A., and Michael J. Perlin. "Guidelines for Group Process," *School Health Review*, 5:37–39, July/August, 1974.

Good, Thomas L., Bruce J. Biddle, and Jere E. Brophy. *Teachers Make a Difference*, New York: Holt, Rinehart, and Winston, 1975.

Hamrick, Michael H. "Give Students a Choice," *School Health Review*, 4:11–14, July/August, 1973.

Hart, Burton B. "Testing a Multimedia Course," *Health Education*, 6:8–9, May/June, 1975.

Keeney, Clifford E. "The Audio-Tutorial Format," *Journal of Physical Education and Recreation*, 46:24, May, 1975.

Lister, Ian. *Deschooling*, New York: Cambridge University Press, 1974.

Mager, Robert E. *Developing Attitudes Towards Learning*, Palo Alto, California: Fearon Publishing Co., 1968.

Malone, Marianne. "Health Fair for the Campus Community," *School Health Review*, 5:18–19, July/August, 1974.

Miller, Dean F., et al.: "The Readability of Junior High School Textbooks," *Journal of School Health*, 64:382–384, September, 1974.

Nolte, Ann, "The Relevance of Abraham Maslow's Work To Health Education," *Health Education*, 7:25–28, May–June, 1976.

Pruitt, B. E. "The Open Contract: A Program of Individual Study," *Health Education*, 6:37–38, November/December, 1975.

Read, Donald A., and Walter H. Greene. *Creative Teaching in Health*, 2nd edition. New York: Macmillan Co., 1975.

Sarason, Irwin G., and Barbara R. Sarason. *A Teacher's Guide to Modeling and Role-Playing Techniques*, New York: Behavioral Publications, 1975.

Schwank, Jeffrey. *Teaching Human Beings*, Boston: Beacon Press, 1972.

Simon, Sidney B., Leland W. Howe, and Howard Kirschenbaum. *Values Clarification*, New York: Hart Publishing Co., 1972.

Sinning, Wayne, E.: *Experiments and Demonstrations in Exercise Physiology,* Philadelphia: W. B. Saunders Co., 1975.

Smith, Charles D., and Samuel Prather. "Group Problem Solving," *Journal of Physical Education and Recreation,* 46:20–21, September, 1975.

Snow, David L. "Behavior Modification Techniques in the School Setting," *Journal of School Health,* 44:198–204, April, 1974.

Staton, Wesley, M. "Monday Morning at the Movies," *Health Education,* 6:27–29, January/February, 1975.

Teper-Singer, Lynn. "The Many Faces of Role-Playing," *Health Education,* 6:34–35, November/December, 1975.

Wiist, William H. "Television Production for a Community Health Project." *Health Education,* 6:39–41, November/December, 1975.

Willgoose, Carl E. *Health Education in the Elementary School.* 4th edition, Philadelphia: W. B. Saunders Co., 1974, Chapter 9.

Chapter 10

Sources of Teaching Aids

The primary purpose of this chapter is to set forth in detail many fine examples of the wide variety of teaching aids especially valuable for health education in the secondary schools. All of these materials are available on request, and a great many are free or relatively inexpensive. In fact, with the exception of certain more costly films and models, no teacher should have difficulty in obtaining most of the items listed throughout the chapter.

APPRAISING THE SOURCES

Good teaching demands a certain amount of preplanning. This includes an investigation of the media and the kinds of learning materials that are available for a particular health topic. The question of which charts, posters, filmstrips, tapes, transparencies, or other aids to use comes up again and again. This requires a certain amount of lead time in which to collect these aids and look them over. In fact, reviewing learning materials is an ongoing activity throughout the year. Before pamphlets, charts, and books on a current health topic are placed with the librarian or on a side table in the classroom they should be seen by two or three teachers, and perhaps reviewed by a student or two to see if they are as good as they seem to be. Films, filmstrips, tapes, and transparencies require the same careful treatment. The appraisal task is more difficult today than it has ever been, simply because of the wealth of materials being distributed. Hundreds of commercial organizations and voluntary agencies with a health related product to promote are anxious to involve school children and youth in general to spread the word. The same may be said for the numerous official public agencies. Therefore, the task of the teacher as a "dispenser of the truth" is a responsible one that is not easily dismissed. Because of the size of the appraisal task, some of the larger schools have a small committee of health education personnel who collect and review health materials. This is a highly recommended practice, for it insures that most new teaching aids will be brought to the proper attention of instructors where they can be embraced as appropriate or dismissed as inadequate.

In reviewing the source materials it is important to see if they are up to date, especially in terms of scientific information. One should ask if the agency is recognized in the health field. Why has the health pamphlet, tape, or transparency been developed? Is the purpose only to sell specific products? What are the qualifications of the author? What do health personnel in the private and public sector think of the material?

OFFICIAL HEALTH AGENCIES

City, county, state, and federal government organizations that have been established by law to accomplish specific health maintenance, promotion, and control generally have a number of free teaching aids. Pamphlets, films, and exhibits are plentiful. New teachers should investigate what is available from their own state's health and education departments.

The federal government has a great number of materials, single copies of which are usually available at no charge. The list is extensive because health is such a multidimensional topic. This is fine, because it is the way health should be seen by secondary school youth. Helpful in this respect are the following agencies:

Department of Health, Education and Welfare, Office of Education, Washington, D.C. 20025.

Superintendent of Documents, U.S. Government Printing Office, Washington, D.C. 20025 (secure a catalog before ordering materials).

National Institute of Mental Health, Barlow Building, Chevy Chase, Maryland 20015.

U.S. Environmental Protection Agency, Office of Public Affairs, Washington, D.C. 20460.

U.S. Public Health Service, HEW, Washington, D.C. 20201 (includes the National Institutes of Health).

The United Nations World Health Organization, Geneva, Switzerland (New York, N.Y. 20006).

VOLUNTARY AND PROFESSIONAL HEALTH AGENCIES

For several years the following nonofficial agencies, dedicated to some aspect of health and disease, have proven to be a real service to secondary school teachers through their source materials and suggestions for teaching about their topic.

Alcoholics Anonymous
P.O. Box 429, Grand Central Annex
New York, New York 10017

American Academy of Pediatrics
1801 Hinman Avenue
P.O. Box 1034
Evanston, Illinois 60204

American Alliance for Health, Physical
  Education & Recreation
1201 16th Street, N.W.
Washington, D.C. 20036

American Cancer Society
219 East 42nd Street
New York, New York 10017

American Dental Association
211 East Chicago Avenue
Chicago, Illinois 60611

American Dietetic Association
18 East 48th Street
New York, New York 10017

American Foundation for the Blind
15 West 16th Street
New York, New York 10011

American Heart Association
44 East 23rd Street
New York, New York 10010

American Hospital Association
840 North Lake Shore Drive
Chicago, Illinois 60611

American Institute of Family Relations
5287 Sunset Boulevard
Los Angeles, California 90027

American Lung Association
51 Sleeper Street
Boston, Massachusetts 02210

American Medical Association
Department of Health Education
535 North Dearborn Street
Chicago, Illinois 60610

American National Red Cross
17th and D Streets, N.W.
Washington, D.C. 20006
(contact local chapters for materials)

American Nurses Association
10 Columbus Circle
New York, New York 10019

American Optometric Association
Department of Public Affairs
7000 Chippewa Street
St. Louis, Missouri 63119

American School Health Association
515 East Main Street
Kent, Ohio 44241

American Social Health Association
1740 Broadway
New York, New York 10019

Arthritis Foundation
23 West 45th Street
New York, New York 10019

Child Study Association of America
9 East 89th Street
New York, New York 10028

Cleveland Health Museum
8911 Euclid Avenue
Cleveland, Ohio 44106

Hogg Foundation for Mental Health
The University of Texas
Austin, Texas 78712

Muscular Dystrophy Associations
of America
1790 Broadway
New York, New York 10019

National Association of Hearing and
Speech Agencies
919 18th Street, N.W.
Washington, D.C. 20006

National Coordinating Council on Drug
Abuse
P.O. Box 19400
Washington, D.C. 20036

National Council on Alcoholism
2 Park Avenue
New York, New York 10016

National Congress of Parents and
Teachers
700 North Rush Street
Chicago, Illinois 60637

National Foundation
800 2nd Avenue
New York, New York 10017

National Interagency on Smoking and
Health
P.O. Box 3654, Central Station
Arlington, Virginia 22203

National League for Nursing
59th Street and Columbus Circle
New York, New York 10019

National Multiple Sclerosis Society
257 Park Avenue South
New York, New York 10010

National Safety Council
425 North Michigan Avenue
Chicago, Illinois 60611

National Society for the Prevention of
Blindness
79 Madison Avenue
New York, New York 10016

National Society for Crippled Children
and Adults
2023 West Ogden Avenue
Chicago, Illinois 60603

Nutrition Foundation, Inc.
99 Park Avenue
New York, New York 10016

Rutgers Center of Alcohol Studies
Rutgers, The State University
New Brunswick, New Jersey 08903

Planned Parenthood-World Population
515 Madison Avenue
New York, New York 10022

Sex Education and Information Council of
the U.S. (SEICUS)
1855 Broadway
New York, New York 10023

Public Affairs Committee
381 Park Avenue South
New York, New York 10016

United Cerebral Palsy Association, Inc.
321 West 44th Street
New York, New York 10036

COMMERCIAL ORGANIZATIONS

Numerous individual commercial organizations and associations of industry promote their health related products through pamphlets, brochures, and posters. Many have invested large sums of money in films, filmstrips, and transparencies which are superb teaching aids. Much of this material is useful in secondary school teaching. Moreover, a number of organizations have very carefully developed appropriate grade level learning materials. Notable along these lines over the years are such groups as the National Dairy Council, the Cereal Institute, Inc., General Mills, Inc., the Florida Citrus Commission, Johnson and Johnson, the Kellogg Company, the National Fire Protection Association, the Procter and Gamble Company, and Tampax, Incorporated.

A partial list of the more reliable commercial organizations and associations of industry is as follows:

Abbott Laboratories
14th and Sheridan Road
North Chicago, Illinois 60064

Blue Cross Association
840 North Lake Shore Drive
Chicago, Illinois 60611

Aetna Life Affiliated Companies
Education Department
151 Farmington Avenue
Hartford, Connecticut 06115

The Borden Company
350 Madison Avenue
New York, New York 10017

American Automobile Association
Traffic Safety Department
1712 G Street, N.W.
Washington, D.C. 20036

Cereal Institute, Inc.
Educational Director
135 South LaSalle Street
Chicago, Illinois 60603

American Meat Institute
59 East Van Buren Street
Chicago, Illinois 60605

Church and Dwight Company, Inc.
70 Pine Street
New York, New York 10005

Athletic Institute
805 Merchandise Mart
Chicago, Illinois 60650

Colgate Palmolive Company
300 Park Avenue
New York, New York 10022

Automotive Safety Foundation
Ring Building
Washington, D.C. 20036

Consumers Union of U.S., Inc.
Mount Vernon, New York 10550

Cream of Wheat Corporation
Box M
Minneapolis, Minnesota 55413

Distilled Spirits Council of the U.S., Inc.
1300 Pennsylvania Building
Washington, D.C. 20004

Educational Activities, Inc.
Box 392
Freeport, New York 11520

Eli Lilly Company
740' South Alabama Street
Indianapolis, Indiana 46206

Evaporated Milk Association
228 North LaSalle Street
Chicago, Illinois 60601

Florida Citrus Commission
P.O. Box 148
Lakeland, Florida 33802

General Mills, Inc.
Education Section
9200 Wayzata Boulevard
Minneapolis, Minnesota 55426

Good Housekeeping Institute
8th Avenue and 57th Street
New York, New York 10019

H. J. Heinz and Company
P.O. Box 57
Pittsburgh, Pennsylvania 15230

Johnson and Johnson
Educational Division
501 George Street
New Brunswick, New Jersey 08903

Kellogg Company
Department of Home Economics Services
Battle Creek, Michigan 49016

Kimberly-Clark Corporation
Educational Department
Neenah, Wisconsin 54956

Kraft Cheese Company
500 Peshtigo Court
Chicago, Illinois 60690

Licensed Beverage Industries, Inc.
155 E. 44th Street
New York, New York 10017

Maltex Company
Burlington, Vermont 05401

Metropolitan Life Insurance Company
Health and Welfare Division
1 Madison Avenue
New York, New York 10010

Money Management Institute
Prudential Plaza
Chicago, Illinois 60601

National Board of Fire Underwriters
85 John Street
New York, New York 10038

National Dairy Council
Program Service Department
111 North Canal Street
Chicago, Illinois 60606

National Fire Protection Association
60 Batterymarch Street
Boston, Massachusetts 02110

National Foot Health Council
272 Union Street
Rockland, Massachusetts 02370

National Livestock and Meat Board
36 South Wabash Avenue
Chicago, Illinois 60603

Paper Cup and Container Institute
Public Health Committee
250 Park Avenue
New York, New York 10017

Pet Milk Company
1401 Arcade Building
St. Louis, Missouri 63101

Personal Products Company
Milltown, New Jersey 08850

Pharmaceutical Manufacturers Assoc.
1155 15th Street, N.W.
Washington, D.C. 20005

Procter and Gamble Company
P.O. Box 171
Cincinnati, Ohio 45201

Schering Laboratories
Kenilworth, New Jersey 07033

Scott Paper Company
Home Service Center
Philadelphia, Pennsylvania 19113

Smith, Kline and French Laboratories
1500 Spring Garden Street
Philadelphia, Pennsylvania 19101

Spenco Medical Corporation
Box 8113
Waco, Texas 76710

Sunkist Growers
P.O. Box 7888, Valley Annex
Van Nuys, California 91409

Swift and Company
Union Stockyards
Chicago, Illinois 60609

Tampax, Incorporated
Educational Director
5 Dakota Drive
Lake Success, New York 11040

The Center for Humanities, Inc.
2 Holland Avenue
White Plains, New York 10603

Travelers Insurance Company
Hartford, Connecticut 06115

Underwriters' Laboratories, Inc.
207 East Ohio Street
Chicago, Illinois 60611

United Fresh Fruit and Vegetable Association
777 14th Street, N.W.
Washington, D.C. 20005

United States Beet Sugar Association
Tower Building
Washington, D.C. 20005

Upjohn Company
7000 Portage Road
Kalamazoo, Michigan 49002

Wheat Flour Institute
Supervisor of Distribution
14 East Jackson Boulevard
Chicago, Illinois 60604

SOURCES OF AIDS FOR MAJOR HEALTH TOPICS

The following listing of teaching aids by media category is far from complete. However, it does represent materials that have been in secondary schools and were found useful in some way.

All sources are designed for the *student* to use. They are organized by major health topics in keeping with the program and activities presented in Chapters 5 through 8.

1. PHYSICAL ACTIVITY, SLEEP, REST AND RELAXATION

a. Pamphlets or Leaflets

A Boy and His Physique, National Dairy Council

Adult Fitness, U.S. Government Printing Office

A Girl and Her Figure, National Dairy Council

Athletics For Girls, American Medical Association

Exercise and Fitness, American Medical Association

Exercise and Fitness, National Education Association (AAHPER)

How to Shape Up and Keep in Shape, Florida Citrus Commission

Learn Safe Boating, American National Red Cross

Obesity Has Many Angles, United Fresh Fruit and Vegetable Association

✓*Personalized Weight Control,* National Dairy Council

✓*Physical Fitness,* U.S. Government Printing Office

✓*Seven Paths to Fitness,* American Medical Association

Sleep and Sports, American Medical Association

✓*Smoking and Heart Disease,* American Heart Association

Step Up to Foot Health, American Podiatry Association

The Challenge of Health Research, Metropolitan Life Insurance Company

✓*To Decrease the Risk of Heart Disease,* Sunkist Growers

✓*What Makes a Good Hobby?* American Medical Association

✓*You Can Reduce,* National Livestock and Meat Board

b. Films*

Better Odds for a Longer Life, American Heart Association

Endocrine Glands, Encyclopedia Britannica Films

✓*Exercise and Health,* Coronet Instructional Films

✓*How the Body Uses Energy,* McGraw-Hill Book Co.

Obesity, Encyclopedia Britannica Films

Playtown U.S.A., The Athletic Institute

✓*Sleep for Health,* Encyclopedia Britannica Films

Sports Medicine, Pharmaceutical Manufacturers Association

Vigor, Sterling Films

Water Safety, Young America Films

Who's Handicapped?, Vision Quest, Lawrenceville, New Jersey 08648

✓*Wonder Engine of the Body,* American Heart Association

c. Filmstrips*

✓*Checking Your Health,* Encyclopedia Britannica Films

Circulatory Control, Popular Science

✓*Mechanics of Breathing,* Popular Science

✓*Our Heart and Circulation,* Popular Science

Sleep and Rest, Popular Science

✓*Sleep for Health,* Encyclopedia Britannica Films

✓*The Body Machine: Muscular System,* Popular Science

d. Posters

Lift With Your Legs—Not Your Back, American Medical Association

✓*Physical Fitness* (9 posters), American Medical Association

✓*Who—Me?,* National Dairy Council

e. Charts

✓*Exercise Chart,* Metropolitan Life Insurance Company

f. Tapes

✓*Weight Control* (J. Mayer), Educational Activities, Inc.

Backache and You, Spenco Medical Corporation

✓*Exercise and Health,* (Bruess-Gallagher), Harper and Row, Publishers

✓*Overweight,* Spenco Medical Corporation

✓*Exercise and Fitness,* Educational Activities, Inc.

g. Records

Basic Concepts Through Dance, Body Image, Educational Activities, Inc.

Listening and Moving, Educational Activities, Inc.

✓*Rhythms for Physical Fitness,* Educational Activities, Inc.

h. Selected Books*

(J) = Junior High Level

(S) = Senior High Level

A Guide to Gymnastics (J, S), F. Musker (Macmillan)

Dance a While (J), J. B. Flood (W. C. Brown)

Exercise, Rest and Relaxation (J), R. T. Mackey (W. C. Brown)

---

*The addresses of film and filmstrip sources may be found on pages 406 to 409.

*Books appropriate for the librarian to make available.

Handbook of Physical Fitness (J, S), D. Cassidy (Macmillan)

Human Growth (J, S), L. F. Beck (Harcourt, Brace Jovanovich)

Obesity (S), G. Christakis (Nutrition Foundation)

Slim Down, G. Rienzo (Vantage)

Square Dance (J), J. B. Flood (W. C. Brown)

2. NUTRITION AND GROWTH

a. Pamphlets and Leaflets

Additives in Our Food, U.S. Public Health Service, FDA

A Guide to Proper Nutrition, H. J. Heinz Company

A Guide to Good Eating, National Dairy Council

A Nutrition Guide, General Mills

Breakfast and the Bright Life, Cereal Institute

Breakfast Cereals in the American Diet, Cereal Institute

Breakfast Cereals in Today's Lifestyles, Cereal Institute

Breakfast Your Way to a Better Day, Kellogg Company

Build a Better You With Fresh Citrus, Sunkist Growers

Cheese to Suit Every State, Kraft Foods

Choose Your Calories Wisely, Kellogg Company

Daily Food Guide, U.S. Department of Agriculture

Diet and Dental Health, American Dental Association

Don't Discount the Minerals in Citrus Fruit, Sunkist Growers

Eat to Live, Wheat Flour Institute

Facts About the Foods You Eat, Cereal Institute

Food for Fitness, U.S. Government Printing Office

Food for Growing Boys and Girls, Kellogg Company

Food Science and How It Began, National Dairy Council

Food to Grow On, National Livestock and Meat Board

Fresh Citrus 'Round the Clock, Sunkist Growers

Fresh Facts for the Consumer, United Fresh Fruits and Vegetable Association

Guide to Natural Cheese, Kraft Foods

Health Foods: Facts and Fakes, Public Affairs pamphlets

How Safe Is Our Food?, U.S. Public Health Service, FDA

If You Think Breakfast Is for the Birds, Cereal Institute

Let's Be Smart About Calories, Sunkist Growers

Meat Snacks for Better Health, National Livestock and Meat Board

Milk: Its Food Value, National Dairy Council

Nutrition Notes, Cream of Wheat

Pick a Breakfast Pattern, Cereal Institute

Recipes for Clock Watchers, Wheat Flour Institute

Recipes for Fat-Controlled Meals, Florida Citrus Commission

Source Book on Food Practices, National Dairy Council

Take a Fresh Look at Citrus, Sunkist Growers

The Food Way to Weight Reduction, National Dairy Council

The Nutrition Ladder, Florida Citrus Commission

The World of Cheese, Kraft Foods

Your Daily Bread and Its Dramatic History, American Bakers Association

Your Food—Chance or Choice, National Dairy Council

Weight Control Source Book, National Dairy Council

Waist Trimmers, United Fresh Fruit and Vegetable Association

b. Films

And Everything Nice, National Dairy Council

Balance Your Diet for Health, United Fresh Fruit and Vegetable Association

Beef for All Occasions, National Livestock and Meat Board

Behind the Smile, National Dairy Council

Eat to Your Heart's Content, American Heart Association

Food, Fads, Facts, Perennial Education

Food—More For Your Money, Alfred Higgins Productions

Food—Green Grow the Profits, Macmillan Films, Inc.

Fundamentals of Diet, Encyclopedia Britannica

How a Hamburger Turns Into You, National Dairy Council

How a Hamburger Turns Into You, Wexler Film Productions

How Red Berry Save White Man From Singing Blues, United Fresh Fruit and Vegetable Association.

Jenny Is a Good Thing, Wexler Film Productions

Nutrition Sense and Nonsense, National Dairy Council

Over the Plate, National Dairy Council

The Eating on the Run Film, Alfred Higgins Productions

Vitamins from Food, Wexler Film Productions

Your Food, McGraw-Hill

c. Filmstrips

Basic Talk on Weight Control, National Dairy Council

Beef—From Store to Table, National Livestock and Meat Board

Beautiful Naturally, Florida Citrus Commission

Breakfast and the Bright Life, Cereal Institute

Food Around the World, National Dairy Council

Fresh Citrus 'Round the Clock, Sunkist Growers

Grains from Farm to Table, Cereal Institute

How to Shape Up, Florida Citrus Commission

Nutrition: Food vs. Health, Sunburst Communications

Nutrition for You, Educational Activities, Inc.

Population and Food, Popular Science

Story of Wheat, Wheat Flour Institute

The Increasing Importance of Grain Foods, Cereal Institute

Why Eat a Good Breakfast?, Cereal Institute

You and Your Food, Young America Films

Your Food—Chance or Choice, National Dairy Council

d. Posters

A Guide to Good Eating, National Dairy Council

Citrus Fruit (8 posters), Florida Citrus Commission

Food Power for Your Family, American Medical Association

Foods, United Fresh Fruit and Vegetable Association

Fresh Fruit 'Round the Clock, Florida Citrus Commission

Nutrition Facts to Guide Your Food Choices, Cereal Institute

Take a Fresh Look at Citrus, Sunkist Growers

The Four Food Groups, Florida Citrus Commission

Who—Me?, National Dairy Council

e. Charts

A Basic Breakfast Pattern, Cereal Institute

Calorie Bar Charts, United Fresh Fruit and Vegetable Association

Food Value Charts, National Livestock and Meat Board

For the Calcium You Need, Evaporated Milk Association

Functions of Food, National Livestock and Meat Board

Good Health Record, Kellogg Company

Grains: Origin of Breakfast Cereals, Cereal Institute

Kernel of Wheat, Wheat Flour Institute

Nutrient Teaching Charts, National Dairy Council

We Work Together, Wheat Flour Institute

f. Transparencies

Four Food Groups, National Dairy Council

Good Health Begins with Good Nutrition (6), Cereal Institute, Inc.

Nutrient Teaching Transparencies, National Dairy Council

g. Tapes

Nutrition and Health (J. Mayer), Educational Activities, Inc.

Weight Control (J. Mayer), Educational Activities, Inc.

h. Slides
How Food Affects You, U.S. Department of Agriculture

i. Experimental Material
Animal Feeding Demonstration, National Dairy Council

j. Comics
The Winning Combination, Swift and Company

k. Selected Books
'(J) = Junion High Level
(S) = Senior High Level
Cook-A-Meal Cookbook (J), G. Clark (W. R. Scott)
A Diet for Living (S), J. Mayer (McKay)
Diet for a Small Planet (S), F. Lappe (Ballantine)
Eat to Live (J, S), D. Hegestead (Wheat Flour Institute)
Eating for Good Health (S), F. Stare (Doubleday)
Fiber for Foods (J, S) B. Kraus (Signet)
Food and Nutrition (J, S), W. Sebrell (Time, Inc.)
Food Becomes You (J, S) R. Leverton (Doubleday)
Food Choice: The Teenage Girl (J, S), M. M. Hill (Nutrition Foundation)
Food Facts for Teenagers (J, S), M. B. Salmon (Charles C Thomas)
Live High on Low Fat (S), S. Rosenthal (Lippincott)
Keeping Food Safe (S), H. Bradley (Doubleday)
Man and the Earth (S), J. B. Hoyt (Prentice-Hall)
Nutrition for Growing Years (J), M. McWilliams (John Wiley)
Overweight: Causes, Cost and Control (S), J. Mayer (Prentice-Hall)
People and Plows Against Hunger (S), H. Black (Marlborough House)
Slim Down, Shape Up Diets for Teenagers (J, S), G. Maddox (Avon)
Still Hungry in America (S), R. Coles (World)
The Food Book (S), J. Trager (Grossman)
The Overweight Society (S), P. Wyden (William Morrow)

The Teenage Guide to Diet and Health (J, S), R. S. Goodhart (Prentice-Hall)
This Hungry World (J, S), W. Aykroyd (Scribner's Sons)
What the World Eats (J), H. H. Webster (Houghton-Mifflin)
Your Diet: Health Is in the Balance (J, S), F. Stare (Nutrition Foundation)

3. DENTAL HEALTH

a. Pamphlets and Leaflets
A Visit to the Dentist, American Dental Association
Between 13 and 18, American Dental Association
Careers in Dentistry, American Dental Association
Dental Health Education, Cleveland Health Museum
Diet and Dental Health, American Dental Association
Food and Care for Dental Health, National Dairy Council
For Good Dental Health Start Early, National Dairy Council
Fresh Oranges for Sound Teeth, Sunkist Growers
How Bright the Smile, Florida Citrus Commission
How Teeth Grow, National Dairy Council
Nutrition, Diet and the Teeth, United Fresh Fruit and Vegetable Association
Orthodontics, American Dental Association
Smoking and Oral Health (G8), American Dental Association
Smoking Impact on Oral Health (G37), American Dental Association.
Toothbrushing, Church and Dwight Co.
Why Gold?, American Dental Association
You and Your Dentist, American Dental Association

b. Films
Henry Plans Ahead, American Dental Association
One in a Million, American Dental Association
Preventive Dentistry, American Dental Association

Project Teeth, American Dental Association

Project Teeth, National Dairy Council

Set the Stage for Dental Health, American Dental Association

Show Down at Sweet Rock Gulch, Modern Talking Picture Service

Teeth: Their Structure and Care, American Dental Association

Why Fluoridation?, American Dental Association

Your Teeth, Young America Films

c. Filmstrips

Save Those Teeth, Encyclopedia Britannica

The Teeth, Encylcopedia Britannica

Tips on Tooth Care, American Dental Association

You and Your Dentist, American Dental Association

Your Teeth and Their Care, Popular Science

d. Posters

Begin Early, National Dairy Council

Consider Nonsmokers—Please Don't Smoke, American Dental Association

Swish and Swallow, American Dental Association

e. Charts

Decay in Six Year Molar, American Dental Association

Development of Human Dentition, American Dental Association

Enamel Fissure Decay, American Dental Association

Speaker's Flip Chart, American Dental Association

f. Transparencies

Functions of the Teeth, Popular Science

Nature's Helping Hand, American Dental Association

Progress of Decay, Popular Science

The Best Years of Your Life, American Dental Association

g. Records

But What About Me?, American Dental Association

Plain Talk About Fluoridation, American Dental Association

Something in Common, American Dental Association

4. BODY STRUCTURE AND OPERATION (INCLUDING SENSES AND SKIN)

a. Pamphlets or Leaflets

Aberrant Cells—The Nature of Cancer, American Cancer Society

About Your Heart and Bloodstream, American Heart Association

A Boy and His Physique, National Dairy Council

A Breast Check, American Cancer Society

A Girl and Her Figure, National Dairy Council

A Girl and Her Figure and You, National Dairy Council

Blood, American National Red Cross

Build a Better You, Sunkist Growers

Chemical Man, Pharmaceutical Manufacturers Association

Color Is Only Skin Deep, American Medical Association

Contact Lenses, American Medical Association

Contact Lenses, American Optometric Association

Cosmetic Surgery, American Medical Association

Good Looks Here and Now, Armour-Dial, Inc.

Facts About Blindness, American Foundation For The Blind

Hearing Is Priceless, American Hearing Society

Kidney Disease, American Medical Association

See It Like It Is, American Optometric Association

Simple Skin Care for the Family, Armour-Dial, Inc.

Something Can Be Done About Acne, American Medical Association

Sunglasses, National Society For Prevention of Blindness

Sunlight and the Skin, American Medical Association

The Aging Skin, American Medical Association

The Cancer Story, American Cancer Society

The Story of Blood, National Red Cross

To Save a Life, American Heart Association

What Is an Optometrist?, American Optometric Association

You Can't Hit It If You Can't See It, American Optometric Association

Your Blood Pressure, American Medical Association

Your Heart and How It Works, American Heart Association

Your Heart Saver, American Heart Association

Wonderful Human Machine, American Medical Association

b. Films

About the Human Body, American Heart Association

About the Human Body, Churchill Films

Breathing Easy, American Lung Association

Breath of Life, American Heart Association

Breast Self-Examination, American Cancer Society

For a Wonderful Life, American Cancer Society

From One Cell, American Cancer Society

Glands and Hormones, Sterling Educational Films

Human Body: Reproductive System, Coronet Films

Laboratory of the Body, American Dental Association

"New" Pulse of Life, Pyramid Films

Of Mind and Men, American Heart Association

On the Line, American Cancer Society

Teen-aged? Have Acne?, Pharmaceutical Manufacturers Association

The Embattled Cell, American Cancer Society

The Heart—How It Works, American Heart Association

The Human Body: Nutrition and Metabolism, National Dairy Council

The Winners, American Cancer Society

Wonder Engine of the Body, American Heart Association

c. Loop Films

Caring for Feet, Popular Science

Caring for Hands and Nails, Popular Science

External Cardiac Massage, BFA Educational Media

d. Filmstrips

Care of the Skin, Encyclopedia Britannica

DNA and You, Warren Schloat Productions

Functions of the Liver, Popular Science

Growing Into Manhood, Guidance Associates

Growing Into Womanhood, Guidance Associates

Growth, Educational Activities, Inc.

How Hormones Control the Body, Popular Science

How Your Ear Works, Popular Science

Human Vision, BFA Educational Media

How We See, BFA Educational Media

Injuries to the Nervous System, BFA Educational Media

Jennie, American Cancer Society

Laboratory of Life, American Cancer Society

Man: The Human Body, Popular Science

Mechanics of Breathing, Popular Science

Reflex and Conditioning, Popular Science

Sense Organs, BFA Educational Media

Sensing, Thinking, Learning, BFA Educational Media

The Body Machine: Muscular System, Popular Science

The Ears, Young America Films

The Eyes, Young America Films

The Human Nervous System, BFA Educational Media

The Nervous System, Popular Science

Why Skin Has Many Colors, Sunburst Communications

e. Posters

Guard Against Heart Attack, American Heart Association

Only One Pair of Ears for Life, American Hearing Society

Physical Fitness Posters, National Dairy Council

Reduce Your Risk of Heart Attack, American Heart Association

Your Heart and How It Works, American Heart Association

f. Charts

Blood as a Medicine, American National Red Cross

Cross Section of the Eye, National Society for the Prevention of Blindness

Human Development, Denoyer-Geppert Co.

Meredith Growth Charts (Male-Female), National Education Association

Your Heart and How It Works, American Heart Association

g. Transparencies

Body Changes at Puberty, 3M Company

Heredity, 3M Company

Human Anatomy, Popular Science

Inherited and Acquired Characteristics, 3M Company

Muscle Contraction, Milton Bradley

Organs of Sense, Popular Science

Reproductive System, Milton Bradley

Respiratory System, Milton Bradley

Skeletal Structure, Milton Bradley

The Human Body, Popular Science

The Skin, Popular Science

h. Slides

Circulatory System, American Heart Association

Coronary Heart Disease, American Heart Association

i. Tape-Cassettes

Coping With Headaches, Spenco Medical Corporation

Exercise for Your Heart, Spenco Medical Corporation

Heart Drawings, American Heart Association

Strokes, American Heart Association

j. Selected Books

(J) = Junior High Level

(S) = Senior High Level

Cells: Their Structure and Function, (J) E. H. Mercer (Doubleday)

Eye and Brain (S), R. Gregory (McGraw-Hill)

Human Growth (J, S) L. F. Beck (Harcourt, Brace Jovanovich)

Molecules to Man (J, S), (Houghton-Mifflin Co.)

New Hope for Your Skin (J, S), J. Lubowe (Dutton)

Sound Waves and Light Waves (S), W. Koch (Doubleday)

Teenage Guide to Healthy Skin and Hair (J), I. Lubowe (E. P. Dutton)

The Human Body (J, S), I. Asimov (Houghton-Mifflin)

The Second Genesis: The Coming Control of Life (S), A. Rosenfield (Prentice-Hall)

To Catch an Angel (S), R. Russell (Vanguard)

Your Heart Has Nine Lives (J), J. Stamler and A. Blakeslee (American Heart Assn.)

5. PREVENTION AND CONTROL OF DISEASE

a. Pamphlets or Leaflets

Answering Your Questions About Cancer, American Cancer Society

Breast Self Examination, American Cancer Society

Cancer Cause and Prevention, American Cancer Society

Cancer of the Lung, U.S. Public Health Service

Cancer of the Uterus, American Cancer Society

Cancer Questions and Answers, American Cancer Society

Diseases We May Catch from Animals, American Medical Association

Family Health Record, American Medical Association

Heart Disease and Pregnancy, American Heart Association

Immunization, American Medical Association

Immunization for All, Public Affairs Pamphlet

Protect Them From Harm, U.S. Public Health Service

The Athlete and Fungus Infections, Schering Laboratories

The Triad of Infection, Eli Lilly Company

To Decrease the Risk of Heart Disease, Sunkist Growers

V. D. Facts You Should Know, Ohio Department of Health

Venereal Disease, U.S. Public Health Service

Viruses, Colds and Flu, Public Affairs Pamphlet

What You Should Know About Rheumatic Fever, American Heart Association

Why Learn About Cancer, American Cancer Society

b. Films

A New Look at the Common Cold, Pharmaceutical Manufacturers Association

Arteriosclerosis, American Heart Association

Better Odds for a Longer Life, American Heart Association

Biography of a Cancer, Carousel Films

Builders of Youth, Schering Laboratories

Clean: Is It Worth It?, Alfred Higgins Productions

Coronary Heart Disease, American Heart Association

Dance Little Children, Hank Newenhouse

Diabetes (History of), Pharmaceutical Manufacturers Association

Dollar Clinics, Churchill Films

Fight Against Microbes, International Film Bureau

From One Cell, American Cancer Society

Heart Attack, Pharmaceutical Manufacturers Association

High Blood Pressure, American Heart Association

How Much Is a Miracle?, Pharmaceutical Manufacturers Association

How to Keep From Catching V D, Jarvis Covillard Associates

Immunization, Pharmaceutical Manufacturers Association

Microorganisms That Cause Disease, Coronet Films

Mosquito and Its Control, Coronet Films

Nervous Tension, Pharmaceutical Manufacturers Association

Phagocytosis: The Body's Defense, Sterling Films

Scientific Method of Action, International Film Bureau

Smoking and Heart Disease, American Heart Association

The Last Case of Polio, Pharmaceutical Manufacturers Association

The Million Club, American Cancer Society

The Pain of Silence, Modern Learning Aids

The Traitor Within, American Cancer Society

The Transplanters, Pharmaceutical Manufacturers Association

Triad of Infections, Eli Lilly Company

Twentieth Century Epidemic, American Heart Association

Half Million Teenagers, Churchill Films

VD Questions, VD Answers, BFA Educational Media

VD Every 30 Seconds, Perennial Education

Walter Reed and Conquest of Yellow Fever, Association Films

What You Should Know About Cancer, Pharmaceutical Manufacturers Association

c. Filmstrips

A Moment of Discovery, American Cancer Society

Antibiotics: Disease Fighting Champions, Popular Science

Battle Report — The War Against Cancer, Popular Science

How Your Body Fights Disease, Popular Science

International War Against Diphtheria, International Film Bureau

Louis Pasteur and the Germ Theory, Metropolitan Life Insurance Company

The Cancer Challenge to Youth, American Cancer Society

The Long Adventure, National Tuberculosis Association

The Salk Vaccine, Popular Science

The Virus Mystery, Popular Science

Unmasking the Germ Assassins, International Film Bureau

d. Posters

Guard the Temperature: It's Vital, Paper Cup and Container Institute

Guard Your Hands for Health Protection, Paper Cup and Container Institute

Guard Your Health, Paper Cup and Container Institute

Guard Your Service, Paper Cup and Container Institute

No Matter Which Itch, Schering Laboratories

Prevention: Your Best Defense, American Medical Association

Sanitation Guidelines for Food Processing, U.S. Public Health Service

The Nation's Health Is in Your Hands, U.S. Public Health Service

VD Can Be Eliminated, American Medical Association

e. Charts

Combat With a Traitor—Cancer, Eli Lilly Company

The Good Seed, Eli Lilly Company

f. Transparencies

Cell Functions, American Cancer Society

Epidemiology, Cleveland Health Museum

Links in the Chain of Infection, Cleveland Health Museum

Malaria, Cleveland Health Museum

Miasmatic Theory of Disease, Cleveland Health Museum

Types of Microorganisms, Cleveland Health Museum

Vectors of Disease, Cleveland Health Museum

g. Plays

Ring Around the Family (Sex Education), American Social Health Association

The Underground Bird (Drug Scene), American Social Health Association

h. Slides

Manifestations of Syphilis, U.S. Public Health Service, Atlanta, Ga.

The Ethical Challenge: Four Biomedical Case Studies, The Center for Humanities, Inc.

The Foot in Athletics, Schering Laboratories

i. Selected Books

(J) = Junior High Level

(S) = Senior High Level

Cells: Their Structure and Function (J), E. H. Mercer (Doubleday)

Control of Disease (J, S), H. Paul (Williams and Wilkins)

Great Adventure in Medicine (S), S. Rapport (Dial Press)

History of Most Important Diseases (S), E. Ackerknecht (Hafner)

I Am a Chronic Cardiac (S), L. Poole (Dodd, Mead)

Immunization for All (J, S), J. Saltman (Public Affairs Pamphlet)

The Climate Is Hope (S), W. Ross (Prentice-Hall)

The Doctor Has a Heart Attack (S), S. Goodstone (Beacon)

The Gift of the Healer (S), E. Dodd (Friendship Press)

The Cancer Story (J, S), American Cancer Society

The Hopeful State of Cancer (S), American Cancer Society

The Plague Killers (S), W. Geer (Scribner's Sons)

The Triad of Infection (S), M. Kory (Eli Lilly and Company)

Venereal Diseases (J. S), H. Cornacchia (Lyons and Carnahan)

Why Me?, W. Gargon (Doubleday)

World Eradication of Infectious Diseases (J, S), E. Hinman (Charles C Thomas)

6. SAFETY EDUCATION

a. Pamphlets or Leaflets

Alcohol and the Impaired Driver, American Medical Association

Artificial Respiration, American Medical Association

Be Your Own Traffic Judge, National Safety Council

Breath Alcohol Tests, American Medical Association

Developing Emergency Medical Service, American Medical Association

Don't Take Short Cuts, U.S. Public Health Service

Fabrics and Fire, Ohio State Department of Health

Family Emergency Almanac, National Safety Council

First Aid for the Family, Metropolitan Life Insurance Company

First Aid Guide, Johnson and Johnson

First Aid Manual, American Red Cross

Freezin' Reasons, National Safety Council

Handle With Care, National Safety Council

How to Bandage, Johnson and Johnson

In Case of Fire, National Fire Protection Association

Invisible Speed Limit, National Safety Council

Manual on Pedestrian Safety, American Automobile Association

Poison in the Backyard, National Safety Council

Read the Label and Live, National Fire Protection Association

Safety Ahoy!, Aetna Life and Casualty Company

Seat Belts Save Lives, National Safety Council

Sunlight and the Skin, American Medical Association

Take Care—Red Cross Home Nursing Care, American National Red Cross

The Open and Shut Case, Aetna Life and Casualty Company

To Save a Life, American Heart Association

b. Films

A Call to Action, American National Red Cross

Accident Scene, International Film Bureau

Another Man's Family, National Fire Protection Association

Are We Fire Safe?, National Fire Protection Association

Bleeding: What to Do, Pyramid Films

Danger in Sports: Paying the Price, Macmillan Films, Inc.

Dead Right, American Automobile Association

Emergencies in the Making, American Automobile Association

Every Second Car, Films Incorporated

Expedite School Eye Safety, National Safety Council

Fireman at Your Door, Aetna Life and Casualty Company

First Aid Now, Pharmaceutical Manufacturers Association

Growing Up Safely, National Safety Council

Health and Safety, Ealing Corporation

Hot Stuff, National Fire Protection Association

How Drinking Affects Driving, Media Five Film Distributors

Milford, U.S.A., American National Red Cross

Mouth-to-Mouth Resuscitation in Junior High School, Pharmaceutical Manufacturers Association

Mr. Finley's Feelings, Metropolitan Life Insurance Company

Playing in the City, National Safety Council

Pulse of Life, New York State Department of Health

Read the Label—and Live, National Fire Protection Association

Recreation Safety, Aetna Life and Casualty Company

Safety With Electricity, National Safety Council

Ski Sense, Aetna Life and Casualty Company

The Curb Between Us, Barr Productions

The Day Bicycles Disappeared, American Automobile Association

The Safest Way, American Automobile Association

The Science of Fire, National Safety Council

Trouble Takes No Holiday, National Safety Council

You Can Take It With You, National Safety Council

Your Clothing Can Burn, National Fire Protection Association

With Safety for All, National Safety Council

c. Filmstrips

External Cardiac Massage, BFA Educational Media

First Aid: Newest Red Cross Techniques, Sunburst Communications

Lifting, Man's Oldest Problem, Aetna Life and Casualty Company

Mouth-to-Mouth Resuscitation, BFA Educational Media

To Fall or Not to Fall, Aetna Life and Casualty Company

d. Posters
Accident Prevention, Eli Lilly and Company
Clean Up for Fire Safety, National Fire Protection Association
Don't Straddle Lanes, American Automobile Association
Exit, National Fire Protection Association
Fire Hurts, National Fire Protection Association
Near Accidents Are Warnings, National Safety Council
Plan Ahead—Prevent Accidents, National Safety Council
Safety Is Always in Season, National Safety Council
Take Care—Not Chances, National Safety Council
Traffic Safety (10 posters), American Automobile Association
Want a Ride Tonight?, National Safety Council
Watch Your Step, National Safety Council
What Did You Expect?, National Safety Council

e. Charts
Be a Hazard Hunter, American National Red Cross
Be an Able Aider, American National Red Cross
Fact Chart—Portable Fire Extinguishers, National Fire Protection Association
First Aid Chart for Athletic Injuries, American Medical Association
First Aid Facts, Johnson and Johnson
GO, GO, GO Slowly, American National Red Cross
Major Contributions to Safety Education, National Safety Council
Time to Learn—Fire Can Burn, American National Red Cross

f. Transparencies
Drowning Prevention Techniques and Water Safety, Popular Science
Electrical Safety, Popular Science

g. Mannequins (half-bodied and full-bodied)
Alderson Research Laboratories, Inc., 729 Canal Street, Stamford, Connecticut 06902
Dyna-Med, Inc., P.O. Box 2157, Leucadia, California 92024
Guardian Safety Equipment Company, 37 East 21st Street, Linden, New Jersey 07037
Laerdal Medical Corporation, 136 Marbledale Road, Tuckahoe, New York 10707
Simulaids, Tinker Road, Woodstock, New York 12498
Uniflex Medical Supply Company, Rockford, Illinois 61101

h. Plastic Replicas
Poison Ivy, Oak and Sumac, Eli Lilly Company

i. Selected Books
(J) = Junior High Level
(S) = Senior High Level
Accident Facts (J), National Safety Council
All About Fire (J), R. Holden (Random House)
Aquatics Handbook (J, S), M. Gabrielson (Prentice-Hall)
Emergency Care and First Aid (S), H. Stephenson (Little, Brown and Co.)
Emergency Medical Guide (J, S), J. Henderson (McGraw-Hill)
First Aid Manual (J, S), American Medical Association
First Aid—Programmed Instruction (J), Johnson and Johnson
First Aid Textbook (J, S), American National Red Cross
Hazardous Materials (S), National Fire Protection Association
Sportsmanlike Driving (S), American Automobile Association (McGraw-Hill)

7. MENTAL HEALTH

a. Pamphlets or Leaflets
Alcoholism Is a Management Problem, Alcoholics Anonymous
How Teens Set the Stage for Alcoholism, American Medical Association

How to Overcome Shyness, American Institute of Family Relations

Just How Adult Are You?, American Institute of Family Relations

Leading Group Discussion, Hogg Foundation for Mental Health

Mental Health and Social Change, Hogg Foundation for Mental Health

Self-Acceptance, Hogg Foundation for Mental Health

Time, Tension and Mental Health, Hogg Foundation for Mental Health

What Happened to Joe, Alcoholics Anonymous

What is Mental Health?, Hogg Foundation

What Makes a Good Hobby, American Medical Association

What is Hypnosis?, American Medical Association

Your Inferiority Complex, American Institute of Family Relations

b. Films

A Family Affair, International Film Bureau

Bertrand Russell Discusses Happiness, Coronet Films

But Jack Was a Good Driver (Suicide), CRM Educational Films

Emotional Development, CRM Educational Films

Facing Reality, McGraw-Hill

False Friends, International Film Bureau

Fear, New York State Department of Education

Flowers on a One-Way Street, Films Incorporated

Frontiers of the Mind, Films Incorporated

Human Relationships, McGraw-Hill

It's Not Fair, CRM Educational Films

Next Time, Film Modules, Inc.

No Reason to Stay, Films Incorporated

Personality, CRM Educational Films

Portrait of a Genius, Films Incorporated

Suicide, CRM Educational Films

Stairway to Light, Films Incorporated

The Measurement of Depression, Pharmaceutical Manufacturers Association

The Right to Die, Macmillan Films, Inc.

Understanding Your Emotions, Coronet Films

What Do You Want Me to Say?, CRM Educational Films

c. Loop Films

Love Story, Popular Science

Moral Values: Points of Departure, Hank Newenhouse

Night Out, Popular Science

The Meeting, Popular Science

d. Filmstrips

About Love: Beginnings, Warren Schloat Productions

Building Self-Confidence, Popular Science

Coping With Conflict, Sunburst Communications

Dealing With Stress, Human Relations Media Center

Getting Along with Your Family, Popular Science

Habits and Learning, Popular Science

How Shall We Live (series), McGraw-Hill

Ideals to Live By, Popular Science

Let's Disagree Together, Popular Science

Living With Dying, Sunburst Communications

Mythology Is Alive and Well, Guidance Associates

Parents are People Too, Popular Science

Psychological Defenses I, II, Human Relations Media Center

Personality: Roles You Play, Sunburst Communications

Scapegoating: Impact of Prejudice, Sunburst Communications

Should You Go to College?, Guidance Associates

Should You or Shouldn't You? And When, Warren Schloat Productions

Striving for Excellence, Popular Science

Values for Teenagers, Guidance Associates

Who Am I: The Search for Self, Glenn Educational Films

Why Work At All?, Guidance Associates

Your Personality, Guidance Associates

e. Posters

Stop Discrimination, Spenco Medical Corporation

Work is Love Made Visible, Spenco Medical Corporation

f. Sound Slides

Man and His Values, The Center for Humanities, Inc.

The Many Masks We Wear, The Center for Humanities, Inc.

Clarifying Your Values, The Center for Humanities, Inc.

g. Tapes-Cassettes

Minds of Men, Hogg Foundation of Mental Health

Up and Around With Drugs, Spenco Medical Corporation

Mysteries Inside Our Heads, Hogg Foundation

Mental Health — 24 Hours a Day, Hogg Foundation

h. Selected Books

(J) = Junior High Level

(S) = Senior High Level

Between Parent and Teenager (S), H. Ginott (Macmillan)

Brave New World (S), A. Huxley (Harper and Bros.)

Conflict and Creativity (S), S. Farber (McGraw-Hill)

Discovering Ourselves (J, S), E. Streaker (Macmillan)

Emotional and Neurological Health (S), R. Jones (Harper and Row)

Emotional Problems of Living (S), O. English (Norton)

Identity, Youth and Crisis (S), E. Erikson (Norton)

Just For Teens (J, S), C. Jones (Harper and Row)

Love and the Facts Of Life (J, S), E. Duvall (Association)

Male Manners (J, S), K. Corinth and M. Sargent (David McKay)

Man Under Stress (S), R. Grinker (McGraw-Hill)

Sex, Love and Person (S), P. Bertocci (Sheed and Ward)

Stop — Time (S), F. Conroy (Viking)

Teenagers and Sex (J, S), J. Pike (Prentice-Hall)

The Art of Loving (J), E. Fromm (Harper & Row)

The Feminine Mystique (S), B. Friedan (Norton)

The Man that You Marry (S), E. Boll (Macrae Smith Co.)

The Successful Teenage Girl (J), G. D. Schultz (J. B. Lippincott)

The Vital Balance (S), K. Menninger (Viking)

Why Wait Till Marriage (S), E. Duvall (Association)

Young People and Sex (J, S), A. Cain (John Day)

8. SMOKING

a. Pamphlets or Leaflets

Be Kind to Nonsmokers, American Lung Association

Breaking the Habit, American Cancer Society

Breathing — What You Need to Know, American Lung Association

Cigarette Quiz, American Heart Association

Cigarette Smoking: Take It or Leave It, American Cancer Society

Health Consequences of Smoking, National Clearinghouse for Smoking and Health

Me Quit Smoking? Why? American Lung Association

Second-Hand Smoke, American Lung Association

Smoke Cigarettes? American Cancer Society

Smoking and Heart Disease, American Heart Association

Smoking and Lung Cancer, U.S. Public Health Service

The Facts About Smoking, U.S. Public Health Service

Where There is Smoke, American Cancer Society

Why Smoke Cigarettes? American Cancer Society

b. Films

As We See It, American Lung Association

Breathing Easy, American Lung Association

Decision for Mike, American Cancer Society

Emphysema — The Facts, American Lung Association

Is It Worth Your Life? American Lung Association

Smoking and Health, U.S. Food and Drug Administration

The Battle to Breathe, American Lung Association

Who Me? American Cancer Society

c. Filmstrips

I'll Choose the High Road, American Cancer Society

The Cancer Challenge to Youth, American Cancer Society

The Physiology of Smoking and Drinking, Sunburst Communications

To Smoke or Not to Smoke, American Cancer Society

d. Posters

Be Kind to Nonsmokers, American Lung Association

Best Tip Yet—Don't Start, American Cancer Society

Break the Habit, American Medical Association

Cigarette Smoke Is Harmful! American Lung Association

Lungs at Work—No Smoking! American Lung Association

Smokers Have Everything, Spenco Medical Corporation

Smoking Can Affect the Two of You, American Lung Association

Smoking is Nothing to Crow About, U.S. Public Health Service

Smoking is Very Debonair, American Cancer Society

Stamp Out Old Age. Smoke! Spenco Medical Corporation

e. Charts

Don't Smoke, American Heart Association

Respiratory Wall Chart, American Lung Association

Smoker's Slide Rule, Spenco Medical Corporation

Smoking and Heart Disease, American Heart Association

f. Kits

Smokers' Self Testing Kit, National Clearinghouse for Smoking and Health

g. Selected Books

(J) = Junior High Level

(S) = Senior High Level

Common Sense About Smoking (J), C. Fletcher (Penguin Books)

Smokers' Testing Kit (J, S), U.S. Public Health Service

Stop Smoking In Five Days (S), R. Tobin (Dell Publishing Company)

Tobacco and Your Health (S), H. Diehl (McGraw-Hill)

9. SEX AND FAMILY LIVING EDUCATION

a. Pamphlets or Leaflets

A Baby Is Born, Cleveland Health Museum

A Breast Check, American Cancer Society

Accent on You, Tampax Incorporated

A Family Grows, Hogg Foundation For Mental Health

Approaching Adulthood, American Medical Association

Baby Care, Johnson and Johnson

Boys Want to Know, American Social Health Association

Chromosome Studies in Spontaneous Abortion, National Foundation

Eating for Your Baby-to-Be, National Live Stock and Meat Board

Drugs and Sex, U.S. Public Health Service

Family Planning, Planned Parenthood-World Population

Finding Yourself, American Medical Association

For Parents-to-Be, National Dairy Council

From Fiction to Facts, Tampax, Incorporated

Growing Up and Liking It, Personal Products Company

How Do You Know You're in Love?, American Institute Family Relations

It's Wonderful Being a Girl, Personal Products Company

Modern Methods of Birth Control, Planned Parenthood-World Population

Nutrition in Pregnancy, United Fresh Fruit and Vegetable Association

Sex-rated Comments, Hogg Foundation

Prenatal Care, American Medical Association

The Miracle of Life, American Medical Association

The Story of Life, American Medical Association

The World of a Girl, Scott Paper Company

Why Girls Menstruate, American Medical Association

Why the Rise in Teenage Syphilis?, American Medical Association

You're a Young Lady Now, Kimberly-Clark Corporation

b. Films

Adolescent Sexual Conflicts, CRM Educational Films

About Puberty and Reproduction, Perennial Education

About Conception and Contraception, Perennial Education

About Sex, Texture Films

Adapting to Parenthood, Polymorph Films

A Far Cry from Yesterday, Perennial Education

A Baby is Born, Perennial Education

Banquet of Life, Planned Parenthood-World Population

Beyond Conception, Hank Newenhouse

Biography of the Unborn, Encyclopedia Britannica

Biology of the Unborn, Encyclopedia Britannica

Birth Control: How?, Films, Inc.

Boy to Man, Churchill Films

Childbirth, Hank Newenhouse

Childbirth, Polymorph Films

Childbirth: The Great Adventure, Hank Newenhouse

Choosing Your Marriage Partner, Coronet Films

Contraception, John Wiley and Sons

Date Etiquette, Coronet Films

Dating: Do's and Don'ts, Coronet Films

Early Marriage, Perennial Education

Endocrine Glands, Encyclopedia Britannica Films

Endocrine Glands: How They Affect You, McGraw-Hill

Engagement — Romance and Reality, McGraw-Hill

Expecting Diet in Pregnancy, National Dairy Council

Family Life, Coronet Films

Family Planning, Planned Parenthood-World Population

Female Cycle, Films Incorporated

Fertilization and Birth, Planned Parenthood-World Population

From Generation to Generation, McGraw-Hill

From Generation to Generation, Planned Parenthood-World Population

Genetics: Chromosomes and Genes, McGraw-Hill

Girl to Woman, Churchill Films

Glands and Hormones, Sterling Educational Films

Going Steady, Coronet Films

Helen in Paris, Personal Products Company

Hope is not a Method, Perennial Education

How Do You Know It's Love?, Coronet Films

How Life Begins, McGraw-Hill

Human Body: Reproductive System, Coronet Films

Human Growth, Perennial Education

Human Heredity, Perennial Education

Human Growth and Reproduction, McGraw-Hill

Human Heredity, E. C. Brown Trust

Infant Feeding and Nutrition, Polymorph Films

It's Wonderful Being a Girl, Personal Products Company

Lavender, Perennial Education

Learning to Live, Popular Science

Life With Baby, McGraw-Hill

Look What's Going Around, Churchill Films

Love and the Facts of Life, Cathedral Films

Love is for the Byrds, Hank Newenhouse

Lucy, Picture Film Distributing Co.

Man and Woman, Popular Science

Marriage, Films Incorporated

Marriage is a Partnership, Coronet Films

Marriage Today, Walt Disney Productions

Martha, Perennial Education

Masters and Johnson Explore Myths About Sex, Focus Education Inc.

Meaning of Engagement, Coronet Films
Menstruation, Films Incorporated
Naturally a Girl, Personal Products Company
Not Me Alone, Polymorph Films
Planned Families, Sid Dairs Productions
Pregnancy and Birth, Films Inc.
Puberty, Hank Newenhouse
Puberty in Boys, Films Incorporated
Purpose of Family Planning, See-Saw Films
Reproduction in Animals, Coronet Films
Sex and Responsibility, Planned Parenthood-World Population
Sex in Today's World, Focus Education
Sexuality and the Teenager, Hank Newenhouse
Talk About Breastfeeding, Polymorph Films
Teenage Pregnancy, Sterling Educational Films
The Family and Marriage, Hank Newenhouse
The Game, McGraw-Hill
The Homosexuals, Carousel Films
The Maturing Female, Sterling Educational Films
The Merry-Go-Round, McGraw-Hill
The Pain of Silence, Modern Learning Aids
The Party, Paulist Productions
The Really Big Family, Films Inc.
The Rose, Films Incorporated
The Trying Time, Perennial Education
There Is No Time for Romance, National Film Board of Canada
The Wonder of a Girl, Scott Paper Company
To Be A Friend, Billy Budd Films
To Be a Man, Billy Budd Films, Inc.
To Be a Woman, Billy Budd Films, Inc.
VD Questions, VD Answers, BFA Educational Media
VD: Self Awareness, American Alliance for Health, Physical Education and Recreation
VD: A New Focus, American Education Films
VD Every 30 Seconds, Perennial Education
VD—Name Your Contacts, Coronet Films

Venereal Disease, Hank Newenhouse
What to Do on a Date, Coronet Films
What About McBride, CRM Educational Films
When Love Needs Care, See-Saw Films
When Should I Marry?, McGraw-Hill
Women (Menstruation), Popular Science
Young, Single and Pregnant, See-Saw Films
Young Marriage, CRM Educational Films

c. Loop Films

Birth, Hank Newenhouse
Childbirth, Popular Science
Engagements, Popular Science
Family Planning Today, Guidance Associates
Fertilization, Hank Newenhouse
Happy Family Planning, Ealing Corporation
Human Birth, Ealing Corporation
Human Growth, Hank Newenhouse
Love Story, Popular Science
Masculinity and Femininity, Guidance Associates
Points of Departure, Ealing Corporation
Sexual Intercourse, Ealing Corporation
Sexual Values in Society, Guidance Associates
The Older Touch, Popular Science
The Newborn Baby, Ealing Corporation
Women (Menstruation), Popular Science

d. Filmstrips

A Basis for Sex Morality, Cathedral Films, Inc.
About Love: Beginnings, Warren Schloat Productions, Inc.
About You: Boys, Warren Schloat Productions, Inc.
About You: Girls, Warren Schloat Productions, Inc.
And They Lived Happily Ever After, Guidance Associates
Beginning to Date, Guidance Associates
DNA and You, Warren Schloat Productions, Inc.
Family Planning Today, Guidance Associates
Getting Along with the Opposite Sex, Popular Science
Going Steady?, Popular Science

Growing Into Manhood, Guidance Associates

How You Get VD, Sunburst Communications

Learning About Living Things (series), Encyclopedia Britannica

Learning About Sex, Guidance Associates

Love and the Facts of Life, Glenn Educational Films

Masculinity and Femininity, Guidance Associates

Methods of Birth Control: A Simplified Presentation, Planned Parenthood

Sex: A Moral Dilemma for Teenagers, Guidance Associates

Sex: Problems and Possibilities, Warren Schloat Productions, Inc.

Should You or Shouldn't You? And When, Warren Schloat Productions, Inc.

The Miracle of Birth, Warren Schloat Productions, Inc.

The Story of Human Life, Educational Activities, Inc.

The Story of Menstruation, Association Films

The Times They Are A-Changing, Warren Schloat Productions, Inc.

Understanding Human Reproduction, Guidance Associates

Understanding Your Love Feelings, Glenn Educational Films

Values for Dating, Sunburst Publications

Venereal Disease, Guidance Associates

What About Marriage? Sunburst Publications

What Do Teens Think About Sex? Family Filmstrips

e. Posters

Beginning the Human Story: A New Baby, Scott, Foresman and Company

For Healthy Happy Children, Planned Parenthood-World Population

Menstruation, Tampax, Incorporated

Smoking Can Affect the Two of You, American Lung Association

The Exploding Metropolis, Planned Parenthood-World Population

The Family Life Cycle, American School Health Association

The Living Hands, Planned Parenthood-World Population

Tragedy in Growth, Planned Parenthood-World Population

Wanted: Every Baby Should Be, Planned Parenthood-World Population

Was I Planned?, Planned Parenthood-World Population

What Happens During Menstruation?, Personal Products Corporation

f. Charts

Human Development Charts, Denoyer-Geppert Co.

Menstrual Cycle, Tampax, Incorporated

Menstruation, Kimberly-Clark

Menstruation, Personal Products Corporation

U.S. Population Growth, Planned Parenthood-World Population

World Population by Area, Planned Parenthood-World Population

g. Transparencies

Achieving Adulthood, Hank Newenhouse

Beginning of Birth, Cleveland Health Museum

Contraception, Landsford Publishing Company

Factors Influencing Sex Drive, 3M Company

Heredity, 3M Company

How Life Begins, 3M Company

Human Reproduction, Growth and Development, Hank Newenhouse

Living Things from Living Things, 3M Company

Reproductive Process with Overlays, Cleveland Health Museum

Sex Education: Understanding Growth and Social Development, Western Pub. Co.

Sperm Formation, Cleveland Health Museum

The Problem of Venereal Disease, Landsford Publishing Company

The Family, 3M Company

Venereal Disease, Popular Science

h. Tapes-Cassettes

About Girls (For Boys), Audio Arts

About Men (For Girls), Audio Arts

Birth (kit), Cleveland Health Museum

Culture and Sexual Intimacy, McGraw-Hill

Contraception and Family Planning, Spenco Medical Corporation

Living with Divorce, Spenco Medical Corporation

Love and Friendship, Sunburst Publications

Premarital Sex Behavior, Hank Newenhouse

Pressures, Sunburst Publications

Sex Ethics, Sex Acts and Human Need, Hank Newenhouse

Sex is Not a Dirty Word, Harper and Row Media

Two Couples in Love, Sunburst Publications

Worth Waiting For, Audio Arts

i. Records

Dr. Finch Talks to Parents—Sex Education, Hank Newenhouse

Love and Sex, Education Corporation

Teaching Children Values, Educational Activities, Inc.

Teenagers Question About Life, Education Corporation

Sex Education: A Part of Family Living, Educational Activities, Inc.

j. Slides

Birth and Gestation, Cleveland Health Museum

Family Life and Sex Education, Denoyer-Geppert Co.

How Babies Are Made, Creative Scope, Inc.

VD Presentation, American Medical Association

k. Models

Baby in Years Jar with Placenta and Cord, Cleveland Health Museum

Betsi Breast Model, OMNI Educational System

Breast Cancer Teaching Model, Spenco Medical Corporation

Female Reproductive System, Hubbard Scientific Co.

Female Torso, Denoyer-Geppert Company

Human Embryo Model, Denoyer-Geppert Company

Male Pelvis Model, Denoyer-Geppert Company

Nine Stages of Birth, Cleveland Health Museum

Seven Month Fetus in Opened Uterus, Cleveland Health Museum

Uterus With Fetus at 4½ Months, Cleveland Health Museum

l. Selected Books

(J) = Junior High Level
(S) = Senior High Level

Andy, P. Wood (Westminster)

Better Than the Birds, Smarter Than the Bees (J), J. Burn (Abington)

Boys and Sex (J), W. R. Pomeroy (Delacorte)

Cheaper by the Dozen (S), Frank Gilbreth (Crowell)

Facts About Sex for Today's Youth (J), S. Gordon (John Day)

Getting It All Together (S), M. Capizzi (Delacorte)

Girls and Sex (J), W. R. Pomeroy (Delacorte)

Homosexuality, (J, S), SEICUS Publications

Human Sexuality (S), J. McCary (Van Nostrand)

Life Can Be Sexual (S), E. Witt (Concordia Publishing House)

Love and Sex and Growing Up (J), E. Johnson (Lippincott)

Love and Sex in Plain Language (J), E. Johnson (Lippincott)

Love and the Facts of Life (J), E. Duvall (Association Press)

Love, Sex and Being Human (S), P. Bohannan (Doubleday)

Marriage is What You Make It (S), P. Popenoe (American Institute of Family Relations)

Masculinity and Femininity (S), B. Miller (Houghton-Mifflin)

Moving Into Manhood (J), W. Bauer (Doubleday)

My Darling, My Hamburger (S), P. Zindel (Harper & Row)

Our Bodies, Ourselves (S), Woman's Collective (Simon and Schuster)

Premarital Sex in a Changing Society (S), R. Bell (Prentice-Hall)

Premarital Sex Standards (S), SEICUS Publications

Sex Before Marriage (S), E. Hamilton (Meredith)

Sex, Love and the Person (S), P. Bertocci (Sheed and Ward)

Somebody Will Miss Me (J), D. Crawford (Croton Pub.)

Sticks and Stones (S), L. Hall (Follett)

The Ability to Love (S), A. Fromme (Farrer, Straus and Giroux)

The Art of Loving (S), E. Fromm (Harper & Row)

The Family in Perspective (S), W. F. Kenkel (Appleton-Century-Crofts)

The Girl that You Marry (S), J. Bossard and E. Boll (Macrae Smith Co.)

The Long Secret (J), L. Fitzhugh (Harper and Row)

The Secret World of the Baby (J), B. Day (Random House)

The Stork is Dead (J), C. Shedd (World Books)

Towards Manhood (J), H. Bundensen (Lippincott)

What Teenagers Want to Know (J, S), F. Levinsohn (Budlong Press)

When You Marry (S), E. Duvall (Heath)

Young People and Sex (J), A. Cain (John Day)

Environmental Quality and Society, American Medical Association

From Dump To Glaring Dump, American Medical Association

Don't Leave It All to the Experts, U.S. Environmental Protection Agency

From Sea to Shining Sea, U.S. Government Printing Office

Man, an Endangered Species, U.S. Government Printing Office

No Laughing Matter, U.S. Government Printing Office

Noise, the Third Pollution, Public Affairs Committee

Primer of Waste Water, U.S. Government Printing Office

Showdown, U.S. Government Printing Office

The Campaign for Cleaner Air, Public Affairs Pamphlet

The Future of Man's Environment, Planned Parenthood-World Population

The Nation's Water Resources, U.S. Government Printing Office

The Third Wave, U.S. Government Printing Office

The U.S. Environmental Protection Agency, U.S. Environmental Protection Agency

Troubled Waters, Metropolitan Life Insurance Company

10. ENVIRONMENTAL HEALTH

a. Pamphlets or Leaflets

Air Pollution, American Medical Association

A Glossary of Air Pollution, American Lung Association

Air Pollution Facts, American Lung Association

Action For Environmental Quality, U.S. Environmental Protection Agency

A Time to Choose: America's Energy Future, Consumer Union

An Environment Fit for People, Public Affairs Pamphlet

Clean Water Is Everybody's Business, U.S. Public Health Service

Controlling Air Pollution, American Lung Association

Also the following agencies:

Conservation Foundation, 1250 Connecticut Avenue, N.W., Washington, D.C. 20036

Environment Magazine, 438 N. Skinker St., St. Louis, Mo. 63130

Isaac Walton League of America, 1326 Waukegan Rd., Glenview, Illinois 60025

National Parks Association, 1701 18th Street, N.W., Washington, D.C. 20036

National Wildlife Federation, 1412 16th Street, N.W., Washington, D.C. 20036

Planned Parenthood–World Population, 515 Madison Avenue, New York, New York 10022

Population Reference Bureau, 1955 Massachusetts Avenue, N.W., Washington, D.C. 20036

Project Man's Environment, National Education Association, 1201 16th Street, N.W., Washington, D.C. 20036

Sierra Club, Mills Tower, San Francisco, California 94104

The Wilderness Society, 729 15th Street, N.W., Washington, D.C. 20005

Zero Population Growth, 367 State Street, Los Altos, California 94022

b. Films

Air Pollution, Encyclopedia Britannica

Air Pollution and Plant Life, U.S. Environmental Protection Agency

A Matter of Time, Conservation Foundation

Banquet of Life, Planned Parenthood-World Population

Beargrass Creek, Stuart Finley Productions

Beyond Conception, Hank Newenhouse

Challenge to Mankind, McGraw-Hill

Environmental Awareness, National Park Service, Washington, D.C.

Five Million, Planned Parenthood-World Population

For All to Enjoy, Conservation Foundation

Man and His Resources, McGraw-Hill

Medicine Man, American Medical Association

Megalopolis: Cradle of the Future, Encyclopedia Britannica

Mosquito and Its Control, Coronet Films

Multiply and Subdue the Earth, Indiana University

Nobody's Children, McGraw-Hill

Our Changing Environment, Encyclopedia Britannica

Our Crowded Environment, Encyclopedia Britannica

Pesticides in Focus, United Fresh Fruit and Vegetable Association

Population Ecology, McGraw-Hill

Pure Waters and Public Health, Modern Talking Picture Service

The Earth and Mankind, Planned Parenthood-World Population

The Great Clean Air Car Race, U.S. Environmental Protection Agency

The House of Man — Our Crowded Environment, Encyclopedia Britannica

The Last Frontier, Department of the Interior

The Question of Values, U.S. Environmental Protection Agency

The First Pollution, U.S. Environmental Protection Agency

The Noisy Landscape, Sterling Films, Inc.

The Proper Place, Association Films

The Third Pollution, Environmental Control Administration

Tom Lehrer Sings Pollution, U.S. Public Health Service

Urban Sprawl, Stuart Finley Productions

Water Pollution, Encyclopedia Britannica

What's New in Solid Waste Management, U.S. Environmental Protection Agency

c. Filmstrips

Environment: Changing Man's Values, Guidance Associates

Land and Man, BFA Educational Media

Man's Natural Environment: Crisis Through Abuse, Guidance Associates

The Litter Monster, Alfred Higgins Productions

The People Problem, Guidance Associates

The Pesticide Problem, BFA Educational Media

The Wisdom of Wildness, Guidance Associates

d. Posters

4½ Million Mothers in Need, Planned Parenthood–World Population

Living Space, Tokyo, Planned Parenthood — World Population

Nutrition Facts to Guide Your Food Choices, Cereal Institute

Sanitation Guidelines for Food Processing, U.S. Public Health Service

The Exploding Metropolis, Planned Parenthood–World Population

e. Sound-Slides

The Science and Ethics of Population Control, The Center for Humanities, Inc.

f. Cassettes

Air Pollution Control (10 Audiocassettes), U.S. Environmental Protection Agency

g. Transparencies

Environmental Balance, Cleveland Health Museum

h. Selected Books

(J) = Junion High Level
(S) = Senior High Level

A Different Kind of Country (S), R. Dasmann (Macmillan)

America the Raped, G. Marine (Simon and Schuster)

From Sea to Shining Sea (S), U.S. Government Printing Office

Human Ecology and Public Health (S), E. D. Kilbourne (Macmillan)

Man, Medicine and Environment (S), R. Dubos (Praeger)

1976: Agenda for Tomorrow (S), S. Udall (Holt, Rinehart, Winston)

On the Shred of a Cloud (S), R. Edberg (U. of Alabama Press)

Problems of Human Environment (S), United Nations

Restoring the Quality of Our Environment (J, S), U.S. Government Printing Office

Since Silent Spring (S), F. Graham, Jr. (Houghton-Mifflin)

The Breath of Life (J, S), D. Carr (Norton)

The Environmental Handbook (S), G. De-Bell (Ballantine)

The Population Bomb (J, S), P. Ehrlich (Ballantine)

The Subversive Science: Essays Toward an Ecology of Man (S), P. Shephard (Houghton-Mifflin)

The Unseen World (S), R. Dubos (Rockefeller Institute Press)

11. ALCOHOL AND DRUGS

a. Pamphlets or Leaflets

Alcohol and Alcoholism, National Institute of Mental Health

Alcoholism Is a Management Problem, Alcoholics Anonymous

Alcohol, Man and Science, Hogg Foundation

Alcohol: Some Questions and Answers, National Institute on Alcohol Abuse

Amphetamines, American Medical Association

Answers to Most Frequently Asked Questions About Drug Abuse, U.S. Public Health Service

Barbiturates, American Medical Association

Before Your Kid Tries Drugs, National Institute of Mental Health

Contradictory Views on Use of Marijuana, Public Affairs Pamphlet

Don't Guess About Drugs, National Institute of Mental Health

Drug Abuse: Escape to Nowhere, National Education Association (AAHPER)

Drugs of Abuse, Food and Drug Administration

Drugs of Abuse, U.S. Government Printing Office

Fighting Illegal Drug Traffic, Smith, Kline and French Laboratories

Forty-Four Questions, Alcoholics Anonymous

Glue Sniffing, American Medical Association

How Teens Set the Stage for Alcoholism, American Medical Association

LSD, U.S. Public Health Service

Marijuana, U.S. Public Health Service

Marijuana: Questions and Answers, U.S. Public Health Service

Narcotics, U.S. Government Printing Office

Narcotics, U.S. Public Health Service

Speed Kills, Metropolitan Life Insurance Company

The Alcoholic, National Council on Alcoholism

The Crutch That Cripples, American Medical Association

The Glue Sniffing Problem, American Social Health Association

The Great Imitators, American Cancer Society

The Up and Down Drugs, U.S. Public Health Service

The New Alcoholics: Teenagers, Public Affairs Pamphlet

To Young Teens On Druggism, Metropolitan Life Insurance Co.

Thinking About Drinking, U.S. Government Printing Office

What We Can Do About Drug Abuse, Public Affairs Pamphlet

What You and Your Family Should Know, National Institute of Mental Health

Young People and A.A., Alcoholics Anonymous

b. Films

Alcohol and You, BFA Educational Media

Alcohol in the Human Body, Sid Davis Productions

Are Drugs the Answer, National Institute of Mental Health

Bennies and Goofballs, U.S. Food and Drug Administration

Bridge from Noplace, National Institute of Mental Health

Cross Country High, Barr Films

Compassion, New York State Education Department

Drug Abuse: A Call to Action, Association Films

Drug Abuse: Everybody's Hangup, National Education Association

Drug Abuse: The Chemical Bomb, National Institute of Mental Health

Drug Addiction, Encyclopedia Britannica

Drugs and the Nervous System, Churchill Films

Drug Education, Ealing Corporation

False Friends, International Film Bureau

Flowers of Darkness, National Institute of Mental Health

Here's Help, National Institute of Mental Health

How Drinking Affects Driving, Media Five Film Distribution

I Am an Alcoholic, McGraw-Hill

LSD, Audiovisual Branch, U.S. Navy, Washington

LSD: Insight or Insanity, Bailey Film Associates

LSD: Lettvin vs. Leary, National Institute of Mental Health

Medicines and How to Use Them, American Medical Association

Narcotics: The Decision. Bailey Films

National Smoking Test, CBS News

Rapping and Tripping, Filmfair Communications

Speed Scene, National Institute of Mental Health

Speedscene: The Problem of Amphetamine Abuse, Bailey Films

Teenage Drinking, CRM Educational Films

The Bottle and the Throttle, Sid Davis Productions

The Circle, National Film Board of Canada

The Distant Drummer (Drugs), National Institute of Mental Health

The Final Factor, American Automobile Association

The Losers, Carousel Films

The Phony Folks (Smoking), Sid Davis Productions

The Trip, Hank Newenhouse

The Trip Back, Sterling Films

Time Pulls the Trigger, Brigham Young University

What About Drinking?, Young America Films

Who Cops Out?, International Film Bureau

Who — Me?, American Cancer Society

World of the Weed, NET Film Service, Indiana University

You Can't Grow a Green Plant in a Closet, Film Distributing Company

c. Filmstrips

Drinking, Drugs and Driving, McGraw-Hill

Drugs and Health, Encyclopedia Britannica

Drugs in Our Society, Cathedral Films, Inc.

Glue Sniffing, Society for Visual Education

LSD, Society for Visual Education

LSD; The Acid World, Guidance Associates

Marijuana, Guidance Associates

Marijuana: What You Can Believe, Guidance Associates

Me, Myself . . . and Drugs, Guidance Associates

Narcotics, Guidance Associates

Narcotics and You, McGraw-Hill

Psychedelics, Guidance Associates

The Drug Threat, Guidance Associates

You and the Law, Guidance Associates

d. Posters

Black Is Beautiful — Black and on Stuff Isn't, National Institute of Mental Health

Brother — Don't Pass It On, National Institute of Mental Health

Don't Blow It with Drugs, National Institute of Mental Health

Don't Get Hooked, Public Health Service

Even the Longest Filter Doesn't Help, Public Health Service

H — Heroin — Permanent Peace, American Medical Association

Sometimes Alcohol Takes Over, American Medical Association

We'll Miss Ya Baby! Congress Has Acted, American Cancer Society

What's Your Brand?, Imagination, Inc., St. Paul, Minnesota 55114

Will They Turn You On, National Institute of Mental Health

e. Transparencies

Alcohol and Inhibitions, 3M Company, Minneapolis, Minnesota

Alcohol Teaching Kit, Cleveland Health Museum

Drugs and Your Body, Popular Science

Drug Information, Hubbard Scientific Company, Northbrook, Illinois 60062

Examination of Smoking, 3M Company

How Safe Are Drugs?, Food and Drug Administration

Personality Factor and Dangerous Drugs, 3M Company

Range of Mood and Behavior Modifiers, 3M Company

Substances That Modify Mood, School Health Education Study, 3M Company

The Use and Misuse of Drugs, Food and Drug Administration

f. Tapes

Hallucinogens, Educational Progress Corporation, Tulsa, Oklahoma 74145

Marijuana, Educational Progress Corporation

Narcotics, Educational Progress Corporation

Stimulants and Depressants, Educational Progress Corporation

Drugs — Abuse and Use, Educational Activities, Inc.

The Psychedelic Experience, McGraw-Hill

The Youth Scene, Educational Activities, Inc.

Tripping Out, Box 285, Sylvania, Ohio 43560

Youth Turns On, Columbia University Press

g. Records

Drugs: How, Why and When, Educational Activities, Inc.

Questions-Answers About Drugs (3 records), U.S. Government Printing Office

The Drug Scene, Educational Activities, Inc.

h. Comics

Hooked, National Institute of Health

Where There is Smoke (Jr. H. S.), American Cancer Society

i. Plays

Leave It to Laurie (Smoking), American Cancer Society

Narcotics and Youth (Drugs), Kiwanis International, Chicago, Illinois 60611

j. Charts

Dial-A-Drug, Spenco Medical Corporation

Dial-A-Drink, Spenco Medical Corporation

k. Selected Books

(J) = Junior High Level

(S) = Senior High Level

Alcohol and Civilization (S), S. Lucia (McGraw-Hill)

Alcoholism and Society (S), M. Chafetz (Oxford University Press)

Alcohol Problems: A Report to the Nation (S), T. F. Plaut (Oxford University Press)

Alcohol: Use, Nonuse, and Abuse (S), C. Carroll (Wm. C. Brown)

Black Market Medicine (J, S), M. Kreig (Prentice-Hall)

Conflict and Creativity (S), S. M. Farber (McGraw-Hill)

Drug Abuse Education Resource Book (S), National Education Association

Drugs and Alcohol (S), K. L. Jones (Harper and Row)

Drugs and People (S), D. Read (Allyn and Bacon)

Drugs from A to Z: A Dictionary, 2nd edition (J, S), R. Lingeman (McGraw-Hill)

How Dry We Are: Prohibition Revisited (S), H. Lee (Prentice-Hall)

Let's Talk About Drugs (J, S), L. Curtis (Tane Press)

Man Against Himself (S), K. Menninger (Harcourt, Brace, Jovanovich)

Marijuana (J, S), E. Bloomquist (Glencoe Press)

Medical Readings on Drug Abuse (S), O. Byrd (Addison-Wesley)

Readings on Drug Use and Abuse (S), B. Hafen (Brigham Young University Press)

Teenage Drinking in the U.S. (S), G. Maddox (John Wiley)

The A. A. Way of Life (S), Alcoholics Anonymous

The Control of Pain (S), F. Prescott (Thomas Crowell)

The Drug Dilemma (J, S), S. Cohen (Mc-Graw-Hill)

The Drug Scene (J, S), D. Louria (Mc-Graw-Hill)

The Junkie Priest (J, S), J. Harris (Complete Pocket Books)

The Lonely Sickness (J, S), E. Whitney (Beacon)

The New Social Drug (S), D. E. Smith (Prentice-Hall)

The Poetry of Rock (S), R. Goldsmith (Bantam)

The Tunnel Back (S), L. Yablonsky (Macmillan)

Thinking About Drinking (J, S), U.S. Public Health Service

Twelve Angels from Hell (S), D. Wilkerson (F. H. Reuell Co.)

Undercover Agent—Narcotics (J, S), D. Agnew (Macfadden)

Utopiates: The Use and Users of LSD-25 (S), R. Blum (Atherton)

What You Should Know About Drugs and Narcotics (J), A. Blakeslee (Association)

What You Should Know About Drugs (J, S), W. Goredetzky and S. T. Christian (Harcourt Brace, Jovanovich)

Why Me? (J, S), W. Gargon (Doubleday)

12. CONSUMER HEALTH

a. Pamphlets or Leaflets

A Way to Cut Your Doctor Bills, American Medical Association

Beware of Health Quacks, American Medical Association

Can We Eat Well for Less?, National Dairy Council

Chiropractic: The Unscientific Cult, American Medical Association

Consumer Union Report on Life Insurance, Consumer Union

Cosmetic Surgery, American Medical Association

Danger: the Cancer Quacks, U.S. Public Health Service

Facts About the Foods You Eat, Cereal Institute

Facts on Quacks, American Medical Association

Fads, Myths, Quacks and Your Health, Public Affairs Pamphlet

Food Facts Talk Back, American Dietetic Association

Food—Misinformation, American Dietetic Association

Fresh Facts for the Consumer, United Fresh Fruit and Vegetable Association

Guides Against Bait Advertising, Federal Trade Commission

Home Freezing of Fruits and Vegetables, United Fresh Fruit and Vegetable Association

How Safe Is Our Food?, U.S. Public Health Service (FDA)

How the Postal Inspection Service Protects You Against Mail Fraud, U.S. Post Office Department

Mechanical Quackery, American Medical Association

Money Management Program, Household Finance Corporation

Read Labels Carefully, U.S. Public Health Service (FDA)

Read the Label, National Fire Protection Association

The Medicine Show, Consumer Union

Toward Better Tomatoes, United Fresh Fruit and Vegetable Association

Weigh All Ingredients Carefully, U.S. Public Health Service (FDA)

What They Say About Chiropractic, American Medical Association

b. Films

A Reason for Confidence, U.S. Public Health Service, Station K, Atlanta

Dialogue with Life, Modern Talking Picture Service

Even for One, Sterling Films

Have a Wonderful Evening, National Fire Protection Association

Man Alive, Lederle Laboratories

Misery Merchants, Arthritis and Rheumatism Foundation

More Food for Your Money, National Dairy Council

Nutrition Quackery, Association Films

Nutrition Sense and Nonsense, United Fresh Fruit and Vegetable Association

Read the Label: Set a Better Table, Modern Talking Pictures

Science and Superstition, Coronet Films

Steering Clear of Lemons, Consumer Report Films

The Consumer Game, Pyramid Films

The Medicine Man, Sterling Films

What Is Disease? Walt Disney

c. Filmstrips

Bras and Girdles, Popular Science

Consumer Tips on Fresh Citrus, Sunkist Growers

Drug Abuse: Everybody's Hang-up, National Education Association

Florence Nightingale, Metropolitan Life Insurance Company

Keeping Foods Safe to Eat, Popular Science

Mechanical Quackery, American Medical Association

Nutrition: Food vs. Health, Sunburst Communications

The Farm Question, Guidance Associates

The Food and Drug Administration: A Nation's Watchdog, Guidance Associates

What Clothes Should I Wear? Popular Science

You the Consumer, Popular Science

So Your Budget Won't Budge, Popular Science

d. Slides

What's New on Labels, U.S. Public Health Service, FDA

e. Transparencies

Applying Health Criteria, 3M Company

Government Agencies and Health, 3M Company

Health Information and Mass Media, 3M Company

Professional Health Specialists, 3M Company

f. Kit

Defenses Against Quackery, American Medical Association

g. Selected Books

(J) = Junior High Level

(S) = Senior High Level

At Your Own Risk: The Case Against Chiropractic (S), R. L. Smith (Trident Press)

Black Market Medicine (S), M. Kreig (Prentice-Hall)

Buyer Beware (J, S), F. Trump (Abington)

Dark Side of the Marketplace (J, S), W. Magnuson (Consumers Union, Mt. Vernon, New York)

Doctors on the Frontier (J), R. Dunlop (Doubleday)

Drugs and Your Body (J), FDA (U.S. Public Health Service)

Innocent Consumer vs. the Exploiters (S), S. Margolius (Pocket Books)

Magic, Faith and Healing (J, S), A. Kiev (Macmillan)

Medical Messiahs (J, S), J. Young (Consumers Union, Mt. Vernon, New York)

Nutrition, Science and You (J, S), R. Leverton (National Science Teachers Assn.)

Nuts Among the Berries (S), R. M. Deutsch (Ballantine)

One for a Man, Two for a Horse (J, S), G. Carson (Doubleday)

Remedies and Rackets (S), J. Cook (W. W. Norton)

Slim Down, Shape Up Diets for Teenagers (J, S), G. Maddox (Avon)

The Bargain Hucksters (J, S), R. Smith (Crowell)

The Consumer Guide to Better Buying (J, S), S. Margolius (Pocket Books)

The Doctor and His Patient (J), S. Bloom (Russell Sage)

The Golden Age of Quackery (J), S. H. Holbrook (Collier)

The Health Hucksters (J, S), R. Smith (Bartholomew House)

The Hidden Persuaders (S), V. Packard (Pocket Books)

The Medicine Show (J, S), Consumer Reports (Macmillan)

The Vulnerable Americans (J, S), C. Gentry (Doubleday)

Toadstool Millionaires (S), J. H. Young (Princeton University Press)

13. WORLD HEALTH

a. Pamphlets or Leaflets

Album of Europe — 31 Countries — One Health, WHO

Growing Up With UNICEF, Public Affairs Pamphlet

Health on Focus, WHO

The World Health Organization, Public Affairs Pamphlet

Twenty Years of Work, WHO

Venereal Disease Is Still a World Problem, American Medical Association

What Did You Have for Breakfast This Morning?, National Dairy Council

b. Films

Assignment Children, Indiana University, Audiovisual Center

A Time of Hope, Pharmaceutical Manufacturers Association

Born Equal, Indiana University, Audiovisual Center

Eternal Fight, Indiana University, Audiovisual Center

False Friends, Pan American Health Organization

Man Alive (WHO), McGraw-Hill

People Like Maria, Pan American Health Organization

Physician to the World, Care, Inc.

Somewhere in India, Indiana University, Audiovisual Center

The Fight to End Malaria, Association Films

To Your Health, Pan American Health Organization

Walter Reed and the Conquest of Yellow Fever, Association Films

Water, Pan American Health Organization

c. Filmstrips

International War Against Diphtheria, International Film Bureau

Population and Food, Popular Science

Unmasking the Germ Assassins, International Film Bureau

d. Magazines

Gazette, Pan American Health Organization, Regional Office of WHO, Washington, D.C. (published quarterly in Spanish and English)

World Health, WHO, Avenue Appia, 1211 Geneva 27, Switzerland

e. Selected Books

(J) = Junior High Level

(S) = Senior High Level

Doctors to the World (J), M. Morgan (Viking)

Eradication of Malaria (J, S), G. MacDonald (U.S. Public Health Service)

Food Wonders of the World (J, S), (UNICEF)

From Witchcraft to World Health (J), S. Leff (Macmillan)

Health and Humanity (S), S. Leff (International Publishers)

Medical Care in Developing Countries (S), M. King (Oxford)

Official Records of WHO (S), (World Health Organization)

Promises to Keep: The Life of Dr. Thomas A. Dooley (J, S), A. Dooley (Farrar, Straus and Giroux)

World Eradication of Infectious Diseases (J, S), E. Hinman (Charles C Thomas)

World Health (S), F. Brockington (Pelican)

14. HEALTH CAREERS

a. Pamphlets or Leaflets

Careers in Dentistry, American Dental Association

Decision for Research, American Heart Association

Dental Health Education, Cleveland Health Museum

Facts About Blindness, American Foundation for the Blind

Health Education as Your Career, National Education Association (AAHPER)

Put Your Talent to Work in the Health Field, National Health Council

Safety Education as Your Career, National Education Association (AAHPER)

Speech Therapy, National Society for Crippled Children and Adults

Students Consider a Career in Podiatry, American Podiatry Association

The Challenge of Health Research, Metropolitan Life Insurance Company

The Physician's Career, American Medical Association

This Is School Nursing, National Education Association (AAHPER)

Wanted: Medical Technologists, Public Affairs Pamphlets

What Is an Optometrist, American Optometrist Association

b. Films

Day of Judgment, Pharmaceutical Manufacturers Association

In Medical Laboratory, American Cancer Society

New Life for Lisa (Nursing), Pharmaceutical Manufacturers Association

Patterns of a Profession, American Dental Association

Portrait of an Internist, Pharmaceutical Manufacturers Association

The Challenge of Dentistry, American Dental Association

c. Filmstrips

A Job That Goes Someplace, Guidance Associates

A New Look at Home Economics Careers, Guidance Associates

Career Planning in a Changing World, Popular Science

Careers in Health, Popular Science

Careers in School Food Service, Guidance Associates

Careers in the Aerospace Age, Guidance Associates

Choosing Your Career, Guidance Associates

Jobs for High School Students, Guidance Associates

Liking Your Job and Your Life, Guidance Associates

Preparing for the Jobs of the 70's, Guidance Associates

Preparing for the World of Work, Guidance Associates

Should You Go to College?, Guidance Associates

Your Job Outlook, Popular Science

d. Posters

Choose a Career in the Medical Field, American Medical Association

e. Selected Books

(J) = Junior High Level
(S) = Senior High Level

A Dozen Doctors (S), D. Ingle (University of Chicago Press)

Great Men of Medicine, (J, S), R. Hume (Random House)

The Doctor and His Patient (S), S. Bloom (Russell Sage)

The Plague Killers (S), W. Geer (Scribner's Sons)

ADDRESSES OF FILM SOURCES

Agency for Instructional Television
Box A
Bloomington, Indiana 47401

Alfred Higgins Productions
9100 Sunset Blvd.
Los Angeles, California 90069

American Education Films
132 Laskey Drive
Beverly Hills, California 90210

Association Films, Inc.
25358 Cypress Avenue
Hayward, California 94544

Audio Arts
Portland, Oregon 97208

Avis Films
2408 W. Olive Avenue
Burbank, California 91506

Bailey Films, Inc.
6509 De Longpre Avenue
Hollywood, California 90028

Barr Films
P. O. Box 5667
Pasadena, California 91107

BFA Educational Media
2211 Michigan Avenue
Santa Monica, California 90404

Billy Budd Films, Inc.
235 E. 57th Street
New York, New York 10022

Brigham Young University
Provo, Utah 84601

Calvin Productions
1105 Truman Road
Kansas City, Missouri 64106

Canadian National Film Board
680 5th Avenue
New York, New York 10019

Capitol Film Laboratories, Inc.
470 E Street, S.W.
Washington, D.C. 20024

Carousel Films
1501 Broadway
New York, New York 10036

Cathedral Films, Inc.
2921 W. Alameda Avenue
Burbank, California 91505

Charles Cahill and Associates
P. O. Box 3220
Hollywood, California 90028

Churchill Films
6671 Sunset Boulevard
Los Angeles, California 90028

Classroom Film Distributors, Inc.
5120 Hollywood Boulevard
Los Angeles, California 90027

CRM (McGraw-Hill) Educational Films
Del Mar, California 92014

Columbia University Press
   (Center for Mass Communication)
562 W. 113 Street
New York, New York 10025

Consumer Report Films
Box XA 22, 256 Washington Street
Mt. Vernon, New York 10550

Coronet Instructional Films
65 E. South Water Street
Chicago, Illinois 60601

Ealing Corporation (BFA)
2211 Michigan Avenue
Santa Monica, California 90404

Educational Activities, Inc.
P. O. Box 392
Freeport, New York 11520

Educational Corporation
P. O. Box 517
Skokie, Illinois 60076

Encyclopedia Britannica Films, Inc.
1150 Wilmette Avenue
Wilmette, Illinois 60091

Environmental Control
   Administration
12720 Twinbrook Parkway
Rockville, Maryland 20852

Eye Gate House, Inc.
146 Archer Avenue
Jamaica, New York 11435

Family Filmstrips
5823 Santa Monica Boulevard
Hollywood, California 90038

Film Distributing Company
Box 373
Mill Valley, California 94941

Filmfair Communications
10946 Ventura Boulevard
Studio City, California 91604

Films, Incorporated
1144 Wilmette Avenue
Wilmette, Illinois 60091

Focus Education Inc.
3 E. 54th Street
New York, New York 10022

Guidance Associates
Pleasantville, New York 10570

Hank Newenhouse
1825 Willow Road
Northfield, Illinois 60093

Human Relations Media Center
22 Clemmons Square
Pound Ridge, New York 10576

Ideal Pictures Corporation
321 W. 44th Street
New York, New York 10036

International Film Bureau, Inc.
322 S. Michigan Avenue
Chicago, Illinois 60604

Jarvis Covillard Associates
P. O. Box 123
Culver City, California 91230

John Wiley and Sons
605 Third Avenue
New York, New York 10016

Knowledge Builders
625 Madison Avenue
New York, New York 10000

Landford Publishing Company
P. O. Box 8711
San Jose, California 95125

Macmillan Films, Inc.
34 MacQuestan Parkway South
Mt. Vernon, New York 10550

Modern Talking Picture Service
45 Rockefeller Plaza
New York, New York 10020

Modern Learning Aids
Box 302
Rochester, New York 14603

Paulist Productions
7575 Pacific Coast Highway
Pacific Palisades, California 90272

Perennial Education
1825 Willow Road
Northfield, Illinois 60093

Picture Films Distributing Co.
43 West 16th Street
New York, New York 10011

Polymorph Films
331 Newbury Street
Boston, Massachusetts 02115

Popular Science
330 W. 42nd Street
New York, New York 10036

Pyramid Films
Box 1048
Santa Monica, California 90406

See-Saw Films
P. O. Box 262
Palo Alto, California 94302

Sterling Educational Films
241 E. 34th Street
New York, New York 10016

Society for Visual Education, Inc.
1345 Diversey Parkway
Chicago, Illinois 60614

Stuart Finley Productions
3428 Mansfield Road
Fall Church, Virginia 22041

Sunburst Communications
Pound Ridge, New York 10576

Teaching Film Custodians
25 W. 43rd Street
New York, New York 10036

Texture Films, Inc.
1600 Broadway
New York, New York 10019

United World Films
221 Park Avenue South
New York, New York 10003

Walt Disney Productions
800 Senora Avenue
Glendale, California 91201

Warren Schloat Productions, Inc.
115 Tompkins Avenue
Pleasantville, New York 10570

Western Publishing Company
830 Third Avenue
New York, New York 10022

Wexler Film Productions
801 N. Seward Street
Los Angeles, California 90038

Young America Films
330 W. 42nd Street
New York, New York 10036

Chapter 11

Evaluation of the Health Instruction Program

Sooner or later nearly every parent and taxpayer wants to know how well the schools are doing their job. Except in a general way it has always been difficult for teachers to answer the inquiry and prove beyond a reasonable doubt that their students have understood, made decisions, and acted on the educational items to which they have been exposed. Nevertheless, there is a strong desire by many teachers to subscribe to the Thessalonian admonition to prove all things and to "... hold fast to that which is good."

THE TREMBLE FACTOR

Seldom are teachers fully aware of the embarrassing and crushing possibilities of failure in their work. Economist Paul Rosenstein-Rodan has named the effect of this knowledge "the tremble factor"; however, it is not faced by a sizable number of teachers. According to John Silber, one of the most effective uses to which the tremble factor has ever been put was in the construction of ancient Rome. When the scaffolding was removed from a completed Roman arch, the Roman engineer stood beneath. If the arch came crashing down, he was the first to know. His concern for the quality of the arch was intensely personal and it is not surprising that so many Roman arches have survived.

It is certainly marvelous that teachers manage to survive, protected from the tremble factor, and even achieve a high level of teaching success. Such occurrences may well be the exception rather than the rule. And this is every bit as true in health teaching as in other subject areas.

MEASUREMENT AND EVALUATION IN HEALTH EDUCATION

Measurement is essentially a process of making comparisons and relating them to personal needs in an effort to find out where one is headed. It answers the questions of how much, how many, and how often; it is concerned with quantities and qualities in evidence. Evaluation, however, goes beyond the mechanics of testing and measuring by looking at the results of measurement in the light of aims and objectives. Moreover, to evaluate is "to set a value on" (Webster)—to determine relative "worth, excellence, or importance." In short, evaluation in education is a process of judging the effectiveness of educational experience.

Health evaluation is employed to determine the health status of students and to properly classify them for participation in school activities. It is used to ascertain the effectiveness of the total school health effort—services, environment, and instruction. More specifically, health evaluation measures both teacher and pupil efficiency by noting the degree of progress toward preconceived health goals. It also provides a basis for grading students and reporting individual student achievements. Finally, one of the most important purposes of evaluation in health education is to discover useful information about student knowledges, attitudes, and practices which may be of value when the health curriculum or course of study is being revised and updated.

It is, however, difficult to demonstrate the effect of good health teaching on human activity. For one thing, the power of the human organism to adapt to the physical and psychological stresses placed upon it is most remarkable. Thus, the person who "practices" poorly frequently goes unrecognized. Then there is the "sleeper effect" in health teaching, in which material learned today may not be applied until months or years later. In addition, the measurement of attitudes and the assessment of feelings are difficult under the best of circumstances.

STAFF AND PROGRAM

The total school health program may be excellent in appearance on paper, but its ultimate success depends upon an efficient staff—from school board members and superintendent of schools to principals, medical director, nurses, food service personnel, health coordinator, and instructional staff.

One way to quantitatively evaluate staff is to follow the procedures of the Texas Education Agency.[1] Standards for two of the health staff categories, school health coordinator and instructional staff, are set forth here to illustrate one method of appraisal.

> The following rating system is provided, which will enable a quantitative evaluation of any part or all of the school health team. The list of functions and responsibilities serves to suggest areas for improvement as well as providing for evaluation of the program. In rating each function or responsibility in terms of compliance, place 1, 2, 3, 4, or 5 beside each, which would indicate the degree of performance or compliance, as outlined below:
> 1 = Guideline is met without exception
> 2 = Guideline is met in most instances (75% or more)
> 3 = Guideline is met reasonably well (55% to 74%)
> 4 = Guideline is met to a limited degree (25% to 54%)
> 5 = Guideline is not met at all

School Health Coordinator

_____ 1. Assists the school administrative personnel in the organization of an advisory school health council.

_____ 2. Interprets for all concerned the objectives and activities of the several phases of the program.

_____ 3. Acts in liaison with health service personnel, school staff members, and community health agencies on behalf of the program development.

_____ 4. Acts in liaison with parent-teacher and child study groups on behalf of home-school cooperation and parental participation in the program.

---

[1]Texas Education Agency, _Suggested Guidelines for Evaluating School Health Team Members in an Optimum School Health Program_ (Rev.), Dallas, Texas: Texas Education Agency, Revised.

_____ 5. Provides a leadership role in planning, implementing, directing, and evaluating the total school health program.

_____ 6. Coordinates reports, records, and findings from all phases of the school health program.

_____ 7. Coordinates the activities of such a program with those in the community—working with health departments, civic and professional organizations, parents, physicians, dentists, private and voluntary health agencies, and school and community health councils.

_____ 8. Keeps abreast of new scientific and medical developments in health-related fields that may enhance the effectiveness of the program.

_____ 9. Keeps all school personnel thoroughly informed on all aspects of the school health program, particularly the role of each person.

_____ 10. Serves as adviser for student groups or committees participating in activities of health programs.

Instructional Staff

_____ 1. Takes leadership role in initiating and participating in developing objectives, policies, plans, and procedures.

_____ 2. Consults and cooperates with other members of the school-community.

_____ 3. Practices continuous daily observation of students regarding physical, mental-emotional, and socio-cultural health status.

_____ 4. Cooperates in the prevention and control of communicable disease.

_____ 5. Observes departures from normal health and possible signs of communicable disease, and refers the child to the appropriate school personnel.

_____ 6. Follows a planned program of procedures and techniques which complement school-community health program objectives.

_____ 7. Provides time for consultation with children, parents, and health team members.

_____ 8. Supports and cooperates with health services and healthful environment phases of the total school-community health program.

_____ 9. Participates in curriculum development activities.

_____ 10. Motivates and assists students in achieving adequacy in health knowledge, attitudes, and practices.

_____ 11. Relates learning experiences to meaningful or expressed student needs and interests which are recognized by the school-community health council or the health committee of his school.

_____ 12. Participates in planning and implementing procedures for health and safety measures.

_____ 13. Exemplifies habits and attitudes which are conducive to a high quality of health.

_____ 14. Seeks out and participates in opportunities for professional growth and development.

_____ 15. Utilizes all available resources for maintaining current health knowledge.

_____ 16. Assumes responsibility for maintaining sanitary, safe, and congenial school environmental conditions in the classroom.

_____ 17. Contributes to planning and implementing research and development phases of the total program.

_____ 18. Participates in the evaluation of the total school-community health program.

_____ 19. Utilizes community resources in providing for the enrichment of the curriculum.

_____ 20. Cooperates in the resolution of individual and group health problems.

_____ 21. Participates in the health appraisal of pupils, providing helpful information to the examining physician.

_____ 22. Provides appropriate supervision to help the child meet his needs if prescribed by a physician and in accordance with the school policy.

_____ 23. Assists in interpreting the school health program to the home and in developing parent-school cooperation.

_____ 24. Serves as a liaison to the librarian for obtaining current health education resource materials for students and faculty.

_____ 25. Takes a leadership role in stimulating students to pursue a career in health related fields.

_____ 26. Acts as a resource person for the health needs of the school.

An exceptionally well-prepared and thorough instrument for examining health instruction efforts, _A Rating Scale for Health Instruction Programs,_ may be obtained from Jule Ann Collins, 80 Kenilworth Court, Lafayette, Ind. 47905.

CURRICULUM EVALUATION

How effective is the curriculum in meeting the needs of both boys and girls at the junior high school level? At the senior high school level? This raises the further questions: How can needs be assessed? How can progress toward fulfilling these needs be measured? In short, how does one determine whether a particular program is adequate?

One way is to employ criteria developed by some reputable body. The _Evaluative Criteria, National Study of Secondary School Evaluation,_ revised in 1974 by the American Council on Education, presents health education criteria in checklist form.[2] These rather extensive criteria may be applied to a local health education program as a self-testing activity or by an outside agency. The criteria pertain to the organization of the health program, the nature of the offerings, the physical facilities, and the direction of learning. In the final category, some searching questions are raised about instructional staff, instructional activities, instructional materials, and methods of evaluation in use.

The appraisal of curriculum content, objectives, materials, and grade placement of learning activities always centers on societal needs. What are the health problems? Is health content current? Are resources up to date? Is health content assessed with particular reference to its interdisciplinary structures? It is in answering these kinds of questions that decisions can be made pertaining to program changes, creativity, and innovations. There are times when programs are so good that further changes should not be made. There are numerous advantages in program flexibility, but because it is sometimes stylish or popular to change content around, there frequently occurs "change for change's sake."

In evaluating curriculum content, both the teacher who is teaching it and the student who is learning it must be viewed in a kind of bond relationship. Teacher attitude alone can disturb what might otherwise have been a favorable health behavior change.

Further evaluations of the health instructional area may involve surveys of parental views, particularly as they are solicited in relation to special topics. This source of information can be quite effective in providing home-community feedback to the schools. In fact, a number of people in the community are in a position to help appraise the health curriculum as they observe youth in such places as recreation centers, churches, part-

_____
[2]May be obtained from NSSSE, American Council on Education, 1785 Massachusetts Avenue, N.W., Washington, D.C. 20036.

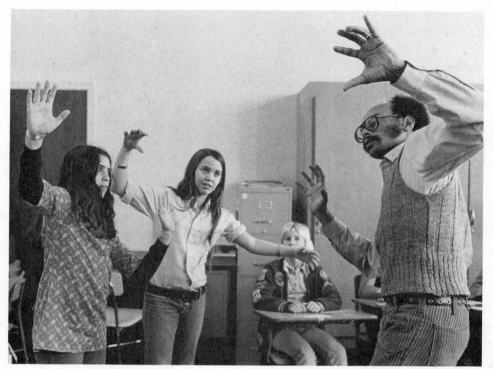

Figure 11–1 How to evaluate role playing as a teaching technique. (Courtesy of National Education Association Publishing and Joe Di Dio)

time jobs, and medical offices. This information, coupled with the personal viewpoints of a number of health and non-health instructors, very often provides a solid dimension affecting the question of whether the program should remain the same or be changed.

APPRAISING KNOWLEDGE

Cognitive evaluations very often need to be broadened. Bloom, Hastings, and Madaus call for progress to be measured by the degree to which individual behavior conforms to the prearranged behavioral objectives.[3] It is significant, therefore, to build into the evaluation process an opportunity for the student to illustrate and demonstrate his or her health understanding in some reasonably organized way. For example, applying concepts through such activities as problem solving, which include analysis and synthesis, approaches the relationships that are practical in bringing about judgmental skills in everyday life.

Bloom's six educational objectives in the cognitive domain can be applied to health teaching as follows:

1. Knowledge

The recall of specifics — methods, processes, theories, structures, or settings. Test for health definitions, terminology, and trends.

Example: Tranquilizers help in mental illness because they:

(1) Stimulate the individual

---

[3] Benjamin S. Bloom, J. Thomas Hastings, and George F. Madaus, *Handbook of Formative and Summative Evaluation of Student Learning,* New York: McGraw-Hill, 1971.

(2) Calm disturbed individuals

(3) Act as a depressant

(4) Both stimulate and depress

2. Comprehension

The lowest level of understanding, where the individual can make use of something without necessarily relating it to other things. Here, an individual demonstrates the ability to translate or paraphrase a communication.

Example: You have heard the following terms used in the classroom and in the community: "ecology," "thermal pollution," "vinyl chloride," "ozone layer," and "breeder reactor." In a short paragraph tell what these terms mean to you.

3. Application

Employing technical principles or abstractions, ideas, and theories in some way. Questions of application call for a show of practical ability where one is able to match some already acquired concept with the phenomenon being considered.

Example: Observe several air pollution photographs and explain how they may or may not be representative of what is seen in some towns and cities today.

4. Analysis

An idea, concept or structure is examined by breaking it down into its parts so that the *relationship* between parts is clear.

Example: The husband of a woman who died of lung cancer claimed that the physician did not provide proper medical care during the several months in which he had the woman as a patient. Why is this accusation unfair?

(1) Lung cancer cannot be cured unless the lungs are removed.

(2) The woman was told several times by the physician to stop smoking, but she paid no attention.

(3) The woman went to the physician too late for the cancer to be brought under control.

(4) The cancer appeared suddenly in the woman the week before she died.

5. Synthesis

All parts and elements are brought together to form a whole. The student is able to work with pieces and make arrangements in such a manner as to create a structure or pattern not there before. Theorizing a firm statement on the basis of data on hand demonstrates the competence to synthesize.

Example: Create a short essay in which you discuss the relationship between nutritional elements and how this bears on human energy levels. There is an explanation of this in the filmstrip *Focus on Nutrition.*

After viewing the filmstrip pause and think about the assignment and plan your remarks.

6. Evaluation

Judgments are made pertaining to the worth of ideas, techniques, and materials.

Example: Of the several routines that one might use to restore breathing, which is the least effective?

(1) Arm lift–back pressure

(2) Mouth-to-mouth

(3) Prone pressure

(4) Barrel rolling

It is the opinion of Glatthorn that evaluation processes can be vastly improved by having the teacher becoming involved in six separate stages of appraisal:[4]

1. Diagnosing: Finding out what the learner knows before the learning begins. A

---

[4]Allan A. Glatthorn, *Alternatives in Education: Schools and Programs,* New York: Dodd, Mead and Co., 1975, p. 170.

diagnostic pre-test employing a large number of relatively easy items is used. Or, a discussion at the opening of the class in which the teacher probes for problems and weaknesses.

2. *Giving feedback:* The learner is given information about strengths and weaknesses and suggestions how deficiencies might be remedied. Feedback is also given to the teacher as the pupil indicates what he liked best and least about the topic.

3. *Judging:* The student and the teacher judge the student's performance by relating it to some set of criteria or achievement standard. Also, the student is taught some self-evaluation skills.

4. *Grading:* A symbol (word, letter, number) is assigned to the results of the evaluation.

5. *Recording:* Noted in writing are all important evidences of pupil achievement, with the student encouraged to add his or her own special accomplishments.

6. *Reporting:* Student progress information is shared with parents and others with the student responsible for helping to prepare the transcript.

CRITERION-REFERENCED MEASURES

There is a marked distinction between tests or procedures designed to compare individuals, and tests designed to measure individual competence in some specific task or domain. The criterion-referenced test yields measurements that are directly related to performance standards, i.e., predetermined tasks. Here learning modules are set up complete with a number of learning activity packages, and a pre- and post-test. In the health education area this evaluation technique can be carried out in connection with the contract method of teaching.

APPRAISING HEALTH ATTITUDES AND BEHAVIORS

For decades Gordon Allport studied, wrote, and struggled with the subject of human attitudes. Throughout this period he made it quite clear that personal feelings are so ingrained, so carefully protected, and even hidden from the holder that a valid measurement of attitudes is most difficult. Moreover, when attitudes are further defined as more than a feeling, as representing a predisposition to act or a potential behavior, it becomes even more difficult to measure them accurately.

Asking pupils how they *feel* about a health idea or practice may yield a reliable answer if the setting is right. Students will respond from the heart when they are truly interested in the topic, and when they feel comfortable with instructor and class members alike. It is when they sense that they are a significant part of a question-discussion situation that they will allow their inner feelings and beliefs to emerge. Under such circumstances — frequently difficult to arrange in today's crowded schools — health attitudes can be appraised. Because such appraisals cannot be accomplished on a mass basis, numerous attempts have been made to create attitude scales, in which the student is asked to respond to a statement or situation by checking off on a continuum his degree of feeling, from the least favorable to the most favorable.

The relationship between feelings and actions is a real one. There is evidence that an individual must strongly agree with a favorable health practice if his behavior is to be changed. People simply do not modify their way of doing things without some emotional or motivational process. Olsen was aware of this when he produced his attitude scale a few years ago.[5] He looked for attitudes in terms of reactions to statements. Note the clear directions given:

The key to the responses remains constant throughout this inventory. The key is as follows:

A. *Strongly Agree*   B. *Agree*   C. *Undecided*   D. *Disagree*   E. *Strongly Disagree*

If you *Strongly Agree* with an item, mark column "A" in the space provided on the answer sheet. If you *Strongly Disagree* with an item, mark column "E" in the space provided on the answer sheet. Some sample items are:

1. Not facing reality is the basis of most problems.
2. Too much fuss is being made over health problems.
3. The best way to relieve tension or stress is to take a tranquilizer.

Bloom points out that in the affective domain, the pupil must progress from a *receiving* state where he or she becomes aware of the health problem to a *responding* state of talking about it. As it is accepted, a state of *valuing* occurs and leads to the internalization of values through *organization*. The peak of the process is *characterization,* in which the individual becomes effective in doing something about the problem.

Not only is attitude measurement helpful in determining health feelings and concerns, but it is also useful as a means of initiating discussion of a topic. This is one of the reasons Vincent gave for creating his scale to measure attitude toward smoking marihuana.[6] The scale is different from most scales in that the statements (rather than the responses) proceed on a continuum from very favorable to very unfavorable. (See Figure 11–2). This simplifies the scoring and makes the test easy to take. The scale values indicated in the column labeled (S) are omitted from the copy of the test that the students use. These values reflect a 5-point continuum: 5 — very favorable; 4 — favorable; 3 — neither favorable nor unfavorable; 2 — unfavorable; and 1 — very unfavorable. The score on the scale is the middle value of those statements to which the student responds. If, for example, he responds to statements 117, 127, 129, 131, and 137, his middle score would be 2.9 — an attitude that is neither favorable nor unfavorable. The scale is considered both valid and reliable, and has been used with eighth, tenth, and twelfth grade students.

What has been said about the difficulties of appraising attitudes applies equally well to the measurement of health behavior. An accurate weighing of health practices is difficult under the best of circumstances. Over the years teachers have been quick to present health facts to their classes and to expect an accurate regurgitation of the facts at testing time. This kind of operation continues despite the fact that numerous studies have shown that little relationship exists between what a pupil knows in an informational sense and what he practices in real life. Obviously, concrete health information is important; it will always be needed. But added to it must be the dimension of personal involvement — the opportunity to *act* on facts during and after formal instruction. Students who have this opportunity are more apt to behave in an optimum way when their health practices are appraised at a later date.

When Schley and Banister experimented with behavior change as a result of health

---

[5]Larry K. Olsen, *Olsen Health Inventory,* Department of Health and Safety Education, University of Illinois, Champaign, Illinois 61820.

[6]Raymond J. Vincent, "A Scale to Measure Attitude Toward Smoking Marihuana," *Journal of School Health,* 40:454–456, October, 1970. See also Vincent's "New Scale for Measuring Attitudes," *School Health Review,* 6:19–21, March/April, 1974.

ATTITUDE TOWARD SMOKING MARIHUANA

Recently increasing publicity has been given to smoking marihuana. The following scale is meant to explore some of your *feelings* toward smoking marihuana. It is *not* meant to test what you know about marihuana. Read each item carefully and *circle* the number opposite each statement with which you agree. Make *no marks* opposite the statement with which you *disagree*.

(S)

4.9	149.	Smoking marihuana is a requirement for successful living.
4.7	147.	Smoking marihuana is necessary if one is to achieve his potential.
4.5	145.	Smoking marihuana is an excellent way to increase one's understanding of the world about him.
4.3	143.	Smoking marihuana is too good a thing to be given up.
4.1	141.	Smoking marihuana can be a helpful way of adjusting to the world around us.
3.9	139.	A person should be allowed to smoke marihuana if he wants to.
3.7	137.	Smoking marihuana can be justified.
3.5	135.	Smoking marihuana is all right in some cases.
3.3	133.	The benefits of smoking marihuana depend entirely upon the individual.
3.1	131.	Smoking marihuana is not necessarily wrong.
2.9	129.	Smoking marihuana is one way of trying to be different.
2.7	127.	Smoking marihuana isn't absolutely bad but it isn't good either.
2.5	125.	I question whether or not it is morally right to smoke marihuana.
2.3	123.	Smoking marihuana is not a necessary part of life.
2.1	121.	Smoking marihuana is an emotional "crutch."
1.9	119.	Smoking marihuana is a foolish thing to do.
1.7	117.	Smoking marihuana is wrong.
1.5	115.	Smoking marihuana is bad.
1.3	113.	Smoking marihuana is a foolish way to try and escape reality.
1.1	111.	Smoking marihuana shows an utter lack of self respect.

Figure 11–2

teaching, they asked their students to cooperate by responding to an anonymous questionnaire.[7] This was considered to be an important part of the course. To find out how the first 14 units in the health science course had effected improvements in student health practices, each student was asked during the fourteenth week to respond anonymously to three statements about each unit previously studied. For example:

Unit 1: Decision making

1. As a result of studying this unit, my attitude toward the improvement of health practices in this area of health is (_____ better, _____ worse, _____ unchanged).

2. As a result of studying this topic, my personal actions and/or activities in the area of health with which this topic deals are (_____ better, _____ worse, _____ unchanged).

3. As a result of studying this topic, I (have, have not) helped someone else improve a personal health practice.

Interestingly, over 90 per cent of the students felt that they improved in one or more of the health practices during the first fourteen weeks of the course, and 84 per cent claimed to have helped someone else improve in a personal health practice. Improve-

---

[7]Robert A. Schley and Richard E. Banister, "Behavioral Change in an Academic Setting: How It Works," *School Health Review*, 1:13–18, November, 1970.

ments most commonly described included the use of seat belts while driving, improvement in eating habits, and a feeling of improved mental health and decision-making ability. The responses of the students were strong, which is probably a tribute to the instructors, particularly since a high percentage of the class felt that the objectives were clearly stated and they appeared to like the topic.

From time to time, health behavior inventories and checklists have been fashioned in order to solicit direct responses from students about what they do or what they see as their problems. The *Johns and Juhnke Health Behavior Inventory,* developed over two decades ago and recently updated, is a simple instrument designed to find out what practices are exercised and to what degree.[8]

More recently, O'Daniels of the University of Kentucky worked out a *Health Problems Inventory* to be used with high school students.[9] On this instrument the student notes his psychological, physiological, and occupational problems. The Inventory appears to be quite practical in discovering a number of mental and physical health practices. The sample of the 190-item battery shown below is responded to on a "never," "rarely," "sometimes," "often," and "always" basis.

121. I use self-medication procedures.
122. I purchase "fad" medical products.
123. I have accidents frequently.
124. I smoke cigarettes.
125. I drink alcoholic beverages.
126. I have frequent minor illnesses (sore throats, colds, etc.)
127. I have frequent headaches.

DESCRIPTIVE SYSTEM WITH VIDEOTAPES

Videotaping in-class and out-of-class events provides a detailed description of events in a natural setting—a setting that can be reviewed and analyzed later. Here, health events are classified into meaningful categories to provide a concise picture of what occurred. What is said, what is asked, and what is done can be appraised, with feedback to the students. Various levels of student interest and behavior are observed on a time basis—receiving information, practicing, reading, assisting others, exploring alternatives, giving information, and so on. With this data bank it is possible to appraise student progress in a dimension that may supplement knowledge testing.

ADDITIONAL APPRAISAL METHODS

There are a number of possible ways to appraise student progress toward health goals, the most popular and probably the least effective of which is the paper and pencil test. Often these tests would be worth more if their results were combined with information gathered in several other ways. Moreover, such appraisals are more meaningful when carried out more often during the time the course is being taught, instead of strictly for grading purposes halfway through and at the end of the course.

Oral questioning is one simple way of finding out what students know and what they have somehow failed to comprehend and act upon. For the teacher with small classes, this time-consuming activity can be most rewarding.

---

[8]Edward B. Johns, Warren L. Juhnke, and Marion Pollock, *Health Behavior Inventory,* Los Angeles, California: Tinnon-Brown Publishing Company, Revised.

[9]Phyllis S. O'Daniels, *Health Problems Inventory.* May be obtained from the author at the University of Kentucky, Lexington, Kentucky 40506.

TEST 1

DO YOU WANT TO CHANGE YOUR SMOKING HABITS?

For each statement, circle the number that most accurately indicates how you feel. For example, if you completely agree with the statement, circle 4, if you agree somewhat, circle 3, etc.

Important: Answer every question.

	completely agree	somewhat agree	somewhat disagree	completely disagree
A. Cigarette smoking might give me a serious illness.	4	3	2	1
B. My cigarette smoking sets a bad example for others.	4	3	2	1
C. I find cigarette smoking to be a messy kind of habit.	4	3	2	1
D. Controlling my cigarette smoking is a challenge to me.	4	3	2	1
E. Smoking causes shortness of breath.	4	3	2	1
F. If I quit smoking cigarettes it might influence others to stop.	4	3	2	1
G. Cigarettes cause damage to clothing and other personal property.	4	3	2	1
H. Quitting smoking would show that I have willpower.	4	3	2	1
I. My cigarette smoking will have a harmful effect on my health.	4	3	2	1
J. My cigarette smoking influences others close to me to take up or continue smoking.	4	3	2	1
K. If I quit smoking, my sense of taste or smell would improve.	4	3	2	1
L. I do not like the idea of feeling dependent on smoking.	4	3	2	1

HOW TO SCORE:

1. Enter the numbers you have circled to the Test 1 questions in the spaces below, putting the number you have circled to Question A over line A, to Question B over line B, etc.
2. Total the 3 scores across on each line to get your totals. For example, the sum of your scores over lines A, E, and I gives you your score on *Health*—lines B, F, and J gives the score on *Example*, etc.

				Totals
___ A	+ ___ E	+ ___ I	=	_____ Health
___ B	+ ___ F	+ ___ J	=	_____ Example
___ C	+ ___ G	+ ___ K	=	_____ Esthetics
___ D	+ ___ H	+ ___ L	=	_____ Mastery

Scores can vary from 3 to 12. Any score 9 and above is *high;* any score 6 and below is *low.*

Figure 11–3

Observation, for the teacher who knows what to look for, can be objective in nature. The frequent claim that observation is loose and subjective can be refuted when specific behaviors are sought. In a mental health unit, for example, one can observe evidence showing a greater awareness of others, a more friendly person, and a pupil who is more willing to help others than he used to be. What can be observed in the lunchroom that may relate to the nutrition lesson? Are the lunches any better coming from home? Is there less food thrown away at lunch time? Is there more interest shown in discussing a particular health topic?

Health check lists and rating scales help to bring increased validity to the observation by sharpening the ability of the observer. They are not usually standardized, but are developed at the local level for local use. There are also scales by which the students rate themselves. A popular example is the *Smoker's Self-Testing Kit,* available in quantity for class use.[10] Here there are four tests, one of which is shown in Figure 11–3.

Health records, both cumulative and anecdotal, can be used more than they have been. When these records are reviewed, the comments of the school nurse may be helpful in understanding something about student practices. Not only are individual anecdotes helpful, but the results of individual case studies sometimes afford a clue or two about the worth of the instructional program.

Student surveys are frequently designed by pupils themselves in order to sample the attitudes of classmates pertaining to a particular health issue. They may also seek to discover adult and student practices. In recent years they have become more popular, as students check their own feelings and actions on such topics as smoking, drinking, use of drugs, and boy-girl relationships. A thorough survey of health practices before and after in-depth study of a major health topic frequently provides a better yardstick of progress toward goals than almost any other means—subject, of course, to the degree of seriousness shown toward this form of appraisal by those being surveyed.

Diaries and similar student writings have value when they can be obtained. Some instructors require pupils to express their innermost feelings on a health issue and then try to tell why they feel as they do.

Parental viewpoints are valuable when they can be obtained. They are more difficult to realize at the junior-senior high school level than in the primary grades. A formal approach is usually necessary to make contact with parents individually or in small groups. In some cases a random sample of parents is drawn from the larger body and a structural interview is arranged and carried out by an instructor in health education.

In addition to the parents, there are a number of people in a town or city who have direct dealings with secondary school youth. They come to know them in ways different from those of parents and teachers. They hear their unsophisticated remarks and see them in action in a number of ways that provide a clue to their general state of mental and physical health. Practices and attitudes around such places as a youth center, a city playground, a church-school discussion group, or some other community gathering spot are indicative of how far-reaching school discussions have been.

Study contracts, as indicated in Chapter 9, are a fine teaching arrangement. They are also a means of evaluating individual pupil progress. Success in meeting a contract specification simply means that the student has done what he set out to do. It is important to look for quality rather than quantity when using contracts to appraise student success in meeting health topic objectives.[11]

---

[10]U.S. Public Health Service, *Smoker's Self-Testing Kit,* Washington, U.S. Government Printing Office, 1974.

[11]See amplification of this point by William L. Yarber, "Put Quality Control into Your Grade Contracts," *School Health Review,* 5:22–24, March/April, 1974.

STANDARDIZED TESTS OF HEALTH KNOWLEDGE, ATTITUDES AND BEHAVIORS

Measurement instruments of health knowledge, attitudes, and behaviors that are standardized, current, and highly serviceable are in short supply. One of the reasons for this is that it is difficult to prepare a standardized test that isn't outdated before long, due to ever-increasing additions of new health knowledge. It is also troublesome to accurately pinpoint the grade level for which a particular test is appropriate. This has caused test makers to prepare tests designed to appraise students all the way from grade 7 through grade 12, with norms established for each grade. The obvious weakness here is that the depth level and word difficulty level fails to be suitable for such a wide range of student maturation. Tests, therefore, should be carefully prepared and standardized on students who are as close as possible in all traits and behaviors associated with age, grade, locality, and general background.

There are always occasions when instructors want to find out what students know, but good health tests must do more than measure knowledge. There are no standardized health tests that embrace all of Bloom's requirements. Some are concerned with knowledge only, and there are others which attempt to tie knowledge and its application together. In the health tests produced by the Educational Testing Service (Princeton, New Jersey), knowledge questions make up only about 20 per cent of the total; the others are as follows: application, 50 per cent; analysis, 20 per cent; and evaluation, 10 per cent. Information about these health tests is available on request.

The health education area is rich in opportunities to build a comprehensive examination which will literally give the student a "workout" in demonstrating his real understanding of health conditions, issues, and values. Preparing appropriate questions for a particular topic is time-consuming. It is far easier to simply write out a true-false question or ask the pupil to set forth certain facts. In this connection it may be better to have fifteen or twenty fully developed appraisal items than a 100-item battery of knowledge type questions. Suppose, for example, the teacher wants to find out how effective the instruction was in consumer health. An answer that is quite meaningful might be provided by setting up an examination along the following lines.

Consumer Health

Knowledge:　What are the several functions of the Food and Drug Administration?

Application:　You have discovered that John and his friend Joe are both confined to their homes with sore throats. Although they have the same physician, he has written a different prescription for each boy. A classmate of yours cannot understand the reason for this. It is up to you to explain it. Write out what you will say.

Analysis:　Study the following statement. Then support it or disprove it. "Newspapers and television frequently advertise health products that are useless."

Synthesis:　Design a plan that will bring all of the health-related personnel in a community together in such a way that their specialized health efforts will be highly effective for all of the citizens.

Evaluation:　Present the arguments, for and against, that are related to the following situation: You have been reading quite a bit about consumer products. Some people say that the government is too easy-going in permitting certain products to be sold, and that industry is only interested in making money. Other people point out that both industry and the government have the welfare of the consumer at heart.

By the time the student has responded to the preceding appraisal items, he will have demonstrated far more in the way of understanding about consumer health than is frequently measured in the more common alternate response and multiple choice type questions. Yet, carefully formulated multiple choice questions can be employed to measure pupil application and evaluation just as well as for specific knowledge.

Among the more recent standardized health and safety tests for secondary school use are the following:

JUNIOR HIGH LEVEL

Colebank, Albert D. *Health Behavior Inventory: Junior High,* Monterey, California: California Test Bureau, Revised. (There are 24 health attitude items, 25 health behavior items, and 50 health knowledge items, for a total of 100 multiple choice questions.)

Cooperative Health Education Test (AAHPER), 1972. Educational Testing Service, Box 999, Princeton, New Jersey 08540.

Kilander, H. Frederick. *Information Test on the Biological Aspects of Human Reproduction,* 3rd edition, Staten Island, New York, 1968. (A 33-item multiple choice test.)

Kilander, H. Frederick. *Information on Drugs and Drug Abuse,* 3rd edition, Staten Island, New York. Revised. (25-question multiple choice.)

Kilander, H. Frederick. *Information Test on Smoking and Health,* Staten Island, New York. Revised. (A 25-item test for junior high school through college levels. Single copies available from Dr. Glenn Leach at Wagner College.)

Kilander, H. Frederick, *Nutrition Information Test,* 5th edition, Staten Island, New York, 1968. (A 33-item multiple choice test with norms set up from junior high school to college. Also available from Dr. Leach.)

Schwartz, William F. *Achievement Test on Syphilis and Gonorrhea,* Durham, N.C.: Family Life Publications, Inc., Revised. (This is the original 25-item venereal disease test set up for programmed instruction, published by the American Alliance for Health, Physical Education and Recreation.)

Secarea-Olsen *Evaluation Instrument for Appraising Health Knowledge of Seventh Grade Students,* Champaign, Illinois, 1974. Available from Larry K. Olsen, Department of Health and Safety, University of Illinois, 61820.

Thompson, Clem W. *Thompson Smoking and Tobacco Knowledge Test,* rev., Mankato State College, Mankato, Minn.

Veenker, Harold C. *Health Knowledge Test for the Seventh Grade,* Lafayette, Indiana: Purdue University. Revised.

SENIOR HIGH LEVEL

Fast-Tyson *Health Knowledge Test,* Kirksville, Missouri, 1975. Available from Charles G. Fast, c/o Northeast Missouri State University 63501.

Johns, Edward B., Juhnke, Warren L. and Pollock, Marion B. *Health Behavior Inventory,* Los Angeles, California: Tinnon-Brown Publishing Company, 1974.

Kilander, H. Frederick. (See Junior High Level listing.)

Kilander, H. Frederick. *Kilander Health Knowledge Test,* 7th edition, Staten Island, N.Y.: Dr. Glenn Leach, Wagner College. Revised. (A popular high school instrument of 100 multiple choice questions.)

LeMaistre, E. Harold, and Pollock, Marion B. *Health Behavior Inventory: Senior High,* Monterey, California: California Test Bureau, Revised. (75 multiple choice items.)

McHugh, Gelolo. *Sex Knowledge Inventory,* rev., Durham, N.C.: Family Life Publications, Inc., 1970.

Pollock, Marion B. *Mood Altering Substances: A Behavior Inventory,* Los Angeles, California: Tinnon-Brown Publishing Company, 1968. (75 multiple choice items.)

Within the category of unpublished theses, dissertations and research articles, there are a number of health measures. A large number of these are informative and concerned with items which should appear in health tests, and how they may be organized; but in terms of test usage they are out of date. They are not listed here. Among the more complete and recent contributions are the following:

JUNIOR HIGH LEVEL

Cook, R. J. *Development of a Sixth Grade Knowledge Test,* unpublished master's thesis, University of Illinois, Urbana, 1973.

Fulton, Martin W. *A Traffic Safety Attitude Scale for 9th Grade Students,* doctoral dissertation, Indiana University, Bloomington, 1965.

Harich, Mary F. *Attitude Changes Among Ninth Grade Girls Following Instruction in the Development of Healthy Sexuality,* master's thesis, University of Maryland, College Park, 1969.

Ladner, Linda Rae. *Knowledge Test on Smoking,* master's thesis, University of Illinois, Urbana, 1968.

Nethers, Gloria Jean. *Knowledge Attitude Test on Nutrition,* master's thesis, University of Illinois, Urbana, 1968.

Vincent, Raymond J. *An Investigation of the Attitudes of Eighth Grade, Tenth Grade and Twelfth Grade Students Toward Smoking Marihuana,* doctoral dissertation, Southern Illinois University, Carbondale, 1968. (See also *Journal of School Health,* Oct., 1970).

SENIOR HIGH LEVEL

Attwood, Madge L. *Construction of an Instrument for Evaluating Drug Abuse Knowledge in High School Students,* master's thesis, University of California, Los Angeles, 1968.

Benson, Bemeda C. *The Construction and Administration of a Knowledge Test Regarding the Use of Alcoholic Beverages for High School Students,* master's thesis, Texas Women's University, Denton, 1967.

Hardt, Dale V. *Development of an Investigatory Instrument to Measure Attitudes Toward Death,* in the *Journal of School Health,* 45:96–99, February, 1975.

Parcel, Guy S. *Development of an Instrument to Measure Attitudes Toward the Personal Use of Premarital Contraception,* in the *Journal of School Health,* 45:157–160, March, 1975.

Seffrin, John R. *A Family Health Knowledge Test,* master's thesis, University of Illinois, Urbana, 1967.

Stauffer, Delmar J. *Consumer Health Knowledge Test,* master's thesis, University of Illinois, Urbana, 1967.

Yeakle, Myrna A. *The Development of a Community Health Knowledge Test for Senior High School Students,* master's thesis, University of California, Los Angeles, 1968.

It is practically impossible to decide upon which health instrument to use without personally examining them. Usually this can be accomplished by visiting the educational tests section of a college or university library, where copies of the standardized health tests are generally kept. Theses and dissertations, however, will usually have to be obtained through an interlibrary loan; or they may already be published in microcard or microfiche form for easy viewing on the appropriate visual reader. Most publishers of standardized health tests and scales will send a sample copy to the teacher who is a prospective user, providing there is no question about the safeguard of the instrument and its scoring key.

LOCAL TESTS AND TEST CONSTRUCTION

It is not the purpose of this chapter to go into a detailed explanation of the wide variety of testing methods, testing practices, test items, and the particulars pertaining to the evaluative criteria behind test instruments. However, a few comments are necessary as one gets ready to prepare a local written examination.

Local health education tests to find out how well pupils understand a topic are helpful in evaluating the teacher's efforts and the students' progress. However, they are usually not much more than screening devices at best. If they have been tried and revised several times they are better. If item difficulty and item analysis procedures have been applied to the test questions, then the tests will be even more valid. It is sufficient to say that good test instruments evolve over a period of time, a time filled with testing, retesting, and revision. Human understandings and practices are much too complicated to be broken down for easy appraisal. However, one should keep trying to measure more accurately, for evaluation, in the end, is a continuous process.

It is an excellent practice in local testing for the instructor to ask himself, "What data do I need in order to make decisions about the program and the students?" The kinds of decisions useful to the instructor pertain to such items as the following:

Determining a fair grade for each pupil.

Being able to tell a student his pattern of strengths and weaknesses, particularly in relation to information acquired, courses of action, and reasons why.

Identifying students who do not have the ability to apply what they seem to know.

Discovering where health instruction content and techniques are weak and in need of improvement.

In general, all test preparation will be fairer and more effective if the following items are kept in mind during the test construction activity.

1. Test content should range from very easy to difficult.
2. Generally, the test should include more than one type of item.
3. It is advisable to include more items in the first draft of the test than will be needed in the final form.
4. Test items should be so phrased that the content, rather than the form of the statement, will determine the answer.
5. All items of a particular type should be placed together in the test.
6. A regular sequence in the pattern of response should be avoided.
7. Trivial, ambiguous, and trick statements should not be used.
8. Concentrate on one idea in a question; try to stay away from partly true and partly false questions.
9. Avoid broad generalizations and the use of words such as never, always, none, and all. Such words arouse doubts in the minds of intelligent students, and are seldom true.
10. When the test is ready to be given, the directions to the students should be clear, complete, and concise.

11. The adoption of a simple scoring procedure should be worked out before the test is given.

A. Free-Response Questions

The essay and short-answer examination with an opportunity to respond freely to a question can be quite objective. Much depends upon how the test questions are worded. They lose their value if they merely call for bits and pieces of information. The strongest point in their favor is that they reveal pupil individuality and thoroughness of preparation. Also, guessing is more difficult than with other types of exams.

EXAMPLES

Essay Question: Comment on the fast rising venereal disease rate in the country as a whole. What are some of the reasons why the rate is much higher in certain states and cities? Support your views with research findings.

Short-Answer Question: In a few sentences express your understanding of the following mental health terms:
alcoholism
psychological stress
mood modifier
personality
psychiatrist
clinical psychologist

B. Multiple-Choice

Students who find difficulty in writing and expressing themselves frequently prefer guided-response or choice questions on an examination. Moreover, it is possible to obtain a rather wide sampling of knowledge in a short time.

A multiple choice item consists of a stem or lead, together with a list of suggested options or alternatives, only one of which is correct or the best answer. Incorrect answers are referred to as foils, decoys, or distractors. A carefully prepared multiple choice question with several options can provide the basis for evaluating course content and critical thinking, provided the instructor adheres to the following points:

1. Preface the questions with a short, clear set of directions.

2. Use questions which are within the appropriate range of difficulty for the intended test population. Those that are answered correctly by less than 10 per cent or more than 90 per cent of the population do not contribute significantly to valid measurement.

3. Pose a single, clearly defined problem in the stem.

4. Make the options consistent with the stem and reasonably similar. In order for the discrimination power of the student to be measured, the choices open to him must be of parallel structure and very much alike. In a five-choice question, at least three choices should be so close that only the student with real understanding will be able to select the most appropriate or best answer. The other options should be plausible and attractive enough to gain the attention of students who are misinformed or inadequately prepared. Care should be taken to guard against a distracting option that unnecessarily calls attention to the best answer. An option, for example, that simply states the opposite of the best answer is inappropriate.

EXAMPLES

Multiple-Choice: Read each question carefully. Select the one item which *best* answers the question. Put the number of the item selected in the space in front of the question.

_____ 4. The most significant medical use of an amphetamine is in:
1. bringing about calmness under pressure
2. treating emotional problems
3. encouraging one to stay awake
4. inducing clear thinking
5. none of the above

_____ 12. The most efficient way to maintain optimum control of weight is to:
1. balance caloric intake to caloric needs
2. eat one light meal every day
3. refrain from eating desserts and between-meals snacks
4. eat more proteins than fats
5. take regular exercise

_____ 42. When a woman becomes pregnant her menstrual period ceases because:
1. no eggs are released from the ovaries during pregnancy
2. the menstrual blood is absorbed into the bloodstream
3. the wall of the uterus is weak
4. the embryo requires the blood for nourishment
5. the male sperm triggers a stop-action in the thyroid

C. True-False

Youth and adults alike seem to respond well to true-false questions. It is difficult to complicate them and they can usually be answered right away. Good questions are straightforward and are as near to true or false as possible. Sweeping generalizations are to be avoided. The instructions are particularly important; the pupil should know that the "partially false" question should be considered "false." It is also important to know whether to guess when in doubt or to leave the question unanswered. In this connection, information about scoring is significant for the pupil. If leaving a question blank counts against him he'll be certain to answer all questions, even if he has to guess (and expect at least a 50 per cent return on his effort). Sometimes, however, an instructor doesn't want the student to guess. He wants him to leave blank those questions he doesn't know; and to make certain guessing is held to a minimum the student may be penalized for getting the wrong answers. The scoring formula of right answers minus two times wrong answers (R-2W) has been used successfully to discourage guessing. It is harsh in many respects, but after students work with it for awhile they begin to be pretty honest in responding to what they know and admitting to what they don't know.

EXAMPLE

True and False: The letters T and F have been placed before each statement given. Draw a circle around the letter T if the statement is *True* and around the letter F if the statement is *False* or *Partially False*.

T   F   6. The average woman is most likely to conceive during the three days before menstruation.

T   F   11. It is possible for mental retardation to be avoided by improving the diet of a newborn infant.

T	F	43.	Anyone who has swallowed a poison should be induced to vomit right away.
T	F	51.	When a physician takes the blood pressure he is measuring the rate at which the heart beats.

D. Affirm—Negate—Neutral

A more sophisticated kind of question is one that permits the student to indicate his doubts as well as his certainties. The honest indecisions of a class can be most helpful to the instructor as he plans to review a lesson or considers course content changes for another year.

EXAMPLE

Affirm—Negate—Neutral: Circle Yes, No or U.

Yes No   U   1. Physicians are subject to periodic re-examinations of their medical knowledge in order to maintain their licenses.

Yes No   U   2. A woman can be a carrier of a venereal disease and be completely unaware of it.

Yes No   U   3. It interferes with the normal digestive process to drink milk immediately after eating citrus fruit.

E. Matching

A popular guided-response item that requires little test paper space and is easy to prepare is the matching question. A "stimulus" column and a "response" column are set up side by side with the stimulus on the left. The response column should have several more items than the stimulus column in order to insure a reasonable degree of difficulty. In the directions, it should be clearly indicated which column is to be matched with which. Matching questions are useful in health items, factors, dates, personalities, and practices.

EXAMPLE

Matching. Which of the sex education terms listed in the left-hand column are identified with the terms in the right-hand column? Consider each separately. Put the number of the sex education term in the parentheses after each item.

1. Progesterone   a. The neck of the uterus   ( )
2. Fetus   b. Microorganism causing syphilis   ( )
3. Cervix   c. The unborn offspring   ( )
4. Egg cell   d. Pregnancy hormone which prepares uterus   ( )
5. Spirochete   for ovum
6. Androgen   e. A yellow mass in the ovary   ( )
7. Clitoris   f. Hormone producing male characteristics   ( )

g. Erectile structure in front of vagina ( )
h. A contraceptive fluid ( )
i. Female reproductive cell, the ovum ( )

F. Fill in or Completion

Leaving blanks in a sentence permits a pupil to fill in what he knows. In completing a sentence he may show his knowledge of a whole concept or involved idea. However, it is very difficult to prepare valid completion questions without writing a rather lengthy sentence. Too often the student has to figure out what the sentence is referring to in order to bring his knowledge to bear. He might know a greal deal about the particular topic, but not know how to recall it because of a poorly described fill-in test question. For these reasons this kind of examination question has very limited use.

VALUE IN PRE-TESTING

Determining what a class of students knows about a major health topic at the start of the lessons makes good sense. Some pre-testing or early appraisal does much to set the stage for a unit of work. It readies the class, particularly if they understand why the pre-testing is being done. Also, pre-testing acquaints the instructor with where the class as a whole is strong, and in which major health area it needs more work. Frequently, time is at a premium, so it would be advantageous to omit a health area in which the class was reasonably strong, and to concentrate effort where the attention is needed.

Pre-testing may take several forms, in which questionnaires, attitude scales, and interviews are employed to find out where the student stands in relation to a health topic. A mixture of opinions, attitudes, feelings, and expressions of interest combine to present the instructor with a fairly good picture of individual and class values pertaining to health practices and health-related items. Such a procedure is not foolproof, because human values are often difficult to tap. However, when a number of pupils take a dim view of a recognized health practice—such as the fluoridation of drinking water or the use of seat belts in automobiles—it is necessary to examine the environmental forces (influences) in the school, home, and community that have helped fashion current health views and values. The dedicated teacher can do no less. In this respect evaluation is an ongoing process which permeates all instructional efforts.

QUESTIONS FOR DISCUSSION

1. Allan Glatthorn says that student decision-making must be efficient, honest, democratic, rational, and unifying. If this is so, how is it possible to appraise readily the extent of decision-making by individual students? (See Glatthorn reference at the end of this chapter.)

2. Why is it that teachers have traditionally done a poor job of determining their personal strengths and weaknesses? Is it because there has been a shortage of supervisors and curriculum specialists? Have they been too involved with day to day activities?

3. Few health instructors take the time to pre-test a class before a unit of work is presented. They sometimes claim that it takes too much time to do this at the start of every major health topic. How do you respond to this point of view?

4. Earlier in the text, the contract approach to learning was discussed along with other methods of teaching. It was pointed out that with this approach, motivation to learn increases as the student becomes involved in the self-direction of his learning and the self-evaluation of his progress. Indicate how you feel about the extent of the self-evaluation. Could this be a better way of appraising student progress than the traditional method of paper and pencil tests?

5. School demonstration projects are usually set up to show how a certain subject matter can be handled with students for the benefit of all concerned. How might it be possible to work into such a project an evaluation dimension — something that would satisfy the school concern for accountability?

SUGGESTED ACTIVITIES

1. Select a major health area in which to appraise student health behavior. Construct a check list of pertinent items that will help you identify pupil strengths and weaknesses. The items included on the checklist should be "behavior" items — active evidences of health understanding.

2. Review the Byrd Health Attitude Scale (Stanford University Press), written a number of years ago. Read it over carefully and change certain statements so that they are up to date. If it was given after such a modification, would the results be useful? Explain your answers.

3. Prepare a five-question essay examination that will measure student concepts having to do with consumer health. Keep in mind that these questions can be quite objective if the instructor is clear about just what it is that he is seeking in the way of an answer.

4. The health education tests developed by Educational Testing Service embrace the Bloom taxonomy and are designed to make the student do more than recall health facts and situations. Obtain copies of the tests and see if you can pick out the questions that call for an application of health knowledge. How do they differ from questions written to permit analysis and synthesis of information?

5. Suggest several ways in which to evaluate a series of lessons on mental health. If possible, ask some health education teachers who teach in the secondary schools to offer a suggestion or two. Is it quite possible that pupils exposed to a mental health lesson manifest no change in personal state of mental health because of the instruction? How may this be remedied?

6. Visit the section of a library where educational tests are stored, and examine the variety of instruments available for measuring health knowledges, attitudes, practices, and so on. How up to date are the tests and test questions? Find out, if possible, where certain of the tests are being used in the vicinity of your school or college.

SELECTED REFERENCES

Anderson, William G. "Videotapes Data Bank," *Journal of Physical Education and Recreation,* 46:31–34, September, 1975.
Beitz, Dennis E. "Health Appraisal In Secondary Schools," *Journal of School Health,* 46:322–324, June, 1976.

Cheffers, John T. F., Edmund J. Amidon, and Ken D. Rodgers. *Interaction Analysis: An Application to Nonverbal Activity,* Minneapolis: Association for Productive Teaching, 1974.

Glatthorn, Allen A. *Alternatives In Education: Schools and Programs,* New York: Dodd, Mead and Co., 1975, Chapter 9.

Good, Thomas L., Bruce J. Biddle, and Jere E. Brophy. *Teachers Make a Difference,* New York: Holt, Rinehart and Winston, 1975, Chapter 6.

Kirchenbaum, H., R. Napier, and S. Simon. *Wad–ja–get?* New York: Hart Publishing Co., 1971.

Nygaard, Gary. "Interaction Analysis of Physical Education Classes," *Research Quarterly,* 46:351–354, October, 1975.

Read, Donald A., and Walter H. Greene. *Creative Health Teaching,* 2nd edition, New York: Macmillan Co., 1975, Chapter 19.

Solleder, Marion K. "Evaluation in the Cognitive Domain," *Journal of School Health,* 42:16–20, January, 1972.

Solleder, Marion K. *Evaluation Instruments in Health Education,* Revised. Washington, D.C.: American Alliance for Health, Physical Education and Recreation.

Vincent, Raymond J. "New Scale for Measuring Attitudes," *School Health Review,* 6:19–21, March/April, 1974.

Willgoose, Carl E. "Providing for Change: New Directions," in *New Directions in Health Education:* (Donald A. Read, editor), New York: Macmillan Co., 1971, Chapter 1.

Yarber, William A. "A Comparison of the Relationship of the Grade Contract and Traditional Grading Methods to Changes in Knowledge and Attitude," *Journal of School Health,* 44:395–399, September, 1974.

Graduated List of Behavioral Objectives for the Major Health Topics, Junior and Senior High School

PHYSICAL ACTIVITY, SLEEP, REST, AND RELAXATION

JUNIOR HIGH LEVEL

Plans a balanced program of physical activity and rest which contributes to general fitness.

Demonstrates how vigorous physical activity increases the efficiency of the cardiorespiratory system.

Explains how daily activities and environmental forces influence energy expenditure and sleep.

Lists the several kinds of recreational activities which supplement and complement other daily activities and influence rest and relaxation.

Takes rest, recreation, and exercise in order to contribute to physical, emotional, and social needs.

Shows how periodic physical examinations and planning of daily activities, including hobbies, help make effective, healthful living possible.

Diagrams the relationship of every part of the body to the well-being of the entire body.

Describes how rest and sleep are needed to enable the body to repair itself, to remove fatigue products, and to enable muscles to relax and replenish their store of fuel.

SENIOR HIGH LEVEL

Explains why the proper time to acquire sound practices to be used in the maintenance of physical fitness is during the adolescent period.

Relates own experiences of physical activity as valuable in helping one cope with the stress, tension, and mental strain sometimes experienced in daily living.

Takes a physical fitness test that has been developed to show how well a person performs physical tasks, how well individuals are prepared for emergencies as well as for daily work, study, and play.

Illustrates how sedentary practices of modern living reduce the effectiveness of body functions.

Analyzes why recreation is a fundamental human need, essential to the well-being and fitness of everyone and why it contributes to mental health by helping to provide a balanced program of living.

Explains individual tolerances pertaining to the requirements for sleep which are related to overall living practices and temperament.

Describes the differences between those social forces that encourage activity rather than sleep, and those factors that influence sedentary rather than active use of time.

NUTRITION AND GROWTH

JUNIOR HIGH LEVEL

Diagrams how the body requires food energy and nutrients to carry on its vital functions, to build new cells for growth and repair, and to supply energy for physical activity.

Describes how state of dynamic balance exists with regard to intake and outgo of food, energy and nutrients in the body.

Observes that people vary considerably in their requirements for food. Body size, rate of growth, heredity, physical activity, and individual metabolic rates all affect caloric needs.

Explains how lack of sufficient nutrients can lead to nutritional deficiency diseases.

Notices that individuals who are growing fast during adolescence show the effect of an inadequate food supply more quickly than others.

Identifies obesity in individuals and notes that it may affect appearance, self-confidence, life expectancy, and relationships with others.

Distinguishes among people that almost everyone follows the same general pattern of growth and development, but there is a wide range of variation within the normal growth pattern; potential for growth is fixed by heredity and modified by environment.

Observes that pleasant surroundings and friends, and good manners, affect the enjoyment of food.

Explains how skeletal age can be measured by a physician, dental age by a dentist, and sexual age by noting the appearance of secondary sex characteristics.

Writes how body build cannot be changed, but fatness may be changed by eating and exercise patterns.

Investigates how the processing of foods and the control of commercial preparations helps protect the consumer.

Lists ways in which food quacks and food faddists can endanger the health of their followers.

SENIOR HIGH LEVEL

Formulates a statement supporting the concept that a nation's productivity ultimately depends on a significant amount of human endurance to work; this applies both in America and in the developing nations of the world.

Discusses the fact that adequate nutrition is important during and before pregnancy to both mother and baby.

Explains how proper nourishment and favorable emotional experiences for the infant may be provided with either breast or bottle feeding.

Demonstrates how widespread malnutrition in the developing nations of the world interacts with disease and other factors to produce reduced life expectancy and poor health for many people; this is not helped by a world population that is growing in geometric fashion.

Reasons that personal, community, and world-wide nutritional health needs may be met by regulating caloric intake and activity, choosing balanced meals, and improving food production and processing.

Analyzes the way in which the homemaker prepares foods and how this influences the quality of nutrition of family members.

DENTAL HEALTH

JUNIOR HIGH LEVEL

Explains that all over the world, teeth are susceptible to decay by certain foods, but most people appear to be indifferent to its consequences.

Documents the fact that appearance, speech, and economic success are related to sound teeth and gums.

Illustrates how proper dental practices will bring freedom from dental discomfort, reduce time and money spent on dental corrections, and improve well-being.

Describes how neglect of teeth may result in dental disorders, which in turn may adversely affect other parts of the body.

Evaluates the literature on the use of fluorides as a very effective way of preventing tooth decay.

Practices individual safety measures to prevent dental accidents.

Compares the increasing number of people requiring treatment for malocclusion with those who do not, and acknowledges that this is partly due to the steadily increasing demand for orthodontic care by better educated people.

Identifies the specialized personnel who treat dental disorders.

SENIOR HIGH LEVEL

Surveys a group of individuals to discover that the prevention and correction of dental disease depends on the motivation of individuals.

Explains how dental decay has plagued both civilized and uncivilized peoples since time began. Writes that only a few people in isolated areas of the world today are not affected by dental decay.

Identifies the variables in tooth decay and gives attention to tooth structure irregularities, alignment, dental plaque, mouth bacteria, acids, foods, saliva, gum disorders, cleansing practices, and emotional tension.

Explains that there is no evidence to support the claim that toothpaste or mouthwash can significantly reduce or destroy mouth bacteria.

Prepares an article stating that the most significant innovation in preventive dentistry is fluoridation of the drinking water in the larger cities and towns, and fluoridization (topical applications) in rural communities where it is not practical to provide controlled fluoridation measures.

Contrasts the several methods of financing dental care.

BODY STRUCTURES AND OPERATION

JUNIOR HIGH LEVEL

Tells how growth and development is a sequential yet unique process determined by the structure and function of the individual.

Describes how hormones secreted by the endocrine glands have an effect on the physical growth and development of the whole body.

Writes confirming the fact that normal function of the body is sometimes interrupted by disease, accidents, or malformation.

Diagrams how a number of vision and hearing disorders can be treated and corrected, and how professional personnel are essential to this process.

Demonstrates how eyeglasses are worn to correct refractive errors; they do not cure the error.

Investigates the validity of the statement that the leading cause of loss of sight among adolescents is injury to one or both eyes.

Initiates and leads a discussion in support of the fact that hearing, like vision, is a function of both the structure and a learning center in the brain.

Explains how the skin protects the body from the outside world, helps regulate body temperature, and provides sensations of touch, pain, warmth, and coldness.

Experiments with the senses of smell and taste which are related, and bring about enjoyment during the act of eating.

PREVENTION AND CONTROL OF DISEASE

JUNIOR HIGH LEVEL

Explains that it is easier and less expensive to prevent diseases than to cure them.

Illustrates how the degenerative, chronic, and constitutional diseases have taken a prominent role in affecting health all over the world.

Discovers that there has been an increase in the health and life expectancy of all age groups due to advances in medical science.

Relates how some diseases are caused by microorganisms such as bacteria, viruses, rickettsia, fungi, and protozoa.

Diagrams how the spread of disease is influenced by both the social conditions and the physical nature of the environment.

Creates a chart which depicts how disease is any condition which interferes with the proper functions of the individual; it may be either communicable or noncommunicable in nature.

Defines the "lines of defense" which help protect the body against disease.

Checks own immunization record and acknowledges that immunization is an important protective measure against certain diseases; it may be acquired naturally by having had the disease, or artificially as a result of medically introduced substances.

Directs fellow students to public health facilities in the community where medical personnel are capable of treating and eradicating venereal disease.

Explains how degenerative or constitutional diseases such as cancer and heart disease cannot be transmitted to others; they may be controlled by individuals, families, and the community.

SENIOR HIGH LEVEL

Shows how chronic disorders such as diabetes, arthritis, cancer, and heart disease have similar general effects as well as unique effects on individuals and society.

Acknowledges that all tissue is vulnerable to cancerous growths.

Explains how varied and complex factors interrelate in the transmission and development of respiratory diseases such as colds, asthma, emphysema, lung cancer, pleurisy, and pneumonia.

Makes known that through early diagnosis of some cancers it may be possible to completely cure or prolong health and longevity.

Tells others that the chief danger from a cold is that it leaves one susceptible to many secondary infections such as pneumonia.

Discovers that although "cold shots" do not prevent the cold, they may reduce the severity, duration, and frequency of attacks.

Expresses the view that individuals have the responsibility to assist in community efforts for control and prevention of disease and disorders.

Shows how history demonstrates that diseases have affected the growth and development of a number of countries; studying these situations gives insight into future health practices.

Observes and describes mononucleosis as an infectious disease of unknown origin, with involvement of glandular tissues; it is prevalent during the spring and fall seasons.

MENTAL HEALTH

JUNIOR HIGH LEVEL

Demonstrates how sound mental health means being on "good terms with yourself," accepting others as they are, and meeting the demands of life as best you can.

Indicates the way personality develops in a continuing process; there are ways to develop a worthy personality.

Shows a delicate balance between self-expression and self-control.

Explains that no one factor is responsible for one's mental health; heredity sets limits, and environment determines levels of attainment.

Describes the manner in which environmental stress can cause physiological reactions which in turn may cause anxiety; a pleasant environment may bring about feelings of calmness and tranquility.

Tells how growing up means facing and carrying through tasks without frequently finding excuses for failure.

Details how teenage popularity is based on many factors; peer pressures sometimes produce stress which individuals can learn to handle; self-respect is a prerequisite for receiving and giving respect to others.

Expresses emotions in an acceptable manner that can be controlled; individuals with problems can be helped.

Outlines how people learn to cope with the changes and complexities of society; problems and frustrations are individual, yet all people of all societies deal with similar problems.

Explains how individuals must assume responsibility for their own health; almost everyone has the capacity for physical, mental and emotional growth.

SENIOR HIGH LEVEL

Describes the complexity of human behavior, and how personality is the composite of one's total being.

Demonstrates how socially useful work gives a person dignity; achievements and improved status add to the self-image.

Illustrates a variety of possible life plans with probable courses; and identifies needs, abilities, and problems that help one to choose a possible life plan.

Explains in detail why mental illness is one of the major health problems of Western civilization; mentally ill persons are being helped in a number of ways.

Names a number of common misconceptions and fallacies concerning mental illness.

Shows how the mentally mature person strives to accept worthiness of all people, regardless of cultural, ethnic, or religious characteristics.

Sets forth several illustrations of psychological stress and how it produces physiological changes which may lead to chronic disease and disorders.

Recalls a number of challenging health careers directly and indirectly associated with the mental health area.

CONSUMER HEALTH

JUNIOR HIGH LEVEL

Discriminates between reliable and unreliable health information and advertising.

Determines that quackery and faddism are dangerous to health because they prevent people from following sound health practices and receiving adequate health protection.

Demonstrates the ways reputable physicians share their ideas, findings, and other pertinent information with the rest of the scientific community. Explains how the quack promises sure and quick cures.

Relates how self-diagnosis and self-treatment can endanger health; they sometimes occur because of fear, false economy, and poorly understood illnesses.

Analyzes how many agencies serve, protect, and inform the health consumer — some of them are UNESCO, the Food and Drug Administration, the Post Office Department, local Health Departments, voluntary health agencies, state health departments, and the Better Business Bureau.

Explains how standards for the processing of foods, drugs, and cosmetics are defined by the Food and Drug Administration. The advertising of these products is of concern to the Federal Trade Commission.

Utilizes magazines that sometimes rate health products; *Parent's Magazine, Good Housekeeping,* and *Consumer Reports* are important to understand.

Discovers that emotional motives for purchasing health products and services may lead to unwise consumer behavior.

Analyzes teen fads, fashions, and other consumer trends having to do with such items as body weight and complexion aids.

Illustrates how teenager buying influence is considerable, both within and outside the family; some of this represents a striving for adulthood.

SENIOR HIGH LEVEL

Discovers that there are a number of important differences between health specialists; the preparation, licensing, and certification of medical and paramedical personnel is very carefully supervised.

Explains how health services, as well as health products such as food, food additives, cosmetics, drugs, and medications are often selected on the basis of hearsay, emotional feelings, past experiences, and social forces and pressures.

Employs sound criteria to help make intelligent choices in providing for professional health care.

Tells how diagnosing and treating illness and injury is the responsibility of qualified personnel.

Explains how expanding knowledge in every area of medicine has made medical specialties a necessity.

Analyzes the ways in which promoters of health products and services capitalize on consumer ambivalence—our expression of both positive and negative feelings about the same object or activity.

Demonstrates the way behavior based on superstitions, ignorance, or prejudice, rather than on scientific evidence, can be expensive and harmful to the health consumer.

Studies various types of hospital systems, each serving its own particular type of function.

Illustrates how medical care is an important part of the national and family budget. Because this care is costly, medical insurance is increasingly necessary.

WORLD HEALTH

JUNIOR HIGH LEVEL

Diagrams how communicable diseases may be spread throughout the world in a matter of hours because of the increased number of people traveling by rapid means of transportation.

Explains how the advanced nations of the world need to cooperate with the developing nations in disease prevention programs designed to control insects, polluted water, and general sanitation.

Demonstrates through documentation how the nutritional needs of the world have become overwhelming as the population has increased; malnutrition is a serious condition everywhere.

Shows the manner in which international health agencies bring modern scientific technology to bear on world health problems.

Illustrates the way the Pan American Health Organization, the United Nations, and the World Health Organization work cooperatively to improve world health.

Examines the way the culture of the people influences the nature and extent of international health problems.

SENIOR HIGH LEVEL

Describes the manner in which total health transcends local, state, national, and international political boundaries.

Analyzes how regional health problems are influenced chiefly by cultural variations, economic differences, key occupations, geography, ecological balance, and technological development.

Demonstrates through research reports that only when the people of a country participate in a health program does it have a chance to be successful.

Depicts how older family members influence younger members; if patterns of behavior are based on superstitions and myths, the progress of world health will be delayed.

Discovers and expresses the view that programs for training health personnel are essential in the underdeveloped regions of the world.

Illustrates the fact that there are diseases which are potentially epidemic that need to be constantly controlled; when a disease is an epidemic there are many cases; when it is pandemic, the cases are spread over a large geographic area.

Details how nutrition and mental health programs are greatly needed throughout the world; drug abuse and emotional disturbances are high on the list of mental health problems.

HEALTH CAREERS

JUNIOR HIGH LEVEL

Clearly explains how there is a growing need for many more professional health workers such as physicians, nurses, dentists, and pharmacists; there is also a need for more allied health personnel.

Gives examples of how earning a livelihood by working in a health career field can be of great service to humanity, and can afford deep personal satisfaction.

Illustrates how academic preparation coupled with personality and interests sets the stage for the selection of an appropriate health career.

Differentiates between the many major fields of medical (M.D.) specialization; there are many more in dentistry, and in nursing.

Describes how hospitals, nursing homes, rehabilitation facilities, and community health centers could not operate without the help of technicians, aides, helpers, and volunteers.

ALCOHOL

JUNIOR HIGH LEVEL

Role plays how various kinds of alcoholic beverages affect the body in different ways.

Writes that there is a relationship between all chemicals which have an effect on the mind—they either stimulate or depress at some level of the brain.

Describes how alcoholic beverages may result in personal and community health and safety problems.

Discusses alcoholism as a disease that has many causes; it affects people in different ways; it can be treated.

Acts out how many adolescents view drinking as "adult" behavior; teenagers tend to imitate adults.

Explains how some young people resort to drinking as a way of meeting the unhappiness of failure.

Demonstrates how alcohol inhibits muscular coordination and judgment.

Documents and tells how the excessive use of alcohol may affect one's ability to keep a job; accident rates increase when workers have been drinking and the ability to concentrate, hear, see, and touch are impaired by alcohol.

Outlines how crime may be an outcome of the use of alcohol and drugs.

SENIOR HIGH LEVEL

Shows how alcohol may be used in a number of ways to benefit as well as adversely affect people.

Illustrates how the economy of the country is affected by alcohol consumption—by industry, taxes, accidents, broken homes, and welfare costs, among others.

Outlines how the rehabilitation of alcoholics calls for community involvement.

Makes the decision to drink or not to drink; a mentally healthy person does not attempt to escape reality by the excessive use of alcohol.

Explains that there is a relationship between alcohol and cirrhosis of the liver, pneumonia, tuberculosis, acute pancreatitis, longevity, and mental well-being.

Talks with people in order to discover that psychological-emotional treatment and rehabilitation are available through Alcoholics Anonymous.

Finds that alcohol research is being carried on by many individuals and organizations; some are voluntary and some are public.

Refrains from drinking prior to school activities (dances, games, etc.) because it is in poor taste and frequently leads to trouble.

DRUGS

JUNIOR HIGH LEVEL

Illustrates that if properly used, drugs are of immense value to mankind.

Explains how the development of better drugs has decreased disease, extended the life span, and improved mental health.

Identifies prescription drugs that can only be legally purchased with a prescription from a medical doctor or a doctor of dentistry who is licensed to prescribe medication.

Tells why only a registered pharmacist is licensed to fill a prescription and why left-over medicine should be discarded.

Names the numerous commercials on television, radio, newspapers, and magazines that are designed to "sell" the public on habitual use of unnecessary drugs, tonics, alkalines, pills, capsules, laxatives, and pain relievers.

Examines the Federal Food, Drug and Cosmetic Act, which is designed to insure the safety and efficacy of drugs reaching the consumer.

Researches the literature to discover that experimentation with drugs can lead to uncontrolled use of drugs; it may also lead to other individual health problems.

Chooses not to use drugs such as the stimulants (amphetamines) for "kicks" since the "side effects" may not be able to be dealt with—excessive nervousness, poor judgment, spasms, tremors, and hallucinations.

Explains how a number of narcotic drugs are used by physicians to treat patients, to deaden pain and induce sleep, and how care is exercised against overuse.

Identifies a number of illegal drugs, all of which are capable of affecting a person's mood and ultimate well-being.

Role plays in order to show that the craving for certain drugs is so intense in the addict that maintaining his drug supply becomes his main concern—leading to crime to support the habit.

SENIOR HIGH LEVEL

Uses drugs as medically directed; to do otherwise is to ignore years of research, testing, and quality control.

Details how it is possible to become addicted to drugs because of mental or social problems, feelings of inadequacy, or a low self-image.

Finds that solving problems by seeking help from friends, counselors, clergymen, or physicians is more constructive than the problem of drug addiction.

Interprets research to show that withdrawal illness is the reaction of the body to the absence of the drug upon which the person has become dependent.

Explains how the U.S. Department of Justice, Bureau of Narcotics and Dangerous Drugs, has agents around the world trying to reduce heroin traffic into this country.

Comments on the fact that the Supreme Court has ruled that drug addiction is an illness, and that the development of programs of compulsory treatment of addicts would serve the health and welfare interests of the country.

Illustrates with examples from the literature why most addicts are described as immature, easily frustrated, and incapable of assuming responsibility; in their rehabilitation, they learn to face up to life's responsibilities without the use of drugs. The helping process is difficult and complex.

Depicts how the economy of the nation is affected by illegal drug production, drug traffic, and drug use.

SMOKING EDUCATION

JUNIOR HIGH LEVEL

Gives up smoking, or cuts down on the amount smoked per day.

Explains how many countries have recognized the relationship between lung cancer and smoking, and some have taken measures to control the use of cigarettes.

Illustrates how no cigarette filter has been developed which can protect the smoker from the cancer-producing agents in tobacco smoke.

Shows that since television advertising has been discontinued, it is more difficult to encourage teenage smoking.

Names individuals, including young people, who start to smoke because they and their friends do not understand the scientific findings, and they are frequently unconcerned with future illnesses resulting from smoking.

Lists the number of reasons why many people have made the decision not to smoke.

Demonstrates how smoking is more injurious to one's health if one smokes rapidly, inhales the smoke, and leaves a short butt end.

Discovers that in addition to lung cancer and other respiratory diseases, smokers have more other diseases than non-smokers.

Portrays in graph form how smoking curtails length of life, and can affect the performance of an athlete, causes chronic bronchitis, pulmonary emphysema, and cardiovascular disease, and is found more commonly in smokers than in non-smokers.

SENIOR HIGH LEVEL

Eliminates smoking, or cuts down on the amount smoked per day.

Draws bar graphs to show how the mortality ratio of cigarette smokers over non-smokers is particularly high for chronic bronchitis, emphysema, cancer of the larynx, peptic ulcers, and heart and coronary artery disease.

Develops useful guidelines to help people who wish to give up smoking.

Examines the role of a personal commitment, and notes that the reasons for smoking are largely psychological and sociological.

Takes part in local agency activity concerned with the health status of Americans and is vigorously involved in anti-smoking programs.

Tells how leading scientific and medical groups in the country acknowledge the health hazards of smoking.

Analyzes why the sale of tobacco is presently essential to the economic well-being of certain areas of the United States.

Looks into the use of statistical evidence as a universally accepted scientific procedure in research.

Explains that although no true "smoker's personality" has been identified, there are distinct personality characteristics associated with smokers.

Constructs a line graph to show that smokers who discontinue the practice have a total death rate considerably lower than that of those who continue to smoke.

Illustrates how the most comprehensive and widely accepted smoking research has been conducted by the U.S. Government.

Sets an example for younger boys and girls, and notes an association between students' smoking and parental patterns.

SEX AND FAMILY LIVING EDUCATION

JUNIOR HIGH LEVEL

Human Behavior

Explains that although complicated by psychological and physiological functions, individual behavior can be controlled.

Self-directs intelligence to the solution of personal problems.

Experiences changes in energy levels and emotions.

Demonstrates that emotional health has a bearing on all behavior and happiness.

Discusses the way personality develops as one works out a smooth relationship between self and others, including friends of both sexes, family, and society.

Acknowledges that although there are different rates of development, there are normal patterns and differences in physical and emotional growth.

Expresses emotions in a variety of situations.

Explains how personal standards of behavior are influenced by how we see ourselves, what we wish to become, and how we interact with the many factors in the environment.

The Family Unit

Verbalizes that because the society is always in a state of change, the roles of the family members will change.

Justifies the fact that as parents and children make adjustments, their family life becomes more healthful and a happier one.

Identifies the essential function of the family to provide identity, security, and love for all family members.

Explains how a variety of families from different cultures make up a particular community. The community, therefore, is only as strong as the quality of the individual family members.

Demonstrates the way families, working together, use a logical approach to find solutions to their problems.

Reproductive Process

Shows how physical development at adolescence is related to heredity and sexual maturity.

Diagrams how the male and the female have a unique reproductive structure and function.

Describes how in the male, the sex drive develops before or concurrently with the maturation of spermatozoa.

Explains that as the sex drive develops, it finds a natural expression through increased interest in associations with members of the opposite sex.

Acknowledges that girls and boys are biologically capable of mating and reproducing a number of years before they are mature enough to be responsible parents.

Outlines the manner in which menstruation occurs normally in the absence of conception and fertilization.

Experiences seminal emissions as a normal occurrence during the growing-up period.

Describes how expressing the sex drive through inappropriate means creates problems for the individual, the family, and society.

Dating

Discovers that men and women, boys and girls learn to understand each other as sexual beings through the age-old custom of dating.

Helps formulate moral standards of conduct that pertain to dating and the making of personal decisions.

Talks over the fact that the quality of boy-girl relationships while on a date is the responsibility of both the boy and the girl.

Practices control and illustrates how controlling the sex drive on a date is best understood and accomplished if the boy and girl both understand themselves biologically and emotionally, and also understand each other.

Accepts responsibility for the welfare of his dating partner as well as his own.

Details the many ways to be popular.

Applies the expression that there is a difference between being "sexy" and being feminine.

Discusses issues pertaining to the statement that human sexuality has to do with what it means to be masculine or feminine.

Shows how premarital sexual experiences frequently result in unwanted pregnancies, venereal disease, and broken boy-girl relationships.

SENIOR HIGH LEVEL

Human Relationships

Demonstrates the manner in which emotional well-being encompasses a wide variety of emotional responses.

Explains in detail how human sexuality is concerned with the qualities of manhood and womanhood.

Illustrates how physiological sex drives differ between males and females, and must be understood if an individual is to appreciate the feelings of companions.

Describes the wide variety of sources and samples of love. Such terms as "young love," "puppy love," "true love," and "sexual love" have different meanings to people with different understandings.

Outlines how going steady has its advantages and its disadvantages.

Expresses an understanding of the fact that because parents are interested in the total welfare of their children, they usually express some attitude toward dating behavior.

Demonstrates self-respect by acknowledging the importance of setting limits for one's behavior while on a date.

Refrains from using too much alcohol, which may create a situation in which responsible sexual behavior is undermined.

Urges others to understand that venereal disease can be controlled in this country if individual cases are reported and treated.

Explains how prostitution is a social problem related to drug addiction, and to the hedonistic philosophy of Playboyism.

Discusses how the "new morality" need not ignore the virtues of respect for individuals and responsibility for one's own actions.

Acts in a given situation by a consideration of both the immediate and the long range consequences of his actions.

Explains that male and female homosexuality has to be understood for what it is; homosexual individuals can be helped through proper psychiatry and counseling.

Preparation for Marriage

Shows how the choice of a marriage partner is influenced by many personal, economic, and societal factors. Understands that these should be thoroughly understood before two people decide to invest their lives and their resources in a joint enterprise.

Differentiates between a meaningful engagement and just going together.

Shows how a mature husband and wife relationship is based on mutual goals, giving of oneself without thought of return, and broad understandings of why the other person feels the way he does.

Analyzes how the premarital medical examination is designed to help a couple start married life in a state of optimal health.

Explains that the more a couple interested in marriage have in common, the better their chances of having a successful marriage.

Applies the statement that a society has to adjust to the problems brought about through overpopulation, divorce, abortion, and unwanted children.

Details family planning and how it means creating a family according to a purposeful design.

Tells how in order to provide for the total well-being of a family, children may be spaced at certain intervals; a large segment of the population employs contraceptive methods as a means of orderly family growth.

Passes along the information that physicians and other qualified advisors assist young people with specific information about family planning methods.

Describes how pregnancy requires the expectant mother to make a number of adjustments in nutrition, personal care, and emotional attitude.

Details the manner in which proper personal health practices, coupled with adequate medical care and vitamin and mineral supplements, enhance the prospective mother's chances of delivering a normal, healthy baby.

Is able to recognize that the birth of a couple's first child frequently requires a major adjustment for the husband and wife.

Expresses the view that the birth of the baby and the growth of the child during its first year helps one to appreciate and have a reverence for life.

Reacts positively to the proposition that one's personal standard of sexual behavior is complicated by a number of alternatives according to the culture, but it is ultimately related to a personal respect for the rights and feelings of others and the responsible actions of mature men and women.

Applies in viewpoint the principle that a society is made whole and livable when the joys of family activity, planning, and fulfillment transcend the immediate gratification of individuals.

Explains how parents have a major influence on the socialization and development of their children.

Practices the worthy use of leisure time and acknowledges its contribution to the full development of the individual and the family as a necessary attribute in modern society.

SAFETY EDUCATION

JUNIOR HIGH LEVEL

Illustrates how new inventions and discoveries create hazards in the environment.

Explains that potential dangers are inherent in many activities; activities such as walking, bicycling, and boating can be made safe or unsafe. With proper precautions most injuries can be avoided.

Demonstrates the way prompt care given in emergencies can save lives and prevent further injury.

Demonstrates how knowledge and practice of safety rules in recreational activities helps to prevent accidents.

Articulates and shows how water safety instruction can prevent needless accidents and develop skills for leisure hours.

Shows why accurate knowledge is important in handling an emergency situation.

Charts evidence to show that accidents are caused by a combination of events, each of which may be subject to human control.

Explains that individuals cannot always live safely by themselves since the attitudes of others affect them.

Acknowledges that the major causes of injuries in the home are falls and fires.

Participates and explains that through the close cooperation of students and school personnel, safety hazards in the school environment can be significantly reduced.

Demonstrates how there should be two persons in a boat for water skiing, one as the operator and the other as the observer.

Explains that the main task of the babysitter is to prevent accidents and injury while providing adequate care for the children.

Tells how the atomic and nuclear weapons are the most destructive weapons ever created by man.

Diagrams the manner in which various kinds of storms are capable of mass destruction of property and injury to people.

Shows a number of ways in which first aid includes only immediate and temporary care until professional assistance can be obtained.

Illustrates a number of rules used in physical education activities that are designed to develop good safety habits.

Explains how smoking in bed is a prime contributor to house fires.

SENIOR HIGH LEVEL

Tells how the application of safety practices in industrial, recreational, and school activities adds to their enjoyment and value by helping to prevent accidents.

Explains that as civilization expands and the environment is further explored, new hazards to man's health are added.

Demonstrates how the application of emergency medical procedures enhances survival when major disasters occur.

Acknowledges that total community planning is needed to establish effective environmental controls which consider all factors affecting man.

Analyzes the great impact of forces involved in automobile accidents; there are usually more than one type of injury, and these are frequently of a complex rather than simple nature.

Shows how penetrating radiation can cause great damage to body tissues.

Illustrates how injuries occurring because of tornadoes, hurricanes, earthquakes, and winter storms include almost every type.

Explains the way an emotionally upset person may present a danger to himself as well as to those around him.

Outlines how violence, which sets the stage for injuries, may be caused by such things as overcrowded living conditions, dehumanized populations, and general fear and distrust of one's fellow man.

Speaks out, and makes clear that safe automobile driving includes the use of seat belts and shoulder straps, abstinence from alcohol, and a respect for the rights of others.

Practices correct sport and recreational skills, coupled with courtesy during the activity, in order to realize more fun and fewer mishaps.

Depicts clearly that the highest liability insurance rates are paid by the 16 to 25 year age group because of their higher accident rate.

Promotes the concept that industries make provisions to promote the physical welfare of their employees by researching such items as the effect of fatigue on production, health, and safety.

Examines the number of safety standards and legal factors in the construction of buildings, roads, bridges, and other structures.

Visits several official and non-official health agencies which are directly concerned with such areas as child safety, automobile safety, industrial safety, and school safety; they advance the concept of public responsibility for the prevention of accidents.

ENVIRONMENTAL HEALTH

JUNIOR HIGH LEVEL

Reveals how the existence of mankind will depend on the ability to interact effectively with the total environment; human ecology is a study of this interaction.

Diagrams on paper how all parts of an environment, living and non-living, are interdependent; their stability and existence are interconnected.

Acknowledges through verbalization that the most constant characteristic of both the living and the non-living parts of any environment is change.

Illustrates by example how all forms of life are characterized by the continuous interaction between heredity and environment.

Explains how individuals and groups are related to each other and their environment; this determines their characteristics.

Shows that the way a person perceives his environment influences the manner in which he uses it.

Arranges an exhibit to show that the process of living involves a continual interplay between the individual and water, air, soil, geography, climate, housing, and other individuals.

Analyzes the sociocultural environments to determine that certain persons have a higher incidence of disease than others; i.e., venereal disease, crime, and communicable diseases among the poor.

Applies the philosophy that the health of a country's population is considered to be a prime factor in its economic growth and development. Poor standards of living and low economy contribute to disease and illness.

Describes how the consequences of using insecticides, pesticides, and other such poisons in an overpopulated society present a number of complex problems.

Explains the way federal, state, and local health agencies interact to create a favorable community environment.

SENIOR HIGH LEVEL

Describes how heredity and all the environments—biological, social, and cultural—help mold the many characteristics and behaviors of an individual.

Sets forth the view that although stabilized by tradition and law, governments are changed by modification of the people's perception of the governmental function.

Tells how the concern for natural resources and technological advancement must be balanced so that all of man's needs may be given proper attention.

Takes part in a project in which medical science, industry, public health, and conservation personnel are actively engaged in research linking population, land areas, and various types of pollution to specific diseases.

Observes that as individuals have consumed the fruits of their environment at random, and increasingly triumphed over climate problems, pestilence, and famine, there has been created an environment which contains new hazards to human health.

Analyzes how an epidemiological study of the characteristics and interactions of disease agent, host, and environmental factors helps to determine the causes of disease, disability, health problems, defects, and death.

Experiences through field study that the impact of economic, demographic, social, cultural, scientific, and technological changes has not only improved man's health, but has also created additional health needs and a number of ecological problems such as pollution, noise, neuroses, and malnutrition.

Demonstrates the way a number of social and cultural changes in the community have an ecological bearing on urban development, air and water pollution, mental illness, alcoholism, drug addiction, accidents, and other problems.

INDEX